I0062110

Roy J. Shephard is a member of the Department of Environmental
Health, School of Hygiene, University of Toronto.
S. Itoh is a member of the Department of Physiology, Hokkaido
University School of Medicine, Japan.

This volume presents in tightly edited form more than ninety
papers from the third international symposium on circumpolar
health, held in Yellowknife in July 1974.

The conference brought together physicians and paramedical
professionals from all the circumpolar nations. They discussed
methods of delivering health care and education to isolated
communities, the epidemiology and pathology of current epidemics, and the many physiological, social, psychological, and
medical problems arising from the sudden acculturation of
indigenous northern peoples to a western life-style.

Physiologists and nutritionists will be interested in the
effects of changes from natural to processed foods and of
diminished levels of physical activity; sociologists and
psychologists in adaptations to rapid social change and the
attendant problems of alcoholism and violence; epidemiolo-
gists in the spread and subsequent control of bacteria, viruses, and parasites previously unknown in northern communities;
physicians in such common northern problems as upper respiratory and ear infections; dental surgeons in the impact of
changing foods on oral health; and geneticists and anthropologists in the potential for study of small communities of a
common basic stock which have lived in isolation for many
centuries.

Many of the problems encountered by white workers in the
north - exposure to cold, venereal disease, unusual rhythms
of light and darkness, responses to isolation, and even relationships between isolated professionals and their univer-
sity-based supervisors - are also discussed.

Proceedings of the 3rd International Symposium,
Yellowknife, NWT

CIRCUMPOLAR HEALTH

Edited by
ROY J. SHEPHARD
Department of Environmental Health, School of Hygiene,
University of Toronto

S. ITOH
Department of Physiology, University of Hokkaido

Published for Health and Welfare Canada,
Medical Services Branch, Northwest Territories Region
by University of Toronto Press,
Toronto and Buffalo

© University of Toronto Press 1976
Toronto and Buffalo
Printed in Canada
Reprinted in 2018

Library of Congress Cataloging in Publication Data

International Symposium on Circumpolar Health, 3d, Yellowknife, Northwest Territories, Can., 1974.
Circumpolar health.

Includes Index.
1. Arctic Medicine - Congresses. 2. Eskimos - Health and
hygiene - Congresses. 3. Lapps - Health and hygiene - Congresses. 4. Indians of North America - Health and hygiene
- Congresses. I. Shephard, Roy J. II. Itoh, Shinji,
1912 -   III. Canada. Medical Services Branch, Northwest Territories Region. IV. Title. [DNLM: 1. Cold
climate - Congresses. W3 IN916VE 1974c / QT160 161 1974c]
RC955.2.157 1974   613.1'11   76-2608
ISBN 0-8020-3333-4
ISBN 978-1-4875-8094-0 (paper)

CONTENTS

viii   Contents

x   Contents

xii   Contents

HEALTH CARE DELIVERY

PUBLIC HEALTH AND ARCTIC ECOLOGY

PREFACE

The circumpolar regions offer one of the last frontiers of
medical science. Until a few years ago the arctic was a
bleak, inaccessible region, penetrated only by a few hardy
souls who could bring no more comfort to the ills of the
indigenous peoples than could be crammed into the ubiquitous
black bag. But the pace of change has been rapid. The indigenous people have largely abandoned their nomadic camps,
coming together in larger settlements with schools, a nursing station if not a hospital, and (generally) regular air
communication with major urban centres. There is now no obstacle (other than the cost of air freight) to taking almost
all the facilities of modern medicine to northern communities.

Much remains to be discovered about the medical problems
of arctic life. Morbidity and mortality remain far higher
than in the south. Problems of a rugged physical environment
are compounded by makeshift housing and sanitation, ig-
norance of the principles of hygiene, sometimes poor nutrition, and often the stress of rapid cultural change. Diseases such as tuberculosis and rheumatic fever, long
controlled in the south, are still a problem in many parts
of the north. Otitis media is widespread. Epidemics of hepatitis, brucellosis, botulism, and encephalitis and a high
incidence of intestinal parasitic infections testify to the
problems of hygiene. Nor is "civilization" an unmixed
blessing for the indigenous peoples. The psychologist's indices of acculturative stress have their parallel in an
alarming toll of alcoholism, suicides, and venereal diseases. Dental health is steadily deteriorating as store
food replaces the traditional diet. Mercury and other pollu-
tants of our industrial society force us to caution the native against eating his normal foods. The rifle and the
snowmobile deplete game reserves and leave the hunter with
a permanent defect of hearing.

This bewildering array of problems must be handled by a
dedicated but pitifully small health care delivery team.
Over the vast distances of the arctic, there are unusual
opportunities to experiment with new approaches - public
health nurses, nursing and dental assistants, with the

emphasis on recruitment of indigenous personnel - possibly
within the framework of native cooperatives. There is also
much scope for thought as to how physicians can be encouraged to work in remote areas, being spared both a sense
of isolation and also a limitation of their freedom by appropriate relationships with visiting consultants.

The north also holds much interest for the pure scientist.
The isolated indigenous populations provide fascinating material for the geneticist and those interested in inherited
disease. The lack of daylight and other temporal cues during
the winter months offers the possibility of distinguishing
exogenous and endogenous circadian rhythms. The bitterly
cold environment challenges man's range of adaptability, providing the physiologist with such questions as control mechanisms, thermogenesis, and cold diuresis, the engineer with
problems of clothing design, and the physician with the occasional need to diagnose and treat frostbite and hypothermia.

The future probably belongs to the public health engineer
and the educator. Through appropriate design of housing and
public buildings, the harshness of the external environment
can be tempered. Given adequate resources, there is no reason
why current problems of water supply, sewage, and garbage
disposal cannot be corrected. But much will depend ultimately
upon the attitudes of the indigenous people - their willingness to accept the advice of the experts and to understand
the reasons behind this advice.

These were some of the themes tackled by the Third International Symposium on Circumpolar Health, held in Yellowknife, Northwest Territories, 8-11 July 1974. The meeting was
much larger than its predecessors in Alaska and Northern Finland. Nearly 400 registrants came from all of the nations
bordering the arctic. The scientific committee accepted more
than 170 papers for presentation, and many were of such a
high quality that it was thought worth while to assemble the
proceedings as a resource volume for all concerned with circumpolar health.

Symposium proceedings fall into at least three broad categories. Type one is the tape transcript. This preserves for
posterity such gems as the chairman's request for a glass of
water, but summarizes a number of the main speeches in two
words, "tape inaudible." Type two is based on unedited manuscripts, seized from lecturers as they leave the rostrum. The
end-product is commonly preferable to the first type of
volume, but nevertheless it still has many shortcomings. The
material from English-speaking contributors is often little
more than a set of poorly phrased lecture notes, with incomplete sentences, inadequate references, and carelessly

documented tables, while some foreign contributions degen-
erate into indecipherable gibberish. Type three is the fully
edited volume. Authors are given a clear statement of the
quality of manuscript required, and an editorial board then
makes careful review of the material for inaccuracies, re-
dundancies, and overlap with other presentations.

This is, we hope, a type three volume. Following the
Yellowknife Conference, authors were invited to submit carefully prepared manuscripts, and more than 90 papers were received in a format judged suitable for publication. Where
appropriate, this information has been further supplemented
by brief "commentaries," based on edited abstracts of other
contributions. Editing the volume has taught us much - not
only about circumpolar health, but also about the personalities of the rugged individualists who work in the north.
Some contributions were literary masterpieces, imbued with a
fine sense of the beauty and the poetry of the arctic. Despite firm instructions, many contributors felt impelled to
exceed the stipulated page limits. In a few instances, the
material was of such interest that leeway was allowed, but
often the editors were forced to make hard decisions and
vigorous use of scissors and paste. A surprising number of
participants painstakingly copied the area of Alaska and the
Northwest Territories, along with other humdrum items of
geography - all apparently from a common and unacknowledged
source! Some saw fit to boast or complain of the hazards and
discomforts we have all endured, waiting at lonely airstrips
for the plane that fails to arrive. One or two were moved to
long diatribes against bureaucracy, the stupidity of the natives, or the arrogance of the whites. A few saw the handling of a simple local problem as a mammoth space-age experiment, and the occasional enthusiast inflated his title of
office and accompanying acknowledgments to two or more
pages! The authors may quarrel with our decision, but these
do not seem matters to commit to perpetuity - unless in a
privately financed volume.

However, in addition to thanking the contributors, two
specific acknowledgments must be made. One is to Dr Otto
Schaefer, who carried the heavy burden of initiating and
supervising the progress of the symposium through to its
successful conclusion. The other is to the Medical Services,
Northern Region, of Health and Welfare Canada, who provided
generous financial support, both for the Yellowknife Symposium and also for the publication of this volume. Both Dr
Schaefer and Northern Regional Medical Services are totally
committed to the task of improving Circumpolar Health, and

if this volume helps forward that objective, they will be
well pleased with the efforts of all who have contributed
to it.

R.J.S.
S.I.

CIRCUMPOLAR HEALTH

CIRCUMPOLAR HEALTH

Keynote address

BILL MUSSELL

I am somewhat overwhelmed by the power of the bodies present
at this particular conference and am impressed with the representation from other countries; perhaps I may take the
liberty of welcoming the visitors to our land. It is significant that I should be asked to speak to this conference.
I am not a medical doctor, nor a medicine man of my tribe in
the traditional sense, although I appreciate what some medicine men can do. After discussions with one of your very
active and aggressive organizers, Dr Schaefer, and consultation with the leaders of my tribe and my family I agreed to
come. What a keynote speaker should do remains a question in
my mind, but I am hoping that the key you have given me will
provide an opportunity for me to share with you some of the
human questions that concern me. One of the greatest difficulties we have had as a minority group is in the area of
listening. I have taught school, I have taught teachers, and
I have worked with a number of people, both in the professional and para-professional areas. One of the things that
has always amazed me is the inability of many people to listen. We are all in the business of communication. There are
all kinds of resource people present, but if we are unable to
listen and ask the appropriate questions we are not going to
leave here with much more knowledge than when we came.
What is effective listening? The North American Indian has
been described in many articles and research papers as "very
quiet." We don't get that much involved. We certainly don't
say very much. But little has been said about the asset of
being able to listen. People do a lot of talking at conferences like this. What we understand is tremendously important. It is an area where a lot of difficulties arise between our people and people from the larger society. What we
are able to recall is also important, and I hope that all of
us will leave with additional knowledge that we can recall

and share with those at home who are expecting us to bring
something back from this particular conference. A common
criticism our people make of outsiders who are delivering
services is that they talk too much and don't listen enough.
Some of our leaders say that we must be very careful of doctors and white people generally because they don't come
across as sincere and honest. On what do we base that judgment? We can play many games with words. Words are cheap.
Feelings to support the message we are trying to communicate
are very significant and the physical action supporting that
which is said and how it is said is even more important. All
three dimensions are closely analysed, particularly by our
elders, when deciding whether or not the person delivering a
service can be trusted. Another difference between our communities and yours is that our chiefs are chosen to serve. They
are not there to direct and tell others what to do and how to
do it. There is a great difference between the governmental
system currently operating across the country and that which
operates in our more traditional communities. This causes
considerable conflict. A chief has to earn the respect of his
people. If he were to assume it, he would be the object of
ridicule. One of the problems we are facing now as a minority
group is that our leadership is trying to combine that which
you have given us, offered us, and demonstrated to us in your
way of operating with that which has characterized our traditional way of providing leadership. The fatality rate in
effect is pretty high.

In terms of delivering services, we are all servants in
one way or another. It is very important that the recipient,
and I am again talking now about my own people, feels and
knows that he is accepted as a person by the deliverer of the
service. Too many of our people return from the office of the
doctor or the government agency knowing that they have not
been accepted. The whole concept of respect breeding respect
comes strongly into play. The spin-off from this kind of
treatment is hostility, not perhaps open hostility, but hostility manifested in other forms such as alcoholism, family
breakdown and the use of drugs. The traditional way of
dealing with it among our people is to be indifferent about
it, but when there is a great deal of indifference there is
no immediate remedy. If there is hostility, you can work with
it. If there is a positive response, we can work with it. But
too often our reaction is one of indifference. Originally,
government officials took this lack of response to signify
approval. This is not the case. No response is even stronger
than saying "no."

What is the Southerner doing at this conference? That is
another question I ask myself. I am a Southerner, a member
of the Skilak tribe. I grew up in the Fraser valley and have
made even briefer trips into the North than some of the researchers who have prepared papers. I questioned the matter
of my coming along these lines, and the thing that I see and
certainly regret is that the problems which have characterized our Southern tribes are being repeated in the North. I
see these same problems and their causes in terms of the way
the government is handling the native people of the North.
It is almost the re-invention of the wheel. The same mistakes
are being made in the North as were made in the South 20, 30,
40, 50 years ago. In remedying or trying to lessen these destructive effects, much depends on the quality of relationship
the worker who is delivering a service can establish with the
recipient. This is tremendously important and has not been
dealt with to any extent at any conference that I have been
able to read about. Teamwork is essential in an office, for
example; if there are not positive relationships among the
people on the team, very little is going to get done. If the
same kind of respect for one another does not exist at the
village level, very little is going to be accomplished. More
papers like the one concerning the relationships between
general practitioners and consultants (page 576) should have
been included in this particular conference. I have worked
with provincial governments, federal governments, and our own
governments, and far too often we spend far too much of our
energy and time dealing with our own internal needs at the
expense of the recipient of the service for which we are employed. When the budgets are published, people look at the
millions of dollars spent on the health of native peoples and
on various other things, and they say "My goodness, look at
all the money! How come we have so many problems?" I venture
to say that too many of the problems are internal. This is
something we must think about, particularly the roles, relationships, and responsibilities that we have in terms of
our employing agencies.
   Destruction of culture has occupied the time of various
people. Certainly aspects of that destruction are your bread
and butter. I like to look at it this way - we all have needs
because we are all human beings, physical, emotional, and mental needs. When an outside force comes into the lives of the
native people, the ways in which these needs must be met are
radically changed. Residential schools have destroyed the
traditional ways of life, particularly in the South. A lot of
talk about family breakdowns, suicides, venereal diseases,

and the like are spin-offs from an impoverished way of
development. If you take people away from their families as
youngsters and put them in institutions, then the product
is institutionalized, having had very little, if any, contact with families over the years. In terms of emotional
growth, this is an extremely serious disadvantage. We can
only grow emotionally through relationships with people who
are more mature than we are. If we happen to be parents who
have children and we are emotionally immature (a word thrown
around a lot by people in social work and psychology), the
chances that our children can go beyond our level are very
slim. Relationships are not readily formed within institutions. Many of today's parents at the village level are products of institutions and have not had the opportunity to
grow because they have not had exposure to the elders of the
community and others who are more mature than themselves.
The result is a people with serious emotional problems.

Training professionals is, I think, an excellent idea.
Those hired as trainers must be able to share what they know
with the trainees - again, the whole communications area. It
has been said, and I have certainly seen examples of this,
that some professionals - doctors, professors, and the like -
are awfully stingy about their knowledge and not willing to
share it. The role of the para-professionals at the community level is a demanding one. Expectations are tremendously high and the kinds of problems that para-professionals
will have to face are much greater than those currently
brought to the attention of the field health nurse. They are
expected to deal with highly involved family conflicts, for
example, and the more a person demonstrates what she or he
can do the greater the demands placed on him.

I was fascinated to read some of the implied expectations
of the native regional corporations, particularly in dealing
with mental health type problems. One paper indicates it
will be possible for some traditional medicine to be instituted. My question is, why wasn't this done many years ago?
It looks like a possibility, only when it becomes something
that belongs to us. One serious question I have is who is
going to pay the bill?

A conference like this should emphasize positives. It is
very distressing to me to see that conferences in all disciplines focus on problems. When I first got involved in
probation work several years ago, I couldn't get over how
negative psychiatric assessments were. I was appalled, to
the extent that I went to some of the psychiatrists concerned and said "Listen, I have a degree in psychology and

I am expected to work with this problem, adult or child. That which you state in your reports is useless to me, because all you are telling me is what is wrong with the individual. I want to know what strengths he has." The response I got was "We haven't developed the tools to measure strengths as yet." I would like to see a conference held on positive things. What qualities do the native people have? What strengths are there within their community? What strengths are there within the various institutions used to deliver services?

I seriously question the value of much of the research in terms of its usefulness to the recipient. I can appreciate that there is pure scientific stuff, understood only by scientists and directed only to scientists. But my concern is the value of this research in the sense that I seldom if ever see it brought back to the people who provided the initial data. It is not that we are disinterested. Effective feed-back is tremendously important. Have enough respect for your informants to share your findings with them. If more of this were done, relationships between researchers and our communities would improve immensely, and there would be desirable spin-offs in the sense that people in the village would benefit directly from the work you have done.

Thank you very much.

CURRENT TRENDS IN ARCTIC MEDICAL RESEARCH

Current trends in arctic medical research in the
Nordic countries with special reference to Sweden

H. LINDERHOLM

Particularly during the present century, many research
workers have been interested in medical problems in the
northern parts of the Nordic countries. Research has been
mostly on a national basis, initiated by government or
single research workers, and a considerable amount of knowledge has been gathered concerning northern Fennoscandia,
Iceland, and Greenland (7).

Throughout the last decades, there has been a trend for
Nordic countries to co-ordinate arctic medical research, in
the belief that research will increase in value if investigations are planned with common goals and use comparable
methods so that the results can be compared between countries. In this way, resources of personnel and equipment
also may be better utilized and the investigations may be
broadened to examine a greater number of variables. Furthermore, by comparing various ethnic groups living in similar
environments, it may be possible to distinguish the significance of environmental contra-genetic factors. It may
finally be easier to interpret the results in a global perspective. We thus believe that a joint, co-ordinated effort
can increase the quality of nordic arctic medical research.

On the initiative of the Nordic Council (an internordic
political reference group), a Nordic Expert Committee
worked out suggestions for co-operation in arctic medical
research in 1959 (7). Subsequent discussions centred on the
value of building an institute for arctic medical research,
and the suggestion emerged of appointing a permanent secretariat to stimulate and co-ordinate research efforts.

The governments of Denmark, Finland, Norway, and Sweden
did not establish the Nordic Council for Arctic Medical
Research (NCAMR) until 1969, when a permanent Secretariat
was organized at Oulu, Finland. The NCAMR may be regarded

as an expression of the wish to co-ordinate arctic medical research in the Nordic countries. The council has its own budget and rules for its activities and the Secretariat at Oulu is headed by a secretary general. It may be regarded as a centre for nordic arctic medical research and it has facilitated both international contacts and contacts between research workers and funding agencies. Documentation is one activity of the secretariat, and an appropriate collection of references and literature is being established as a service to research workers in this field.

The NCAMR arranged the Second International Symposium on Circumpolar Health in Oulu in 1971. The council has also published a catalogue of current arctic medical research in the Nordic countries (6), presented at the Oulu symposium and continuing with a 1973 supplement (1). These surveys show that research in the Nordic countries covers most fields of arctic medical research known from international symposia and the literature (cf. also 4).

The NCAMR has stated the urgent need for increased research in arctic and subarctic areas with respect to: (1) special features of disease and health care; (2) problems associated with changes in population distribution and social structure (urbanization); (3) the adaptation of man to arctic conditions; and (4) genetic problems of ethnic minorities in areas where isolation is rapidly disappearing.

Within these fields of research, the council has organized workshops and conferences, and has also initiated research projects. Examples of conferences include those held at Godthåb, Greenland, in 1972 (9) and Berlevåg and Kirkenes, Northern Norway, in 1973 (8). Workshops include those on "Lactate malabsorption" (Helsinki, 1972 (5)), "Coronary heart disease in the Arctic" (Oulu, 1973 (11)), and "Light and darkness, biological rhythms and living conditions in the Arctic" (Kiruna, 1974 (12)). Projects initiated include an investigation of lactate malabsorption among Lapps in northern Finland (10) and an epidemiological study of diseases in the northern parts of the Nordic countries.

Most of these activities have been reported in the *Arctic Medical Research Report,* a publication edited by the NCAMR. The journal also includes scientific papers on arctic medical research, and it may be obtained from the secretariat at Oulu, Finland.

Other organized activities include a contribution to the "International biological program, human adaptability" (IBP/HA) project. A nordic team carried out broad population

studies on the Lapps of northern Finland from 1966 to 1971
(3). More recently, the research workers engaged in this
project have directed their interest to Iceland and, together with Icelandic scientists, have started a broad
population and epidemiological study of "Icelanders in a
changing world." National organizations also exist, such as
the Danish Association for Medical Research in Greenland.
In Finland, the IBP/HA research group has been particularly
active.

Sweden has no national organizations for arctic medical
research, but a considerable part of the research effort,
particularly in genetics, population biology, and epidemiology, is concentrated at the University of Umeå, the most
northern Swedish university. Findings were demonstrated at
the Ecology Symposium at Luleå in 1971 (2), a satellite
meeting of the Second International Symposium on Circumpolar Health held in Oulu. In Gothenburg, an IBP/HA group,
including odontologists, has shared in studies of Lapps in
northern Finland and has also contributed to the project
"Icelanders in a changing world." Other projects concerning
infectious diseases, cold physiology, and military research
are going on in Stockholm and elsewhere in Sweden.

SUMMARY

Co-ordination of arctic medical research in the Nordic
countries is facilitated by the Nordic Council for Arctic
Medical Research (NCAMR). This organization was established
by the Nordic governments in 1969, with a permanent secretariat at Oulu, Finland. It may be regarded as an expression of the belief that such joint activities are
fruitful and increase the efficiency and scientific value
of the research undertaken. The council has pointed out
fields of research needing investigation, and by organizing
scientific meetings, conferences, and workshops, it has
tried to stimulate and co-ordinate research. Both international and national groups and individual research workers
are supported by the council in their contacts with funding
agencies. The council also edits the *Arctic Medical Research
Report*.

REFERENCES

1. "Arctic medical research in progress in the Nordic
   countries. Supplementary list 1973," Nordic Council for
   Medical Research Report, 5: 1-56 (1973)

2. Bylund, E., Linderholm, H., and Rune, O., "Ecological problems of the circumpolar area, Lulea, Sweden," to be published (1974)
3. Lewin, T., and Hedegård, B., "The internordic IBP/HA studies of the Skolt Lapps in northern Finland 1966 to 1969," Proc. Finn. Dent. Soc., 67, Suppl. 1: 9-12 (1971)
4. Linderholm, H. "Arctic medicine in the Nordic countries. Aspects of the scope of arctic medicine and some current research problems," World Med. J., 4: 75-9 (1973)
5. "Nordic workshop on lactose malabsorption, Helsinki, August 26-27, 1972," edited by Leena Hansson and Ilmari Palva, Nordic Council for Arctic Medical Research Report, 3: 1-19 (1973)
6. Nordisk arktisk medicinsk forskning. Projektkatalog with English summary. (Nordiska samarbetskommittén för arktisk medicinsk forskning, 1971)
7. Nordiskt samarbete om arktisk medicin (Betänkande av Nordiska expertutskottet för arktisk medicin, Stockholm, 1961)
8. Roundtable conference between the Nordic Council for Arctic Medical Research and representatives of the Health Services in northern Norway and northern Finland at Berlevåg and Kirkenes, March 1973. Nordic Council for Arctic Medical Research Report, 4: 1-24 (1973)
9. "Rundabordskonference mellem nordisk samarbejdskomite for arktisk medicinsk forskning og repraesentanter for det grønlandske sundhedsvaesen, Godthåb 3-6 sept 1972," by B. Harvald, Nordic Council for Arctic Medical Research Report, 2: 1-8 (1972)
10. Sahi, T., Eriksson, A.W., Isokoski, M., and Kirjarinta, M., "Lactose malabsorption in Finnish Lapps," in Third International Symposium on Circumpolar Health, July 8-11, 1974, Yellowknife, NWT, Canada, Abstracts of Papers, p.18
11. Workshop on coronary heart disease in the Arctic, Oulu, 26-27, October 1973, Nordic Council for Arctic Medical Research Report, 7: 1-66 (1974)
12. Workshop on light and darkness, biological rhythms and living conditions in the Arctic. Kiruna, Sweden, 26-27 April 1974, Nordic Council for Arctic Medical Research Report, 10 (in press, 1974)

Current trends of medical research in Greenland

B.J. HARVALD

Medical research in Greenland encounters special problems.
The population is scattered over an enormous area. Climatic
and geographical factors make travelling difficult, dangerous, and expensive. Transport and installation of scientific
equipment is complicated or impossible. Forwarding of
samples is slow. The language barrier limits contact with
the native population.

The ideas behind many Greenlandic research projects have
arisen from casual clinical observations during field work.
Instances include epidemiological, genetic, and socio-
medical studies, dealing with glaucoma (3), congenital malformations (1, 7, 12, 13), diabetes (6, 14), lactase deficiency (4), venereal diseases (17), and tuberculosis (8, 9,
11, 15).

In other cases, the research has consisted of an application of new technology to a Greenlandic population sample,
either from the Thule or Angmassalik districts, where the
populations are still pure Eskimo, or from the mixed populations of West Greenland. Some studies of this type have
drawn exclusively on Greenlanders living in Denmark or on
Greenlandic blood- or serum-samples, sent to laboratories in
Denmark for independent reasons. In this type of study the
idea for the project has been generated by highly developed
laboratories in Denmark. Examples include the blood- and
sero-typing studies (5) of the Copenhagen forensic institute,
the transplantation antigen studies (10) of the Aarhus
tissue typing laboratory, the serum lipid studies of the
laboratory of clinical chemistry in Aalborg (2), and the β-
hepatitis antigen studies (16) of the laboratory of clinical
chemistry at the Bispebjerg Hospital, Copenhagen.

Medical research in Greenland has access to the same
facilities as research in Denmark, but it has been realized
by the Danish Medical Research Council that special encouragement is currently needed, since the opportunity still
exists in Greenland to study a unique ethnic group that re-
tains its own cultural pattern while under a totally Danish
health care system. Greenland also allows observation of the
direct socio-medical implications and consequences of a very
fast-moving process of urbanization and industrialization.
From both points of view, there is a strong factor of urgency.

TABLE 1
Resources for medical research in Greenland

Project	Resources
Idea	
Problem formulation	Scientific Advisory Service of Danish
Choice of method	Medical Research Council
Protocol	
Budget	Danish Medical Research Council
Financial support	Other funds
Travelling	Ministry for Greenland
Scientific field work	Greenland Health Service
Preparation	Danish Society for Medical Research in Greenland
Publishing	Nordic Council for Arctic Medical Research

Available resources at different steps of project processing are summarized in Table 1. In problem formulation, choice of method, and elaboration of protocol, assistance is offered by the scientific advisory service of the Danish Medical Research Council. On application, the research worker is referred to one of about 40 consultants, paid by the Research Council for a maximum of 10 hours per consultation.

Most financial support is derived from the Danish Medical Research Council, which during its six years of existence has given a high priority to medical research in Greenland. Travel expenses have to a certain extent been covered by the Ministry for Greenland and travelling has been facilitated by the local health service in Greenland.

The Danish Society for Medical Research in Greenland was founded in 1970 with the special purpose of promoting and co-ordinating research activities. The society has some sixty members, most of them actively engaged in medical research in Greenland. The society offers a mechanism for fostering contact between research workers, for discussion of plans and results, and for getting advice on the practical organization of field work in Greenland. The society generally arranges meetings three of four times a year, and the executive board maintains a consultative function throughout the year.

A rough distinction can be drawn between results of arctic medical research that have general applicability and findings that are of interest only for the Arctic. In the former case, there are usually no problems of publication in international journals, but in the latter case it may prove difficult to reach the right audience through ordinary channels. Here the report series of the Nordic Council for Arctic Medical Research has filled a gap. The report series is published in English and accepts both short papers and monographs of up to 100 pages. The layout is quite unpretentious. Reports are distributed internationally without cost to most centres of arctic medical research and are also available to individual scientists on request.

The total annual costs of medical research in Greenland are currently Cdn $100,000 to 150,000. This estimate includes not only the direct financial support of concrete projects, but also the university and hospital resources used for such projects and the Danish share of the costs of the Nordic Council for Arctic Medical Research.

SUMMARY

A survey is given of the organization and facilities for medical research in Greenland. The estimated annual costs are at present Cdn $100,000 to 150,000.

REFERENCES

1. Andersen, S., and Rønn, G., "Incidental findings following mass radiography in Greenland," Ugeskr. Loeg., 132: 777-9 (1970)
2. Bang, H.O., and Dyerberg, J., "Plasma lipids and lipoproteins in Greenlandic West coast Eskimos," Acta med. scand., 192: 85-94 (1972)
3. Clemmesen, V., and Alsbirk, P.H., "Primary angle-closure glaucoma (a.c.g.) in Greenland," Acta ophthal., Copenhagen, 49: 47-58 (1971)
4. Gudmand-Høyer, E., and Jarnum, S. "Lactose malabsorption in Greenland Eskimos," Acta med. scand., 186: 235-7 (1969)
5. Gurtler, H., Gilberg, Aa., and Tingsgaard, P., "Blodtypefordelingen i Grønland," Dansk Med. Selsk., 1: 21 (1973)
6. Harvald, B., "Disease prevalence in Greenland," Acta socio-med. scand., Suppl., 6: 203-5 (1972)

7. Harvald, B., and Hels, J., "The incidence of cardiac malformations in Greenlandic Eskimos," Acta med. scand., 185: 41-44 (1969)

8. Horwitz, O., "Epidemiology of tuberculosis in Greenland," Acta socio-med. scand., Suppl., 6: 232-9 (1972)

9. Iversen, Erik, "Epidemiological basis of tuberculosis eradication II. Mortality among tuberculosis cases in the general population of Greenland," Bull. Wld. Hlth. Org., 45: 667-87 (1971)

10. Kissmeyer-Nielsen, F., Andersen, H., Hauge, M., Karen E. Kjerbye, Mogensen, B., and Svejgaard, A., "HL-A types in Danish Eskimos from Greenland," Tissue Antigens, 1: 74-80 (1971)

11. Krebs Lange, P., "Morbilli and tuberculosis in Greenland," Scand. J. resp. Dis., 51: 256-67 (1970)

12. Rønn, G., and Andersen, S., "Dextrocardia in Greenland," Acta radiol. Stockh. 12: 161-3 (1972)

13. Rønn, G., and Andersen, S., "Diaphragmatic hernias in Greenland," Scand. J. thor. cardiovasc. Surg., 5: 284-5 (1971)

14. Sagild, U., Littauer, J., Sand Jespersen, C., and Andersen, S., "Epidemiological studies in Greenland 1962-1964. I. Diabetes mellitus in Eskimos." Acta med. scand., 179: 29-39 (1966)

15. Stein, K.P.S., Krebs Lange, P., Gad, U., and Wilbek, E., "Tuberculosis in Greenland," Arch. Environ. Health, 17: 501-6 (1968)

16. Østergaard Hansen, A., Skinhøj, P., and McNair, A., "Hepatitis og hepatitisassocieret antigen (HAA) i Gronland," Dansk Med. Selsk., 1: 72 (1973)

17. Aagaard Olsen, G., "Sexual norms under the influence of altered cultural patterns in Greenland," Acta psychiat. scand., 49: 148-58 (1973)

Commentary

"Current trends in arctic medical research in Finland," by H. Forsius (Department of Ophthalmology, University of Oulu, Oulu, Finland). Most of the work in progress in Finland in the field of arctic medical research is organized by the northernmost faculty of medicine in the country, at Oulu.

The Department of Public Health is supervising work on
special features concerned with morbidity and mortality (S.
Näyhä and A. Harni) and is studying a series of children
born in northern Finland in 1966 (P. Rantakallio), which has
been followed since the time of their mothers' pregnancies.
The Department of Internal Medicine is studying the primary
prevention of coronary heart diseases in northern Finland
(J. Takkunen), and the Department of Dermatology is
attempting to trace genetic skin diseases and is studying
the effects of extremes of light and cold on the skin. One
project in the Department of Pediatrics concerns the effect
of variations in daylight on school attendance and the
Department of Criminal Pathology is involved in a project
studying the relationship between alcohol consumption and
death by misadventure (J. Hirvonen). From 1966 to 1971 the
Nordic Human Adaptability section of the International Biological Program carried out extensive research into the
original reindeer-herding population, the Lapps, in Finland,
most of the results of which are still to be published.
Topics covered are genetics, immunology, pediatrics including child psychiatry, nutrition, sociology, odontology,
demography, and ophthalmology. The same research group,
under H. Forsius and A. W. Eriksson (Folkhalsan Institute
of Population Genetics, Kauniainen), did field-work in 1974
on the influence of the Lapps on the populations of southern
Lapland.

BIORHYTHMS, COLD PHYSIOLOGY, AND PATHOLOGY

Seasonal variations in daily patterns of urinary excretion by Eskimo subjects

MARY C. LOBBAN

Three years ago, at the Second International Symposium on
Circumpolar Health held at Oulu, Finland, I described alterations which appeared to be taking place in the daily
rhythms of renal excretion in Eskimo subjects as the life-
style of the people changed and their social environment
became more southernized. The lack of rhythmicity observed
in Eskimo subjects in the 1950s (1) at Wainwright, Alaska
(71°N), had been replaced by a variety of daily patterns of
urinary excretion of water and electrolytes for Eskimos
both in the western Northwest Territories of Canada (Inuvik,
69°N, and Tuktoyaktuk, 70°N) and in the east (Hall Beach,
70°N). When compared with the daily excretory patterns of
subjects from temperate zones, most of these newly developed
rhythms did not show good temporal synchronization, particularly in the continuous daylight of mid-summer (2), but at
other seasons of the year there were definite indications of
"day" and "night" excretory rates. It was obvious that further recordings of Eskimo daily excretory patterns should be
made at different seasons of the year, using a larger population sample. In 1973, I was given the opportunity to spend
all four seasons of the year with the Eskimo people of Pond
Inlet (72°N, eastern Northwest Territories), where I was
able to study different age groups under spring (L/D),
summer (L/L), autumn (L/D), and winter (D/D) conditions.

METHODS

Each subject - child, adult, or aged - agreed to void urine
at frequent intervals into labelled, wide-mouthed polythene
bottles over a period of 36-40 hours, the volume and time
of each voiding being recorded in the field. A small quantity of each sample was preserved under toluene in a hard

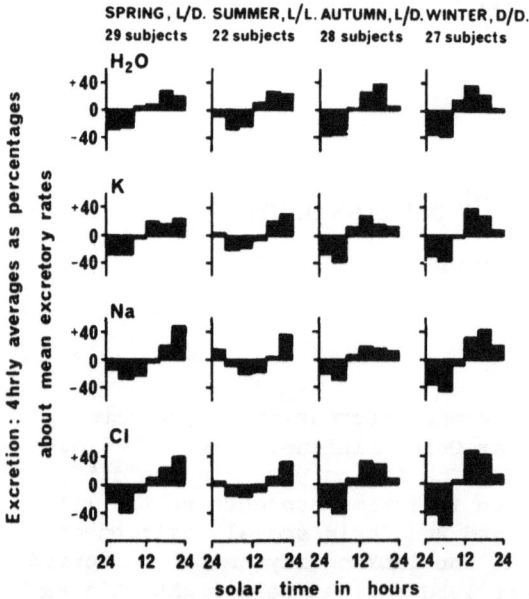

Figure 1   Daily rhythms of renal excretion in adult Eskimo subjects, Pond Inlet, NWT, in the four seasons

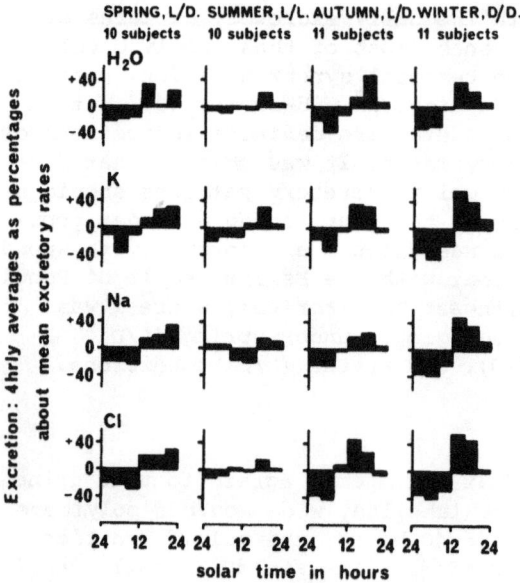

Figure 2   Daily rhythms of renal excretion in aged Eskimo subjects, Pond Inlet, NWT, in the four seasons

glass tube for subsequent laboratory analysis of potassium
and sodium content (by flame photometry) and chloride content (by electrometric titration). Urine collections were
made for the same subjects at all four seasons of the year.

RESULTS

The daily patterns of renal excretion for water, potassium,
sodium, and chloride (averaged values for the group) for
adult Pond Inlet Eskimo subjects are presented in Figure 1.
Some degree of rhythmicity is indicated for each of the
urinary constituents at all four seasons of the year. When
compared with the patterns of excretion usually encountered
in subjects from temperate zones, all periods of peak excretion are late, and in summer (L/L) they are very late,
leading to a temporal reversal of the excretory rhythm.
In winter (D/D), however, despite the absence of an L/D external environment, both temporal synchronization and the
daily peak-to-trough range of the excretory patterns are
well maintained.
    Daily patterns of renal excretion for aged Pond Inlet
Eskimo subjects are indicated in Figure 2. A greater seasonal variation occurs for this group than for the adults. In
spring (L/D) water excretion is irregular, but the electrolytes all show late peaks, as for the adults. Autumn and
winter recordings show, surprisingly enough, a fair degree
of temporal synchronization, the winter patterns having a
good peak-to-trough range. Summer recordings are irregular,
desynchronized both from clock time and from one another,
and are poorly developed.
    The seasonal daily patterns of renal excretion for Pond
Inlet school children, shown in Figure 3, are perhaps the
most satisfactory of all. In spring and autumn, when the
synchronizers of the natural environment (L/D) coincide
with the social synchronizer of regular school hours, good
temporal synchronization and reasonable peak-to-trough
ranges are evidenced by all urinary constituents. In winter
(D/D), when the children are still attending school, the
best-developed and synchronized rhythms of all are seen,
but in summer, when environmental fluctuations in lighting
are absent and school is not in session, the daily rhythms
are irregular, desynchronized, and of very low peak-to-
trough range.
    A rhythm may become temporally desynchronized without
losing its degree of development, and vice versa, i.e.,
good peak-to-trough ranges may be observed at unusual times,

SPRING, L/D. SUMMER, L/L. AUTUMN, L/D. WINTER, D/D.
19 subjects   17 subjects   19 subjects   18 subjects

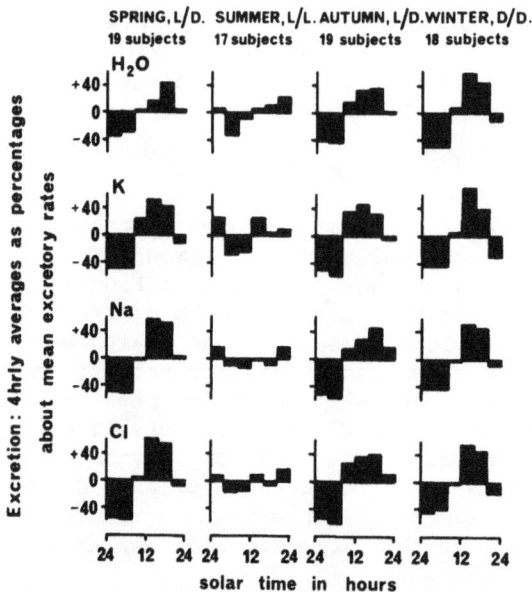

Figure 3   Daily rhythms of renal excretion in Eskimo children, Pond Inlet, NWT, in the four seasons

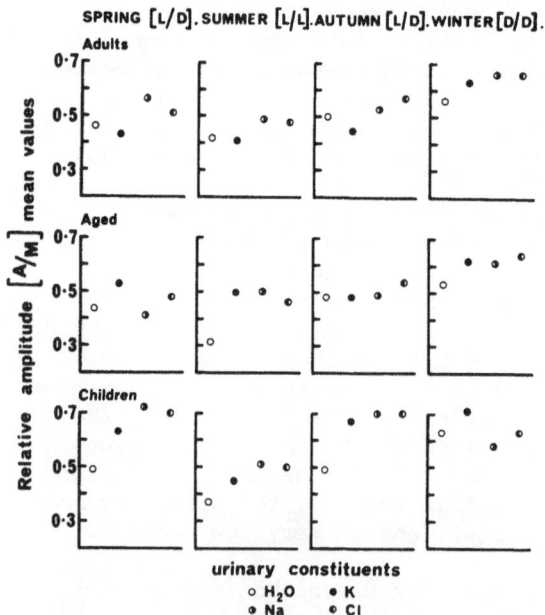

SPRING [L/D]. SUMMER [L/L]. AUTUMN [L/D]. WINTER [D/D].

Figure 4   Relative amplitudes of daily rhythms of renal excretion in Eskimo subjects, Pond Inlet, NWT, in the four seasons

or good temporal synchronization may occur in the presence
of very low peak-to-trough ranges. A more precise measure
of the degree of development of an excretory rhythm lies in
the calculation of its relative amplitude. The relative amplitudes of all the daily rhythms of renal excretion for all
three age groups are shown in Figure 4. Adult and aged subjects demonstrate little difference in the relative amplitudes of the four urinary constituents for spring, autumn,
and summer, although temporal desynchronization occurs in
the summer daylight. In the darkness of winter, however, the
rhythms are better developed than at any other season. For
the children, spring, autumn, and winter rhythms all show
high relative amplitudes; however, in summer the values drop
dramatically for all four urinary constituents, indicating a
true qualitative difference from the other seasons, when the
children are at school.

DISCUSSION

The daily patterns of renal excretion of Eskimo subjects in
all age groups now show rhythmic fluctuations at all four
seasons of the year. The children, subject to the action of
the dual synchronizers of regular school-times (social) and
the annual light/dark seasonal fluctuations (environmental),
show the most striking departures from the lack of daily
rhythmicity found in earlier Eskimo recordings and the
largest differences between the seasons of the year (3). In
spring and autumn, when the light day/dark night environment
and the Eskimos' activity patterns reinforce each other,
some degree of rhythmicity is found in all three age groups,
and it is difficult to determine the relative importance of
environmental and social synchronizers in the development
and maintenance of the daily renal rhythms. Likewise in
summer, the continuous daylight of the natural environment,
the freedom of the children from school, and the general
relaxed atmosphere of the holiday season all come together
to allow an extremely irregular pattern of activity, with
eating and sleeping throughout the 24 hours of the day: at
this season, renal rhythms may become reversed (in the
adults and aged) or almost totally disrupted (in the children). In the darkness of mid-winter, however, when environmental and social synchronizers are in opposition, well-
developed rhythms of very good temporal synchronization are
found in all three age groups: it is clear that in a
modern Eskimo settlement, with artificial lighting and
heating and the children attending school, it is the social
synchronizers that exert the greatest effect.

Pond Inlet provides a beautiful arctic setting, where old skills and traditions still exsit alongside the new, modern life-style which is being brought in from the south. Although the land still plays a considerable part in the life of the Pond Inlet Eskimo, modern conditions would appear to be bringing about not only social but also biological changes in the people. Some degree of rhythmic flexibility is still evidenced by the seasonal variations in the people's daily rhythms of renal excretion, and we must hope that the benefits of a modern life-style, with its dependence upon clock-time, do not eventually change the Eskimo's physiology too much and make him less adaptable to the demands of his arctic environment.

ACKNOWLEDGMENT

I wish to express my most grateful thanks to the people of Pond Inlet for their enthusiastic and good-humoured co-operation in this work.

SUMMARY

The urinary excretion of water and electrolytes was followed in 59 Eskimo subjects living in the North Baffin settlement of Pond Inlet (72°N) in spring, summer, autumn, and winter, 1973. Seasonal variations in the daily patterns of excretion were observed, and in both summer and winter these were more closely related to the life-style of the subjects than to the seasonal light/dark variations in the natural environment. It would appear that the recent and marked changes in the social environment of the Eskimo have been accompanied by biological changes in the people themselves. We must hope that these changes do not eventually destroy the flexibility of the Eskimos' physiology, so that the people are no longer able to adapt to the peculiar demands of the arctic environment.

REFERENCES

1. Lobban, Mary C., "Daily rhythms of renal excretion in arctic-dwelling Indians and Eskimos," Quart. J. exp. Physiol., 52: 401-10 (1967)
2. Lobban, Mary C., In O.G. Edholm and E.K.E. Gunderson (eds.), Polar Human Biology (Chichester, England: Heinemann Medical Books Ltd., 1973), pp. 306-14

3. Lobban, Mary C., "Seasonal variations in daily patterns of renal excretion in modern Eskimo children," J. interdiscipl. Cycle Res. (in press)

The relationship between physiological and
biological mechanisms of human adaptation

V.P. KAZNACHEYEV

Studies on the physiological and biological mechanisms of human adaptation are fundamental to the development of efficient measures of public health control and prophylaxis of diseases. The data obtained to date concern mainly particular systems of homeostatic regulation (Slonim, 1969; Mirrakhimov, 1972; Itoh, 1974). However, it may prove fruitful to treat data in the framework of integrated theories (Barbashovs, 1960: Danishevsky, 1968: Slonim, 1969; Avtsin, 1972; Parin, 1973). Parin's definition of the norm as the dynamic state of a living system which favours maximum adaptivity (1973) is implicit in this approach.

Although individual adaptive mechanisms are now amenable to measurement, it is difficult to assess the state of the total organism and to make long-term predictions therefrom. Interrelated ergometric, psychological, and biorhythmic estimates of adaptation yield meaningful information. No less knowledge is gleaned from research at the molecular and submolecular levels (Figure 1). Under certain ecological conditions it is possible to distinguish specific and non-specific mechanisms of adaptation at each of these levels. A wide range of ecological factors act on the organism, mainly through analysers and regulatory systems, but also directly at the tissue, cellular, molecular, and other levels.

This range of ecological factors is of great importance in studies of the adaptive processes of man living in the Far North. In addition to mediated factors (psycho-emotional strain, biorhythms, hyper- and hypo-kinesia, temperature), there are other factors (nutrition, microelements) that have a more direct effect. Factors related to geomagnetic and cosmic influences deserve particular emphasis. They

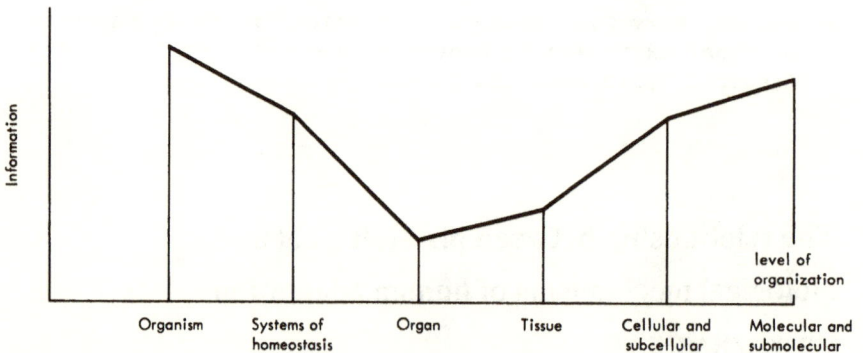

Figure 1   Dependence of relative value of information on the level of organization

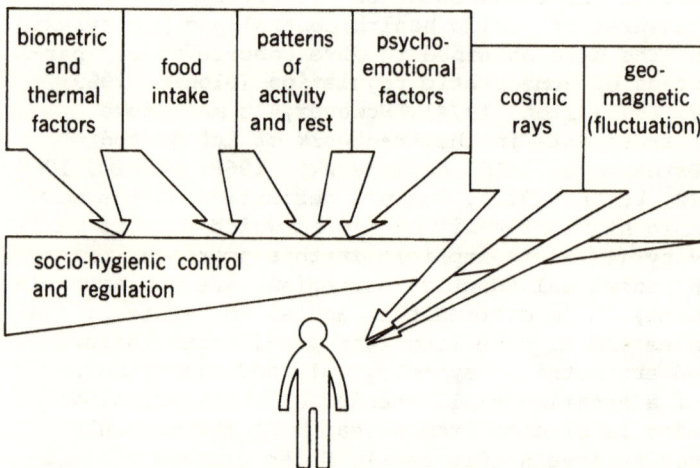

Figure 2   Ecological factors involved in adaptation to high latitudes and possibilities for control

operate directly at the cellular, molecular, and subcellular levels. Differentiation of these factors should help to solve problems of health control and enhance man's ability to adapt himself to technological and social changes. However, the control of factors that act directly will remain a challenging problem for some time (Figure 2).

The idea that geomagnetic, solar, and cosmic factors play an important role in human physiology was suggested by Chijevsky (1915-30). He demonstrated that many physiological and biological phenomena are closely related to cycles of solar activity. To elaborate his idea further would be to say that the development of the biosphere and noosphere (Vernadsky, 1965) heralds the era of noocosmogenesis, the development of the noocosmos. Adaptive processes may be of two types. Specific reactions may be conditioned by a factor that is also very specific and pertains exclusively to a given environment such as the presence of specific infection, or an absence of gravitational field (weightlessness). Specificity may also arise through a unique combination of environmental factors which per se are not specific. As a rule, the two types of specific mechanism act together and lead to complex adaptive processes. To gain insight into this complexity and disentangle the various individual components is a formidable problem.

Data will be presented on the specificity of human adaptation to conditions in high latitudes. Adaptation is manifested at molecular and submolecular levels and is related to the effects of geomagnetic and cosmic factors characteristic of these latitudes. Based on the results obtained, the hypothesis is suggested that conditions in high latitudes produce a specific "syndrome of polar tension." The significance of this syndrome in the pathology of adaptive processes will be discussed.

SOME DEFINITIONS

Environmental conditions that conform to the geno- and pheno-typic requirements of a biosystem at a given point of time are defined as adequate conditions. Inadequate conditions are those which, at a given point of time, do not conform to the geno- and pheno-topic needs of a biosystem.

Adaptation

(a) In terms of thermodynamics, adaptation may be described as the maintenance of the optimum non-equilibrium state of a biosystem under inadequate environmental conditions. Adaptation provides maximum work efficiency (Bauer, 1935), and thereby helps the self-perpetuation and survival of the biosystem.
(b) In terms of cybernetics, adaptation may be referred to as a process of self-preservation, brought about by auto-regulation at the functional level under inadequate environmental conditions. It is the choice of a functional strategy that provides optimum attainment of the ultimate goal of a biosystem.

(c) In terms of biology, adaptation may be regarded as the process of maintaining and developing the biological features of a species, population, or ecosystem despite inadequate conditions.

(d) In terms of physiology, adaptation may be regarded as a process maintaining the functional state of individual homeostatic systems and the organism as a whole, thereby ensuring its integrity, development, work capacity, and maximum longevity under inadequate environmental conditions.

Specificity of adaptive processes may be conferred by interactions with (a) unique environmental factors or (b) combinations of non-specific environmental factors.

THE ECOLOGICAL STRUCTURE OF HIGH LATITUDES

The most important non-specific factor is the cosmic rays emitted by the solar system. Cosmic rays of different wavelengths react in different ways with matter and are subjected to scattering, absorption, and other conversions (Rossi, 1966). As a result, at high latitudes the earth's geomagnetic field oscillates mainly under the effect of secondary magnetic radiation (Pertsov, 1973). These oscillations of the geomagnetic field and their distribution over the earth's surface depend on the structural features of the magnetic sphere of the earth (Pushkov and Silkin, 1966). The lower the magnetic latitude, the more energy a particle requires to reach the earth's surface. A primary particle can reach the earth at the equator only if it has energy of not less than 14.9 billion electron volts, whereas at a magnetic latitude of ±30° the corresponding value is 10 billion electron volts (Figure 3).

Clearly, the intensity of primary and secondary radiation that reaches the earth's surface increases with the magnetic latitude. This may induce changes in the physical and chemical properties of such model systems as water (Kislovsky, 1971), colloids (Piccardy, 1971), biological systems (Danishevsky, 1968), and the earth's atmosphere (Mustel, 1971).

Cosmic and electromagnetic fields interact with elements of the biosphere at the molecular and submolecular levels (Presman, 1968). Magnetic and electric properties of biological systems undergo severe alterations; their molecular structures enter into a metastable state, and the number of free radicals of water, such as OH', H^+, OOH' (Kislovsky, 1971), and of other compounds increases. Intense cosmic radiation at high latitudes also enhances the ionization of

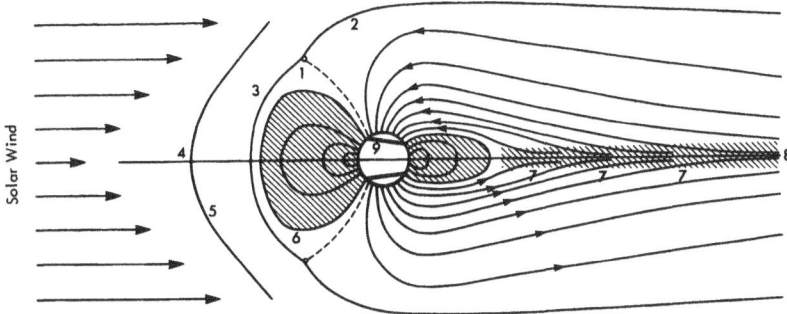

Figure 3   Schematic meridional cross-section of the earth's magnetic sphere (1, neutral points; 2, magnetic points; 3, transition area; 4, geomagnetic equator; 5, shock wave; 6, areas of radioactive capture; 7, areas of particle acceleration; 8, neutral layer; 9, zones of aurora polaris)

oxygen, thereby activating free radical processes in the cellular membranes of respiratory organs (Tappel, 1973).

PRIMARY BIOPHYSICAL EFFECTS UNDER HIGH LATITUDE CONDITIONS

There is now substantial evidence to support the idea that the functioning of many biological systems is accompanied by the formation of free radicals. Free radicals usually arise in systems which are susceptible to oxidation-reduction conversions (electron transport, oxygen activation, etc). These processes occur in mitochondrial membranes, in the endoplasmic reticulum, and in cytoplasmic oxidases and oxygenases.

An increase or a decrease in the level of free radicals can be initiated by many agents. Most studies have been directed to the elucidation of factors that increase the level of free radicals in cells capable of stimulating free peroxidation of lipids in cellular membranes. These include, among other factors, irradiation with X-rays and ultraviolet light, poor nutrition, vitamin E deficiency, chemical toxins, and oxygen toxicity. Exposure to these factors increases the content of free radicals, facilitates their interactions with fatty acids, and results eventually in lipid peroxidation damage of biomembranes, subcellular organelles, and the enzymes they contain.

In the course of evolution a number of protective systems have evolved to prevent the development of chain radical processes:
(1) Non-enzymic antioxidant systems: naturally occurring antioxidants, tocopherol, sterols, and others.

(2) Enzymic antioxidant systems, including peroxide dismu-
tase, NADPH-generated systems, glutathione reductase,
glutathione peroxidase

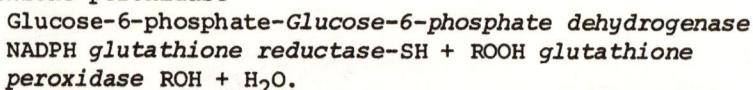

   Glucose-6-phosphate-*Glucose-6-phosphate dehydrogenase*
   NADPH *glutathione reductase*-SH + ROOH *glutathione*
   peroxidase ROH + H_2O.

These cycles of enzymic reactions prevent the series of
chain reactions initiated by free radicals in biomembranes
(Vladimirov and Arachkov, 1972).
(3) Adaptive changes may also occur in the biomembrane
structure, resulting in an elevated content of saturated
fatty acids (Tsyrlov, 1972).

   The results of our studies carried out on normal subjects residing in the Far North and middle latitudes
(Kulikov, Mishin, and Liakhovich, in preparation) have
suggested that under conditions where free radicals are
activated, the changes have a sequential pattern.

   Phase I is associated (Figure 4) with the accelerated
generation of peroxide radicals, increased content of fatty
acid hydroperoxides in membranes, decreased level of natural
antioxidants, and decreased resistance of erythrocyte membranes to the damaging effect of superoxide radicals (O_2).

   Phase II is characterized (Figure 5) by a stabilization
of the level of oxygen radicals and fatty acid hydroperoxides, possibly as a result of increased activity by
enzymic antioxidant systems.

   Phase III is characterized (Figure 6) by a slower generation of superoxide radicals and a decreased content of
fatty acid hydroperoxides, with increased resistance of membrane structures to factors activating lipid peroxidation
(Tsyrlov et al., 1972).

   These results are consistent with the view that factors
specific to high latitudes can have profound effects on
the state of biosystems which are characterized, first and
foremost, by changes at the molecular level. These changes
may act in the same way as primary noise sources in a
communications system (in the sense of information theory)
and trigger a whole set of metabolic reactions at the
cellular, tissue, and finally the whole-body level as man
adapts to high latitude conditions.

SOME METABOLIC ASPECTS OF ADAPTATION TO HIGH LATITUDE
CONDITIONS

The presumed direct damaging effects of cosmic and geomagnetic disturbances on biological membranes prompt a

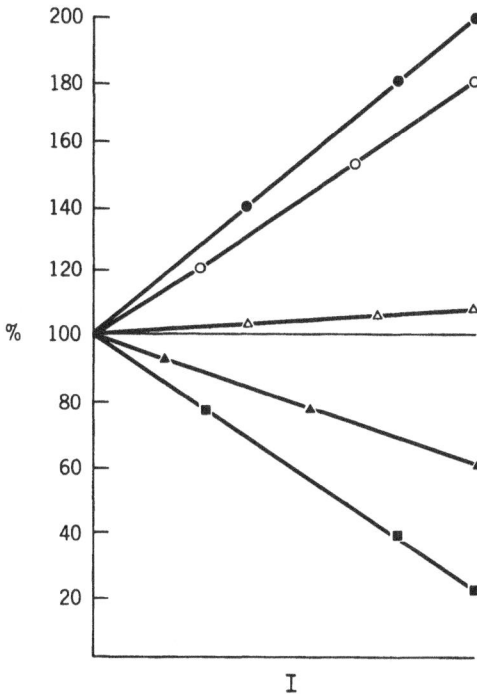

Figure 4   Dynamics of free-radical reactions and their control system in man under high-latitude conditions and in
experimental animals, phase 1 (O, rate of O_2 production;
●, fatty acid hydroperoxide content; ■ , antioxidant activity; Δ , enzymatic antioxidant system activity; ▲ , erythrocyte
membrane stability)

fresh look at metabolic changes in adaptation processes.
Lipids, carbohydrates, and proteins differ in their adaptive
value as sources of free energy and synthetic materials.
Harper (1969) has emphasized that during work glucose is not
the main substrate either in the liver or in most other
tissues (with the exception of neural and adipose tissues
for which glucose is absolutely necessary). Ketone bodies
and fatty acids are the predominant fuels for these tissues.
The studies of Krebs et al. (1970) have demonstrated that
the redox potential of liver cells changes similarly under
various stresses (starvation, diabetes mellitus, heavy
physical exercise); in each of these situations, metabolic
fuel is supplied mainly by the oxidation of fatty acids.
There is reason for believing that this oxidation has other
advantages. Quite likely the capacity of intensifying lipid

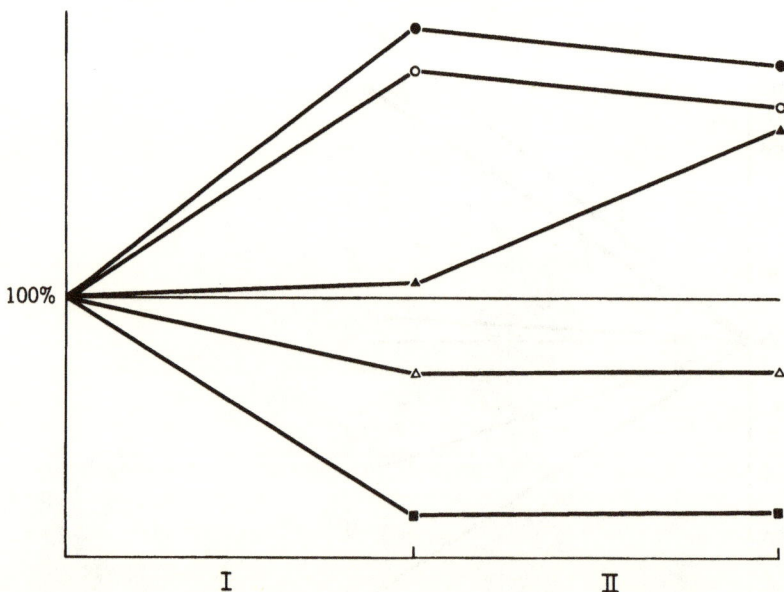

Figure 5 Dynamics of free-radical reactions and their control system in man under high-latitude conditions and in experimental animals, phase I-II (●, ROOH; O, O_2^-; ▲, membrane stability; △, enzymes; ■, AOA)

TABLE 1
Results of free radical level studies in persons in the Far North
(superoxide-dismutase, measured by erythrocyte enzyme quantity causing
50 per cent delay of adrenaline oxidation)

	Donors in middle latitudes	Donors in the Far North	
		Moderate manual labour	Manual labour
ROOH	0.134 ± 0.01	0.274 ± 0.02	0.314 ± 0.05
Antioxidant activity, non-enzymatic	235 ± 18.1	51 ± 5.0	-37 ± 4.0
Glutathione reductase	1.7 ± 0.08	1.7 ± 0.05	2.2 ± 0.07
G-6-P dehydrogenase	0.7 ± 0.04	0.73 ± 0.04	1.16 ± 0.05
Erythrocyte membrane stability	22 ± 0.63	13 ± 0.17	20.4 ± 0.63

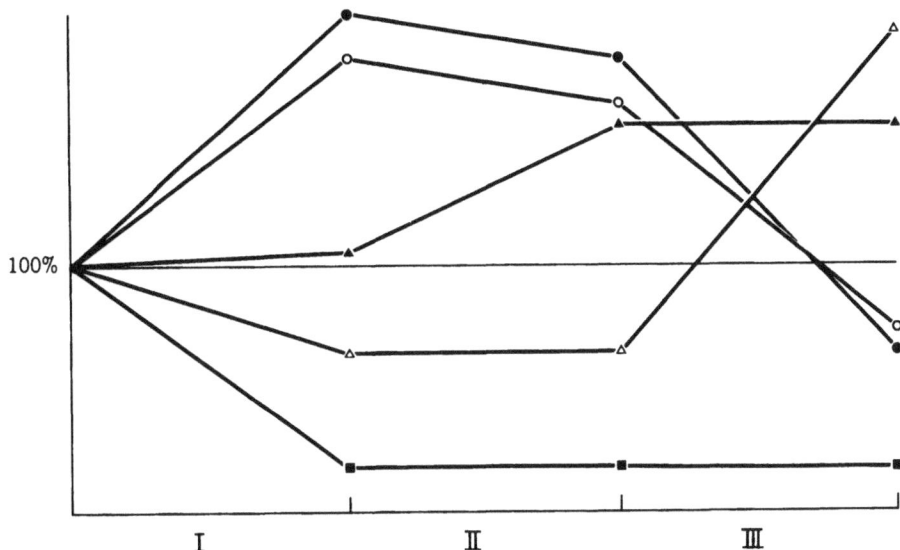

Figure 6   Dynamics of free-radical reactions and their control system in man under high-latitude conditions and in experimental animals, phase I-II-III ($\bullet$, ROOH; O, O_2^-; $\triangle$, enzymes; $\blacktriangle$, membrane stability; $\blacksquare$, AOA)

TABLE 2
Dynamics of free radical reactions in man under Far Northern conditions

Parameters	Phase I	Phase II	Phase III
Superoxide anion-radical of oxygen (O_2^-)	180	160	70
Fatty acid hydroperoxides	200	180	60
Antioxidant activity (non-enzymatic)	20	20	20
(enzymatic)	100	150	150
Membrane stability	60	60	100

metabolism under unfavourable conditions may have evolved because it participates directly in the repair of damaged cellular constituents. This is of particular importance when primary damage is being inflicted by cosmic and geomagnetic disturbances. Specific structural alterations at the molecular level may have adaptive value for newcomers to high latitudes.

Our investigations demonstrated that the blood level of free fatty acids was increased in men who moved from

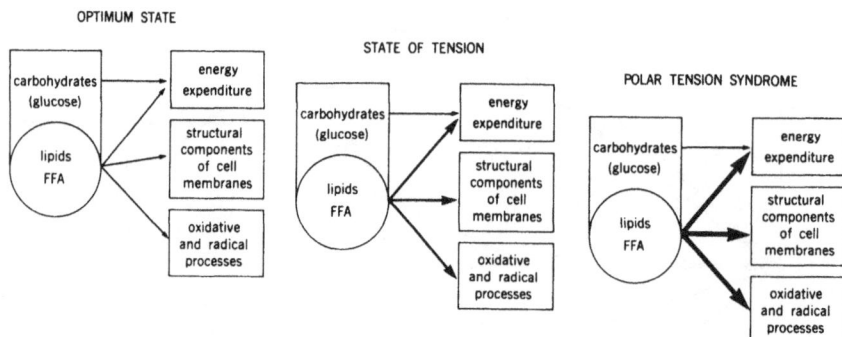

Figure 7   Distribution of metabolic carbohydrate and lipid flows under high-latitude conditions

TABLE 3
Dynamics of carbohydrate and lipid metabolism under high-latitude conditions in man for various periods of residence (mean and standard deviation)

	Blood sugar (mg%)	Total lipids	FFA	11 oxycortico-steroid (μg%)	Phospho-lipids
1-2 months	82.6 ± 5.1	701±24	519±24	25.1± 0.6	188±7.05
	p* > 0.05	p<0.01	p<0.01	p < 0.01	p < 0.01
6 months	65 ± 5.9	544±38	544±38	22± 1.2	197±7.05
	p <0.05	p<0.01	p<0.01	p < 0.01	p < 0.01
1 year	73 ± 7.2	503±74	503±74	24.7± 0.9	162±4.7
	p< 0.05	p<0.01	p<0.01	p < 0.01	p < 0.01
1.5 years	72 ± 4.0	440±30	440±30	24.8± 0.8	204±16.4
	p< 0.05	p<0.01	p<0.01	p < 0.01	p < 0.01
2 years	91 ±6.3	458±33.7	458±33.7	24.8± 0.7	179±4.7
	p>0.05	p<0.01	p<0.01	p < 0.01	p < 0.01
Men in Novosibirsk	92 ± 6.0	245±21.2	245±21.2	19.8± 0.47	181±11.7

* All probabilities calculated relative to men permanently resident in Novosibirsk.

elsewhere to work in the Far North (Panin, 1973). This increase was particularly marked in winter and could not be attributed merely to alterations in diet (Table 3, Figure 7). These observations are consistent with those of Timofeeva et al. (1974), who studied the metabolism of native athletes (Yakuts) and athletes who had lived in Yakutia for more than three years. According to these workers, blood sugar values are much lower in newcomers, especially in the winter season. Another interesting finding was that the basal metabolic rate in athletic newcomers was decreased relative to statistical standards established for populations

of the European part of the USSR, whereas in athletic Yakuts
the rate was increased. It is pertinent to recall the rare
occurrence of diabetes mellitus among Eskimos, who exhibit,
however, glycosuria and tolerance of oral glucose load
(Schaefer, 1968).

Taken together, these observations seem to indicate that
aboriginal populations of the North show a shift of energy
metabolism towards increased lipid utilization. What is normal for aborigines of the North may constitute a precondition
for the development of pathological processes in newcomers
adapting to high latitude conditions.

The observed preferential oxidation of fatty acids in aborigines and in men adapting to conditions in the North may be
determined by the need to compensate for (1) molecular and
energy shifts due to continuous exposure to disturbing environmental factors (cosmic and geomagnetic); (2) high energy
expenditures to meet acute demands, such as unfavourable cosmic conditions or increased physical and psychoemotional
strain.

As mentioned above, social and hygienic measures may blunt
the sharp edge of the effects of weather, deficient nutrition, excessive energy expenditure, and psychoemotional
strain. Thus studies of cosmic and geomagnetic disturbances
that have primary effects on biosystems deserve new emphasis;
at present, it is difficult to control these harmful agents.

SOME FEATURES OF ADAPTATION TO HIGH LATITUDES

The general impression is that specific mechanisms play a
central role in the adaptation of man to high latitudes.
The initial changes occur deep in cellular structural constituents exposed to cosmic and geomagnetic disturbances;
these changes extend in such a way as to alter the information flow and energy characteristics of the cells.

Our studies (Kaznacheyev et al., 1967) have established
that superweak electromagnetic fields transmitting information within a cell and between cells are of importance in
cell activities. Experiments have demonstrated that cells
attacked by exogenous agents emit light signals with frequencies in the visible band adjacent to the ultraviolet
band. When they reach isolated cultures of normal cells,
these signals are detected. The culture receives instructions on how the pathological process has developed and by
reproducing the destructive sequence, its own cells die. If
an additional light source is introduced in the course of
the experiment, the transmission of biological information
is inhibited.

In the light of these data, it may be thought that cosmic and geomagnetic disturbances mediated through free radical processes can modify intra- and extra-cellular conditions. At the quantum level, cosmic and geomagnetic disturbances mediated through free radical processes can modify intra- and inter-cellular relationships.

It is not clear at what stage of the putative processes receptor-reflex mechanisms are established; nor have we traced the afferent pathways and trigger mechanisms of regulatory neuroendocrine and related functions as yet. There is no doubt, however, that the latter are eventually decisive in the development of adaptive processes. The various gamma-non-specific adaptive mechanisms have been dealt with extensively in the literature (Barbashova, 1960; Tikhomirov, 1965; Meerson, 1973). It may be thought that the spatial and temporal patterning of these non-specific mechanisms are quite peculiar in prepolar and polar regions. Diverse as they may be, they are the result of the interaction of multiple non-specific reactions which have been amply studied as separate entities.

Attempts to incorporate all the components of strain and tension at the quantum, submolecular, and molecular levels into a dynamic whole have culminated in the idea that these components in their entirety create a specific state of tension. Recalling Bauer (1935), one may say that the state of stable equilibrium is modified in cells and that their entropy tends to increase. Such shifts lead to drastic functional and structural impairments. Counteracting mechanisms are mobilized in cells, tissues, and the organism as a whole to dampen and stabilize processes which are increasing the entropy. Critical here, as our data seem to indicate, are the conversion of energy sources maintaining and promoting antioxidant activity, on the one hand, and genetic mechanisms assuring the synthesis of naturally occurring antioxidants, on the other hand. All of these mechanisms operate concomitantly with various other adaptive responses oriented towards the maintenance of steady flows of energy and information.

To explore these possibilities, 2,400 normal adults of the northern regions of the European part of the USSR were investigated. The survey was made at different seasons of the year, and measured many non-specific variables of adaptation (Table 4). The most important adaptive functions have medium and strong correlations with the index of magnetic tension.

TABLE 4
Effect of earth's magnetic field (K-index) on some components of the
syndrome of polar tension, correlation analysis for 1,600 subjects
(cited from Neverova and Andronova)

Physiological variable	Correlation
17-ketosteroid excretion	Very strong
Adrenaline excretion	Medium
Cholinesterase activity	Medium
Urinary vitamin B_1	Strong
Mean weighted skin temperature	Strong
Blood flow rate	Strong
Cardiac output	Medium
Maximum blood pressure	Medium
Pulse pressure	Medium
Pulse	Medium
Hemoglobin concentration	Medium
Blood oxygen capacity	Medium
Erythrocyte sedimentation rate	Medium
Minimum blood pressure	Weak
Systolic blood volume	Weak
Mean dynamic pressure	Weak
Peripheral resistance	Weak
Thrombocytes	Weak
Blood coagulation	Weak
Erythrocytes	Weak, insignificant
Leucocytes	Weak, insignificant

Comparisons of these data with the results of our biophysical studies suggest that the core of the adaptive
spectrum under high latitude conditions is biophysical in
nature. Acceptance of this suggestion helps us to understand
many of the conditions described in the literature such as
polar dyspnoea, psychoemotional lability, astenization,
manifestations of peculiar hypoxia, and increased oxygen
debt. It also makes comprehensible why the adaptation period
may last for 1.5 to 2 years or even longer (Barbashova,
1960; Kandror, 1968: Avtsin, 1972: Neverova et al., 1972;
Mirrakhimov, 1972; and Bichikhin, 1974).

There is reason to unify all the clinical manifestations
on the common basis of pathogenic specificity and to regard
the state of man exposed to high latitude conditions as one
of very specific tension (Figure 8), the "polar tension
syndrome." This syndrome includes all the pathogenic features which reflect specific and non-specific mechanisms of
adaptation directed towards the stabilization of cellular
constituents whose regime has been modified by cosmic and
geomagnetic disturbances.

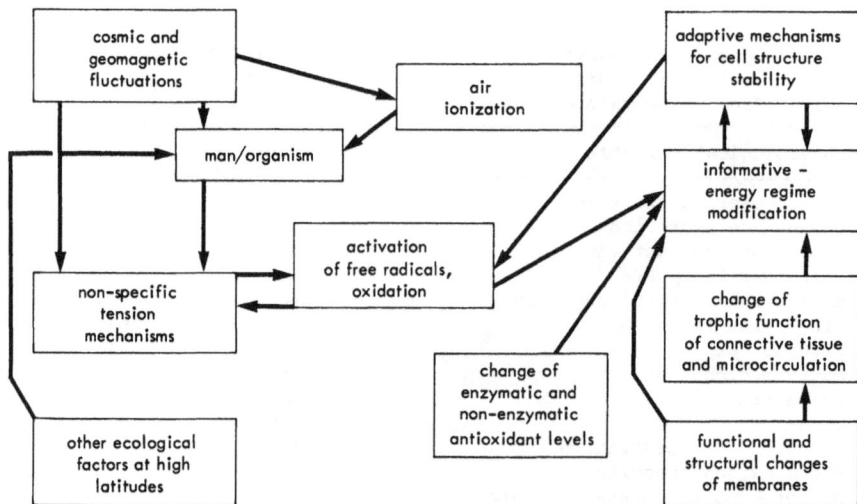

Figure 8   Elements of pathogenic structure of "polar tension syndrome"

The data we have obtained, along with those in the literature, indicate that any marked tension in man or animals is characterized by significant changes at the level of free radical processes and by mobilization of mechanisms of adaptation and compensation. Changes at this level are one of the limiting steps in sequential events providing reliable biosystems. However, changes occurring under tense states are generally mediated by external factors, whereas changes associated with the "polar tension syndrome" are the result of the direct geomagnetic and cosmic perturbations of biostructures. This constitutes the basic difference between the aetiology and pathogenesis of the polar syndrome and other states of tension. The "polar tension syndrome" is associated with alterations of peroxide processes due to: (1) direct influences of geomagnetic and cosmic disturbances of biostructures; (2) mediated metabolic shifts resulting from specific combinations with other ecological factors encountered at high latitudes. This syndrome does not refer to a pathological condition but rather characterizes the specificity of the adaptive process, its general trend. What then is the "biosocial cost" (Avtsin, 1972) of the syndrome? To what extent will it tax health in the near or distant future? Will readaptation produce different pathological states with their own specific and general pathological states?

The proposed approach to high latitude adaptation opens
new vistas. A promising line of research will be the study
of aborigines of the Far North to discern how selection has
genetically fixed processes of adaptive value under the specific cosmic, geomagnetic, and other peculiarities of these
regions. Search for methods of individual selection, systematic predictions of response, and disease prophylaxis in
high latitudes are all needed. The concept formulated may
provide the framework for an extensive program of basic and
applied research in environmental physiology.

SUMMARY

The problems of adaptation are considered in thermodynamic,
cybernetic, biological, and physiological terms. The typical
biological system is a spatio-temporal cosmic structure that
converts flows of energy to self-maintenance, with the
development of increasing negative entropy, and the maximi-
zation of external work. Evidence is presented that cosmic
and electromagnetic fields interact with the biosphere at
the molecular and submolecular levels, particularly through
the formation of free radicals. The application of these
concepts to the development of an optimum adaptation to high
latitudes is discussed.

Mechanisms of human cold adaptation

K.E. COOPER

Not long ago, the terms adaptation, acclimatization, and
acclimation were redefined. Adaptation has come to mean the
general anatomical, physiological, biochemical, or behavioural characteristics of an animal which favour its survival in a specific environment. Acclimatization (12) is
used to describe the physiological changes induced by complex factors such as seasonal and climatic changes, while
acclimation describes the changes induced by a single environmental factor, as in the controlled experiment. Many
authors use the term adaptation to refer to genetic or
racial characteristics, but I shall use it rather more
generally as a process by which an animal with built-in

adaptive abilities for one climate may so change its responses that survival in a different harsh environment is favoured. As we shall see, the term acclimation may be a mis-
nomer, because of the near impossibility of inducing a
change in one environmental factor without seriously modifying others.

Changes that occur in any animal on transposition from
one climate to another presumably arise in response to some
form of stimulus from the environment. The stimulus may be
a direct sensory input determined by specific or non-
specific nerve endings in exposed parts of the body, or it
may be a more complex input. For example, a relatively
sedentary individual moving to employment in the Arctic may
find that the process of keeping alive involves not only
exposure to cold but also a considerable increase of energy
expenditure. When walking from place to place, possibly
against strong winds, he will wear very much heavier clothing,
and will work at a rate sufficient in conjunction with the
added clothing to enable him to feel warm. Inevitably, this
changes his energy expenditure and his food intake. Training
of his body muscles will also result. Consequently, there is
an input from the increased muscular activity, and an input
from the cerebral cortex and other central mechanisms as well
as that coming from nerve endings in exposed skin. The
adaptation that may take place when a man moves from a temperate to a cold region is thus not just an adaptation to
cold, but involves a very much more complex series of inter-
plays requiring modifications of physique and behaviour. In
contrast to many mammals, man can adjust his microclimate
during cold exposure by the use of clothing and by building
shelters. Thus with certain exceptions in primitive desert-
dwellers (where the cold exposure is nowhere as severe as in
the Arctic), man spends little time with a wide area of body
surface exposed for sensory input. Under some conditions,
one would look particularly at the hands, the face, and
possibly the feet as areas where local adaptive changes
might develop, as for example, the hands of the Gaspe fishermen (2, 6, 11, 20, 22, 26). In addition, specific responses
such as the cold pressor response elicited by stimulation of
peripheral nerve endings in exposed parts might undergo an
adaptive change which probably is better called habituation
(7, 8, 17, 22).

The metabolic response to cold may take the form of frank
shivering, an increase of muscle tension, or heat production
which is not dependent on muscle activity (frequently called
non-shivering thermogenesis). In some species, including newborn of man, part of this non-shivering thermogenesis takes

place in areas containing brown fat or brown adipose tissue,
but there is no doubt that there can be considerable non-
shivering thermogenesis in tissues other than brown fat. In
the study of metabolic changes during exposure to cold,
Canada is proud to have played an important part (4, 12, 13,
14, 15, 24), particularly in terms of defining sites and
mechanisms of the generation of heat during non-shivering
thermogenesis. In 1962 (28) the whole role of the adrenal
cortex and medulla in metabolic acclimation to cold in the
rat seemed well defined, but things have become less clear
since then.

Webster (29) has reviewed the current situation extremely
well. In a table, he summarizes the roles of catecholamines,
the thyroid, and the adrenal cortex in the process of acclimation to cold in laboratory rats. There is universal agreement that, in the initial exposure to cold, catecholamine
excretion, secretion, and synthesis are all elevated, and
that during continuous exposure to cold these three factors
decline towards the baseline for animals kept in a warm room.
One problem is that so many experiments have been done on
animals that are still growing. In consequence, the surface
area to weight ratio of the animals changes during the period
of the experiment, and hair may also grow so that the animal
effectively has less cold exposure towards the end of the experiment than it did at the beginning. Nevertheless, one
effect of noradrenaline has remained clearly valid, namely
that over the first three to four weeks of exposure to continuous cold (0 to 5°C) the thermogenic effect of injected
noradrenaline increases and persists throughout the cold exposure. Whether or not this is so in man remains to be
worked out. In looking at the animal model (as Webster points
out, it is difficult to know which animal to look at), there
is an increase of thyroid weight and TSH secretion is elevated during cold exposure but the problem is compounded by an
increase of appetite and food intake (13) in the cold. The
majority of animal foods are rich in iodine. Thus we have now
cited two examples of the apparent alteration of one climatic
or environmental factor compounding a series of changes;
there is not the single stimulus to end product relationship
of a possible increased secretion of a hormone during cold
acclimation. Animal work suggests (23) that increased tolerance to severe cold can be independent of non-shivering
thermogenesis. Shivering itself seems in animals to start at
lower environmental temperatures if the animal is cold acclimated than if the animal is warm acclimated. A great deal
more study is required to determine whether this is so in

man, though my experience after five years in the Calgary
winter leads me to suspect, without objective evidence, that
this may be true.

In animals which possess brown fat, non-shivering thermogenesis is elicited fully before shivering comes into play;
non-shivering thermogenesis may depend more on the relationship between skin temperature and spinal cord temperature
than on that between skin temperature and hypothalamic
temperature (3). Relationships showing the threshold sensa-
tion for non-shivering thermogenesis based on receptors in
the skin and hypothalamus, or in the skin and spinal verte-
bral canal, have been shown by Bruck (3); the effect of acclimation on this relationship is to lower the subcutaneous and
cervical temperatures at which cold-acclimated animals produce non-shivering thermogenesis. Apart from the human baby,
it is unlikely that this effect can be extrapolated to man.
Even in the case of the human baby, considerable work would
have to be done to establish such a hypothesis, and it is
doubtful whether the necessary measurements could be justi-
fied ethically. However, there is evidence (5) that exposing
men to cold 8 hours a day for 31 days causes an increase of
heat production which, during the process of acclimation, is
accompanied by a diminished intensity of shivering. This
would suggest that some form of non-shivering cold thermogenesis was developing. Studies of spinal man by Spalding
would seem to indicate that during cold exposure there was
no non-shivering thermogenesis in the muscles below a cervical cord transection. If spinal cord cooling can induce non-
shivering thermogenesis in man, it is probable that connec-
tions with the rest of the brain are necessary.

It is likely that Spalding's patients were cold acclimated, since they moved around in relatively light clothing in
British wards and in the open air. Thus an intact nervous
system above the cervical cord seems necessary for the
development of non-shivering thermogenesis during cold exposure. Human metabolic rate shows no systematic change if
measured with man in the thermoneutral zone of environmental
temperature. Apart from the investigations of Joy (18)
there is little evidence that infused noradrenaline affects
heat production to an extent that would be of great significance during cold acclimation. However, the effect of phenoxybenzamine on warm and cold acclimation in sheep (29) is
of interest; sheep and man have many similarities, and in
sheep at least phenoxybenzamine may inhibit shivering by
interfering with fusimotor nervous control of muscle
spindles. This leads to the suggestion (29) that there may

be some form of cold thermogenesis other than shivering in sheep, and indicates it would be worthwhile looking further at man for evidence of non-shivering thermogenesis.

Considerable work has been done in the last few years by the Japanese (16, 17). Studies have been made on different parts of the Japanese islands, using the Japanese mainland people as more sophisticated individual controls. In one island (Hokkaido), the Ainu people are persistently exposed to cold, with poor accommodation, very poor heating, poor clothing and quite severe cold stress, particularly in the winter. These people have lower free fatty acid (FFA) levels than the non-Ainu Japanese controls. The basal metabolic rate of the Ainu differs from that of the non-Ainu Japanese in being negatively correlated to the plasma FFA, and it is suggested that the turnover rate of plasma free fatty acid is increased markedly in the Ainu. In addition, stimulation of fat metabolism in the Ainu produces an elevation of plasma ketone bodies, and there is a linear correlation between energy metabolism and plasma ketone body levels. It seems that in this particular ethnic group free fatty acid is rapidly converted to ketone bodies in the liver. In this way, the Ainu differs very much from the Eskimo who has high free fatty acid and low ketone body levels in the plasma. A small dose of noradrenaline produces a marked elevation of oxygen consumption, plasma FFA, and ketone bodies in the Ainu, whereas in the non-Ainu Japanese controls these variables were virtually unaffected. Differences between the Ainu, the mainland Japanese, and the Eskimo may be related to really severe cold stresses which are not suffered by the other groups, and to dietary factors. Itoh and his colleagues (16, 17) have described regional changes in the fatty acid composition of subcutaneous fat during cold adaptation. Fatty acids in the forearm and leg tend to become more of the mono-unsaturated type. This may have a mechanical effect on movements of the extremity.

It is interesting to consider these changes in the light of the hard to interpret philosophy of O'Connor (27) that peripheral thermoregulatory responses might be related, under different conditions, to changes in the fatty acid composition of the intestitial spaces and cell membranes. One must again consider the hypothesis of Hammel (10) that, whereas metabolic habituation in people who eat well would lead to a more rapid increase of metabolic rate and a lower tissue insulation due to a relatively large blood flow to the extremities, a hypothermic-tissue insulative response could occur in those who suffer cold exposure and food

shortage. The aborigine can sleep while shivering and can endure a fall in body and peripheral temperature to a much
greater extent before shivering commences than can non-
aborigine controls.

We should now consider changes of peripheral blood flow
in the extremities of persons habitually exposed to cold,
such as fishermen in cold regions. The phenomenon of cold
vasodilatation has been studied intensively. There has been
continuous argument as to the mechanism of cold-induced
vasodilatation in the extremities of man. It can occur independently of the nerve supply to the blood vessels of the
exposed digit, but the state of the body heat content influences the extent of cold vasodilatation. A person who is
cold, with a low central temperature, experiences cold vasodilatation but to a lesser extent than somebody who is warm.
The most attractive hypothesis seems that of Keatinge (19)
who has shown that at low temperatures arterial smooth
muscle becomes unresponsive to noradrenaline. Cooling of
sheep carotid arteries below 10 to $12^{o}C$ blocked both the
electrical and the mechanical response to noradrenaline.
Nevertheless, very strong electric shocks or depolarization
with potassium-rich solutions cause large slow contractions
of the arteries. It would appear, therefore, that the acto-
myosin system was able to contract, albeit more slowly at
$5^{o}C$ than at $35^{o}C$, and that something in the excitation-
contraction coupling mechanism failed at the low temperature
to which these arteries had been exposed.

The story then would be that when the hands are plunged
into cold water there is a reflex vasoconstriction mediated
by the noradrenergic nerves; since there is little thermal
insulation in the fingers, there is very rapid cooling of
the smooth muscle to the point where it no longer responds
either to nerve-ending derived or circulating catecholamines. As the smooth muscle relaxes, a large blood flow
again passes through the vessel. This warms up the smooth
muscle and once again it becomes sensitive to noradrenaline, whereupon it contracts. The slow waves of the Lewis
"hunting reaction" could thereby be explained in a simple
way. Studies of cold-induced vasodilatation must include
extremely careful control of the state of the body heat at
the time of cold immersion; if the first wave of dilatation
is more rapid, this may indicate some local change in the
arterial smooth muscle rather than in the central neuro-
genic response. Keatinge (19) noticed that the ulnar vein
of a bullock, which presumably at the time of year when the
animal was killed had been carrying considerable quantities

of cold blood, responded to noradrenaline both mechanically and electrically at temperatures between 6 and 7°C. Again, the ear arteries of the rabbit, which are always colder than their femoral arteries, respond to noradrenaline down to temperatures of 6 to 7°C whereas the femoral artery loses its response at about 12°C (9). It is therefore important that studies on the peripheral arteries of mammals be repeated after exposure and acclimation to heat, to thermoneutral environments, and to cold, examining whether any consistent pattern of behaviour of the excitation-contraction coupling response to noradrenaline can be worked out. Furthermore, in any studies of cold vasodilatation in man there should be very precise information concerning the state of heat storage and overall body thermal conditions.

Cold pressor test has been compared in people indigenous to cold areas, people from more temperate climates who have been acclimated to cold, and people who are neither acclimated nor acclimatized to cold. Many measurements have been made on Gaspe fishermen (22) and others who habitually exposed their limbs to cold (1, 2, 7, 17, 20, 21). Most of these studies demonstrated habituation, with a reduction in the blood pressure response on immersing the hands or feet in iced water. However, Brown and his colleagues (2) showed that in one group of Eskimos, immersing the hand and forearm in cold water caused a greater elevation of blood pressure than in the control white man. It may be that these Eskimos were not habituated because of the extremely good clothing they wear. A very intensive study of the Ainu people and the fishermen of Hokkaido in the Japanese islands again shows evidence of habituation (17), with the females responding less vigorously to the cold pressor test than the males.

We turn now to more diffuse considerations. We would expect the sensory processing of a cold exposure to include memory, emotional, and other responses, and the reticular activating and limbic systems might well be involved in central nervous system organization of this sensory processing. Our Japanese colleagues (16) have shown changes in components of the electro-encephalogram relating to the hippocampal and amygdala regions during cold exposure, particularly in the two cycle per second frequencies. If memory and emotion are involved in habituation to intense cold, which is not only a normal sensory phenomenon but also aversive, then limbic system structures might well be involved.

We have seen, then, evidence for changes in physiological performance of people from temperate climate who are either

habituated to cold, or who are indigenous to cold regions
and have suffered cold exposure from birth. The evidence
seems to favour the concept (10) that body responses as a
whole depend on a combination of cold and food supply. There
are additional factors which have not been discussed, such
as the dietary requirements of people living in the cold and
the proper balance of diets, including the proportions of
fat, carbohydrate, and protein, and the vitamin intakes, all
of which seem undefined at present.

While there is evidence of changes at the tissue level,
for example in arterial smooth muscle, there may be more
subtle factors arising in the whole body responses to cold.
A possible involvement of the limbic system and of those
parts of the nervous system concerned with habituation should
make us think in terms of the plasticity of central nervous
system processing, allowing adaptation of man to a hostile
climatic situation. It is also possible that sensory inputs
can be modified at the peripheral level by changes in skin
thickness, damage to peripheral nerves, and vascular changes
induced by the thermal conditions. As Mackworth (25) showed,
deterioration of two-point discrimination in a cold hand is
less marked in cold-acclimated than in warm-acclimated man,
and this difference has a vascular basis. There may also be
mechanisms, analogous to those which the proponents of the
gate theory of pain have proposed, modifying the sensory input on its way to the central processing apparatus; such
modifications would then determine both the sensory experience and metabolic/endocrine responses to cold exposure.
Central nervous system conditioning, in a Pavlovian sense,
where the reward is better performance and the punishments
unpleasant thermal sensations and hunger, may again play a
part in acclimatization. It seems true that the old concept
that a few specifically localized parts of the nervous
system were involved in temperature regulation and acclimatization has to be discarded. It is necessary to look at
the sensory processing of the central nervous sytem as a
whole as it modifies the effector mechanism, both neural
and endocrine, through the control of both energy metabolism
and heat balance.

SUMMARY

Cold adaptation is reviewed with particular reference to
man. Evidence of adaptation at the cellular level is presented, together with evidence concerning the role of endocrine secretions in modifying cold exposure responses. The
role of diet and body composition is discussed in relation

to chronic cold exposure. Changes in heat conservation and loss via the peripheral circulation are reviewed, and possible alterations of brain control mechanisms for heat conservation and production in chronic cold exposure are examined with particular reference to the activity of non-hypothalamic regions such as the limbic system in modifying direct and behavioural adaptations to cold. Finally, the possibility of genetic or racial adaptations to cold is examined.

REFERENCES

1. Belding, H.S., in Burton, A.C. and Edholm, O.G. (eds.), *Man in a Cold Environment* (London: Arnold, 1955), p. 190
2. Brown, G.M., and Page, J., *J. appl. Physiol.*, 5: 221-227 (1952)
3. Bruck, I., in O. Lindberg (ed.), *Brown Adipose Tissue* (New York: Amer. Elsevier Co., 1970), p. 117
4. Cottle, M., and Carlson, L.D., *Endocrinology*, 59: 1-11 (1956)
5. Davis, T.R.A., *J. appl. Physiol.* 16: 1011-1015 (1961)
6. Elsner, R.W., Nelms, J.D., and Irving, L., *J. appl. Physiol.*, 15: 662-666 (1960)
7. Glaser, E.M., Hall, M.S., and Whittow, G.L., *J. Physiol. (Lond.)*, 146: 152-164 (1959)
8. Glaser, E.M., and Shephard, R.J., *J. Physiol. (Lond.)*, 169: 592-602 (1963)
9. Glover, W.E., Strangeways, D.H., and Wallace, W.F.M., *J. Physiol. (Lond.)*, 194: 78-9 (1968)
10. Hammel, H.T., in D.B. Dell (ed.), *Adaptation to the Environment* (Washington: Am. Physiol. Soc., 1964), p. 413
11. Hampton, I.F.B., *Fed. Proc.*, 28: 1129 (1969)
12. Hart, J.S., *Rev. Can. Biol.*, 16: 133-174 (1957)
13. Heroux, O., in E. Bagusz (ed.), *Physiology and Pathology of Adaptation Mechanisms* (Oxford: Pergamon Press, 1969), p. 347
14. Himms-Hagen, J., in G. Weber (ed.), *Advances in Enzyme Regulation*, col. 8 (Oxford: Pergamon Press, 1970), p. 131
15. Horvath, S.M., Radcliffe, C.E., Hutt, B.K., and Spur, G.B., *J. appl. Physiol.*, 8: 145-148 (1955)
16. Itoh, S., Ogata, K., and Yoshimura, H., *Advances in Climatic Physiology* (New York: Springer Verlag, 1972)
17. Itoh, S., *Physiology of Cold-Adapted Man*, Hokkaido Univ. Med. Library Series, vol. 7 (Sapporo, Japan: Hokkaido University, 1974)

18. Joy, R.J.T., *J. appl. Physiol.*, 18: 1209-1212 (1963)
19. Keatinge, W.R., *Survival in Cold Water* (Oxford: Black-well, 1969)
20. Krog, J., Folkow, B., Fox, R.H., and Anderson, K.L., *J. appl. Physiol.*, 15: 654-658 (1960)
21. Krog, J., Alvik, M., and Lund-Larsen, K., *Fed. Proc.*, 28: 1135 (1969)
22. LeBlanc, J., Hildes, J.A., and Heroux, O., *J. appl. Physiol.*, 15: 1031-1034 (1960)
23. LeBlanc, J., *J. appl. Physiol.*, 17: 950-952 (1962)
24. Leduc, J., *Acta physiol. scand.*, 53: Suppl. 183 (1961)
25. Mackworth, N.H., *J. appl. Physiol.*, 5: 533-543 (1953)
26. Nelms, J.D., and Soper, J.G., *J. appl. Physiol.*, 17: 444-448 (1962)
27. O'Connor, J.M., *Irish J. Med. Sci.*, p. 27   (1943)
28. Smith, R.E., and Hoejer, D.J., *Physiol. Rev.*, 42: 60-142 (1962)
29. Webster, A.J.F., in Robertshaw, D.   (ed.), *Environmental Physiology*, MTP, International Rev. Science, vol. 7 (London: Butterworth, 1974)

Regional sweating in Eskimos and Caucasians*

O. SCHAEFER, J.A. HILDES, P. GREIDANUS, and D. LEUNG

Sweat-gland response to pharmacological stimulation was studied in 37 Eskimo men and 21 Caucasian controls. The two groups differed significantly with respect to the mean numbers of activated sweat-glands on various body surface areas. Eskimos showed greater numbers of active glands, and sweated earlier and more profusely on the face, but had reduced sweat-gland count over most test sites on the trunk and extremities, where sweating appeared relatively late and was very scant.

The degree of reduction in regional sweating response of the Eskimo men relative to Caucasian controls was approxi-

*   This is a summary only. The paper is published in more complete form, including details of methodology, in the October 1974 issue of the *Canadian Journal of Physiology and Pharmacology*.

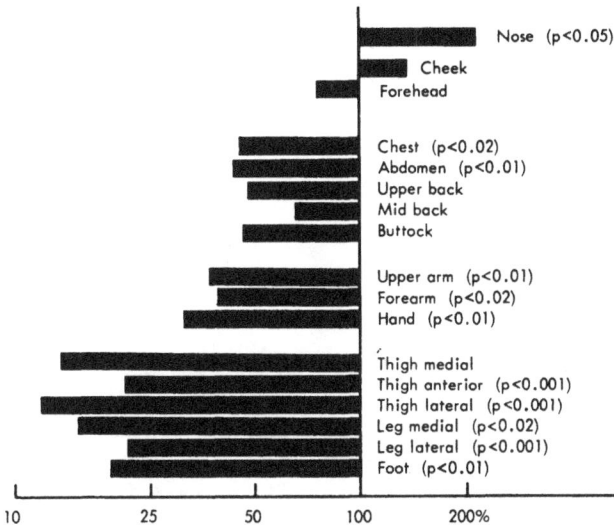

Figure 1   A semilog scale is used to express the relationship between the regional sweat-gland response of 17 male
adult Eskimos and of 20 Caucasian controls who provide the
standard (100%). Note that Eskimos had higher sweat-gland
counts only in the perioral areas of the face, but lower
counts in all other body regions, and markedly so in the
lower extremities

mately 1:2 on the trunk, 1:3 on the upper extremity, 1:4 on
the lower extremity, and 1:5 on the feet, paralleling the
distance from the body core and the danger of freezing.
   On the cheeks and nose, the Eskimos responded with
greater numbers of activated sweat-glands and earlier and
more profuse sweating than Caucasian controls. The difference reached statistical significance only for sweat-gland
counts on the nose, but on the forehead - traditionally
covered down to the eyebrows by a thick frontal hair cur-
tain - Eskimo men had a slightly lower mean sweat-gland
count than Caucasians (Figure 1).
   If we relate sweating on the trunk and limbs to sweating
on the face, and compare body/face ratios for the two races
(Figure 2), we find even greater regional disparities than
the direct comparisons mentioned above. Thus, the direct
comparison of activated sweat-glands on the dorsum pedis,
in Eskimos 7.0 and in Caucasians 36.7, equalled 1:5, but
if related to the mean of their three facial test scores
this would become 7.0/76.3 : 36.7/60.7 or 1:6.6. If we

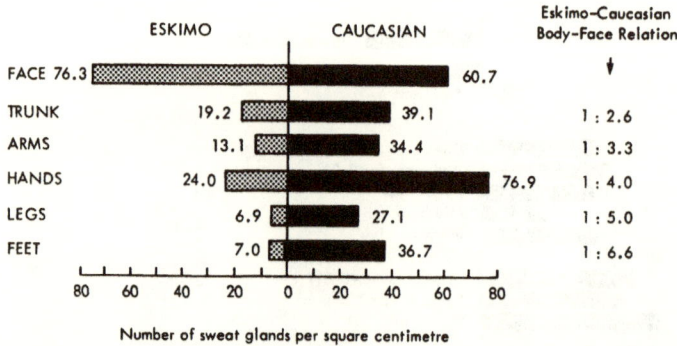

Number of sweat glands per square centimetre

Figure 2   The lower sweat-gland response of Eskimos in the trunk and extremities becomes even more striking when expressed relative to the facial sweat-gland response. A comparison of these relations in Eskimos and Caucasian controls reveals that the relative reduction in Eskimos varied from 1:2.6 over the trunk to 1:6.6 over the feet, if the relation between the sweat-gland density on face and body sites in our Caucasian controls is taken as standard (1:1)

TABLE 1
Mean counts of active sweat-glands per cm^2 in 17 Eskimo and 20 Caucasian men (mean and standard error)

Body area	Eskimos	Caucasians	Ratio E/C	Significance of difference between means
1 (forehead)	67.2 ± 14.1	89.4 ± 13.7	0.75	n.s.
2 (cheek)	68.4 ± 13.6	50.1 ± 5.4	1.37	n.s.
2A (nose)	93.2 ± 12.3	42.7 ± 17.8	2.18	$p < 0.05$*
3 (upper arm, lat.)	11.5 ± 5.0	31.2 ± 5.3	0.37	$p < 0.01$**
4 (forearm, ant.)	14.8 ± 4.3	37.7 ± 7.2	0.39	$p < 0.02$*
5 (hand, dorsal)	24.0 ± 7.3	76.9 ± 13.1	0.31	$p < 0.01$**
6 (chest, above nipples)	18.8 ± 6.7	41.8 ± 5.8	0.45	$p < 0.02$*
7 (abdomen, level umbilicus)	24.4 ± 6.8	56.5 ± 7.6	0.43	$p < 0.01$**
8 (back, over scapula)	17.0 ± 6.4	35.7 ± 6.9	0.48	n.s.
9 (back, lumbar)	24.7 ± 7.4	37.2 ± 6.6	0.66	n.s.
10 (buttocks)	11.3 ± 4.2	24.3 ± 5.8	0.47	n.s.
11 (thigh, lat./post.)	2.8 ± 0.8	24.8 ± 4.1	0.12	$p < 0.001$***
12 (thigh, ant.)	6.6 ± 2.6	31.4 ± 4.8	0.21	$p < 0.001$***
13 (thigh, med./post.)	7.3 ± 3.7	15.4 ± 4.7	0.47	n.s.
14 (leg, lateral)	9.5 ± 5.0	42.7 ± 7.3	0.22	$p < 0.001$***
15 (leg, med.)	7.8 ± 4.2	21.0 ± 3.4	0.37	$p < 0.02$*
16 (foot, dorsal)	7.0 ± 3.4	36.7 ± 8.9	0.19	$p < 0.01$**

relate mean counts at the peripheral test sites to those over the nose as representative of perioral sweating rather than using the means of all three facial test sites, the corresponding ratio becomes 7.0/93.2 : 36.7/42.7 or 1:11.4, which further highlights the regional disparity between Eskimos and Caucasian controls.

Reduction of sweat-gland response in heavily clothed parts of the body, and particularly in the most peripheral and frost endangered legs and feet, is well suited to the macro- and micro-climatic conditions of traditional Eskimo life and clothing. This may represent an example of morphological or functional adaptation to vital priorities of life in the Arctic. The increase of sweat-gland response on the exposed areas of the face is somewhat less impressive and may leave the Eskimos with a heat dissipation problem, perhaps assuming greater importance under the changed micro-climatic conditions of modern Eskimo life.

Is cold-diuresis a pressor diuresis?*

L.R. WALLENBERG and P.O. GRANBERG

The observation that exposure to low ambient temperature is accompanied by increased production of urine is about one hundred years old. In the 1940s and 1950s, studies were published on man, reporting that in cold the urinary output of sodium was also enhanced - a cold-induced natriuresis (2, 3). No real cause of the latter was found. The role of antidiuretic hormone (ADH) was discussed, since injections of small amounts of ADH prevented the cold diuresis (1). It was considered that exposure to cold reduced the secretion of ADH, which could well explain the increased output of water in the urine.

We decided to re-investigate the cold-induced diuresis, using modern methods of renal physiology, including studies in strong antidiuresis and strong water diuresis in

* Parts of this paper have been accepted for publication in vol. 34 of Scand. J. clin. lab. Invest.

order to control ADH activity and keep it constant throughout the experiment. Most previous authors had found an increase of arterial blood pressure in the cold. None of them,
however, discussed the possible significance of this finding
for cold-induced natriuresis. Recent literature suggests
that the transport and uptake of sodium is controlled by
physical forces, particularly the arterial perfusion
pressure in the kidney (4). The aim of our investigation was
thus to see whether cold-induced natriuresis could be caused
by changes of arterial blood pressure.

METHODS

Volunteer human subjects were exposed to moderate cold,
using air at $+15^{\circ}C$ on a closed hypothermic operating table.
The subjects took part in two experiments each, one in hydropenia and one in water diuresis. Standard clearance techniques were used, with constant infusion of inulin and para-
amino-hippuric acid. The blood pressure was measured with a
manometer on one arm.

Eighteen observations were obtained from nine subjects.
In one half of the experiment there was a constant and maximal ADH secretion, and in the other half practically no ADH
activity. Thus, the subjects served as their own controls.

Experiment I

With the technique used, no change of urinary flow was observed during exposure to cold. The phenomenon, previously
referred to as cold-diuresis, did not appear when ADH secretion was kept constant. Fractional excretion of sodium increased some 40 to 50 per cent during cold, both in hydropenia and in water diuresis. Since the glomerular filtration
rate was unaffected, the increased sodium excretion was most
probably caused by a reduced tubular sodium reabsorption.

The arterial blood pressure increased between 17 and 24
mm Hg during cold exposure. There was a significant relationship between the increased sodium excretion and the rise of
arterial blood pressure during both hydropenia and water
diuresis (Figure 1).

In water diuresis, the clearance of free water was
assumed to represent tubular reabsorption of sodium in the
distal tubules. Thus, the expression $C_{H2O} + C_{Na}$ represents
the delivery of sodium to the distal tubules and the expression $C_{H2O}/(C_{H2O} + C_{Na})$ represents the fractional distal

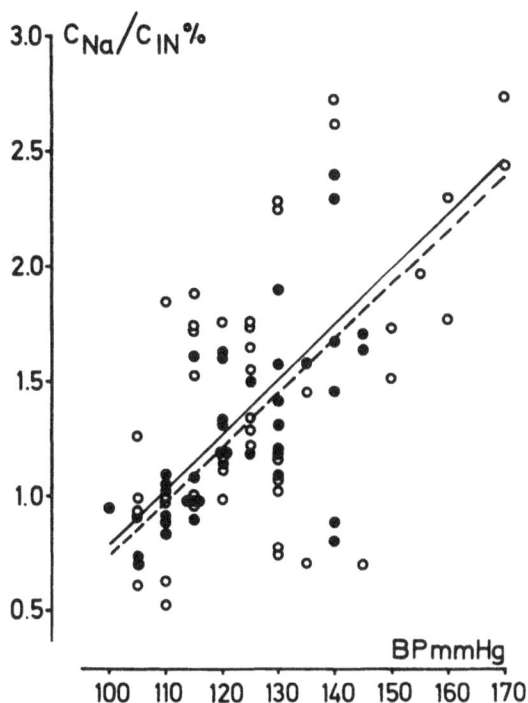

Figure 1 Relationship between the changes in fractional
sodium excretion (C_{Na}/C_{In}) and arterial systolic blood
pressure (BP mm Hg) following 60 minutes of cold exposure at
+15°C for nine subjects in hydropenia (●) and in water diuresis (O)

tubular sodium reabsorption. We found a significant decrease
in the fractional distal reabsorption of sodium and an inverse relationship between the cold-induced blood pressure
rise and fractional distal reabsorption of sodium.

The main results were identical in the two groups of experiments indicating that ADH is of minor importance for
human cold-induced natriuresis.

Several authors have shown that the reabsorption of
sodium and fluid is related to the oncotic pressure of blood
in the tubular capillary. Lewy and Windhager (7) showed that
the rise in the oncotic pressure of peritubular capillary
blood facilitated a net movement of fluid from the tubules
to the capillary lumen. There was a possibility that the
relationship we found between sodium excretion and the use
of blood pressure during cold exposure could be explained
by a transmission of the arterial hydrostatic pressure to

the peritubular capillaries, thereby increasing the hydrostatic gradient against which sodium was reabsorbed. This
would result in a reduced reabsorption of sodium.

Experiment 2

One way of testing this finding was to increase the oncotic
pressure in the peritubular capillaries. A new group of
volunteers undergoing water diuresis was exposed to cold for
one hour. During the exposure, they were infused with hyper-
oncotic human albumin solution, 0.4-0.5 g/kg body weight.

The results were compared with those from a non-infused
control group. Cold exposure was accompanied by the same
blood pressure rise in the infused group as in the control
group. The glomerular filtration rate was unchanged in both
groups but the cold-induced fractional sodium excretion was
almost completely inhibited in the infused group. The significant relationship between blood pressure rise and sodium
excretion in the control group was no longer present in the
albumin-infused group. These facts favour the suggestion
that sodium reabsorption in cold is balanced by hydrostatic
and oncotic pressures within peritubular capillary blood.

The results seem to indicate that only the distal convoluted tubules participated in the cold-induced human natriuresis. We decided to study the proximal tubules also.
We did this by estimating tubular reabsorption of solute-
free water $T^C_{H_2O}$. In hydropenia, this factor represents the
amount of solute-free water reabsorbed from the distal
tubules and collecting ducts. Sodium is presumed to be
actively pumped out of the ascending limb of the loop of
Henle, which is impermeable to water. This creates a hypertonic gradient in the medulla, which moves water out of the
collecting ducts in the presence of ADH. The more that
sodium is actively transported out of the ascending limb of
the loop, the higher the hypertonic gradient will be to
draw water from the collecting ducts, and the higher will be
$T^C_{H_2O}$. Thus, we used $T^C_{H_2O}$ as an index of sodium reabsorption in the ascending limb of the loop of Henle, which is
dependent on the delivery of filtrate from proximal tubules.
This active reabsorption of sodium can be increased by an
increased delivery from proximal tubules, as has been demonstrated by several authors (5, 6). If we could demonstrate
an increased $T^C_{H_2O}$ during cold, it would be a strong indication that the reabsorption of sodium was reduced in the
proximal tubules also during cold.

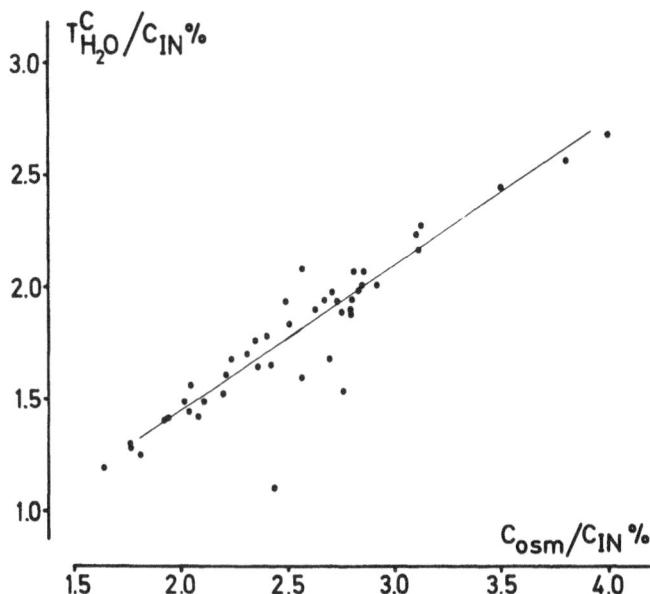

Figure 2   Relationship between the free water reabsorption
($T^C_{H_2O}$) and clearance of osmoles (C_{Osm}) for nine hydropenic
subjects during 60 minutes of cold exposure. Each subject is
represented by five dots: one in each of three control
periods at room temperature, one after 30 minutes in the
cold, and one after 60 minutes in the cold

Experiment 3

Again, volunteers were exposed to cold for one hour, this
time in hydropenia.

The results from this series show that clearance of osmoles was increased significantly during cold exposure, as
was the tubular reabsorption of solute-free water, T^C_{H2O}.
In Figure 2 the significant relationship between the increase in excretion of osmoles and T^C_{H2O} is shown. The more
osmoles - predominantly sodium - that came down from proximal
tubules, the higher was the reabsorption of sodium in Henle's
loop. It was obvious that cold exposure seemed to reduce tubular reabsorption along the entire convoluted tubule, but it
appeared that the reduction in the proximal tubule was compensated by an increased reabsorption in the loop of Henle.

CONCLUSIONS

If cold exposure is performed in hydropenia and water diuresis, no changes of urinary flow, previously referred to as

cold diuresis, are found. The cold-induced rise of blood
pressure seems to interfere with tubular sodium reabsorption, possibly by raising peritubular capillary hydrostatic
pressure, thereby increasing the hydrostatic gradient
against which sodium is transported. The result is a natriuresis. This can be inhibited by raising the peritubular
capillary oncotic pressure through the infusion of hyper-
oncotic albumin solution. The reduction in reabsorption of
sodium affects both proximal and distal tubules. However,
the proximal reduction is compensated by an increased me-
dullary reabsorption of sodium. Under these circumstances
the extent of human cold-induced natriuresis seems to
approximate that of the suppressed reabsorption in the distal tubules.

SUMMARY

Changes in arterial blood pressure, fractional sodium excretion and osmolar clearance, free water reabsorption and distal tubular reabsorption of sodium were studied in healthy
volunteers during a cold stress of $+15^{\circ}C$ for one hour, both
in maximal hydropenia and in maximal water diuresis. During
cold exposure, there were significant increases in blood
pressure, sodium excretion, osmolar clearance and free water
reabsorption, with a significant decrease in distal tubular
reabsorption of sodium. A significant relationship was found
between the cold-induced rise of arterial blood pressure and
fractional sodium excretion, both in hydropenia and in water
diuresis. With the technique used, no changes in urinary
flow - previously referred to as cold diuresis - were found
during the cold exposure. The significance of arterial renal
perfusion pressure for human cold-induced natriuresis and
the site of action of the mechanism are discussed.

REFERENCES

1. Bader, R.A., Eliot, J.W., and Bass, D.E., "Hormonal and
   renal mechanisms of cold diuresis," J. appl. Physiol.,
   4: 649-58 (1952)
2. Bass, D.E., and Henschel, A., "Electrolyte excretion
   during cold diuresis," Fed. Proc., 13: 8 (1954)
3. Conley, C.L., and Nickerson, J.L., "Effects of temperature change on the water balance in man," Am. J.
   Physiol., 143: 373-89 (1945)
4. Dresser, T.P., Lynch, R.E., Schneider, E.G., and Knox,
   F.G., "Effect of increases in blood pressure on pressure

and reabsorption in the proximal tubule," Am. J.
Physiol., 220: 444-7 (1971)
5. Earley, L.E., Kahn, M., and Orloff, J., "The effects of
infusions of chlorothiazide on urinary dilution and concentration in the dog," J. clin. Invest., 40: 857-66
(1961)
6. Goldberg, M., McCurdy, D.K., and Ramirez, M.A., "Differences between saline and mannitol diuresis in hydropenic
man," J. clin. Invest., 44: 182-92 (1965)
7. Lewy, J.E., and Windhager, E.E., "Peritubular control of
proximal tubular fluid reabsorption in the rat kidney,"
Am. J. Physiol., 214: 943-54 (1968)

Renal function after core and surface rewarming of hypothermic dogs

J.F. PATTON

Peritoneal dialysis is an effective method of core rewarming following induced hypothermia and, when compared to
surface rewarming, results in an earlier return towards prehypothermic cardiovascular function (9). Renal function is
affected markedly by a reduction of core temperature (8,
10). The glomerular filtration rate and renal blood flow are
decreased in both dog and man at body temperatures below 33-
34°C (6, 7). In addition, renal function remains depressed
following surface rewarming (3) and acute renal failure,
chronic renal insufficiency, elevated blood urea levels, and
a pronounced decrease in urine output have been described
following cases of accidental hypothermia (1, 5).

The present study was undertaken to evaluate the effects
of core rewarming by peritoneal dialysis on the post-rewarming renal function of the dog.

METHODS

Female mongrel dogs weighing 16-25 kg were anaesthetized
with thiamytal sodium. The oesophageal temperature was
monitored continuously with a Yellow Springs telethermome-
ter and thermistor. Catheters were placed into the left

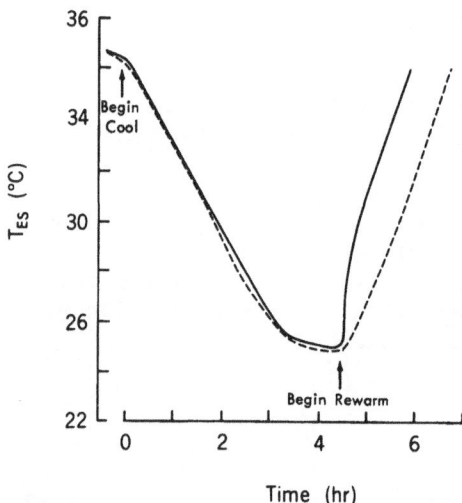

Figure 1   Mean oesophageal temperature during cooling, hypothermic stabilization, and rewarming (—— peritoneal rewarm,
--- external rewarm)

femoral vein (for infusion of test substances) and into the
left femoral artery (for blood sampling). The ureters were
catheterized through a midline incision for the collection
of urine.

Duplicate 15-min renal clearance tests were performed,
using standard clearance techniques during a normothermic
control period, at a core temperature of 25°C, immediately
upon rewarming to 36°C and at 12 hr after rewarming. Solutions of creatinine for the determination of glomerular
filtration rate (GFR) and para-aminohippurate (PAH) for the
determination of the renal blood flow (RBF) were infused in
5 per cent mannitol at a constant rate of 2.47 ml/min.

Animals were cooled to an oesophageal temperature of
25°C by an Omnitherm hypothermic machine with blankets
through which water was circulated at 6 to 8°C (Figure 1).
The animals were maintained for one hour at 25°C while
steady-state clearance measurements were made and then rewarming was initiated. Eight dogs were rewarmed externally
by circulating water at 40 to 42°C through the blankets.
The mean time for rewarming in this group was 132 minutes,
the rate being 5°C/hr.

An additional eight dogs were rewarmed, using peritoneal
dialysis by inserting a catheter into the left paraverte-
bral gutter through a small midline incision. Standard
commercial dialysis tubing and K+-free peritoneal dialysis

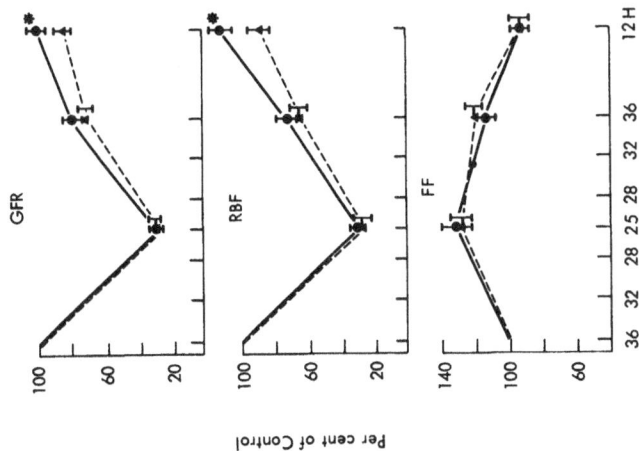

Figure 2 Changes in GFR, RBF, and filtration fraction (FF) as a percentage of control (--- ER, —— PD, *p < 0.05)

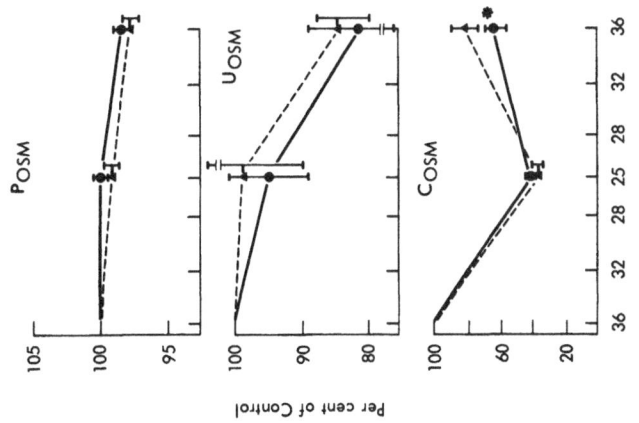

Figure 3 Changes in plasma and urinary osmolarity and osmolar clearance as a percentage of control (--- ER, —— PD, *p<0.05)

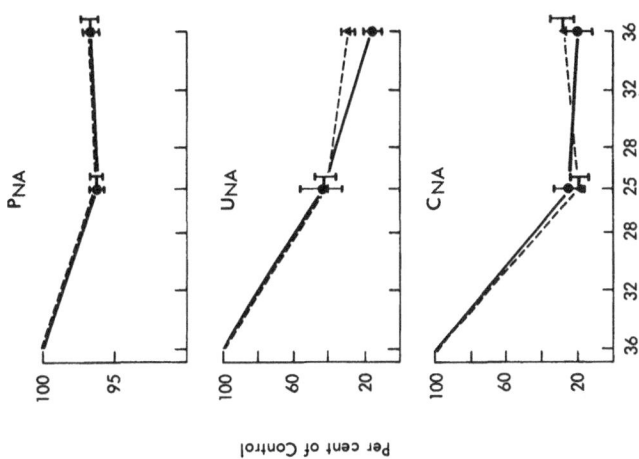

Figure 4 Changes in plasma and urinary sodium and sodium clearance as a percentage of control (--- ER, —— PD)

solutions were used. Two litres was rapidly instilled at a
temperature of 40 to 42°C by gravity flow and immediately
removed by siphoning into a reservoir. A mean volume of 13
litres was required to raise the core temperature to 36°C.
The mean time for rewarming was 92 minutes, with a rate of
7.2°C/hr.

RESULTS

Figure 2 shows the changes in GFR, RBF, and filtration
fraction (FF) as a percentage of normothermic values. During
hypothermia, both the GFR and RBF decreased to approximately
30 per cent of the prehypothermic levels. However, the fall
in PAH clearance was greater than the simultaneous decline
of GFR, so that the filtration fraction increased 20 per
cent during this period.
     Immediately upon rewarming, both the GFR and RBF were
still significantly depressed, although slight improvement
was seen in the peritoneally dialysed group. The failure of
these variables to return to prehypothermic levels despite
a normal core temperature is most likely due to active
vasoconstriction during the rewarming period. By 12 hours
after rewarming, the GFR and RBF had returned to control
values in the peritoneally dialysed group, but remained
significantly depressed in the externally rewarmed group.
     Alterations in the plasma and urinary osmolality and the
osmolar clearance during hypothermia and immediately after
rewarming are shown in Figure 3. During hypothermia, there
was little change in the plasma or urinary osmolalities,
the decrease of osmolar clearance to 40 per cent of control
being mainly the result of a decrease in urine volume which
occurs at this time. Upon rewarming, the osmolar clearance
returned to 62 per cent and 82 per cent in the dialysed and
externally rewarmed groups, respectively. This reflects a
slightly greater increase of urine flow in the externally
rewarmed group than in the dialysed group.
     Figure 4 shows the changes in the plasma Na+, urinary
Na+, and Na+ clearance. There were no differences between
the peritoneally and externally rewarmed groups upon restoration of normothermia. The marked decrease in the Na+
clearance during hypothermia reflects a decrease of both
urine flow and urinary Na+ concentration, suggesting that
the filtered load of Na+ is decreased as a result of the
decreased GFR. After rewarming, the Na+ clearance was relatively unchanged from that of the hypothermic period, due
to the continued low Na+ excretion. This occurred despite

the fact that the urine flow was increased and the filtered
load of Na+ was increased by the increased GFR.

DISCUSSION

Acute renal failure is one of the most common post-rewarming
complications resulting from accidental hypothermia (5).
Because of its simplicity, peritoneal dialysis is the method
of choice in uncomplicated cases of acute renal failure and
it has been used in the post-rewarming management of the
patient in renal failure caused by accidental hypothermia
(2). However, heretofore, its impact as a method of rewarming has not been evaluated in terms of renal function.
    The data show, as previously reported (9), that peritoneal
dialysis is an efficient means of rewarming, rapidly trans-
ferring large quantities of heat to the core and leading to
a more rapid return of core temperature than that seen with
conventional external rewarming.
    Furthermore, peritoneal dialysis resulted in a return to
normothermic values of both the GFR and RBF within 12 hours
of rewarming, while renal function failed to return to control levels in the externally rewarmed group. This latter
finding substantiates previous reports on post-rewarming
renal function using external or surface methods (3). The
recovery of the GFR and RBF in the dialysed group undoubtedly reflects the over-all improvement in cardiovascular
function seen at this time in previous experiments (9). The
cardiac output and arterial blood pressure are both significantly improved following peritoneal rewarming, and the
marked elevation in the total peripheral resistance which is
seen during hypothermia is restored more completely to normothermic levels in animals rewarmed by peritoneal dialysis
(9). All of these variables would tend to improve the renal
blood flow, intraglomerular hydrostatic pressure, and the
glomerular filtration rate.
    Peritoneal dialysis is a technique that does not require
highly trained personnel or expensive or complicated equipment and can be initiated without delay (4). However, this
procedure is not without some complications, the most common
of which is hypovolaemia, resulting in dehydration and
hypernatremia (2). In the use of hypertonic dialysis solutions, the movement of water is generally faster than that
of electrolytes, so that rapid exchanges of fluid may remove
a disproportionate amount of water, causing concentration of
extracellular electrolytes. In the present study, despite
the use of hypertonic fluids with rapid exchange to maximize

heat transfer, no evidence of hypovolaemia, hypernatremia, or hyperosmolality was seen. This was most likely due to the relatively small number of fluid exchanges necessary to restore normothermia.

In conclusion, the potential for peritoneal dialysis, because of its heat transfer and dialysing capabilities and its ability to restore renal function, appears to be considerable as a form of treatment in cases of accidental hypothermia.

SUMMARY

Peritoneal dialysis (PD) has been shown to be a more effective means of rewarming than surface rewarming (SR). PD is also a common form of therapy for acute and chronic renal failure, conditions which frequently occur following SR of individuals suffering from deep hypothermia. Dogs were cooled to an oesophageal temperature (T_{es}) of 25°C with a hypothermic blanket. Clearances of creatinine (for measurement of glomerular filtration rate), para-amino-hippurate, PAH (for measurement of renal blood flow), and osmolar (C_{OSM}) and sodium (C_{Na}) clearances were measured before cooling (control), at the end of cooling (HYP), immediately after rewarming (REW) and 12 hours after REW (12H). The rate of REW was greater with PD (7.2°C/hr) than SR (5.0°C/hr.). GFR, RBF, C_{OSM}, and C_{Na} decreased to 29%, 26%, 37%, and 20%, respectively, of control values during HYP. GFR and RBF returned to 101 per cent and 111 per cent of control in the PD group and to 83 per cent and 85 per cent in the SR group by 12H. The data indicate that, when compared to SR, PD results in a significant improvement of GFR and RBF.

REFERENCES

1. Gil-Rodriquez, J.A., and O'Gorman, P., "Renal function during profound hypothermia," Brit J. Anaesth., 42: 557 (1970)
2. Jones, J.H., "Peritoneal dialysis," Brit med. Bull., 27: 165-9 (1971)
3. Darim, F. and Reza, H., "Effect of induced hypothermia and rewarming on renal hemodynamics in anesthetized dogs," Life Sci., 9: 1153-63 (1970)
4. Mattocks, A.M. and El-Bassiouni, E.A., "Peritoneal dialysis: A review," J. pharm. Sci., 60: 1767-82 (1971)

5. McKean, W.I., Dixon, S.R., Gwynne, J.F., and Irvine,
   R.O.H., "Renal failure after accidental hypothermia,"
   Brit. med. J., 2: 463-4 (1970)
6. Morales, P., Carbery, W., Morello, A., and Morales, G.,
   "Alterations in renal function during hypothermia in
   man," Ann. Surg., 145: 488-99 (1957)
7. Moyer, J.H., "The effect of hypothermia on renal function and renal damage from ischemia," Ann. N.Y. Acad.
   Sci., 80: 424-34 (1959)
8. Page, L.B., "Effects of hypothermia on renal function,"
   Am. J. Physiol., 181: 171-8 (1955)
9. Patton, J.F. and Doolittle, W.H., "Core rewarming by
   peritoneal dialysis following induced hypothermia in
   the dog," J. appl. Physiol., 33: 800-4 (1972)
10. Walker, A.W., Smith, G., and Frazer, S.C., "Renal res-
    ponses to hypothermia," Clin. chim. Acta, 14: 462-74
    (1962)

Cases of paradoxical undressing by people exposed to severe hypothermia

B. WEDIN

The literature records a few cases where people who have
died from exposure have been found in a totally undressed
or partially undressed state (1, 3, 4). Gormsen (2) related
two cases: a 30-year-old woman who had completely undressed
and a 15-year-old boy who wore only a shirt and a vest.

The local records of the Swedish police have now been
searched for further cases of paradoxical undressing among
individuals suffering from severe hypothermia. A few Norwegian cases have also been investigated. The investigation
has extended over the last 10 years, and has revealed 36
cases, 25 men and 11 women. Two earlier female cases are
also reported, because of their value as illustrations of
the behaviour of victims of extreme hypothermia.

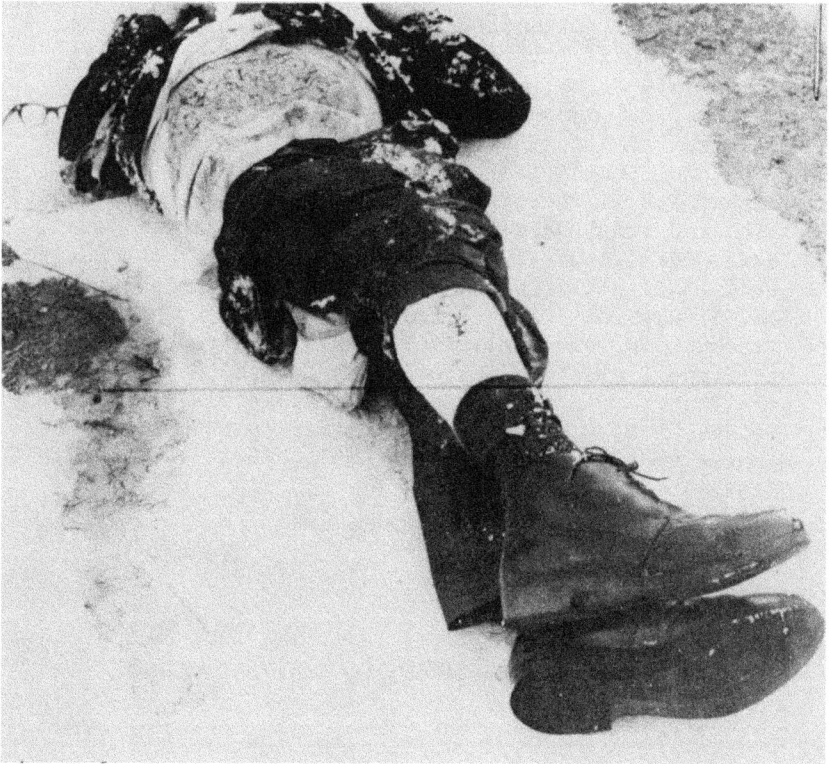

Figure 1

CASE REPORTS

Case 1

On 25 March 1969, a 78-year-old man was found dead beside a
wood pile in the southernmost part of the country (Figure
1). The previous day he had been reported missing from a
nursing home. The distance between the home and the place
where he was found was about 5 km. The ground was covered
with a few decimetres of snow. The temperature had varied
between $+3^{\circ}$ and $-5^{\circ}C$, with periods of sunshine as well as
rain and sleet.

    The dead man had trampled around in the snow and then
sat down in the place where he was found. After he had lain
down in the snow he had kicked his feet about several times.
He lay prone, slightly on his right side. The picture shows
the corpse after it had been turned over. The snow had
melted where his body had been lying, especially under his

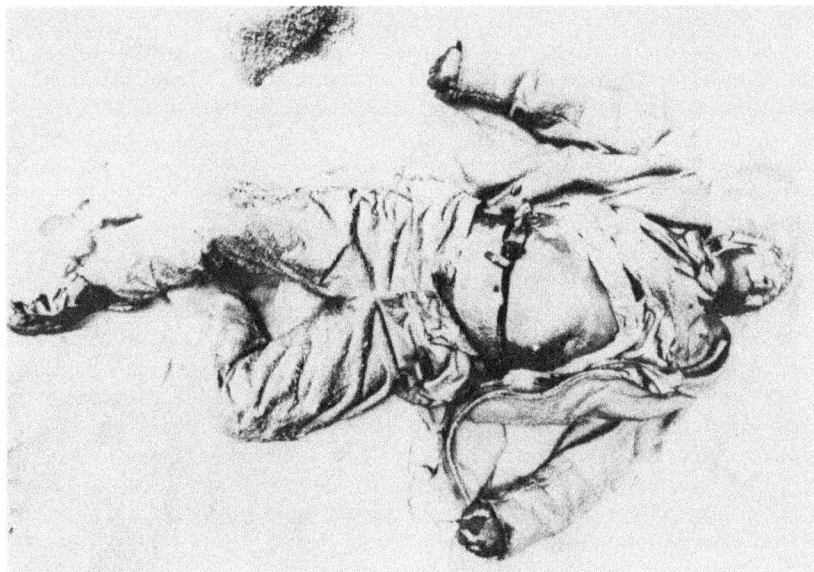

Figure 2

chest and abdomen. No evidence of alcohol was found in his blood or urine.

Case 2

On 25 January 1966, a 69-year-old man was found lying dead in a park in central Stockholm (Figure 2). During the previous 24 hours or so the temperature had varied between -8° and -12°C. A small amount of snow had fallen.

   The man was lying on his back in the snow with his arms slightly spread away from his body. His knees were about 20 cm apart, and his right leg was crossed over the left one. His head was lying lower than his body and had evidently sunk into the snow when it melted. His eyes were frozen shut. On both sides of his body the snow had been pressed down to a depth of half a metre. On the right side of the body clawlike marks could be seen in the snow as if he had been crawling. Around his feet there were kick marks on both sides. The dead man wore a winter coat which was completely undone and had been laid open in the front. Under his winter coat he wore a cardigan with six buttons, with only the last one buttoned. Under the cardigan was a shirt with only the top button done up. Both his cardigan and shirt were pulled out of his pants and up around his

chest, exposing his skin. The two top buttons of his trousers
were undone and the trousers were open. The body was exposed
from the hips to the chest. The intracardiac blood alcohol
level was 0.9 g/ℓ and the urine alcohol level 2.3 g/ℓ.

Case 3

On 6 November 1970, a 62-year-old diabetic man was found
dead about 100 m from his cabin. He was last seen alive two
days earlier. The temperature had varied between +4° and
-7°C, and the ground was partially covered by snow.

He had been on his way to get water from a pump 100 m
from the cabin. He had fallen but managed to get up again.
On his way back from getting the water he had fallen once
more. When he got up he did not resume his course but
wandered around in the area where his body was found. He
stepped down into a ditch and continued walking in it. He
climbed out of it at least five times but at last fell into
the water and crawled in it.

The man was found kneeling in the ditch with his head
resting against its side. The fingers of his right hand
were firmly wrapped around a branch of a small tree. This
man too had trampled around the area where his body was
found. His trousers were found 3-4 m from the body. His
underwear was removed so that his buttocks and part of his
thighs were exposed. An autopsy revealed chronic inflammation of the pancreas and cardiosclerosis.

Case 4

On 14 November 1972, a 45-year-old man was found in a
parking area at a port in southern Sweden. The temperature
during the night had varied between +2° and +6°C. The previous evening he had been very drunk and almost incapable
of walking, and had stumbled several times. One witness had
seen him fall and not rise from the asphalt. His overcoat
was pulled up over his head and his pants were pulled down
to his knees. The intracardiac blood alcohol level was 1.5
g/ℓ and the urine alcohol level 2.6 g/ℓ.

Case 5

On 6 April 1971, a 56-year-old married woman disappeared
from her home. In spite of her husband's good income and
good position in the community, she had been found pil-
fering recently and was very depressed. Three days later
she was found dead in exposed conditions, almost totally

naked. The temperature during those days had varied between +1° and +8°C. She had tried to commit suicide both by slitting her wrist with a pair of scissors and by strangling herself. No alcohol or barbiturates were found in the body but there were some other pharmacological substances.

She wore only a fur coat, blouse and brassiere. The coat and blouse were pulled up to her shoulders, and the rest of her body was naked. Boots, stockings, long trousers, underwear, and girdle were found beside the body, as well as a fur hat and gloves.

Case 6

The morning of 1 February 1966, a 52-year-old married woman was found lying dead outside a store. She was a known alcoholic. The temperature during the night had varied between +2° and -8°C. There had been minimal snowfall that morning. The snow at her feet had been trampled down over an area about 30 by 40 cm. The woman had been standing with only stockings on.

The evening before, the woman had been in the store with a man. Her hat, shoes, and handbag were all found on the ground, removed in a tidy fashion. The upper edge of her underwear was pulled down 30-40 cm, and the top three hooks of her corset were undone. She was lying on her back. The upper torso was lying on the fur coat, which had apparently been cast carelessly on the ground, and she had either lain or fallen down upon it. There were no signs of a fight or of her having vomited. Analysis showed a 1.3 g/ℓ intracardiac blood alcohol level and a 2.9 g/ℓ urine alcohol level. Barbiturates were found in the blood and liver.

Case 7

On 18 December 1968, a 50-year-old married woman was found dead outside a restaurant in Stockholm (Figure 3). During the night, the temperature had been -14°C, and the ground was covered in snow. She had walked from the building up a small hill, rolled down it, and then crawled farther on in the snow.

She was lying prone with her face turned and her body in a position as if she were sleeping. Her arms and part of her thighs were unprotected by clothing. Her face rested on her fur coat. Her dress and slip were drawn up around her waist. Her knickers and girdle remained in place. Analysis showed an intracardiac blood alcohol level of 2.4 g/ℓ and a urine alcohol level of 3.3 g/ℓ.

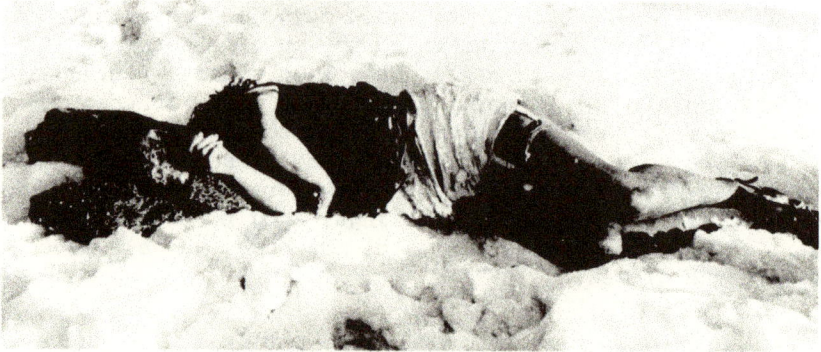

Figure 3

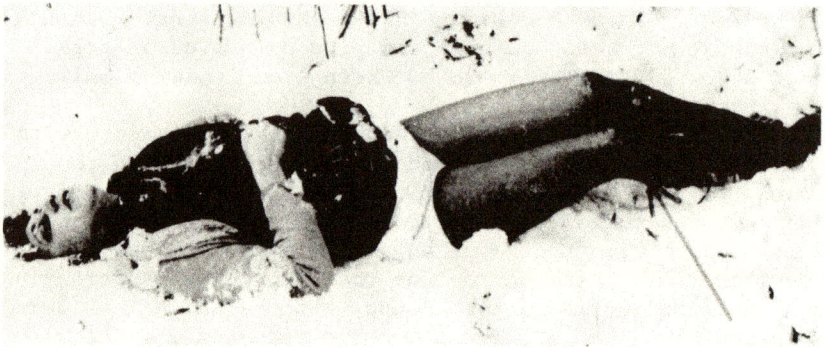

Figure 4

Case 8

On 9 December 1969, a 37-year-old married woman was found
dead in a garden (Figure 4). After a quarrel with her husband, the woman had left their shop the evening before.
The temperature during the night had varied between -7°
and -15°C. The dead woman had been complaining of fatigue
and a cold for several days. She was six or seven months
pregnant. It was learned from neighbours that she was over-
worked and depressed, and during the previous afternoon she
had been seen crying several times. The cause of her depression was the fact that her husband was an alcoholic and
that he would soon be sent to prison. She may also have
believed she had cancer.

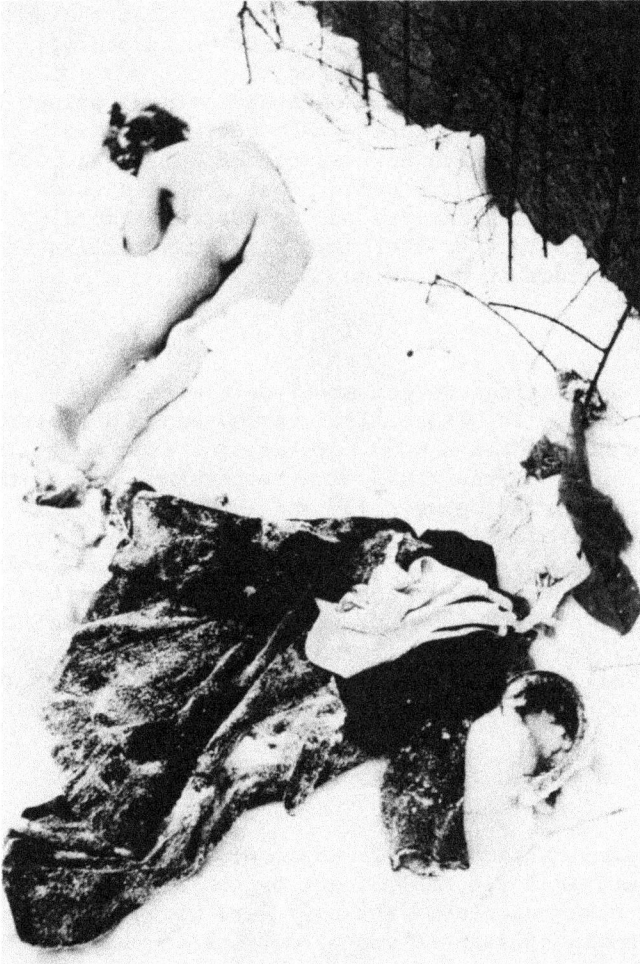

Figure 5

Chemical analysis showed an intracardiac blood alcohol
level of 1.6 g/ℓ, a urine alcohol level of 2.8 g/ℓ,
salicylic acid and the presence of caffeine but no barbiturates or meprobamate.

Case 9

On 20 February 1955, a 37-year-old married woman was found
dead in a park near the Stockholm City Law Courts (Figure
5). The temperature was -10°C. There were no signs of vio-

lence, and the condition of the snow showed that she had
been alone. The woman had removed all of her clothing, without damaging it, and was quite naked.

About ten years earlier the woman had been a patient in
a mental hospital. Two or three years before her death she
had attempted suicide with an overdose of pills. She had
been under medical care for cancer, but was said to be
healthy again. She was anxious and depressed. According to
the forensic pathologist, the woman was found to have been
under the influence of pethidine.

Case 10

Paradoxical undressings do not occur only with low temperatures and snow. On 10 October 1965, a 34-year-old unmarried
woman was found dead in a wood not far from Stockholm. The
leaves were still on the trees. The temperature during the
day before had varied between +3° and +9°C.

The woman was completely naked except for a brassiere.
One of her shoes was lying about 80 m from the place where
she was found, and her long trousers were 10 m from the
body. The rest of her clothing, consisting of stockings,
coat, jumper, and watch, was lying between the trousers and
the body. A diazepin substance was found in the urine, and
in the stomach and intestines a substance resembling chlor-
promazin was found.

Case 11

At about 3 p.m. on Saturday, 18 May 1968, Tage and Kim,
two boy-scouts aged 12½ and 13, set out on a hike. The
weather was cool but clear. The boys were given a compass
and a map showing distances and directions to the place in
the woods where they were to spend the night. When the boys
reached their destination it began to rain. Having no tent
or other means of protection, they prepared to spend the
night in their sleeping bags on the ground beneath some
evergreen trees. They tried to start a fire for warmth, but
the kindling was wet so they could not even cook the raw
meat and potatoes they were carrying in their knapsacks.
Before they set out, their knapsacks were inspected in
order to ensure that cooked food was not included. Three
"hot dogs" were taken from Kim and a package of a dried
fruit preparation from Tage. Tage removed his wet trousers
before getting into his sleeping bag, but Kim had brought
no change of clothes with him, so he was forced to lie in

his wet trousers during the night. The rain turned into
sleet. The boys had trouble getting to sleep, and when two
scout leaders visited them at about 11 p.m., the boys told
them that their sleeping bags were getting wet inside. They
remained awake until about half-an-hour after midnight.

At about 3 a.m. Tage woke up and found Kim awake, and
the sleet still falling. The sleeping-bags were soaked, but
the boys stayed in them until 5:30 a.m. The snow beyond the
shelter of the evergreens was 10 cm thick. The boys, feeling
rather tired, left their sleeping place in their wet
clothes, without having anything to eat. As they had no
covering for the map, it began to fall apart in the sleet.
They lost their way and wandered around in the woods the
entire day. When it began to get dark they came to a field.
Kim's speech was now slurred and he said he felt dizzy and
very tired. Tage helped him stumble along for about an hour.
By now Kim could not speak. He tried, but what he said was
unintelligible to Tage, although he could apparently understand in part what Tage said to him.

Kim's deterioration became more and more rapid. When the
boys finally stopped, Tage suggested that Kim get into his
sleeping-bag, but Kim did not seem to understand what Tage
said to him. He began crawling back and forth in a ditch
beneath a barbed-wire fence. Tage tried to help him out of
the ditch, but failed because Kim resisted. At last Tage
leaned Kim against a pole. He then succeeded in removing his
own pants and getting into his sleeping-bag. When the police
found him next day at about 1 p.m. he stood up by himself
and walked to their car. He saw his friend Kim lying in the
ditch, and heard from the policemen that Kim was dead. He
himself was immediately taken to hospital, and rapidly recovered.

Kim was lying supine on a rock. His left shoulder and
head were bent back over the edge with his left arm extended and fist clenched. Both legs were in the water in the
ditch. His belt was removed from all but two of the belt
loops, and his trousers were down to his knees.

I quote from the police report: "On account of the un-
natural position of the body" and the fact "that the
trousers were undone and partially removed so that the
thighs were exposed down to the knees," a sexual crime was
suspected. While waiting for criminal investigators to
arrive, the area was sealed off by policemen and dogs
(Figure 6). The boy's body was left in the ditch until the
investigating policemen and doctor arrived, which took about
2 hours for the police and about 4 hours for the doctor.

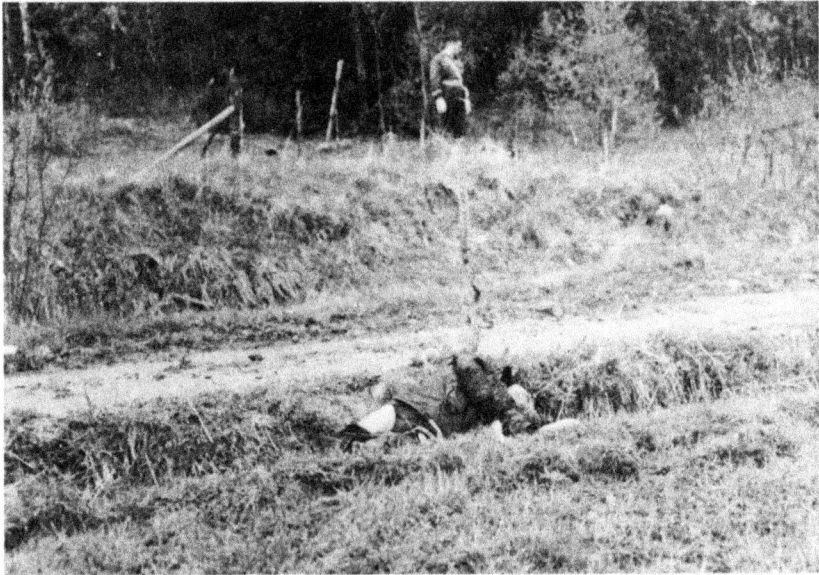

Figure 6

The development of Kim's hypothermia under natural conditions is probably one of the most detailed cases known.
Already on the second day after his rescue, Tage was carefully interrogated by a detective inspector, and the inter-
rogation was taped. This perspicacious boy had thoroughly
observed the behaviour of his comrade, especially the
development of tiredness and the progressive falling off of
his physiological and psychological functions.

CONCLUSIONS

The cases reported, especially the last one, are illustrations of the risk that disorder of the clothing can be
precipitately interpreted as being the result of a sexual
attack. A police officer is not competent to diagnose death,
as he does not have the necessary medical training or equipment. Not even a medical practitioner is always able to decide at the site of the tragedy whether an overcooled person
is actually dead, or only apparently so. If death is not
absolutely certain, the patient should be brought under medical treatment as quickly as possible.

ACKNOWLEDGMENT

The cooperation of the National Swedish Police Board is acknowledged with thanks.

SUMMARY

Cases of paradoxical undressing by individuals suffering
from severe hypothermia were found by a search of the
Swedish police records. A few Norwegian cases have also been
investigated. A total of 25 male and 11 female cases were
found. Among the men 12 of the cases were over 60 years of
age, and 7 of the women were over 50 years old. Cases were
reported from all parts of both countries, and during all
months except July and August. However, 24 of the 36 cases
occurred during the months of November to February. For 11
cases the temperature was lower than -10°C, for 7 it was be-
tween -10° and -5°C, for 7 between -5° and 0°C, and for 11
cases over 0°C. An overcooled person, even if showing no
apparent signs of life, should be brought under medical
treatment immediately.

REFERENCES

1. Garry, R.C., "Control of the temperature of the body,"
   Medicine Sci. Law 9: 242   (1969)
2. Gormsen, H., "Why have some victims of death from cold
   undressed?" Medicine Sci. Law 12: 200 (1972)
3. Norwegian Medico-Legal Board, Annual Report of the Norwegian Medico-Legal Board for 1969.
4. Vejlens, G., Nord. Kriminaltekn. Tidsskr., 22: 141 (1952)

Commentaries

"Renal response and lipid change during cold acclimation of
rodents," by G.E. Folk, Jr. and J.J. Berberich (Department
of Physiology and Biophysics, University of Iowa, Iowa City,
Iowa, USA). Early work in our laboratory established that
hibernators (hamsters) demonstrate conspicuous evidence of
cold acclimation by the seventh day of cold exposure
(Farrand and Folk). Recent studies by gas-liquid and thin-

layer chromatography of hamster subscapular brown adipose tissue (BAT), perirenal white fat (PWF), and inguinal white fat (IWF) indicate that the level of oleic acid is elevated in BAT, PWF, and IWF by day 6 of an 18-day cold exposure. PWF and IWF appear to become more unsaturated than BAT during this same time period. These results correlate well with the changes in food and water consumption and body weight. Some of these indicators of cold acclimation were sought in studies on lemmings. Collared lemmings (*Dicrostonyx*) and brown lemmings (*Lemmus*) were exposed to cold in a summer photoperiod (22L:2D). Cold acclimating responses were measured: i.e., changes in body and organ weight, food consumption, body temperature, adrenal steroid secretion, and renal function (control temperature $17^{\circ}C$). Arctic rodents complete the major components of cold acclimation in six days, rather than the four weeks reported for some species by other authors. A pronounced cold diuresis of markedly dilute urine is maintained by both species (ml/day in *Dicrostonyx*: control 13.5 ± sd 5.1; cold-exposed 34.2 ± sd 5.7). This is equivalent to excretion of 50 ℓ/day in man. Urine values of sodium, potassium, chlorine, pH, glucose, and osmolality will be reported for the conditions of ambient temperature 3 ± $2^{\circ}C$, for $-40^{\circ}C$, and under dehydration. (Sponsored by the Arctic Institute of North America with the approval and financial support of the Office of Naval Research.)

"Physiological responses to cooling of the face," by J. LeBlanc (Laboratories d'Endocrinologie climatique, Faculté de Médecine, Université Laval, Quebec, Canada). Past studies have shown that face and hand cold-water immersion tests ($4^{\circ}C$) are very useful for evaluating the individual responses to cold and for assessing the degree of adaptation. Field conditions are sometimes quite different, and there the evaluation of the environment by the windchill scale, which is based on sensory perception, has been used with success. However, it seemed important to evaluate the cold environment in terms of physiological measurements which can be qualified and to relate these to sensory perceptions. Indeed, cooling of the extremities or the face gives different local and systemic cardiovascular responses which are themselves modified by the degree of muscular activity of the subject. Exposure of the face, the primary sensing zone for the environment, has been tested at different temperatures

(-20° to +40°C) and wind speeds (0 to 40 mph). Skin temperatures (nose, forehead, cheek), pulse, and subjective evaluation were recorded on three groups of subjects: athletes,
mailmen (spending 5 to 6 hours outdoors per day), and control subjects with minor outdoor exposure and untrained.
Unexpectedly, high levels of activity had little effect on
the rate of cooling of the face and the bradycardia observed
with high winds persisted even when the subject was engaged
in heavy exercise.

"Adaptive changes in rats reared in cold for successive
generations," by S. Itoh, K. Moriya, and H. Maekubo
(Department of Physiology, Hokkaido University School of
Medicine, Sapporo, Japan). Wistar rats were reared at 5°C
for more than ten generations. The rectal temperature of the
adapted rats was lower than that in controls. When they were
exposed to cold at -20°C the rectal temperature did not decrease at least for 100 min. Non-shivering thermogenesis was
elevated, as indicated by less decrease in rectal temperature when exposed to cold after curare treatment. However,
the mechanism of non-shivering thermogenesis in the adapted
rats was thought to be the same as in cold-acclimated rats
exposed to 5°C for a short period of time. Norepinephrine
infusion caused a marked elevation of the rectal temperature
in the adapted rats, but less increase in plasma FFA and no
increase in blood sugar. Since the plasma beta-hydroxybuty-
rate level rose to a similar extent in both the adapted rats
and the controls, the release of FFA from the fat store may
not be reduced, but the turnover of plasma FFA is likely to
increase in the adapted rats. Cold exposure at -15°C also
induced less increase in the plasma FFA in the adapted rats,
although it caused pronounced elevation in the plasma beta-
hydroxybutyrate concentration. The results are to considerable extent compatible with observations on Ainu which have
been reported previously.
    Desaturation of adipose tissue glycerides occurred pro-
gressively during prolonged exposure to cold. The proportion
of palmitic acid decreased, while that of palmitoleic, linoleic, and linolenic acids increased. The composition of
fatty acids released in vitro from epididymal fat pads of
the cold-adapted rats was not largely different from the
pattern observed in control rats. However, since the composition of fat tissue glycerides differed significantly between the two groups, the difference in double bond indices

between FFA released and tissue glycerides was considerably
larger in the cold-adapted rats. Preferential release of
saturated fatty acids from the fat store was assumed to
occur in the adapted rats.

"Seasonal patterns of sleep stages and secretion of cortisol
and growth hormone during 24-hour periods in northern
Norway," by Elliot D. Weitzman, Andries S. deGraaf, Jon F.
Sassin, Tormar Hansen, Ole B. Godtlibsen, and Leon Hellman
(Department of Neurology, Montefiore Hospital and Medical
Centre, Albert Einstein College of Medicine, Bronx, New
York and Sentralsykehuset, Tromso, Norway). Life within the
Arctic Circle carries with it exposure to marked seasonal
changes. Extreme shifts in the proportion of light to darkness during the course of the year is a prominent feature in
these areas, ranging between the polar night and the midnight sun. There is abundant evidence that these fluctuations affect plants and animals but very little precise information about the degree to which humans are affected.
Numerous complaints are heard among the general population
of all age groups about disturbances in their sleep pattern,
especially during the dark period of the arctic winter. The
present experiment was designed to investigate not only
seasonal variation in sleep but also alterations in the secretion of cortisol and growth hormone of seven young men in
relation to the different seasons in a subarctic region. A
group of seven healthy male subjects were studied in regard
to sleep stages and 24-hour plasma cortisol and growth hormone patterns during the four seasons of the year in an
arctic environment (Tromso, Norway). During each seasonal
period polygraphic recordings were made on three consecutive nights. Over the last 24 hours blood samples were
collected every 20 minutes with an indwelling venous catheter.

No difference in the amount of total sleep or the percentage of time spent in each sleep stage was found for any
of the yearly seasons. A small but statistically significant
increase in mean plasma cortisol concentration and amount
secreted during 24 hours was found for the autumn and winter
seasons, as compared with the spring and summer. However, no
difference in the circadian curve of cortisol hormonal
pattern was found. All subjects secreted growth hormone
shortly after sleep onset at night and no difference was
found as a function of season of the year.

"Reducing whiteout effects," by M.F. Coffey (Canadian Forces Northern Region, Yellowknife, NWT). Whiteout is a natural phenomena where there is a critical loss of depth perception, the product of a diffused shadowless illumination caused by cloud and a uniformly mono-coloured white surface. These conditions occur most frequently in polar regions but also may take place in more southerly regions especially where there is lack of vegetation and contrast. Whiteout is a critical hazard in the operation of aircraft, as well as for the vehicle driver, and is to some extent of concern for the man on foot. Safety devices minimize the effect; these include the use of specially tinted goggles, coloured dispensible markers, special training, and recently the use of special flying aids such as low light television and the infrared systems. The effect may be similar to high-altitude myopia.

"Protection against extreme cold - 10 clo of insulation?" by R.F. Goldman (US Army Research Institute of Environmental Medicine, Natick, Mass., USA). Assuming a sleeping man has a heat production of 0.8 Met ($\approx$40 kcal/m^2 hr), with 25% lost by evaporation, there remains only 30 kcal/m^2 hr to be lost by radiation and/or convection if the heat balance of the body is to be maintained. The clo unit of insulation is defined as allowing 5.55 kcal/m^2 hr of heat loss for each centigrade degree of difference between the temperature of the ambient air and the average skin surface temperature. Assuming a minimum mean body skin temperature of 32°C for comfort, one can calculate the insulation required to prevent excess heat loss at any ambient temperature. Such calculations for arctic and subarctic environments are depressing, with the required insulation frequently far beyond that available: at -20°C almost 10 clo is required for a sleeping man to stay in thermal balance. The insulation provided by any protective ensemble, including sleeping systems, is readily measured using a heated copper manikin. Recently developed extreme cold, "Arctic," sleeping systems provide about 7 clo of insulation (sleeping with winter underwear and socks), compared with the 4.3 clo provided by the US Army's bulky, multiple layer, arctic uniform. A sleeping hood adds about 0.3 clo, a wool shirt and lined pants another 0.25 clo, a field coat with liner about 0.5 clo, a quilt about another 1.0 clo, and, finally, special reflective mittens and booties adds a further 0.4 clo to produce a total of between 9.3 and 9.9 clo, depending on the basic sleeping system used and its size. The relationship

between these copperman clo and the heat debt incurred was
re-evaluated with 10 men resting at -34°C in 12 different
sleeping systems ranging from 5 to 9 clo. A reasonably
linear relationship was found between the mean heat debt
after 3 hours and clo insulation over the range 5 to 9 clo;
at this temperature increase in clo insulation reduced the
body heat debt by about 15 kcal. Promising improvements in
protection investigated include auxiliary heating and new,
permeable reflective insulations. These approaches are
applicable not only in sleeping systems, but to protective
clothing in general.

"Thermographic (infrared) evaluation of frostbite," by M.P.
Hamlet (US Army Research Institute of Environmental Medicine,
Natick, Mass., USA). Thermography has been widely used to
evaluate diseases that affect the vascular supply of a particular portion of the body including breast adenocarcinoma,
Raynaud's disease, metastatic tumours, placenta previa,
arteriosclerosis obliterans, and vasoconstriction. Changes
in the vascular supply are accompanied by an increase or a
decrease in temperature. This temperature change is often
projected to the surface, where infrared imaging devices can
be used to measure small temperature differentials. Prior
work at this institute and others indicates that the injury
of frostbite is twofold: first, the physical destruction of
cells and organelles due to ice crystal formation, and
second, the rapid and severe loss of nutritive blood flow to
the frozen extremity. Frostbite research has been hindered
by the inability to reproduce the injury consistently in an
animal model. Clinical medicine has been hindered by an inability to determine the severity and extent of the injury
early in the course of frostbite therapy. Early infrared
thermographic devices were slow to produce an image and the
photographs were in shades of grey which are difficult for
the eye to differentiate. A thermal imaging device allows
evaluation of fourth-degree frostbite lesions produced in an
animal model. The device produces multicoloured photographs
that depict surface temperature differences and allows an
early determination of the line of demarcation and subsequently sloughing.

"Electrical response of nerve to freezing injury," by H.C.
Marshall and R.F. Goldman (Arctic Medical Research Laboratory (USARIEM) Alaska, Ft Wainwright, AK, and US Army Re-
Search Institute of Environmental Medicine, Natick, Mass.,
USA). To investigate the effects of superficial freezing injury upon peripheral nerve response, the fingers of eight
male volunteers were placed in a chamber having an air
temperature of -15°C, a wind speed of 6.8 m/sec, and a
relative humidity of 35-45 per cent. Four of these subjects
had experienced prior exposure to the same conditions and
four were new subjects. Exposure was for 15 minutes, or
until the superficial skin froze. The hand was then rapidly
rewarmed in a circulating water bath at 40°C for 15 minutes.
Skin temperature and nerve response were monitored throughout. Results showed those having prior experience to be more
resistant to frostnip than new subjects and more resistant
than they had been upon initial exposure. They maintained
higher skin temperatures than did new subjects. In two subjects, a distal nerve response still could not be obtained
four days after exposure. In two subjects there was evidence
of a paradoxical response, during the rewarming cycle, in
which the latency of one of the action potential components
decreased temporarily, then increased again and gradually
returned toward normal. In no case did the nerve response
return to normal after 15 minutes of rewarming. Indications
are that nerve is a most sensitive tissue to cold injury,
and that cold damage is not immediately reversed by rapid
rewarming. Differences between new subjects and those having
prior frostnip experience may reflect either adaptation or
the superimposition of a psychological stress upon the
physical effects of cold injury.

"Circadian and seasonal hormone cycles in Caucasian males in
the arctic and subarctic," by Betty Anne Philip and Donald
E. Roberts (Arctic Health Research Center and Arctic Medical Research Laboratory, Fairbanks, Alaska). Paper not submitted.

"Biorhythmologic study of man's adaptation to the conditions
of the Far North," by M.G. Kolpakov (Institute of Cytology
and Genetics, USSR Academy of Sciences, Siberian Branch, and
Institute of Clinical and Experimental Medicine, USSR Academy of Medical Science, Siberian Branch, Novosibirsk, USSR).
Paper not submitted.

FITNESS AND WORK PHYSIOLOGY

Working capacity of circumpolar peoples

R.J. SHEPHARD and A. RODE

This section focuses on physical fitness, work physiology studies, and their relation to problems of body composition and energy balance. The behaviour of both indigenous circumpolar populations and "white" immigrants from more southerly latitudes is discussed.

"FITNESS" OF INDIGENOUS CIRCUMPOLAR POPULATIONS

Many investigators have suspected that the vigorous physical activity needed for survival in the Arctic might have a beneficial effect on physical fitness, both through an immediate training response, and in a longer-term evolutionary sense through elimination of weaklings.

However, attempts to confirm this hypothesis have not been uniformly successful. Erikson (5) concluded from respiratory recovery curves that Eskimos were superior to white servicemen, and Rodahl (11), using a treadmill recovery test, found Eskimos had 3.5 times the score of airmen, and 1.5 times the score of acclimatized arctic soldiers. On the other hand, several expeditions from Scandinavia using the bicycle ergometer (1,2,7,8) have reported aerobic powers of only 44 to 53 mℓ/kg min in young Eskimo and Lapp men - values that would not be particularly remarkable in a southern Canadian city (20). The end-point of the bicycle ergometer tests was generally voluntary exhaustion rather than an oxygen plateau, and some authors have admitted freely that their data may have underestimated the true aerobic power of their subjects by as much as 20 per cent. In one study of the Lapps (1), attention was also drawn to the limitation imposed by use of the bicycle ergometer, and substantially higher oxygen consumptions were recorded during cross-country skiing.

THE PROBLEM OF SAMPLE SELECTION

The majority of samples previously studied are small relative to the groups of 223, 308, and 163 circumpolar residents discussed in this symposium. Physiologists and physicians at last seem to be coming to grips with the practical
problems of epidemiology and sampling bias; for too long
it has been assumed that any Eskimo is typical of his race.
In fact, even with the major studies for the International
Biological Program (IBP), some bias was present in most of
the populations examined (21). It is indeed difficult to
apply classical epidemiological methods, since nomadic
people move rather freely from one geographic district to
another, and even from one family to another. One team of
investigators may emphasize medical care, and attract the
sick. Another may emphasize fitness, and attract the
healthy. Unless scientists remain in a settlement for a
long time, they will miss many of the fitter members of the
community since they will be away on long hunting trips,
and a hasty survey may examine mainly unemployed alcoholics
and welfare recipients.

BIAS IN CANADIAN STUDIES

Our 1970-71 sample comprised about 70 per cent of the Igloolik villagers. Nevertheless, it differed in several important respects from the sample seen by the medical team.
Further, it must be stressed that Igloolik is but one arctic
community, and other settlements show very different figures
for the prevalence of disease, malnutrition, alcoholism, and
employment opportunities.

Igloolik is a small and stony island near the tip of the
Melville Peninsula. The region was settled originally because for much of the year open water permitted caribou and
walrus hunting by boat. Over the past ten years, it has developed as a small regional centre of some 500 people, with
two stores, a nursing station, a graded school, two churches,
and a biweekly air service to Frobisher Bay. About a third
of the food requirements are still met by hunting (page 106),
and nutrition is generally good. The influence of the two
churches remains strong, and alcoholism is not the problem
it has become in larger towns such as Frobisher Bay.

MAXIMUM OXYGEN INTAKE DATA

In all populations, the best single measure of cardiorespiratory fitness is the directly measured maximum oxygen

TABLE 1
Direct and indirect measurements of maximum oxygen intake (12).
Data on Igloolik Eskimos classified according to the quality of
effort made by the subjects (f_h = maximum heart rate, R = respiratory
exchange ratio; oxygen intake in 1/min STPD)

	Age	f_h	R	Direct	Indirect	$\triangle$
Men						
Good	23	185	1.14	3.46	3.74	0.28 ± 0.43
Fair	27	179	1.05	3.10	3.39	0.29 ± 0.54
Poor	24	176	0.97	3.27	3.88	0.61 ± 0.47
Girls						
Fair	14	173	1.04	1.91	2.49	0.58 ± 0.51

intake (19,20). In Igloolik, we measured this directly on
36 men and teenage girls. It was not possible to determine
blood lactate levels on our sample, but we graded subjects
in terms of their apparent motivation in performing a step-
test - "good," "fair," or "poor" (Table 1). There was a
gradation of both the maximum attained heart rate and the
maximum respiratory exchange ratio (R) according to this
classification. In those making a "good" effort, the R
value was much as in the "white" community, but perhaps
because of a good level of cardiorespiratory fitness, the
maximum heart rate was lower than in young "white" men.

We compared the directly measured values with those predicted by the Åstrand-Ryhming nomogram (3), and found the
indirect, predicted values were 8 per cent higher. This
could reflect partly the low maximum heart rate of the fit
Eskimos, and partly the non-competitive nature of Eskimo
society, with attendant difficulties in reaching a true
maximum oxygen intake.

Taking the submaximal data for our entire sample of 223
Eskimos, and adjusting this downwards by 8 per cent to
allow for a possible overestimation, the results nevertheless remain substantially higher than figures for both the
"white" population (20) and for other circumpolar groups
such as the Ainu (6) and the Wainwright (10) and Upernavik
(8) Eskimos (Figure 1). The aging curve for the Igloolik
group shows a relatively slow deterioration to middle age,
but a rapid loss of physical condition thereafter; this
may reflect the societal custom of offering the choice of
the hunt to grandparents.

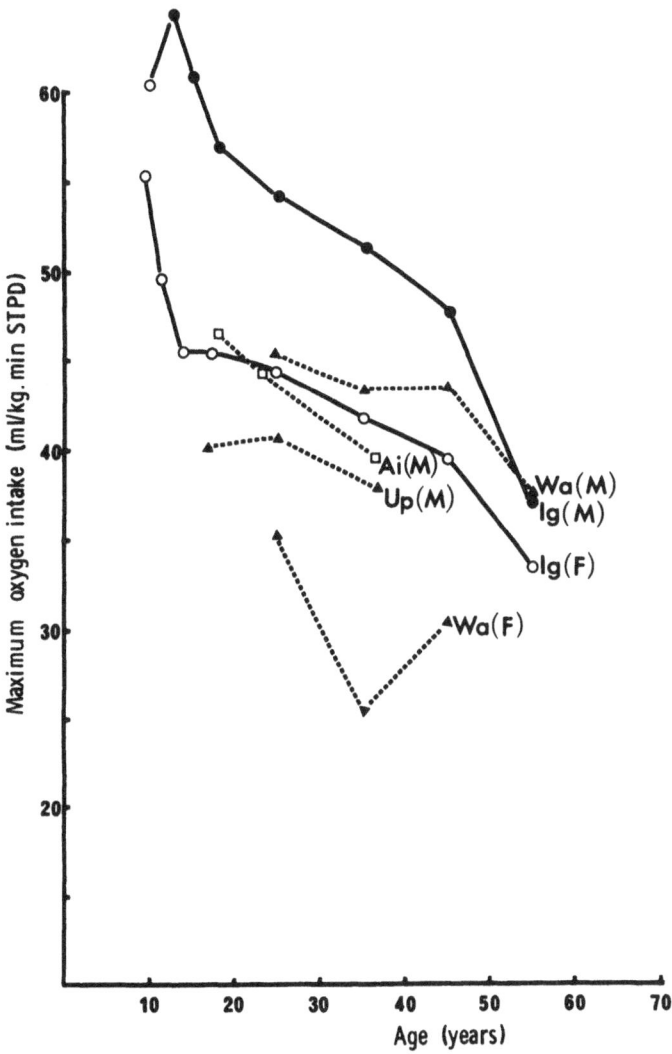

Figure 1   Maximum oxygen intake of Igloolik Eskimos, predicted by Åstrand nomogram and corrected downwards by 8
per cent; comparative data from Ainu (Ai), Wainwright (Wa),
and Upernavik (Up) Eskimos (courtesy of *Human Biology*,
ref. 22)

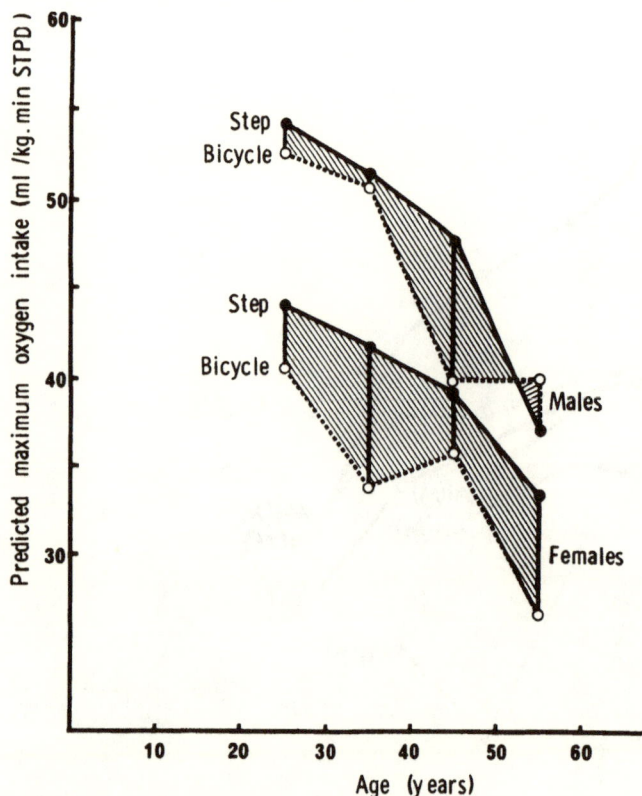

Figure 2   Discrepancy between aerobic power predicted from step-test and bicycle ergometer data on Igloolik Eskimos (14)

PROBLEMS OF EXERCISE METHODOLOGY

To check the validity of our methodology, we carried out a comparable range of fitness tests on the "white" community at Igloolik (21). Readings for maximum oxygen intake and skinfold thicknesses in the "white" group were much as in southerly communities but, perhaps because of the need to walk through deep snow (p. 113), leg strengths were good. The mechanical efficiency of stepping for both Eskimos and "whites" was also as demonstrated previously in the south (14).

It is perhaps worth emphasizing that the bicycle ergometer proved a less satisfactory tool than the step, at least in Igloolik. None of this community had previously encountered any form of bicycle, and the pattern of riding

was clumsy, with a correspondingly poor mechanical efficiency. The supposed advantage of the bicycle ergometer - a
uniform mechanical efficiency from one community to another
- was definitely not realized. Although there has been one
report of normal efficiency values for a small sample of
Kalahari bushmen, the majority of published data on the Eskimo support the relationship we have found between oxygen
cost and work load (21).

The contribution of the use of a bicycle ergometer to
the apparent normality of aerobic power in some circumpolar
groups can be seen from the discrepancy in values yielded
by the two test modalities (Figure 2). If we had relied
upon the bicycle ergometer, particularly in the women, we
should have substantially underestimated maximum oxygen intake.

SEASON AND ACCULTURATION

The body composition of the Eskimo is discussed elsewhere
(p. 91). We may note here that most studies have shown
very low skinfold readings. Nevertheless, the Igloolik
Eskimos have a substantial excess weight relative to ac-
tuarial standards (23); this is lean tissue.

Many physiologists have ventured to the Arctic only in
the comfort of July and August. We judged it important to
examine seasonal differences in fitness and body composition (13). Aerobic power was remarkably similar in the
summer and winter seasons, but in the winter there was a
small, statistically significant increase of skinfold
readings. The energy cost of summer and winter activities
is compared in other papers (pp. 106, 119); for the Eskimo,
hunting is somewhat less frequent during the winter months,
but more energy is needed to traverse snow-covered
surfaces.

Acculturation is associated with a marked gradient of
aerobic power from the frequent hunter through the partially acculturated Eskimo to the settlement worker who has
accepted relatively permanent commercial or government employment (Table 2). Equally, a negative correlation can be
demonstrated between aerobic power and an arbitrary index
of acculturation that Dr Ross McArthur has derived from
such indicators as mastery of the English language and the
number of cooking utensils in the home. Conversely,
McArthur's index is positively correlated with the thickness
of subcutaneous fat.

TABLE 2
The influence of acculturation on selected indices of cardiorespiratory fitness (12, 21).   Hunters are classified + to +++ on the frequency of hunting expeditions; other Eskimos are rated as urban or partially acculturated (Inter.) (age in years, height in cm, weight in kg, $\dot{V}_{O_2}$(max) in ml/kg min STPD, skinfolds in mm, leg extension strength in kg)

| | Urban | Inter. | Hunter | | |
			+	++	+++
Age	35	30	29	31	21
Height	165	166	165	161	167
Weight	70	66	67	67	61
$\dot{V}_{O_2}$(max)	50	57	59	59	67
Skinfold	7	6	5	6	5
Leg Strength	81	85	81	77	79

Such findings do not necessarily prove that settlement life has caused a deterioration of cardiorespiratory fitness. It may be that those with a poor genetic endowment have chosen to seek government work, while those with a higher level of fitness continue to follow the traditional life-style. However, our impression from seeing the Eskimos, talking with them, and participating in some of their hunts is that the physical demands of the chase have been an important causal contribution to the levels of fitness encountered in the hunters.

Among the female Eskimos, aerobic powers are somewhat higher in those who have one or more children (21). This may relate to carriage of the child on the back in the traditional "amauti" - certainly a valuable stimulus to personal fitness. However, acculturation may again play a role, since more of the young and unmarried girls have been educated in southerly communities, and have leared to adopt the social patterns of "white" teenage girls.

CHRONIC DISEASE AND FITNESS

A number of previous studies have failed to consider the possible impact of chronic respiratory disease upon cardiorespiratory fitness. Data for Igloolik Eskimos with a history of chronic respiratory disease (generally tuberculosis) can be represented as percentage deviations from figures for healthy Eskimos of comparable age (Table 3). The systemic effects of chest disease are shown by a small

TABLE 3
The effects of chronic respiratory disease upon selected indices of
fitness (12, 21). Data expressed as percentage deviations from normal
values for Igloolik Eskimos of comparable age

Age	Height	Weight	$\dot{V}_{O_2}$		Skinfold	Grip	Leg ext.
			L./min	ml/kg.min			
Men							
20-29	-1.5	-10.9	-12.1	-21.2	-19.7	-6.5	+ 2.2
30-39	-1.9	- 9.5	-14.7	-24.1	- 6.2	-2.1	+18.1
40-49	-0.3	-11.3	-12.7	-22.8	- 8.7	+6.3	- 9.0
50-59	+1.5	- 6.2	-13.0	-10.6	-52.5	-1.3	- 7.7
Women							
20-29	+1.9	- 4.9	+ 2.4	+ 7.0	+13.7	-5.9	- 8.2
30-39	-3.2	+ 6.0	-14.2	- 9.0	+69.3	-1.3	- 3.6
50-59	-1.2	-15.3	+ 1.3	-13.9	-49.3	-9.1	+ 3.8
All	-0.7	- 8.5	- 9.0	-12.1	+ 7.6	-2.8	- 5.8

diminution of standing height, a substantial diminution of
body weight and muscle strength, and in the men (but less
obviously in the women) a loss of subcutaneous fat. In the
context of the present chapter, the most important observation is the 10 per cent diminution of aerobic power; thus,
if we had included diseased subjects in the Igloolik
sample, we would have substantially underestimated the
aerobic power of the community. Twenty-eight of our sample
had a history of primary tuberculosis and/or hilar calcification; cardiorespiratory function in this group was close
to 100 per cent of the age-related normal values. A further
17 had a history of secondary or advanced tuberculosis, and
3 had emphysema and/or chronic bronchitis, with extensive
fibrosis. These last 20 cases, 9 per cent of our sample,
accounted for most of the functional loss seen in Table 2.

THE OXYGEN TRANSPORT CHAIN

The behaviour of individual links in the oxygen transport
chain (20) of the Igloolik Eskimo was much as might be anticipated in a population composed of individuals who were
fitter then sedentary "white" city dwellers, but were by no
means typical international endurance athletes.
    Contrary to the earlier findings of Dr. Beaudry (4), the
one-second forced expiratory volume of the healthy Igloolik
male Eskimo was at the anticipated level for "white" subjects of comparable age, height, and smoking history, while
values for females were 12 per cent greater than predictions

(15). Vital capacities were 10 per cent above predictions
in men and 18 per cent above predictions in women. The
residual volume was relatively normal in relation to total
lung volume, as were the resting and exercise pulmonary diffusing capacities (page 320).

Maximum cardiac outputs and arteriovenous oxygen
differences were estimated by a CO_2 rebreathing method
(16). The cardiac stroke volume at 70-75 per cent of maximum oxygen intake was very normal, declining from 126 ml
in young adult men to 114 ml in the elderly. Corresponding
figures for the women were 78 and 70 ml. Maximum arteriovenous oxygen differences ranged from 133 to 151 ml/l and
showed no significant age or sex trends over the adult
span.

Haemoglobin levels were normal, with remarkably few examples of clinical anaemia. Blood volumes for settlement
workers were high normal figures, but results for hunters
were somewhat lower, perhaps because they were still
suffering from cold dehydration at the time of testing
(page 113). Cardiac volumes were essentially normal, although the results may have been biased downwards, since
the only available films were on patients examined by the
medical team.

Thus, all terms in the oxygen transport line seem in
keeping with the high normal figures demonstrated by
measurement of maximum oxygen intake.

GROWTH OF FITNESS

Other sections of this volume look at specific aspects of
growth and development. In the context of cardiorespiratory fitness, one may question the traditional wisdom of
using a full longitudinal survey, particularly in a community that is undergoing rapid cultural change (Figure 3). The
result "growth" curve may reflect not only growth, but also
the superimposed effects of acculturation (18). This may
speed the development of some anthropometric characteristics, but could well slow the development of working capacity. A cross-sectional survey is cheaper, but can be
biased in an opposite sense; older children have been exposed to a harsher environment than those who are younger.
The optimum approach seems to combine a cross-sectional
study and longitudinal observations made over a short time
span, the so-called semilongitudinal study (see further,
page 230).

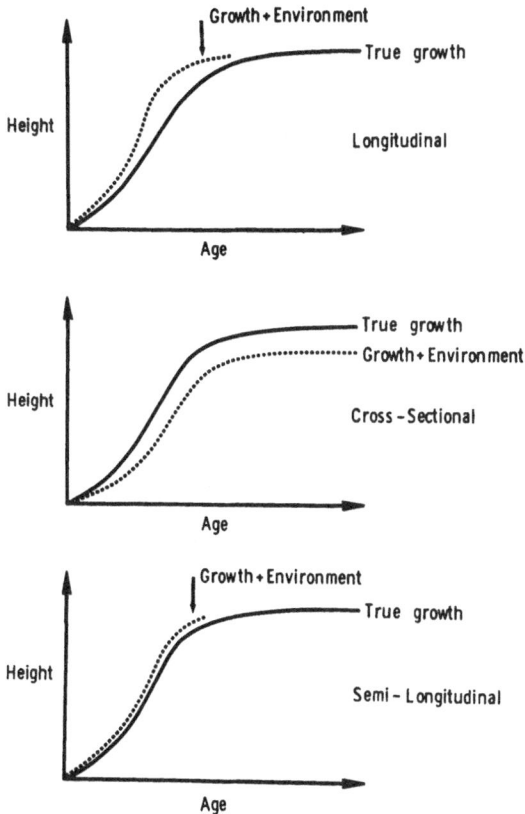

Figure 3   A comparison of longitudinal, cross-sectional, and semilongitudinal studies of growth and development (18), to illustrate possible discrepancies between the true growth curve and that observed from the combined effects of environmental change and growth

The IBP physiology group used a semilongitudinal approach in Igloolik, and found some small differences in the apparent timing of growth spurts between cross-sectional and longitudinal observations. In the boys, a high aerobic power was well maintained throughout adolescence (17). The girls started with an aerobic power almost equal to that of the boys, but deteriorated rapidly with the onset of puberty. The leg and grip strength of the boys also developed much more than that of the girls over the pubertal period. Nevertheless, the girls were stronger than those in "white" communities; their average strength exceeded that of the boys between 11 and 14 years, and they reached a plateau of strength later than "white" girls. We would conclude that, because of continuing physical demands, their potential fitness was realized more fully than that of city-dwellers.

COLD EXPOSURE AND WORKING CAPACITY

While at rest, the Eskimo may have some difficulty in conserving body heat, owing to the harsh arctic climate; on the other hand, hard physical work can subject a heavily insulated person to heat stress. One interesting adaptation of the Eskimo to this problem (page 91) seems to be the replacement of an irremovable layer of subcutaneous fat by the variable protection of several layers of caribou clothing. In the Canadian soldier (page 113), if not his U.S. counterpart (page 119), one factor limiting potential performance is the danger of degrading the insulation of arctic clothing by the accumulation of sweat. A second significant adaptation of the Eskimo is thus an altered distribution of sweat-gland activity (page 46); during vigorous work, as during carbachol administration, sweat accumulates on the face rather than the trunk and limbs (where it would be expected in a "white" person).

Some bronchospasm might be anticipated as a result of the inhalation of bitterly cold arctic air. Our data for the Igloolik Eskimos (p. 320) show rather low $FEV_{1.0}$/FVC ratios. However, this is attributable to an increase of forced vital capacity rather than a deterioration of one-second forced expiratory volume, and it is thus unlikely that we are demonstrating a chronic response to cold. Drs Schaefer and Hildes (page 327) have a clinical impression of a high incidence of pulmonary hypertension, with associated electro-cardiographic evidence of right branch bundle block. If there are no associated clinical abnormalities, a partial right bundle block could be a normal expression of well-developed cardio-respiratory fitness (9). Nevertheless, we examined exercise electrocardiograms from 13 Eskimos where the medical team found a resting right branch bundle block (complete in 6, and incomplete in 7). Unfortunately, the phenomenon was best seen in leads AVR, V4R, V1, and V2, whereas the exercise electrocardiograms were taken in the CM5 position. However, two cases showed evidence of bundle block during effort, and in 3 of the remaining 11 cases there was a suspicion of QRS broadening.

CONCLUSIONS

The picture of the Igloolik Eskimo that emerges from our
studies is thus of an individual with a high but not an
athletic level of cardiorespiratory fitness. Many factors
have contributed to this development. Genetic studies
(page 219) suggest a relatively isolated community, where it
is conceivable a favourable mutation may have developed.
Episodic starvation and disease may have added the weight
of evolutionary pressure. A high protein diet may have
helped conserve a compact body form, and thus a high aerobic power per kilogram of body weight. Nevertheless, much
of the difference between the Igloolik Eskimo and the white
city-dweller could be explained as a response to the greater
physical demands of arctic life. The 35% difference of
working capacity between the most active hunters and the
settlement workers supports the suggestion that where fitness is observed, this is related to vigorous physical activity. Unhappily, hunting is a declining interest of the
community, and it may thus be possible to make a more rigorous test of our hypothesis by repeating our investigations
when the villagers no longer attempt to sustain their trad-
ditional life-style.

ACKNOWLEDGMENT

The work of this laboratory has been supported in part by
a research grant from the Canadian National Research Council.

SUMMARY

The authors have completed detailed studies of 223 Eskimos
living in the Canadian arctic community of Igloolik, using
standard methods developed for the International Biological
Program. This material is reviewed in the general context
of the working capacity of indigenous and immigrant circumpolar populations. The aerobic power of the Eskimos is substantially greater than in "white" immigrants, and the native peoples also have an extremely small amount of subcutaneous fat. Genetic isolation, a high protein diet, episodic
malnutrition, disease, vigorous physical activity, and repeated cold exposure can all modify fitness levels; the main
determinants of the high maximal oxygen intake per unit of
body weight in Igloolik seem to be a low percentage of body
fat, periodic intense activity, and the evolutionary pressures of a harsh environment and poorly controlled disease.

REFERENCES

1. Andersen, K.L., Elsner, R.E., Saltin, B., and Hermansen, L.,"Physical fitness in terms of maximal oxygen intake of nomadic Lapps,"U.S. Air Force Arctic Aeromedical Laboratory, Tech. Rept. AAL TDR 61-53 (Fort Wainwright, Alaska, 1962)

2. Andersen, K.L., "Racial and inter-racial differences in work capacity," J. biosoc. Sci., Suppl. 1: 69-80 (1969)

3. Åstrand, I., "Aerobic work capacity in men and women with special reference to age," Acta physiol. scand., 49: Suppl. 169 (1960)

4. Beaudry, P.H., "Pulmonary function of the Canadian Eastern Arctic Eskimo," Arch. env. Health, 17: 524-28 (1968)

5. Erikson, H., "The respiratory response to acute exercise of Eskimos and whites," Acta physiol. scand., 41: 1-11 (1958)

6. Ikai, M., Ishii, K., Miyamura, M., Kusano, K., Bar-Or, O., Kollias, J., and Buskirk, E.R., "Aerobic capacity of Ainu and other Japanese on Hokkaido," Med. sci. Sports, 3: 6-11 (1971)

7. Karlsson, J., "Maximal oxygen uptake in Skolt Lapps," Arctic Anthropol., 7: 19-20 (1970)

8. Lammert, O., "Maximal aerobic power and energy expenditure of Eskimo hunters in Greenland," J. appl. Physiol. 33: 184-8 (1972)

9. Mitrevski, P.J., "Incomplete right branch bundle block (lead V_1) in athletes," Med. sci. Sports, 1: 153-5 (1969)

10. Rennie, D.W., di Prampero, P., Fitts, R.W., and Sinclair, L., "Physical fitness and respiratory function of Eskimos of Wainwright, Alaska," Arctic Anthropol., 7: 73-82 (1970)

11. Rodahl, K., "Physical fitness," J. Am. geriatr. Soc., 6: 205-9 (1953)

12. Rode, A., and Shephard, R.J., "The cardio-respiratory fitness of an arctic community," J. appl. Physiol., 31: 519-26 (1971)

13. Rode, A., and Shephard, R.J., "Fitness and season. An arctic study," Med. sci. Sports, 5: 1970-3 (1973)

14. Rode, A., and Shephard, R.J., "On the mode of exercise appropriate to an arctic community," Int. Z. angew. Physiol., 31: 187-96 (1973)

15. Rode, A., and Shephard, R.J., "Pulmonary function of Canadian Eskimos," Scand. J. resp. Dis., 54: 191-205 (1973)
16. Rode, A., and Shephard, R.J., "The cardiac output, blood volume, and total haemoglobin of the Canadian Eskimo," J. appl. Physiol., 34: 91-6 (1973)
17. Rode, A., and Shephard, R.J., "Growth, development and fitness of the Canadian Eskimo," Med. sci. Sports, 5: 161-9 (1973)
18. Rode, A., and Shephard, R.J., "Growth and development in the Eskimo," Proceedings of 2nd Canadian Workshop on child growth and development, Saskatoon, Nov. 1972
19. Shephard, R.J., Allen, C., Benade, A.J.S., Davies, C.T.M., di Prampero, P.E., Hedman, R., Merriman, J.E., Myhre, K., and Simmons, R., "The maximum oxygen intake - an international reference standard of cardio-respiratory fitness," Bull. World Health Org., 38: 757-64 (1968)
20. Shephard, R.J., Endurance Fitness (Toronto: University of Toronto Press, 1969)
21. Shephard, R.J., "Work physiology and activity patterns," in: IBP Synthesis Volume Circumpolar Peoples, F. Milan (Ed.) (Cambridge U.K.: University Press, 1975), in preparation
22. Shephard, R.J., "Work physiology and activity patterns of circumpolar Eskimos and Ainu. A synthesis of IBP data," Human Biology, 46: 263-94 (1974)
23. Build and Blood Pressure Study (Chicago, Ill.: Society of Actuaries, 1959)

On the body composition of the Eskimo

R.J. SHEPHARD and A. RODE

A number of authors have commented on the low skinfold readings obtained upon Eskimo populations (3,4,6). It was thus thought desirable to determine body composition by an independent method, and to examine relationships between skinfold readings and this estimate of body fat. Our subjects were 74 adult Canadian Eskimos (33 males aged 15-39 years and 41 females aged 15-59 years).

Methodology

The thickness of the three skinfolds recommended to the International Biological Program - triceps, subscapular, and suprailiac - was determined by Lange skinfold calipers. Height and weight were measured by standard techniques, and body water was estimated by a deuterium dilution procedure (5). Blood volumes were determined on a separate occasion by carbon monoxide uptake method (7).

Percentage Body Fat

None of the group were grossly obese (Table 1). Only one man had more than 20 per cent fat, and only eight women more than 30 per cent fat; nevertheless, average values were rather larger than might have been expected from skinfold readings.

There was no increase of body fat with age in the male Eskimos; indeed, the 30-39 year old age group tended to a lower percentage of body fat and a higher percentage of fat-free solids than the younger men. This may reflect greater acculturation of the younger Eskimos. Skinfold readings also showed little increase with age, but there was a clear separation of hunters (average thickness 5.0 mm) and "acculturated" Eskimos (average thickness 6.7 mm).

TABLE 1
Body composition of Igloolik Eskimos

Age (years)	N	Height (cm)	Weight (kg)	Average skinfold (mm)	Bodyfat (%)	Fat-free solids (%)
Males						
15-19	11	163.1	61.6	5.5	12.7	23.4
20-29	12	165.8	69.3	5.8	15.3	22.7
30-39	10	166.7	71.4	6.2	11.8	23.6
Females						
15-19	9	155.0	54.0	9.6	19.4	21.6
20-29	12	157.5	57.8	9.2	19.8	21.5
30-39	10	153.0	55.3	11.6	26.0	19.8
40-59	10	152.9	58.6	8.8	25.5	20.0

The women had a higher percentage of body fat than the men, and in general the older women were fatter than those who were younger. However, the eight fattest had a rather uniform age distribution, two coming from each of the age groups shown. The decrease of lean tissue in older women was small and statistically insignificant.

Body Water and Blood Volumes
Since the changes in the percentage of body water were relatively small over the adult span, results were pooled in order to test the relationship between blood volume and body water (Table 1). In the male Eskimos, the two variables were unrelated. In the females, the equation fitted by the method of least squares was: body water = 13.2 + 3.55 (blood volume), with an $F_{1,28}$ ratio of 7.67 and a correlation coefficient of 0.61.

Skinfold Thicknesses and Body Fat
The majority of previous authors have related skinfold readings to body density, as determined by underwater weighing. In the present instance, it was simpler to seek direct relationships between body fat and skinfold readings. For female Eskimos, the relationship is as follows, for a linear equation:

$$\% \text{ body fat} = 12.8 - 0.245\,(T) + 0.690\,(SS) + 0.475\,(SP), \quad (1)$$

and for a semi-logarithmic equation

$$\% \text{ body fat} = -13.2 + 24.2\left[\log_{10}\Sigma(T + SS + SP)\right], \quad (2)$$

where T is the thickness of triceps skinfold in mm, SS is the thickness of subscapular skinfold in mm, and SP is the thickness of suprailiac skinfold in mm.

In the male Eskimo, the two types of variable were unrelated. In the female Eskimos, coefficients of correlation were small but statistically significant, with respective values of 0.37, 0.47, and 0.44 for the triceps, subscapular, and suprailiac folds. Equation (1) accounted for the largest percentage of the variance in the body fat (25 per cent). This equation was significant at the 5 per cent level, with $F_{3.28} = 2.97$, and offered a small advantage relative to equations based on the triceps fold alone, or a combination of triceps and subscapular folds. The semilogarithmic equation accounted for less variance (19.6 per cent) than the three-term multiple regression equation but, because there was only one independent variable $[\log_{10}\Sigma(T + SS + SP)]$, the statistical significance was greater ($F_{1,30} = 7.32$ with a p of almost 0.01).

TABLE 2
Total body water, lean solids, and total lean tissue relative to height

		Body water (1/cm)		Lean solids (g/cm)		Total lean tissue (kg/cm)	
		Whites	Eskimo	Whites	Eskimo	Whites	Eskimo
Males	20-39	0.225	0.267	69.1	97.8	0.293	0.366
Females	15-50	0.179	0.207	70.3	75.2	0.252	0.279

Problems of Body Hydration
The main weakness of the deuterium oxide approach is uncertainty regarding tissue hydration in the Eskimo. The
white person who works out of doors in the Arctic suffers
a substantial dehydration because of increased respiratory
loss, heavy sweating and/or increased urinary flow, exhaustion of glycogen reserves, and an inadequate intake of
fluids. If the Eskimo behaved in the same manner, the
assumption that lean tissue contained 73.2 per cent water
might be seriously in error. However, our figures for
blood volume (Table 2) are above the average levels for the
"white" population and give no evidence of dehydration.
Other investigators have also commented on the large blood
volumes of the Eskimo (1,2), suggesting that this may represent a physiological adaptation to repeated and severe
cold exposure. Blood volumes in the settlement men were
larger than in the hunters. This result may have been obtained because the hunters were seen within one or two days
of their return to the village and rehydration was incomplete. The fact that blood volume was related to body water
in the female but not in the male also points to this conclusion. If other tissues too are dehydrated then the
deuterium dilution method could overestimate body fat in
the hunters.

Lean Tissues
Our average figures for body water are similiar to those
reported for sedentary "white" subjects (Table 1). However,
a substantial difference becomes apparent if results are
related to standing height (Table 2). The mass of lean
solids and the total lean tissues are also substantially
greater in the Eskimo.

    In essence, the traditional Eskimo has carried the same
weight of muscle as a "white" person on shorter legs. However, the current generation of adolescents is rapidly

approaching "white" stature, and it will be interesting to
see whether the advantage of lean body mass persists when
the difference of standing height has been eliminated.

Distribution of Body Fat
Despite the evidence of skinfold readings, our deuterium estimates suggest that the percentage body fat of the Eskimo
is of the same order as that seen in moderately fit "white"
subjects. Possibly, the relative distribution of fat between the skin and deeper tissues is modified in the Eskimo.
At first glance, this would seem a negative adaptation to
the arctic environment. However, if hard work is to be performed for survival, it is preferable for insulation to be
provided by larger layers of removable clothing rather than
by a fixed fat depot. Further, if much of the energy need
must be met from rather sporadic meals, it is desirable
that the labile fat stores should be elsewhere than in the
path of heat exchange.

Practical Value of Skinfold Readings
Field testing of nutritional status will inevitably rely
upon simple measures of height, weight, and skinfold thickness. It is thus disappointing to find such slender correlations between skinfold readings and deuterium dilution
estimates of body fat. However, it is perhaps fair to stress
that the higher coefficients of correlation reported in many
"white" series have been obtained at the expense of an artificially selected population containing an unusual proportion of obese subjects. Since less than a third of the body
fat of a thin person is in the subcutaneous region, high
coefficients cannot be expected.

   With growing affluence and inactivity, obesity may soon
become as much a problem for the Eskimo as for the "white"
North American. This view is supported by the recent increases in skinfold thickness in Alaskan Eskimo (page 122)
and the negative age trend in the Igloolik males. Thus
skinfold readings will become progressively more useful to
the health care delivery team as the obesity of the population increases.

ACKNOWLEDGMENT

This work has been supported in part by a research grant
from the Canadian National Research Council.

SUMMARY

The body composition of 74 adult Eskimos (33 males, 41
females) has been determined by a deuterium oxide dilution
method. The figures for lean mass are comparable with
those for the "white" population when reported on an absolute basis, but are larger if expressed per unit of standing
height. Percentages of body fat (average 13.4 per cent in
males, 22.6 per cent in females) are at least as high as
those encountered in many series of college students, despite very low skinfold readings; the possibility is suggested that body fat has a different regional distribution in
the Eskimo. Blood volumes as measured by a carbon monoxide
method are in the high normal range (95.7 ml/kg in the
males, 91.0 ml/kg in the females); however, lower values in
hunters (83.6 ml/kg) than in settlement Eskimos (94.6 ml/kg)
suggests that dehydration may be incurred during hunting
trips. If so, the deuterium method may overestimate the body
fat of the hunters.

Blood volumes are related to body water in the females,
but not in the males. Perhaps because skinfold readings are
so low, there is no relationship between skinfold thickness
and body fat in the male Eskimos. In the females, the best
equation accounts for only 25 per cent of the variance in
the data: % body fat = 12.8 - 0.245 (triceps, mm) + 0.690
(subscapular, mm) + 0.475 (suprailiac, mm).

REFERENCES

1. Baugh, C.W., Bird, G.S., Brown, G.M., Lennox, C.S., and
   Semple, R.E., "Blood volumes of Eskimos and white men
   before and during acute cold stress," J. Physiol., 140:
   347-58 (1958)
2. Brown, G.M., Bird, G.S., Boag, L.M., Delahaye, D.J.,
   Green, J.E., Hatcher, J.D., and Page, J., "Blood volume
   and basal metabolic rate of Eskimos," Metabolism, 3:
   247-54 (1954)
3. Elsner, R.W., "Skinfold thicknesses in primitive people
   native to a cold climate," Ann. N.Y. Acad. Sci., 110:
   503-14 (1963)
4. Jamison, P.L. and Zigura, S.L., "An anthropometric
   study of the Eskimos of Wainwright, Alaska," Arctic
   Anthropol., 7: 125-43 (1970)
5. Novak, L.P., "Total body water in man," Per-Erik E.
   Bergner and C.C. Lushbaugh (ed.) in Compartment, pools,
   and spaces in medical physiology, technical editor

E.B. Anderson. U.S. Atomic Energy Commission, Division
of Technical Information; available from Clearinghouse
for Federal Scientific and Technical Information,
National Bureau of Standards, U.S. Dept. of Commerce,
Springfield, Va., 1967
6. Rose, A. and Shephard, R.J., "Cardio-respiratory fitness
of an Arctic community," J. appl. Physiol., 31: 519-26
(1971)
7. Rode, A., and Shephard, R.J., "The cardiac output, blood
volume, and total haemoglobin of the Canadian Eskimo,"
J. appl. Physiol., 34: 91-96 (1973).

The maximal oxygen uptake in adult Lapps and Skolts

S. SUNDBERG and K.L. ANDERSEN

Physical working capacity has been assumed to be of great
significance in traditional arctic populations. The maximal oxygen uptake is one of the most important determinants
of an individual's physical working capacity, and this
measure has been adopted for use in the International Biological Program for the study of adaptation to different
environmental conditions. Some information is available on
the maximal oxygen uptake of people living in cold habi-
tats. The physical working capacity of nomadic Lapps was
studied by Lange Andersen et al., who described sex and
age differences. They found that the nomadic Lapps had a
physical working capacity superior to that of other arctic
or sedentary people (1). Karlsson has reported data for
the maximal oxygen uptake of Skolts at Nellim in Finland,
and found that their fitness was lower than that of the nomadic Lapps (2). This presentation represents an extension
of Karlsson's study, and is particularly concerned with
studies of adult Lapps and Skolts from the Inari rural
community in northern Finland. These people are no longer
nomads.

The aims of the present study were: (1) to describe
interindividual variations of maximal oxygen uptake in a
random sample of adult Lappish and Skoltish men and women
in relation to age, and (2) to analyse the effects of

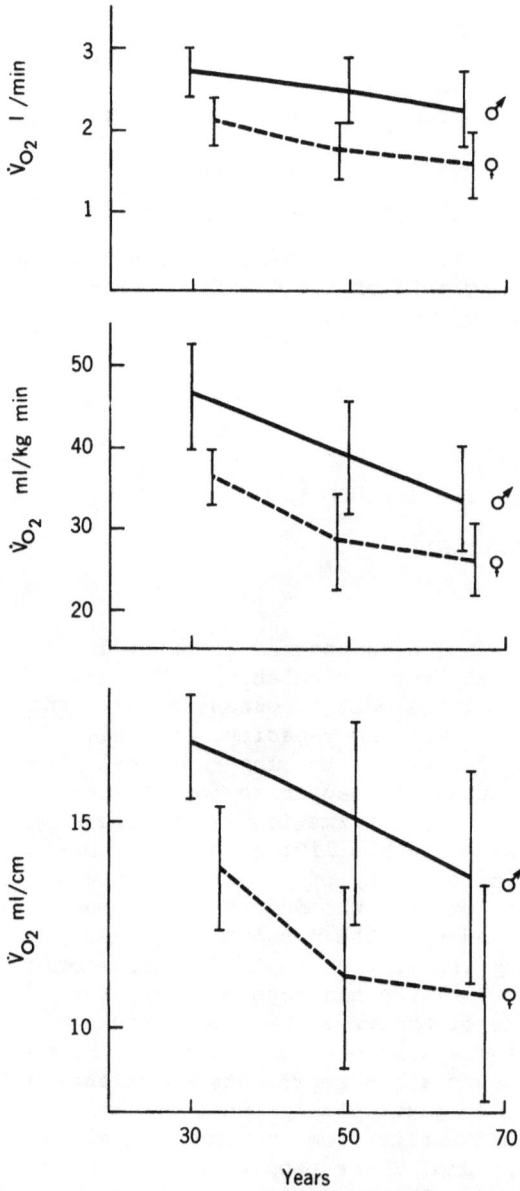

Figure 1   Highest recorded oxygen uptake in relation to age

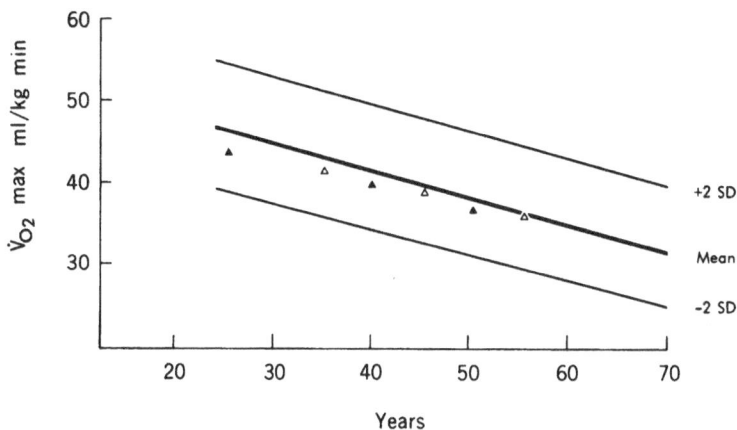

Figure 2   Comparison of oxygen uptake with Norwegian citizens (males):△, Hermansen (1964);▲, Benestad (1970)

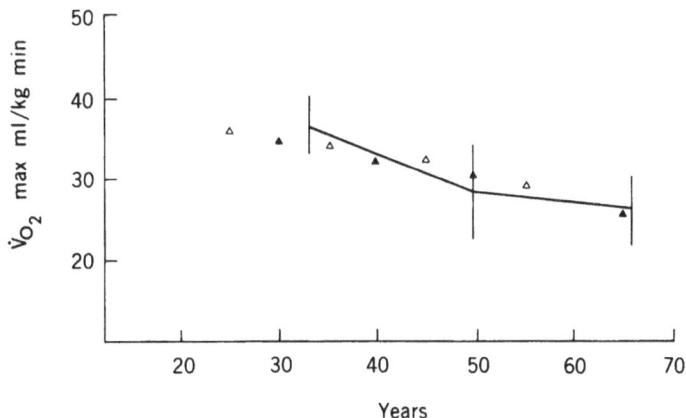

Figure 3   Comparison of oxygen uptake with Norwegian citizens (females):△, Hermansen (1964);▲ , Benestad (1970)

genetic and environmental differences on man's physical working capacity.

The maximal oxygen uptake was measured on 163 Finnish Lapps and Skolts over the age of 20 years (85 men and 78 women). The direct method was used, with exhaustive work on a bicycle ergometer. Before the exercise test, a conventional 12-lead resting-ECG was recorded, and the resting arterial blood pressure was measured. The subjects exercised on a mechanically braked bicycle ergometer at a pedalling rate of 50 revolutions per minute. Two submaximal loads of 6 minutes duration each and one maximal load of

3 minutes duration were used. Heart rate was recorded by ECG. Expired air was collected in Douglas bags, with immediate gas analysis by the Scholander method.

The maximal oxygen uptake was higher in men than in women, and decreased almost linearly with age in both sexes. It showed considerable interindividual variation, the coefficient of variation being 15-18 per cent in men and 8-18 per cent in women. In men the maximal oxygen uptake per kg of body weight was 46 mℓ/min kg at the age of 30 years, decreasing to 33 mℓ/min kg at the age of 70 (Figure 1). In women the corresponding values were 37 and 26 mℓ/min kg respectively. In two Norwegian populations studied by the same method the values were of the same order of magnitude in both sexes (Figures 2 and 3).

The male sector of the population was also compared with other arctic populations. The values did not differ much from each other and it is doubtful if there are any true differences. All these populations seem to have almost the same maximal oxygen uptake. The only exception are the nomadic Lapps of Norway as studied by Lange Andersen, with a maximal oxygen uptake that is 5-8 mℓ/min kg higher in all age-groups than the non-nomadic Lapps and Skolts studied by us (Figure 4). One possible explanation for this difference is that these nomadic Lapps have a higher degree of habitual physical activity than the more sedentary people living in the same area, and therefore a higher maximal oxygen uptake.

Rode and Shephard (3) studied traditional Canadian Eskimos of Igloolik by a different method. They found values almost 10 mℓ/min kg higher than ours in both sexes and in all age-groups. Many of these Eskimos were active hunters still living a traditional life, while others were more "urbanized."

Apparently, only populations with a high degree of habitual physical activity have a maximal oxygen uptake superior to other surrounding technologically developed or traditional communities. In studying the physical working capacity of populations from different ethnic origins, one is struck by similarities rather than by differences. It seems as if a rather high level of habitual physical activity has to be reached by a population before it develops a maximal oxygen uptake superior to that of other populations.

Health of arctic fishermen   101

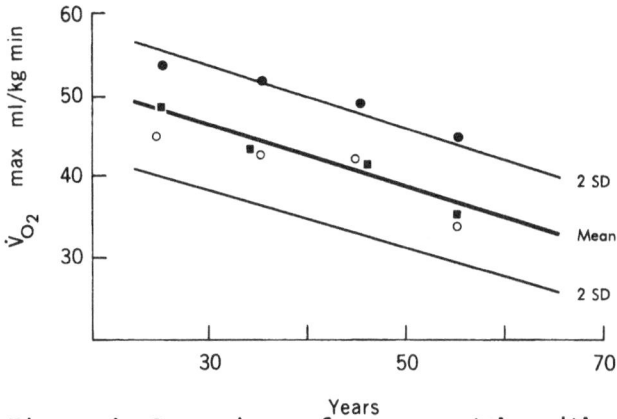

Figure 4   Comparison of oxygen uptake with other arctic or subarctic populations (males):●, Nomadic Lapps,O , Eskimos, Alaska;■, Skolts (Karisson)

REFERENCES

1. Andersen, K.L., Elsner, R.E., Saltin, B., and Hermansen, L., "Physical fitness in terms of maximal oxygen intake of nomadic Lapps," Fort Wainwright, Alaska: U.S.A.F., Arctic Medical Laboratory, Tech. Rept. AAL TDR-61-53 (1962)
2. Karlsson, J., "Maximum oxygen uptake in Skolt Lapps," Arctic Anthropol., 7: 19-20 (1970)
3. Rode, A. and Shephard, R.J., "Cardiorespiratory fitness of an arctic community", J. appl. Physiol., 31: 519-526 (1971)

Health of arctic fishermen as related to occupational work capacity

P. FUGELLI

In many rural municipalities of northern Norway, fishing is the only possible occupation. In such areas, the doctor is confronted with special socio-medical problems when a fisherman becomes partially or totally disabled by disease.

TABLE 1
Distribution of incapacitating disease in fishermen by diagnostic category

Diagnostic group	No. of incapacitated fishermen	%
Cardiovascular diseases	28	46.7
Mental disorders	20	33.3
Injuries, sequelae	4	6.7
Nervous system	3	5.0
Locomotor system	2	3.3
Tuberculosis, sequelae	2	3.3
Metabolic diseases	1	1.7
Total	60	100.0

This paper looks at three questions of importance to evaluation of disability, pensioning, and rehabilitation: (1) What is the prevalence of incapacity among fishermen, and which diseases are responsible? (2) To what extent do impairing diseases reduce the physical working capacity of fishermen? (3) What is the energy requirement of different types of fishing?

The investigation has been carried out on the islands of Vaerøy and Røst, just north of the Arctic Circle and approximately 60 miles from the Norwegian mainland. Some 1,800 people live in this area, and fishing is the major industry. In 1972 the population included 297 fishermen between 17 and 70 years of age. The fishermen were submitted to a clinical screening examination and a socio-medical evaluation of incapacity with the related medical background.

PREVALENCE OF INCAPACITY

A total of 60 fishermen suffered from disease that reduced their earning capacity by 50 per cent or more (Table 1). The prevalence of disability (20 per cent) was remarkably high compared with the figure for Norway as a whole (6 per cent). Diseases of the cardiovascular system were responsible for almost a half of the disabilities; 21 of the 28 patients in this group suffered from coronary heart disease. This is in keeping with the remarkably high prevalence of coronary heart disease in the area as a whole (1). One-third of the diagnosed disabilities were due to mental disorders.

TABLE 2
Maximal oxygen intake of Norwegian fishermen

Diagnostic group	No. of persons	Age $\bar{x}$ yr	Max. O_2 intake, 1/min ($\bar{x}$)	Max. O_2 intake, ml/kg $\bar{x}$ min ($\bar{x}$)
Mental disorders	49	47.7	2.6	34.1
Cardiovascular diseases	12	62.4	1.8	26.0
Digestive system	12	47.2	2.6	34.5
Locomotor system	9	51.7	2.9	37.4
Injuries, sequelae	5	49.4	2.8	36.7
Miscellaneous	16	53.3	2.5	33.2
Total	103(82)	50.7	2.5	33.2
Persons without chronic disease	159	38.9	3.0	41.0

PHYSICAL WORKING CAPACITY

During June of 1972, the maximum oxygen intake was estimated
for 241 Vaerøy men between 17 and 70 years of age (Table 2).
In 44 cases direct measurements were made, while in the remaining cases indirect methods of estimation were used.
Eighty-two of these men suffered from 103 chronic diseases
in all. Maximal oxygen intake was reduced among patients
with cardiovascular diseases, about a half of the disabled
fishermen. Patients with mental disorders did not have a
markedly reduced physical working capacity. The same tendency is evident if we analyse maximal oxygen intake for the
disabled persons. Thirty-nine of the 241 men were 50-100 per
cent incapacitated. Table 3 shows the maximal oxygen intake
for different groups of disabling diseases (16 were direct
measurements and 23 indirect estimations).

ENERGY REQUIREMENTS OF FISHING

To evaluate the degree of disability and the possibility of
rehabilitation, it is necessary to know also the energy
requirements of fishing. Three physiological field studies
were carried out on 24 fishermen in 1971 and 1972 to determine the energy requirements of different types of fishing.
These investigations were under the direction of Rodahl
during the Lofoten fishing season (January-April) and included four common types of Norwegian coastal fishing:
hand-line, long-line, net, and Danish seine (3, 4).

TABLE 3
Maximal oxygen intake in fishermen with incapacitating disease

Diagnostic group	No. of persons	Age x̄ yr	Max. O_2 intake, l/min (x̄)	Max. O_2 intake, ml/kg x min (x̄)
Mental disorders	24	48.5	2.4	33.0
Cardiovascular diseases	8	61.3	1.7	23.5
Metabolic diseases	2	60.5	1.5	18.9
Nervous system	2	56.5	2.2	28.2
Injuries, sequelae	2	44.0	3.4	41.1
Cancer	1	54.0	1.6	26.7
Total	39	52.0	2.2	30.4
Persons without incapacitating disease	202	40.6	3.0	40.0

The mean work load of the coastal fisherman is rather high, corresponding to an oxygen uptake of 0.9 to 1.0 litre per minute (Table 4), equivalent to uphill walking with a 5 per cent incline and a speed of 3.5 to 4.0 km/hr (2). In spite of the varying incidence and duration of the different activities, the average work load over the entire working day is remarkably similar for all four types of coastal fishing, the oxygen consumption of 1.0 ℓ/min corresponding to 34-39 per cent of the maximal aerobic power of the subjects. Considering the long working day, this implies that the older fishermen especially are working at close to the permissible physiological limit. In our screening material, 23 persons between the ages of 60 and 70 years did not have any incapacitating disease. The average maximal oxygen intake of this group of healthy old men was 2.3 ℓ/min (30.7 mℓ/kg min). Working as they are with an average energy output close to the upper tolerable limit, it is not

TABLE 4
Energy requirements of different types of fishing

	No. of subjects	Estimated oxygen intake (l/min STPD) Mean	Range	Per cent of maximal aerobic power Mean	Range
Hand-line	7	0.9	0.5-1.6	37	20-60
Long-line	8	0.9	0.5-1.4	34	25-45
Net	6	1.0	0.8-1.2	35	25-50
Danish seine	3	1.1	1.0-1.4	39	35-45

difficult to understand why their working capacity is easily
disturbed by disease.

SOCIO-MEDICAL SERVICE FOR THE FISHERMEN

The major group of incapacitated fishermen are suffering
from cardiovascular diseases, and their markedly reduced
physical working capacity suggests that rehabilitation within the fishing industry is in most cases unrealistic. If rehabilitation programs are to be tried, hand-line fishing is
probably the most suitable type of operation for those with
medical or physical handicaps, since on the whole it imposes
the lightest work load on the fishermen. Another decisive
factor is that the hand-line fisherman can operate on his
own, whereas in other types of fishing each man must keep up
with the rest of the team. Furthermore, the hand-line fisherman has greater freedom to choose to stay ashore if the
weather is rough.

In patients incapacitated by mental disorders, the
physiological status seems such as to permit rehabilitation.
At least we can state that the physical working capacity per
se does not constitute a decisive hindrance to rehabilitation of these patients.

Our findings would seem to justify the offering of a
lower pensionable age to fishermen relative to other occupations. Considering the high energy requirements of coastal
fishing, it is reasonable that the age of pensioning for
Norwegian fishermen today is 65 years compared with 67 years
for the population in general.

SUMMARY

In some coastal communities of northern Norway, fishing is
the only possible occupation. This confronts the doctor with
special socio-medical problems when a fisherman becomes incapacitated. The present investigation considers three main
aspects of the problem: (1) the prevalence of incapacity
among the fishermen on two islands of northern Norway, (2)
the extent to which different diseases reduce physical
working capacity, and (3) the energy requirements in different types of fishing. Sixty fishermen suffered from incapacitating disease, a high prevalence of 20 per cent. Heart
diseases were responsible for almost one-half of the disability and one-third was due to mental disorders. Patients
suffering from heart disease had a markedly reduced physical
working capacity. Their maximal oxygen intake was on average

1.8 l/min compared with 3.0 l/min for healthy persons. The mean work load in coastal fishing was rather high, corresponding to an oxygen uptake of 0.9-1 l/min or 34-39 per cent of maximal aerobic power. The socio-medical implications of these results are discussed.

REFERENCES

1. Fugelli, P., "Prevalence of coronary heart disease in different parts of Norway," Nordic Council for Arctic Medical Research Report, 7: 10-13 (1974)
2. Givoni, B. and Goldman, R.F., "Predicting metabolic energy cost," J. appl. Physiol., 30: 429-33 (1971)
3. Rodahl, K. et al., "Circulatory strain, estimated energy output and catecholamine excretion in Norwegian coastal fishermen," Ergonomics (in press)
4. Åstrand, I. et al., "Energy output and work stress in coastal fishing," Scand. J. clin. lab. Invest., 31: 105-13 (1973)

Energy balance of an Eskimo community

R.J. SHEPHARD and G. GODIN

The balance between the energy demands of human existence and the energy resources available to a community can be critical for survival, particularly in the harsh environment of the Arctic. The question now assumes a new importance, as sociologists debate the possibility of conserving the traditional Eskimo life-style in the face of the enlarged settlements required for education and primary health care.

Problems of Methodology

A complete energy balance study on a community of 500 people is a formidable undertaking, and our investigation of the Igloolik settlement (1,3) did little more than explore the type of approach that would be appropriate given much larger resources of personnel and equipment.

With regard to energy expenditure measurements, thousands of different tasks are performed each day. In many cases, the caloric cost of such activities is well known for temperate "white" communities. Can one reasonably assume the same figures will apply to arctic residents - particularly Eskimos? Often, this is a dangerous assumption. Although a task may be superficially familiar, the Eskimo may have less or different equipment than his "white" counterpart. Because of a shortage of furniture, for example, many household tasks are performed from a squatting or a kneeling position. In some instances, there are differences of body size (2); the cost of most activities in the "white" population is adjusted to conform to Food and Agriculture Organization standards (65 kg in men, and 55 kg in women). While such weights are not unrealistic for the current generation of Eskimos, differences in the relative length of the trunk and the limbs may alter the efficiency of many types of activity (see, for example, the mechanical efficiency of cycling, page 78). Undetected visual problems may increase clumsiness. Finally, there is uncertainty regarding the level of basal metabolism (BMR). Previous authors found 13-33 per cent augmentation of BMR and attributed this to a combination of cold adaptation, a high protein diet, and anxiety during testing (1). Our own measurements of oxygen consumption during such activities as sitting and standing did not differ from those anticipated in the "white" community. We would thus conclude that if the Eskimos once had a high BMR, this has been lost with lesser cold exposure, reduction in the protein content of the diet, and greater familiarity with the "white" man and his insatiable desire for scientific data. Nevertheless, our calculations of energy balance have been based on two limiting assumptions: (a) no increase of BMR and (b) a 30 per cent increase of BMR.

Data Collection
The oxygen cost of tasks peculiar to the Eskimo community has been measured by a Kofranyi-Michaelis respirometer (4), and other data on energy expenditures have been derived from pulse rate and ventilation measurements, film, and diary records (5). Unfortunately, many of the most characteristic Eskimo activities were performed at distances of 50-150 miles from the village. In order to collect quite small amounts of data, it was thus necessary to make long and arduous journeys by dog or skidoo-hauled sled.

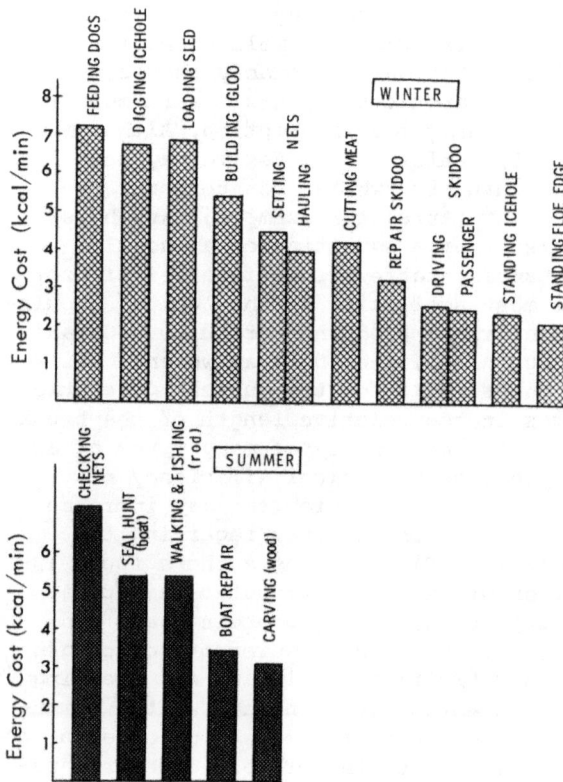

Figure 1 The energy cost of selected summer and winter activities of hunters at Igloolik (3)

Hunting Activities

The energy cost of some hunting activities is illustrated in Figure 1. In the winter, control of a team of 12 or more fierce and hungry dogs can involve an expenditure of over 7 kcal/min. Apparently leisurely fishing must be preceded by digging an ice-hole at a cost of 6-7 kcal/min. The evening rest must be prefaced by building an igloo at 5-6 kcal/min. In the summer, likewise, expenditures of 6-7 kcal/min may be developed, particularly in fishing, when canoes are paddled around the nets against a strong wind.

Settlement Activities

Within the village, the settlement workers generally have lighter tasks, although again there can be quite heavy

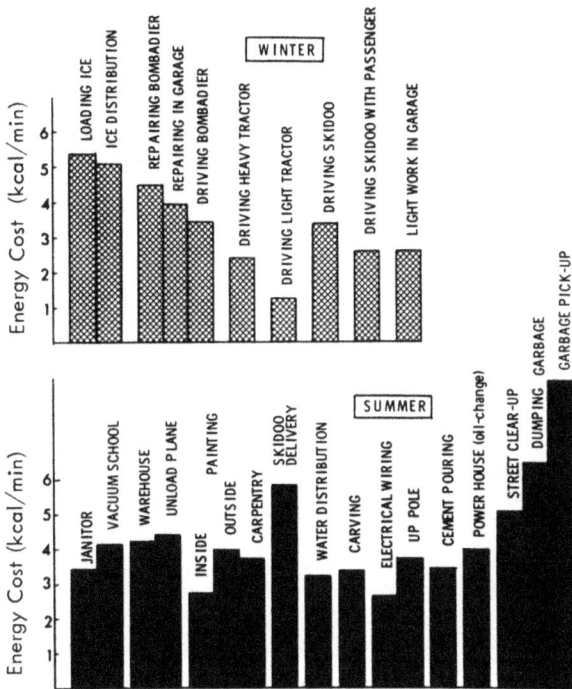

Figure 2   The energy cost of selected summer and winter activities of settlement workers at Igloolik (3)

work (Figure 2). During winter, there is distribution of household water in the form of ice-blocks, and in the summer, the clearance of nine months accumulation of garbage.

The women also work harder than city-dwelling housewives. There are few electrical appliances even within the settlement, and for six or eight weeks of the year all the tasks of child-rearing must be performed by using improvised equipment in a summer tent-camp at the edge of the ice floes. The scraping and preparing of skins and the sewing of winter clothing also fall to the women, and most tasks are performed while carrying a sturdy 20 or 30 pound infant on the back.

Energy Expenditures of Hunters
Some energy balance studies have spoken cheerfully of studying a typical week-end day and a typical working day. However, in Igloolik, life is governed not by the Roman

TABLE 1
Over-all annual energy expenditure (1, 3) of Igloolik villagers (the
first column of the caloric expenditures assumes a normal basal metabolism, the second a 30% increase)

	N	Days	Daily kcal	Yearly kcal x 10^{-6}
Men				
Hunters	29	161	3,670→4,110	17.1→19.2
		204	2,500→3,000	14.8→17.7
Labourers	25	204	3,350→3,800	17.1→19.4
		161	2,500→3,000	10.1→12.1
Sedentary	86	365	2,500→2,900	78.5→91.0
Elderly	7	365	2,300→2,700	5.9→6.9
Children				
0- 5	51	365	635→750	11.8→14.0
5-10	47	365	1,390→1,600	23.8→27.4
10-15	34	365	2,300→2,700	28.5→33.5
Women				
Married	81	365	2,400→2,700	71.0→79.8
Single	37	365	2,300→2,600	31.1→35.1
Elderly	3	365	1,990→2,300	2.2→2.5
Children				
0- 5	62	365	635→750	14.4→17.0
5-10	45	365	1,390→1,600	22.8→26.3
10-15	27	365	1,840→2,200	18.1→21.7

calendar but by the winds and the seasons. At certain times
of the year, sled journeys to the traps on Baffin Island
are impossible. At other periods, use of the whaleboat or a
canoe is appropriate. Game and the associated activities
show a regular annual rhythm. Thus, the annual energy expenditure can only be ascertained by a team which is prepared to live in the community for a year or more.

Combining information from our oxygen consumption
measurements, film, and diary records, we have estimated
the daily cost of twelve different types of hunting
(1, 3). There is a considerable range, from leisurely
watching for seals at the floe edge (2,530 kcal) to the
vigour of carrying a caribou on the back (3,900 kcal),
digging iceholes (4,040 kcal) and paddling a small canoe
(4,440 kcal), but the average for the 12 types of hunt
(3,670 kcal) is substantial, particularly when related to
the small size of the Eskimo.

Energy Expenditure of the Settlement
The food yield of hunting has been estimated (Table 2) from
game records, average carcass weights, and reported analyses
of carcasses (1,3). Details could perhaps be disputed, but

TABLE 2
Annual caloric yield of hunting as estimated from game records for the
Igloolik settlement (1, 3)

	N	Weight (kg)	Total (kg x 10^{-3})	Edible (%)	kcal x 10^{-6}
Bear	16	700	11.2	40	5
Seal					
Ringed	3,648	50	182.4	25	58
Bearded	55	250	13.8	27	5
Walrus	150	700	105.0	26	32
Caribou	800	70	56.0	40	22
Fish	5,000	5	25.0	50	22
Total					144

the over-all food provided from natural resources (144 X
10^6 kcal/year) plainly accounted for only about 30 per cent
of the energy expenditure of the settlement. The deficit
was made good by store purchases - flour, sugar, canned
milk, and soft drinks, with disastrous effects upon the
dental health of the community (page 414). Nevertheless,
haemoglobin readings suggest the present balance between
traditional and western food assures a reasonable protein
intake (see further, pages 78, 106).

The future stability of the community is more problema-
tical. Until recently, the population was kept in check by
sustained breast feeding and a very high infant mortality
(220/1,000 for the period 1960-69). With provision of primary health care, this problem is being progressively
corrected, and even when plotted on a logarithmic scale,
the population now shows an alarming rate of increase.

Such pressures are exacerbated by diminishing game resources, the high cost of gasoline, and concentration of
villagers in regions remote from traditional hunting areas.
In short, we have the sad picture of a community that is
rapidly getting out of balance, with all that this implies
for health, nutrition, self-respect, and human fulfilment.
It is perhaps not surprising that some of the Igloolik
villagers are choosing to reject the "advantages" of civilization, and are returning to smaller settlements in more remote areas where their traditional life-style can be con-
served.

SUMMARY

The social anthropology, activity patterns, and energy balance of "primitive" communities are discussed in reference to data obtained at Igloolik, a settlement of 534 Eskimos in the Canadian arctic (69°, 40' N). Twenty-nine of 147 men were active hunters; estimated energy expenditures varied with the type of hunt, with a probable average cost of 3,670 kcal for each of three days per week. Some 25 men were employed by governmental and commercial agencies for an average of four days per week at a cost of 3,150 kcal per day. The remaining 93 men described themselves as hunters, but were largely sedentary. The Eskimo housewives had less electrical and mechanical equipment than city-dwellers, and frequently carried children on their backs; their daily energy expenditures averaged 2,500 kcal. The nutritional status of the community was good, with 31 per cent of the dietary needs met from the hunt. The energy balance of the village was nevertheless precarious, particularly in view of the logarithmic expansion of population within the settlement.

REFERENCES

1. Godin, G., and Shephard, R.J., "Activity patterns in the Canadian Eskimo," in O. Edholm and E.K. Gunderson (eds.) Polar Human Biology (Cambridge, U.K.: Heinemann, 1973)
2. Godin, G., and Shephard, R.J., "Body weight and the energy cost of activity," Am. Med. Assoc. Arch. env. Health, 27: 289-93 (1973)
3. Godin, G., "A study of the energy expenditure of a small Eskimo population," M.Sc. thesis, University of Toronto, Toronto, Ontario
4. Kofranyi, E., and Michaelis, H.F., "Ein tragbarer Apparat zur Bestimmung des Gasstoffwechsels," Arbeitsphysiol., 11: 148-50 (1949)
5. Weiner, J.S., and Lourie, J.A., Human Biology: A Guide to Field Methods (Oxford, U.K.: Blackwell, 1969)

Changes in body composition during an arctic winter exercise

C. ALLEN, W. O'HARA, and R.J. SHEPHARD

Canadian Forces regularly conduct training exercises in the Canadian Arctic and sub-Arctic. These manoeuvres usually consist of self-contained cross-country movements from an air strip, lasting up to two weeks.

In order to accustom personnel to living and working under adverse conditions where mechanized support may not be available, the cross-country movements are carried out on foot, with all necessary life support equipment being carried or towed on toboggans. The smallest functional group consists of 9 or 10 men, with one toboggan carrying a tent, food and fuel for 3 days. When fully loaded, this toboggan weights 160-180 kg and is moved by a three man team, two in front and one behind. In addition, each man carries a weapon and a rucksack containing his own personal equipment, the total load being some 30 kg.

The present data were gathered from observations on 55 participants in an exercise based on Churchill, Manitoba (week one), and Frobisher Bay, NWT (week two). The cross-country patrols covered 25 km over 12 hours at Churchill and 44 km over 16 hours at Frobisher Bay. Snowshoes were either worn or carried, depending on the terrain. Temperatures ranged from -39°C to -14°C with a mean of -29°C. Mean maximum daily windchill was 2,032 $kcal/m^2$ hr.

The purposes of the investigations were to assess the adequacy of the normal pre-packaged field ration for this type of operation and to monitor any changes in body composition. The field ration is available in seven different menus, averaging 3,600 kcal and providing 16 per cent protein, 32 per cent fat, and 52 per cent carbohydrate.

METHODS AND MATERIALS

Subjects

The subjects were 55 healthy infantrymen (6 tent groups), ranging in age from 19 to 37 years (mean 23 years). Three tent groups (27 men) were used for the energy expenditure studies.

Energy Expenditure

The energy expenditure measurements were taken with a Kofranyi-Michaelis respirometer. This was fitted with an insulated case and a modified harness enabling it to be attached to a military back pack. Timed volumes were recorded and aliquot samples were transferred to glass syringes for later laboratory analysis of oxygen and carbon dioxide concentration. All representative tasks, either on the trail or in camp, were sampled with repeat determinations made as often as possible. The data were extrapolated to cover the 24-hour day by reference to diaries maintained by the subjects and "on the spot" observations by the investigators.

Body Composition

Body composition was assessed by monitoring weight and skinfold thickness changes on four occasions; before the exercise, between weeks I and II, immediately after the exercise, and one week post-exercise. The same calibrated scale was used throughout. Skinfold thicknesses were measured by the same observer using the same Lange skinfold calipers. Two separate measurements were made at each of three sites on the dominant side; triceps, subscapular, and suprailiac.

A standard urinalysis reagent strip was used to indicate the presence and concentration of protein and ketones. These tests were done with one tent group only, as frequently as conditions permitted.

RESULTS AND DISCUSSION

Energy Expenditure

Pulling the toboggan was the most demanding task, and the servicemen generally agreed that the man in the second position did more than a third of the work. Our data support this observation (Figure 1).

During the period of the cross-country patrols, the daily energy expenditure was 3,484 kcal. Making allowances for excreta of 150 kcal/day and food wastage of 200 kcal/day there is a negative caloric balance of approximately 250 kcal/day.

Body Composition

The initial mean body weight was 74.8 kg. During the exercise, there was a decrease of 1 kg, with a return to

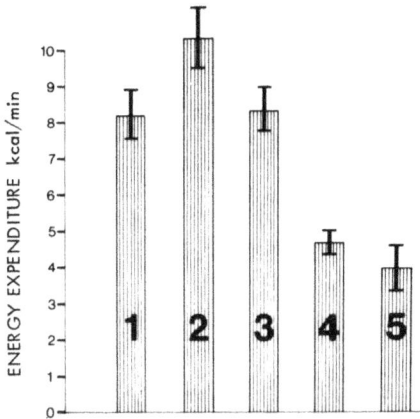

Figure 1   Comparative energy expenditures for patrol activities and tent routines, mean and standard deviation (1,
toboggan pulling, lead position; 2, toboggan pulling,
second position; 3, toboggan pulling, third position,
steering; 4, trail walking, with snowshoes and pack; 5,
tent routine)

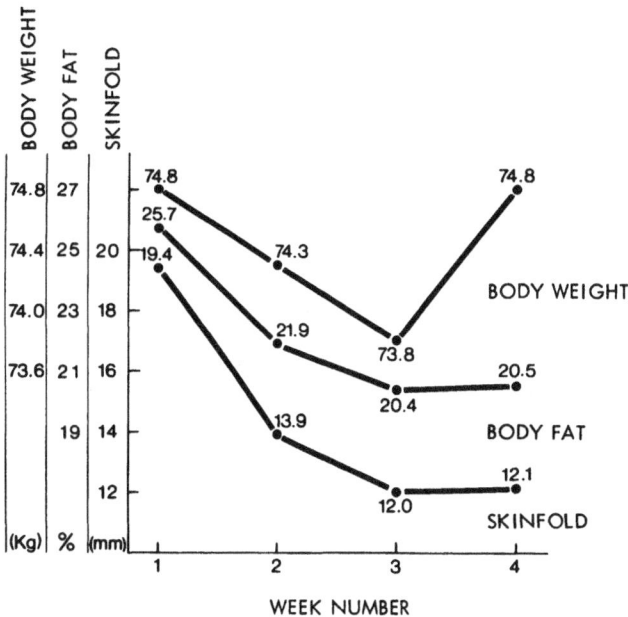

WEEK NUMBER

Figure 2   Changes in body weight, percentage body fat, and
skinfold thickness during the four-week field trial (mean
values for 52 men)

the original value within one week after the exercise
(Figure 2). Skinfold thicknesses showed a greater change,
decreasing from 19.4 mm (average of three sites) to 12.0 mm,
a decrease of 38 per cent. The decreases were not uniform,
ranging from 28 per cent for the subscapular region to 32
per cent for the triceps and 52 per cent for the suprailiac
(Figure 3). During the fourth week, i.e., post-exercise, the
skinfold thicknesses remained essentially unchanged.

The skinfold measurements were converted into density
and percentage body fat using formulae from Durnin (personal
communication) and Brozek (1) respectively. The percentage
body fat decreased from an initial figure of 25.7 to 20.4
by the end of the exercise (Figure 2). These values are
equivalent to 19.2 and 15.0 kg of fat respectively, and imply a loss of 4.2 kg during the exercise. In the same
period, the body weight decreased 1.0 kg. Thus, if the fat
prediction formulae are appropriate, there must have been a
3.2 kg increment in other fluids and tissues, particularly
muscle protein.

While the physical activity experienced during this
exercise was not particularly severe, it was heavier than
many forms of military and industrial work, and was
apparently sufficient to produce a training effect. The
predicted aerobic power, also monitored during this period,
increased by 10 per cent. Since there was no measurable dehydration (average daily fluid intake was 2 litres) and
there was a positive training effect, it seems most likely
that the 3.2 kg discrepancy between fat loss and body weight
loss can be accounted for by a concomitant increase of
muscle tissue.

Urinalysis
Urinalysis showed a high incidence of proteinuria and ketonuria (Figure 4). Not unexpectedly, proteinuria was most
common during the more strenuous parts of the exercise,
with "moderate" concentrations occurring only at the end
of the working day. Ketonuria occurred with equal frequency in both phases of the exercise.

SUMMARY

The effects of long-range arctic winter patrols on body
composition were examined in 55 infantrymen during a two-
week winter arctic exercise. Each man carried 30 kg of
clothing and equipment, and for a third of the patrol time
assisted in pulling a 180 kg cargo toboggan. The men

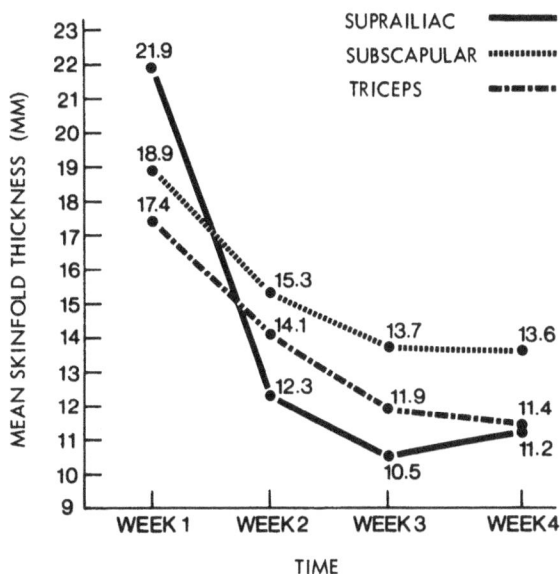

Figure 3 Changes in individual skinfold thicknesses over the four-week field study (mean values for 52 men)

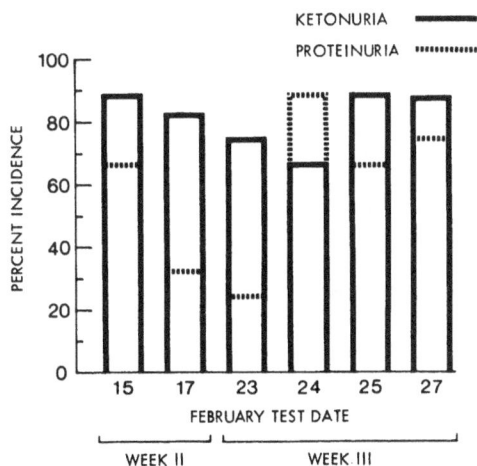

Figure 4 Percentage incidence of proteinuria (results include trace values) and ketonuria in nine subjects

covered 69,000 metres in 2 weeks. Rations issued were
approximately 3,600 kcal/day. Energy expenditures were
monitored by observation, diary, and Kofranyi-Michaelis
meter, the average being 3,484 kcal/day. There was a small
negative caloric balance (250 kcal/day). The mean decrease
in body weight was 1.0 kg. Skinfold thickness decreased by
38 per cent, equivalent to a 5.4 per cent loss of body fat
(4.2 kg), so that a 3.2 kg increment of muscle protein was
likely. Urinalysis showed an unusually high incidence of
proteinuria and ketonuria.

REFERENCE

1. Brozek, J., Grande, F., Anderson, J.T., and Keys, A.,
   "Densitometric analysis of body composition: revision
   of some quantitative assumptions," Ann. N.Y. Acad. Sci.,
   110: 113-40 (1963)

Commentaries

"Comparison of values for maximal oxygen intake obtained in
cross-sectional and longitudinal studies," by Lars Hermansen and Kåre Rodahl (Institute of Work Physiology, Oslo,
Norway). Maximal oxygen intake is perhaps the most widely
accepted parameter for estimation of the individual's
physical performance capacity. Most population studies describing the variation in maximal oxygen intake with
age have been performed as cross-sectional studies. The aim
of the present investigation was to compare the results obtained in cross-sectional and longitudinal studies of the
same population. Altogether 308 subjects aged 10 to 16
years participated. Of these, 28 female and 30 male subjects were studied twice a year during the period from
April 1968 to April 1970. The mean values for maximal
oxygen intake were higher than in other studies reported
in the literature. The mean values for maximal oxygen intake in the longitudinal study were approximately the same
as those obtained in the cross-sectional study.

"Metabolic energy cost and terrain coefficients of walking on snow," by R.F. Goldman, M.F. Haisman, and K.B. Pandolf (US Army Research Institute of Environmental Medicine, Natick, Mass., USA). Terrain coefficients for light and heavy brush, swamp, and sandy level terrains were derived in a previous study (Soule and Goldman, 1972) as empiric coefficients to fit the measured data to a basic treadmill energy cost prediction equation (Givoni and Goldman, 1971). The present study aimed to produce a terrain coefficient for snow of various depths. Ten subjects each walked at two speeds, 0.66 and 1.11 m/s (1.5 and 2.5 mph), on a level treadmill and on a variety of snow depths. Expired air was sampled, using a Max Planck gasometer, during minutes 4-9 and 10-15 of the 15 minute walks. Snow profiles (i.e., snow depth, footprint depression, density, temperature, and hardness) were constructed for the various walks. The ratio of the energy cost of walking at the same speed on the treadmill increased linearly with increasing depth of footprint. At a 17.0 cm depth of footprint, the energy cost roughly triples. Thus, at this snow depression, energy expenditure at 1.11 m/s with about 9 kg of clothing and respirometer weight had reached the rather high levels of about 900 kcal/hr. This is certainly well above the value of 425 kcal/hr ± 10% described as self-paced "hard work" for various terrains and loads (Hughes and Goldman, 1970). Clearly, greater snow depressions (>17.0 cm) should slow walking speed to below 1.1 m/s. The energy cost of walking on snow may also depend on the specific characteristics of the snow. Snowfalls with markedly different physical characteristics were encountered at approximately 16 cm snow depression, the hardness of one being about three times that of the other. At a speed of 1.11 m/s the energy cost of the harder and crusted snow was about 70 kcal/hr greater than that of the fluffier snow, despite similar footprint depths. The least fit (and also heaviest subject) could only complete 8 minutes of the walk at that speed at the greater hardness. Markedly different gaits were observed for these two conditions, with higher leg lift and more static work required at greater hardness. The energy cost of walking on snow in this study agrees fairly well with that reported by Ramaswamy et al. (1966) for Indian soldiers, but lies above the data of Heinonen et al. (1959) at a snow depression of 15 cm.

NUTRITION AND METABOLISM

A review of recent nutritional research in the arctic

H.H. DRAPER

Nutritional research in the Arctic in recent years has been
stimulated by several factors. Rapid erosion of aboriginal
cultures has prompted efforts to obtain baseline data on
the nutritional status of population isolates still under
the influence of traditional diet. In addition, there has
been an increased realization that significant malnutrition
exists among the populations of generally affluent societies, and that within such societies malnutrition is most
prevalent among minorities subjected to rapid cultural
change. Such is the situation of most of the native peoples
of the arctic region. There has been a further realization
that an understanding of the impact of modernization on the
health of these peoples may be of value in dealing with the
nutritional problems of industrialized societies. Arctic
research also has been stimulated by funds appropriated by
national governments for the International Biological Program.

This review will deal briefly with several major subjects of recent nutritional research in the arctic region.

DIETARY AND BIOCHEMICAL STUDIES

Recent dietary surveys have been conducted on a number of
circumpolar populations. In general, they attest to the
pervasive inroads of commercial items into the native food
chain. Studies in 1967-72 among the Ainu, once a highly
carnivorous people, revealed no food habits that differed
substantially from those of Japanese inhabitants of the
same geographical region (Koishi, Okuda, Matsudaira,
Takemura, and Takaya, personal communication). The Ainu
diet consisted largely of rice and raw or cooked vegetables. It provided somewhat less protein and fat, and
hence more carbohydrate, than the Japanese diet, a fact

attributed to a lower economic status rather than to a
racial or cultural preference. The Ainu were leaner than
their Japanese compatriots as judged by skinfold thickness
measurements and Rohrer's index.

Dietary records taken in the northern Alaskan Eskimo
village of Wainwright in 1971 and 1972 (Bell, Raines,
Bergan, Draper, and Heller, unpublished data) showed that
about 44 per cent of the calories consumed by adults were
derived from indigenous foods (mainly land and sea mammals).
At Point Hope, where acculturation is more extensive, the
corresponding figure was 22 per cent. The values for children (24 per cent and 8 per cent, respectively) reflect a
greater preference for processed foods among the young
generation. Protein provided 35 per cent of the calories in
the adult diet at Wainwright, fat 43 per cent, and carbohydrate 32 per cent. In the diet of children, the analogous
values were 18, 39, and 43 per cent. These values reflect a
trend towards the indices for the current U.S. mixed diet
(12, 41, and 47 per cent).

Biochemical assessment indicated that the Alaskan Eskimo
food supply was generally adequate in essential nutrients.
Blood and urine levels of thiamine, riboflavin, vitamin A,
and vitamin C were (with a few exceptions) within the normal range. Vitamin E concentrations in blood plasma were at
least equivalent to those of the general U.S. population
(Wo, Wei, and Draper, unpublished data). Anaemia was the
main sign of undernutrition. Obesity was a significant
finding, especially among adult females, and dental caries
was rampant. In the southwestern villages of Kasigluk and
Nunapitchuk, commercial foods clearly predominated and nutritional status resembled that of an industrialized urban
population of low social status.

Studies on Canadian Eskimos residing in four northern
settlements, carried out as part of a national nutrition
survey, provided evidence of multiple nutritional defi-
ciences (8). Clinical signs of scurvy, anaemia, low serum
folate levels, and low vitamin A intakes were major findings. Obesity was reportedly prevalent. The nutritional
status of Eskimos living in this region was found to be inferior to that of Indians, which in turn was inferior to
that of the general Canadian population.

A survey of Canadian Eskimos living in the Northern Foxe
Basin of the Northwest Territories, carried out under the
auspices of the International Biological Program, yielded
significantly different results (18). The nutritional status of Eskimos in this region was found to be adequate with

respect to most nutrients except folic acid. A high prevalence of substandard serum folate levels found in these and
other populations surveyed recently, usually in the absence
of haematological symptoms, indicates a need to re-evaluate
the biochemical criteria of folate deficiency.

Obesity is a relatively recent finding in Eskimos. Its
assessment by such variables as the ponderal index is complicated by the unusual stature of traditional Eskimos
(short legs, long trunk, plump appearance) which can give a
false impression of obesity. Auger (personal communication)
found little change with adult age in body weight or skinfold thickness among Eskimos at Fort Chimo in Quebec, whereas progressive changes were seen among Métis of the same
region. Nevertheless, true obesity is evident among the
residents of urban centres in southern Alaska, and there is
little reason to believe that Eskimos are not susceptible to
this condition.

Bang and co-workers (3) have investigated the relation of
diet and blood lipid profiles in the Eskimos of northwest
Greenland. According to estimates made in 1974, 26 per cent
of their dietary calories were derived from protein (over
twice the value for the Danish population), 37 per cent from
fat, and 37 per cent from carbohydrate. Values of 44, 47,
and 8 per cent, respectively, were reported for the same
region in 1914. Seal and whale meat constituted the main
sources of protein and fat; bread and sugar were the main
sources of carbohydrate. The distribution of calories in
the diet of this population is similar to that of northern
Alaskan Eskimos (Bell et al., unpublished data).

Hasunen and Pekkarinen (personal communication) conducted a dietary survey among Finnish and Norwegian Lapps in
1970. Among Skolt Lapps of the Sevettijärvi community of
northeastern Finland, protein contributed about 16 per cent
of total calories and fat 29-36 per cent. The predominant
occupation of these Lapps is reindeer herding, and some unusually high intakes of vitamin A from reindeer liver were
recorded. Twenty-five per cent of the men consumed 12,000-
53,000 IU of vitamin A per day in winter, an intake which
extends into the toxic range. In contrast, intakes of calcium and B vitamins tended to be low. In Norwegian Lapps,
protein contributed about 15 per cent of dietary calories
and fat approximately 40 per cent. Vitamin C, thiamine,
and riboflavin were regarded as the primary nutritional
inadequacies. Extraordinary intakes of vitamin A (over
62,000 IU per day) were recorded also for some Norwegian
Lapps.

The diet of the aboriginal population of the Chukchi National Okrug of the USSR was evaluated by Astrinskii and Navasardov (1) and by Zaitsev (20) during the period 1959-63. Reindeer meat was the staple food of the tundra Chukchi, whereas sea mammal meat was the staple of the coastal Chukchi (20). Fat constituted 56-58 per cent of the dietary calories and carbohydrate provided 28 per cent. The average daily consumption of reindeer meat in the tundra settlement of Kanchalan was 700 grams and the average protein intake was 141 grams. Plasma vitamin C levels (0.2-0.4 mg %) were considered low, although they meet most current Western standards. The Chukchi share with other circumpolar peoples a fondness for confectionery. Hepatomegaly, a condition previously reported in other arctic populations, was observed in 113 out of 278 adult subjects (20). This enlargement may be a response to the heavy metabolic demands imposed on the liver by the high protein diet for gluconeogenesis and urea synthesis. Census statistics indicate that in 1926-27 meat, fat, and fish constituted 93-97 per cent of the diet   (1). By the time of the 1959-61 survey, meat and fat consumption had declined over 50 per cent and bread constituted 41 per cent of the diet.

BLOOD LIPIDS

The influence of diet on the composition of blood lipids has been investigated recently in several arctic populations. These studies have had the general objective of evaluating the role of nutrition in the low incidence of hyperocholesterolaemia, cardiovascular disease, and diabetes which have been characteristic of these populations.

Bang and co-workers (3) found that, in addition to having lower plasma cholesterol levels than Danes, Eskimos of northwest Greenland had much lower levels of pre-β-lipoproteins and triglycerides. The average triglyceride concentrations (g/ℓ) were 0.44 in Greenland Eskimos and 1.08 in Danes. As evidence of the influence of environment rather than genetics on these variables, the triglyceride level in Eskimos living in Denmark was 0.99 g/ℓ (3). Cholesterol intake (Bang, Dyerberg, Hjøme, personal communication) was higher in Eskimos than in Danes (245 vs 139 mg per 1,000 kcal). Bang et al. suggested that the low plasma cholesterol levels seen in Greenland Eskimos may be attributable to the high proportion of polyunsaturated fatty acids in their traditional diet of fish and sea mammals. Low plasma triglyceride levels may be a factor in their extremely low incidence of diabetes mellitus.

Analysis of the esterified fatty acids of blood lipids of Greenland Eskimos disclosed a higher proportion of palmitic, palmitoleic, and timnodonic acids and a lower concentration of linoleic acid than in Danes (Dyerberg, Bang, and Hjørne, personal communication). The concentration of total polyunsaturated acids was somewhat higher in Danes. Timnodonic acid (eicosapentaenoic acid), which is found in only negligible amounts in Western populations, constituted up to 16 per cent of the esterified fatty acids of Eskimos. Whether these differences are significant factors in the lower incidence of hypercholesterolaemia and cardiovascular disease in Eskimos is unclear. However, they raise the possibility that two highly unsaturated fatty acids present in the native diet, timnodonic acid and eicosahexaenoic acid, may have some unusual influence on cholesterol metabolism.

Bjorksten, Aromaa, Eriksson, Maatela, Kirjarinta, Fellman, and Tamminen (personal communication) determined the serum cholesterol and triglyceride levels of 11,626 Finns and 828 Lapps during the period 1969-71. No marked differences such as those found between Danes and Greenland Eskimos (3) distinguished Finns and Lapps. Lipid levels in Lapps resembled those in rural Finns, Greenland Eskimos living in Denmark (3), and most other Nordic populations. Age-adjusted mean serum cholesterol concentration in adult Finns was about 260 mg/100 ml, one of the highest values recorded for any population in the world.

Feldman and associates (7) carried out a study of cholesterol metabolism in Point Hope, Alaska, Eskimos. The mean serum cholesterol concentration recorded for a sample of children and adults was 221 mg/100 ml. Relative to U.S. normal values, serum triglycerides were low (69 mg/100 ml), free fatty acids were high (34 mg/100 ml), and pre-β-lipoproteins were low (<35 mg/100 ml). Cholesterol intakes ranged from 420 to 1,650 mg per day. High school students consuming a standard mixed diet providing 177-520 mg cholesterol daily had low serum cholesterol levels (137 mg/100 ml), with serum triglyceride levels near the U.S. norm. A study utilizing ^{14}C-cholesterol indicated that both cholesterol absorption and cholesterol synthesis proceeded with constant efficiency over a wide range of cholesterol intakes (420-1650 mg per day). Absorption efficiency was calculated to be unusually high (about 50 per cent) and the amount of cholesterol absorbed had no effect on the amount of cholesterol synthesized (841 mg per day). These investigators concluded that Eskimos have a much larger capacity

for cholesterol absorption than U.S. whites, and that an
increase in the amount of cholesterol absorbed results in a
proportional elevation of serum cholesterol concentration.
A maximal suppression of endogenous cholesterol synthesis
(36 per cent) was effected by 420 mg or more of dietary
cholesterol per day. The ability of the Eskimo to maintain
normocholesterolaemia was attributed to a modest cholesterol
content in his indigenous diet.

Eskimos residing in northern and southwestern Alaska exhibited a gradient in plasma cholesterol concentrations and
blood pressures which was associated with increasing degrees
of nutritional and social acculturation (Bell et al., unpublished data). The incidence of hypercholesterolaemia in
adults ($\geq$ 260 mg/100 ml) was 11-12 per cent at Wainwright
and Point Hope (northern coastal villages) and 42 per cent
at Kasigluk and Nunapitchuk (southwestern inland villages).
Hypertension ($\geq$ 160 systolic or $\geq$ 95 diastolic) was found
in 5, 13, and 23 per cent of adults, respectively, at Wainwright, Point Hope, and Kasigluk plus Nunapitchuk. In
children aged 7-16 years, the incidence of hypercholesterolaemia ($\geq$ 230 mg/100 ml) was essentially zero at Wainwright
and Point Hope and 19 per cent at Nunapitchuk. A rural-
urban gradient in serum cholesterol concentrations and blood
pressures also has been observed by Maynard in a large
sample of Alaskan Eskimo men (11). The long-standing picto-
gram of low blood cholesterol levels and blood pressures in
Eskimos is no longer valid.

Plasma lipid profiles in the Ainu were investigated by
Itoh (9) as part of a comprehensive study of the physiology of cold-adapted man. No substantial differences were
seen in the concentration of most blood lipids in Ainu and
non-Ainu Japanese except for free fatty acids, which were
markedly lower in the Ainu. This difference was attributed
to better cold adaptation in the Ainu. Small doses of noradrenaline, which produced no response in the Japanese,
caused marked increases in plasma free fatty acids and
oxygen consumption in the Ainu. No essential difference was
found in the composition of plasma free fatty acids between
the two groups.

SUGAR TOLERANCE

Glucose

Several recent studies have been carried out to determine
whether modernization has affected the well-known

resistance of Eskimos to diabetes mellitus. Mouratoff and
Scott (14) observed that although clinical diabetes in
Eskimos residing in southwest Alaska is still rare, more
Eskimos were intolerant of glucose in 1972 than was the
case ten years earlier. Also, a higher proportion of the
population was overweight. It was concluded that the unusual tolerance of Eskimos for glucose does not have a
genetic basis, but may be associated with a high level of
physical activity and physical fitness. Glucose tolerance
tests on smaller samples of northern Alaskan Eskimos performed by S.A. Feldman (personal communication) and by Bell
and co-workers (4) yielded uniformly normal plasma glucose
and insulin responses.

In contrast to these findings on Alaskan Eskimos, over
half of a sample of Canadian Eskimos tested in a hospital
setting were observed to exhibit an abnormal plasma glucose response to an oral glucose load (19). The exaggerated
plasma glucose response was accompanied by a prolonged rise
in insulin titre which appeared to be caused by a delay in
insulin release. Whether this phenomenon is representative
of the normal response to dietary carbohydrate in these
subjects, or to some characteristic of the hospital environment, is unknown.

Unlike Alaskan Eskimos, Alaskan Aleuts of the Pribilof
Islands have an incidence of diabetes mellitus approaching
that of the Pima Indians of Arizona, who have the highest
reported incidence in the world. Two hours after a 75 g
carbohydrate load, plasma glucose concentrations $\geqslant$ 160 mg/
100 mℓ were observed in 22 per cent of males and 35 per
cent of females (5). High serum triglyceride levels were
also prevalent.

A comparison of glucose tolerance in Ainu and non-Ainu
Japanese was carried out by Kuroshima and associates (10).
No differences were found in plasma glucose, insulin, or
growth hormone response to a glucose load.

Lactose
Circumpolar populations share with other populations lacking a long tradition of dairying a limited tolerance for
dietary lactose. Extensive studies by Sahi and associates
indicated that the incidence of intolerance to a 50 g oral
lactose load was 17 per cent in Finnish-speaking adult subjects born in Helsinki as opposed to 34 per cent in Finnish
Lapps (17). This disparity was attributed to a difference
in the time span of milk consumption in the two populations
(about 3,000 years in Finns and 300 years in Lapps). Low

intestinal lactase activity appeared to be transmitted by
a single recessive autosomal gene (16). The enzyme appears
to be not inducible by dietary lactose.

Standard 50 g lactose load tests yielded evidence of intolerance in 54 per cent of Greenland Eskimos of various
ages (13), 80 per cent of adult Alaskan Eskimos and Indians
(6), and 70 per cent of Eskimo school children (4). However, administration of graduated oral doses revealed that
19 out of 20 adult Alaskan Eskimos were asymptomatic after
a 10 g load (equivalent to a cup of milk) and 55 per cent
after a 20 g load (4). This finding supports the view that
many subjects who are intolerant to a 50 g lactose load
(an amount necessary to induce a rise in plasma glucose
which can be reliably estimated) can, nevertheless, tolerate nutritionally significant quantities of dairy foods.
Such foods are major sources of protein, calcium, and riboflavin in the mixed diet, and their continued use in
feeding programs in underdeveloped countries is recommended
by the Protein Advisory Group of the United Nations (15).

Sucrose
Recent investigations have revealed a novel racial-ethnic
form of primary sucrose deficiency among Greenland and
northern Alaskan Eskimos. The symptoms (diarrhoea, abdominal
cramps, and flatulence) are similar to those of lactose
deficiency. However, in contrast to lactose intolerance,
sucrose intolerance is present from birth.

The incidence of intolerance was found to be 10.5 per
cent in a sample of 190 Greenland Eskimos, some of whom
had been referred to a hospital for treatment of diarrhoea
(13). The incidence in the entire population of Wainwright,
Alaska, estimated on the basis of test results and anecdotal evidence, appears to be 2-3 per cent. A conspicuous
familial pattern of intolerance was observed in the Alaskan
subjects (4). Although sucrose intolerance is less prevalent than lactose intolerance, its consequences for those
affected are more serious. Sucrose intolerance imposes
multiple restrictions on food selection from the modern
dietary, whereas lactose intolerance can usually be
managed by moderating the intake of a small number of
foods. Limited screening of children in the Bethel region
of southwest Alaska, where berries have contributed some
sucrose to the aboriginal diet for centuries, revealed no
evidence of sucrose deficiency. It is possible that this
anomaly is limited to the Arctic region where the carnivorous diet imposed no selection pressure favouring sucrose
tolerance.

BONE METABOLISM

Mazess and co-workers have observed that, beyond the age of 40, the rate of loss of bone mineral in northern Alaskan Eskimos (12) and in Canadian Eskimos (personal communication) is greater than that in U.S. whites. Adult animals and humans fed experimental diets simulating the traditional Eskimo regimen (high protein, high phosphorus, and low calcium) also exhibit an accelerated loss of bone. Whether the high incidence of osteoporosis in Eskimos is attributable to their high protein intake per se, to a high intake of phosphorus which is associated with this protein, to a low intake of calcium, or (more likely) to a combination of these factors, is not yet established.

ACKNOWLEDGMENT

The author is grateful to those investigators who have made available the unpublished results used in this review.

REFERENCES

1. Astrinskii, D.A. and Navasardov, S.M., "Consumption of food products by the indigenous population of the Chukchi National Okrug," Problemy Severa, 14: 204-8 (1970)
2. Bang, H.O., Dyerberg, J., and Nielsen, Aase Brøndum, "Plasma lipid and lipoprotein pattern in Greenlandic west-coast Eskimos," Lancet, 5 June 1971, 1143-6
3. Bang, H.O. and Dyerberg, Jørn, "Plasma lipids and lipoproteins in Greenlandic west coast Eskimos," Acta med. scand., 192: 85-94 (1972)
4. Bell, R. Raines, Draper, H.H., and Bergan, J.G., "Sucrose, lactose and glucose tolerance in northern Alaskan Eskimos," J. clin. Nutrition, 26: 1185-90 (1973)
5. Dippe, S.E., Bennett, P.H., Dippe, D.W., Humphry, T., Burks, J., and Miller, J., "Glucose tolerance among Aleuts on the Pribilof Islands." Abstracts of Third Intern. Symp. on Circumpolar Health, Yellowknife, NWT, Canada, 8-11 July 1974
6. Duncan, I.W., and Scott, E.M., "Lactose intolerance in Alaskan Indians and Eskimos," Am. J. clin. Nutrition 25: 867-8 (1972)
7. Feldman, S.A., Ho, Kang-Jey, Lewis, L.A., and Taylor, C.D., "Lipid and cholesterol metabolism in Alaskan Arctic Eskimos," Arch. Pathology, 94: 42-58 (1972)

8. Forbes, A.L., "Nutritional status of Indians and Eskimos as revealed by Nutrition Canada," Abstracts of Third Intern. Symp. on Circumpolar Health, Yellowknife, NWT, Canada 8-11 July 1974

9. Itoh, S., Physiology of Cold-Adapted Man (Hokkaido University Medical Library Series, Vol. 7, 1974)

10. Kuroshima, A., Itoh, S., Azuma, T., and Agishi, Y., "Glucose tolerance test in the Ainu," Int. J. Biometeor., 16: 193-7 (1972)

11. Maynard, J.E., "Coronary heart disease risk factors in relation to urbanization in Alaskan Eskimo men," Abstracts of Third Intern. Symp. on Circumpolar Health, Yellowknife, NWT, Canada, 8-11 July 1974

12. Mazess, R.B., "Bone mineral content in Wainwright Eskimos: a preliminary report," Arctic Anthropology, 7: 114 (1970)

13. McNair, A., Gudmand-Høyer, E., Jarnum, S., and Orrild, L., "Sucrose malabsorption in Greenland," Brit. med. J. ii: 19-21 (1972)

14. Mouratoff, G.J., & Scott, E.M., "Diabetes mellitus in Eskimos after a decade," J. Am. Med. Assoc., 226: 1345-6 (1973)

15. Protein Advisory Group, "PAG Ad Hoc Working Group on milk tolerance-nutritional implications," Protein Advisory Group Bull., 2: 7 (1972)

16. Sahi, T., Isokoski, M., Jussila, J., Launiala, K., and Pyorala, K., "Recessive inheritance of adult-type lactose malabsorption," Lancet, 13 October 1973

17. Sahi, T., "Lactose malabsorption in Finnish-speaking and Swedish-speaking populations in Finland," Scand. J. Gastroenterol.   9: 303-8 (1974)

18. Sayed, J., Schaefer, O., Hildes, J.A., and Lobban, M.A., "Biochemical indices of nutrient intake by Eskimos of Northern Foxe Basin, NWT," Abstracts of Third Intern. Symp. on Circumpolar Health, Yellowknife, NWT, Canada, 8-11 July 1974

19. Schaefer, O., Crockford, P.M., and Romanowski, B., Normalization effect of preceding protein meals on 'diabetic' oral glucose tolerance in Eskimos," Canad. Med. Assoc. J., 107: 733-8 (1972)

20. Zaitsev, A.N., "Food consumption of the people of the far north and its effect on health," Problemy Severa, 14: 198-203 (1970)

Biochemical indices of nutrition of the Iglooligmiut

JUDITH E. SAYED, J.A. HILDES, and O. SCHAEFER

Until the recent Nutrition Canada survey, dietary studies
of Eskimos have been conducted mainly by observation of
food habits, per capita calculations of distribution from
grocery outlets, and by estimation of foods available from
hunting. Problems of dietary surveys of Eskimos are compounded by their traditional practice of nibbling on frozen
or dried fish and meat at irregular intervals. To complement data collected during a dietary survey of the Iglooli-
muit (Milne, personal communication), serum and 24-hour
urinary excretions were assayed for constituents that reflect recent dietary intake. The results of the analysis of
the urinary excretion have been presented elsewhere (7).

METHODS

Venous blood was drawn from about 250 Eskimos in Northern
Foxe Basin, NWT. The sera were aliquoted and stored at
-20° C until assayed. In addition to the clinical biochemical assays, vitamin A was measured fluorometrically as
retinol (1) and folacin activity was measured microbiologi-
cally. Where applicable, criteria of the recent Nutrition
Canada survey (5) were applied in evaluation of the biochemical data.

RESULTS AND DISCUSSION

Protein

Urinary excretion of urea nitrogen and serum concentrations
of albumin reflected generally adequate protein intakes by
the population groups represented. The serum albumin in
males is illustrated in Figure 1; the distribution of
serum albumin among women was similar. Only 7 of 236 subjects were hypo-albuminaemic.

Vitamins
Urinary excretion of thiamin, riboflavin, and N-methylnico-
tinamide reflected high consumption of these B vitamins (7).
On the other hand, only 4 of 82 sera had acceptable levels
of folacin activity; the remaining subjects appeared to

ALBUMIN (g/100 ml)

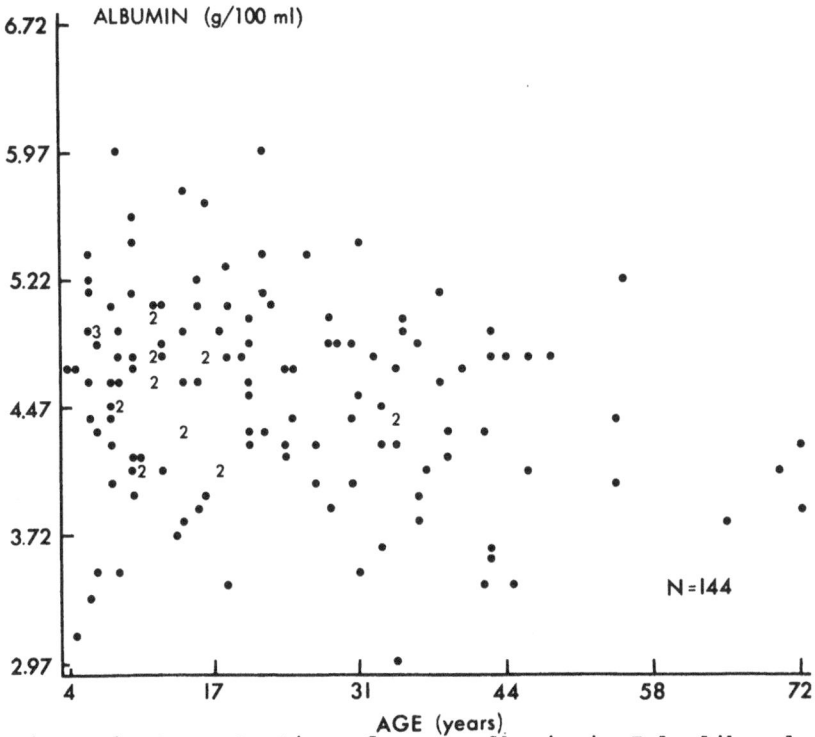

Figure 1   Concentration of serum albumin in Igloolik males

have deficient dietary intake of folic acid. Serum vitamin A levels were variable (Figure 2); no one had less than 60 μg per cent retinol while 20 per cent of the men and 10 per cent of the women had serum retinol concentrations in excess of 220 μg/100 ml. The implications of high serum retinol concentrations are uncertain - the subjects were not necessarily fasting. Review of physical examinations of these individuals gave no indication of clinical evidence of hypervitaminosis A.

Minerals
Based on urinary and blood data, consumption of minerals appeared to be marginal or low. Of the 92 adult males, 34 (37 per cent) had haemoglobin levels less than 14 g/100 ml (Figure 3), while only 3 of 46 adult women had haemoglobin concentrations below 12 g/100 ml.* Of the 121 children and adolescents investigated, 15 had haemoglobin concentrations below the Nutrition Canada standards for age and sex.

*See note on next page.

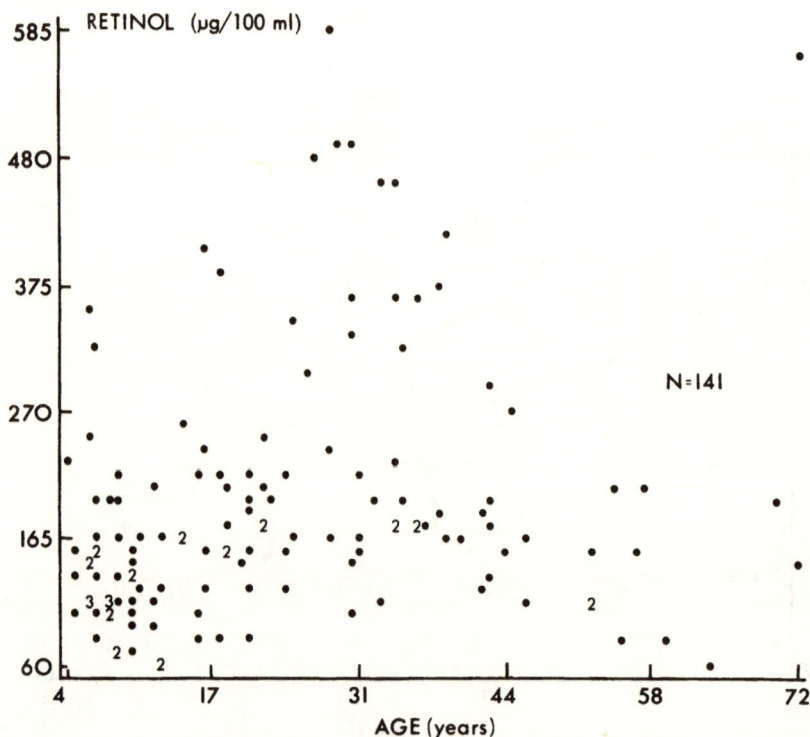

Figure 2   Concentration of serum retinol in Igloolik males

The apparent marginal intake of iron for adult men was reflected also in concentration of serum iron; 61 per cent of
112 adult males had less than 60 μg/100 ml, while 45 per
cent of 87 adult women and 38 per cent of 89 children exhibited unacceptably low concentrations of serum iron. The
criteria of assessment were those employed in recent nutrition surveys (4,7) and their applicability to all population groups is largely theoretical.

The results of assays for biochemical indices of the
nutrient intake of the Iglooligmiut are comparable to those
of Nutrition Canada (5) and to those of Alaskan Eskimos
(2,3,6). However, more meaningful assessment of dietary

* Editor's note: A sample of male and female Iglloolig-
miut from the Northern Foxe Basin were tested independently by Rode and Shephard (J. appl. Physiol., 34: 91-6, 1973).
They found few cases of clinical anaemia and normal average values.

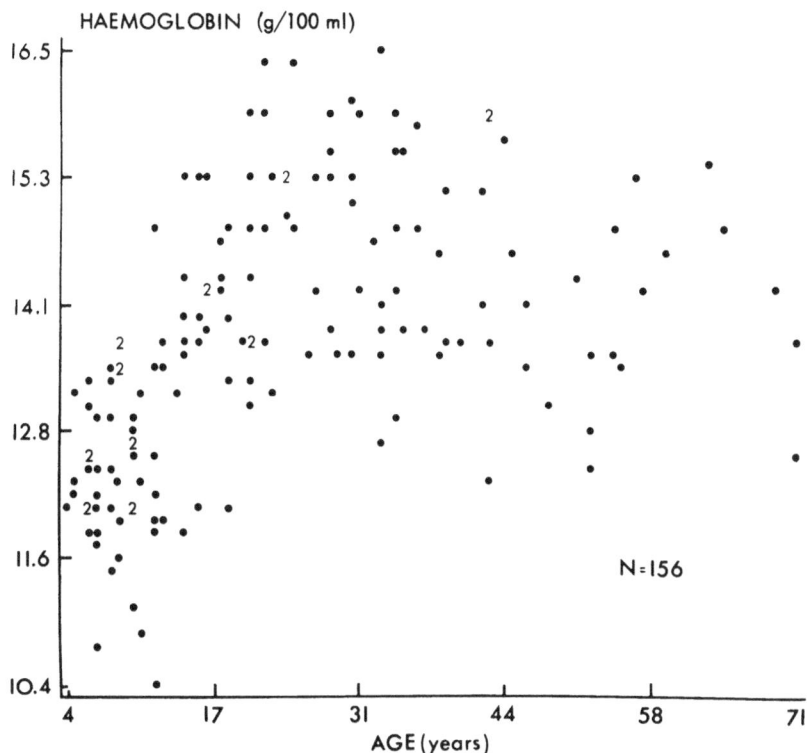

Figure 3   Concentration of haemoglobin in Igloolik males

habits can be achieved only when considered together with
the process of acculturation which affects the availability
of both traditional and imported foods.

SUMMARY

Serum and 24-hour urinary excretions from Eskimos of the
Northern Foxe Basin were assayed for constituents that reflect dietary intake. Levels of these constituents reflected a generally adequate intake of protein, thiamin, riboflavin, niacin, and vitamin A. On the other hand, consumption of folic acid, calcium, and magnesium appeared to be
low. The mean concentrations of haemoglobin and of serum
iron were 14.5 g per cent and 84 μg per cent, respectively, in adult males and 13.3 g per cent and 74 μg per cent
in adult females. According to the criteria used by Nutrition Canada one-third of the men but few women were at

risk of iron-deficiency anaemia. These data reflected
dietary consumptions similar to those of other Eskimo populations and suggest careful consideration of the effect of
acculturation upon diet and consequent nutritional status.

REFERENCES

1. Hansen, L.G. and Warwick, W.J., "A fluorometric micro-
   method for serum vitamins A and E," Am. J. clin. Pathol.,
   51: 538 (1969)
2. Heller, C.A., "The diet of some Alaskan Eskimos and
   Indians," J. Am. Dietet. Assoc., 45: 425 (1964)
3. Mann, G.V., Scott, E.M., Hursh, L.M., Heller, C.A.,
   Youmans, J.B., Consolazio, C.F., Bridgeforth, E.B.,
   Russels, A.L., and Silverman, M., "The health and nutritional status of Alaskan Eskimos," A survey of the Inter-
   departmental Committee on Nutrition for National Defense-
   1958," Am. J. clin. Nutr., 11: 31 (1962)
4. Nutrition. A National Priority. A report by Nutrition
   Canada to the Department of Health and Welfare (Ottawa:
   Information Canada 1973)
5. Sauberlich, H.E., Goad, W., Herman, Y.F., Milan, F.,
   and Jamison, P., "Biochemical assessment of the nutritional status of the Eskimos of Wainwright, Alaska,"
   Am. J. clin. Nutr., 25: 437 (1972)
6. Sayed, J.E., Lobban, M., Hildes, J.A., and Schaefer, O.,
   "An investigation of urinary excretion of vitamins,
   minerals, and nitrogen by settlement Eskimos," Proc.
   Canad. Fed. Biol. Sci., 16: 269 (1973)
7. Ten State Nutrition Survey, 1968-70, IV. Biochemical.
   U.S. Department of Health, Education, and Welfare,
   Center for Disease Control (Atlanta Georgia, DHEW
   Publication, No.(HSM), 72-8132, 1972)

The dietary intake of Finnish Skolt children

K. HASUNEN and M. PEKKARINEN

In recent years, the importance of child nutrition to
present health and future development has been emphasized
increasingly. However, to date there have been few investigations of the dietary intake of Finnish children. The
present paper reports data on Finnish Skolt Lapp children,
comparing findings with studies on children in other parts
of Finland and drawing conclusions regarding the influence
of diet on general health.

Field work was undertaken in the winter and summer of
1970, at Sevettijärvi, the Skolt community in northeastern
Finland. About 120 children up to 19 years of age were
examined, including those living at home and residents of
two schools. The nutritional analysis was carried out by
the exact weighing method. The nutrient content of the diet
was calculated from food composition tables, available information from the food industry and the results of nutrient analyses performed by the Department of Nutrition of
the University of Helsinki. The main results of the winter
studies have already been reported (4). We shall present
here some characteristics of the summer diet and the findings will be compared with the recommended dietary allowances in three selected age groups.

RESULTS

In summer, the consumption of food was less than in winter.
The intake of energy varied from 1,070 to 1,970 calories.
The children got 11 to 15 per cent of the total calories
from proteins and 28 to 38 per cent from fat. The summer
diet provided 3.8-9.5 mg iron. Because of the low energy
intake, the income of B group vitamins was low, too. The intake of vitamin C was 17-34 mg per person per day. These
figures include only the intake of nutrients of natural
foods. Most of the children received preparations such as
iron supplements and cod liver oil or A-D-vitamin concentrates, which contributed to the total intake of these nutrients. A further variable not taken into account was
possible losses in cooking.

The mean daily intake of energy and proteins has been
compared with the recommendations of FAO/WHO (2) and the

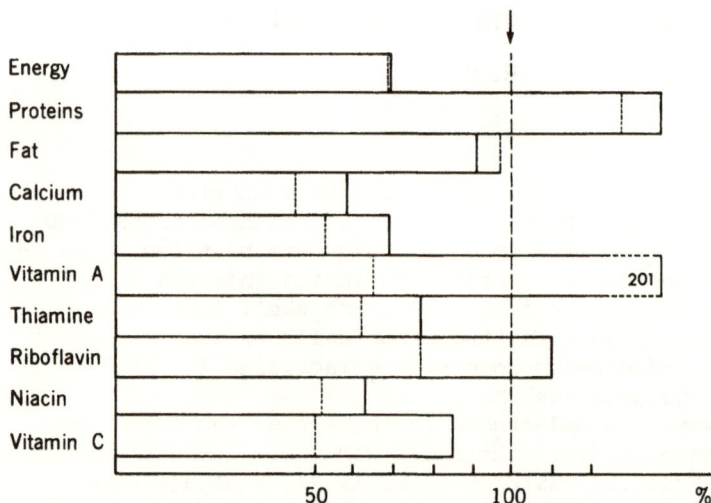

Figure 1 Mean energy and nutrient intakes of Skolt children aged four to six years, expressed as a percentage of
recommended allowances (N = 14, winter, solid line; N = 12,
summer, broken line)

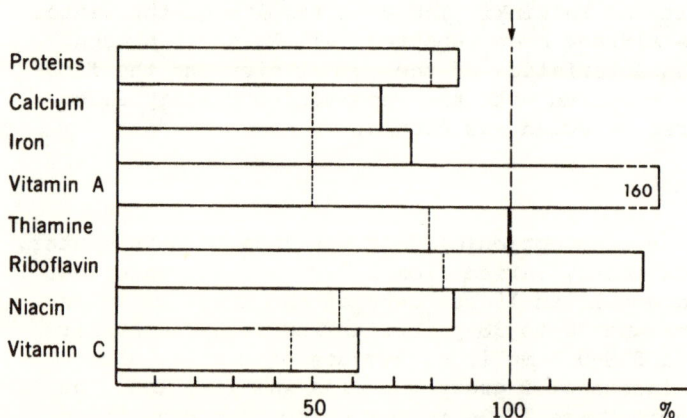

Figure 2 Mean intake of nutrients per 1,000 kcal, expressed as a percentage of recommended allowances, for
Skolt Lapps aged four to six years (N = 14, winter, solid
line; N = 12, summer, broken line)

income of other nutrients with figures proposed by Food and
Nutrition Board, National Research Council (3).
    Figures 1, 3, and 5 present the mean daily intake of

nutrients as a percentage of recommended allowances. The broken line indicates the adequacy of the summer diet, the unbroken one that of winter diet, and the arrow the recommended level. The mean daily intake of fat is expressed as a percentage of the mean recommendation proposed by the Swedish National Institute of Public Health, i.e. 30 per cent of the energy intake (6). Vitamin A is cited as mg retinol equivalents from preformed vitamin and carotene according to FAO/WHO (1).

The need of adequate nutrition is most pronounced in the age group from four to six years. Nevertheless, less attention has been paid to the proper quality of diet at this age than during infancy. Healthy nutrition requires an adequate supply of essential nutrients in spite of the frequent decrease in appetite and lack of interest in food at this age. Among children aged 4-6 years (Figure 1) the intake of both calories and of nutrients was less than accepted norms. In spite of the relatively low caloric intake, the recommended values for proteins were attained. The mean daily intake of calories was about the same in summer as in winter. Nevertheless, the intake of all other nutrients was considerably lower in summer than in winter. Intakes of calcium, iron, thiamine, and vitamin C were far from optimal.

Because of the low intake of both calories and nutrients, it seemed worthwhile to investigate whether the cause was the low energy intake. We recalculated the figures per 1,000 calories (Figures 2, 4, 6) and compared the results with recommendations made by the Swedish National Institute of Public Health (6); their proposals are about the same as those recommended by NRC.

The poor intake of certain nutrients in the age group from four to six years was not due solely to the low intake energy (Figure 2). The contribution of proteins to the total energy was 12-13 per cent, i.e. about 80 per cent of the optimal level. However, the low total intake of thiamine was caused by the low level of food energy.

About half of the children investigated in winter were living in a boarding school. The school provided two hot meals, breakfast and a snack in the evening. The intake of nutrients in the age group from 7 to 9 years was substantially better than that of younger children (Figure 3). In winter the mean values of most nutrients were well above the recommended allowances and much higher than in the summer. Only the contents of food energy and niacin were low. We have not calculated the amino acid content of the Lapp diet. It is known that 60 mg tryptophan is equivalent

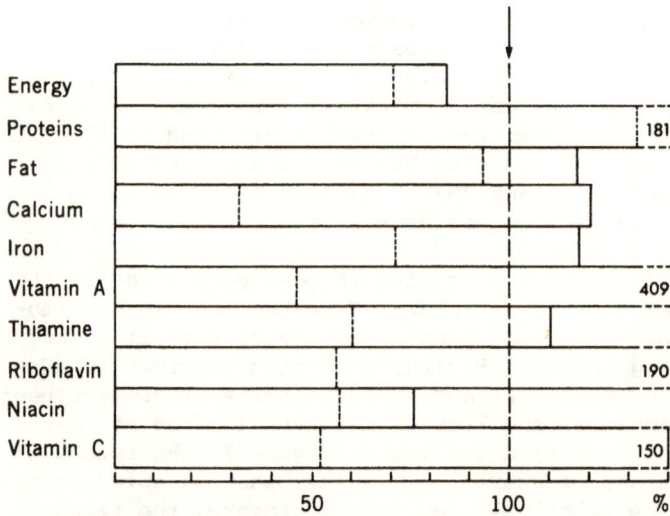

Figure 3 Mean energy and nutrient intake as a percentage of recommended allowances, for Skolt Lapps aged seven to nine years (N = 29, winter, solid line; N = 20, summer, broken line)

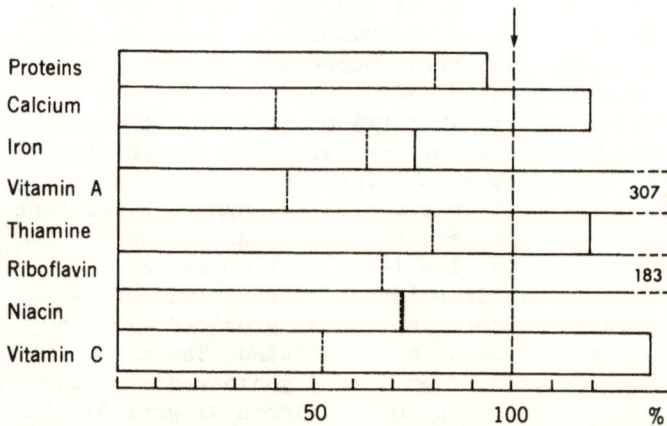

Figure 4 Mean intake of nutrients per 1,000 kcal as a percentage of recommended allowances, for Skolt Lapps aged seven to nine years (N = 29, winter, solid line; N = 20, summer, broken line)

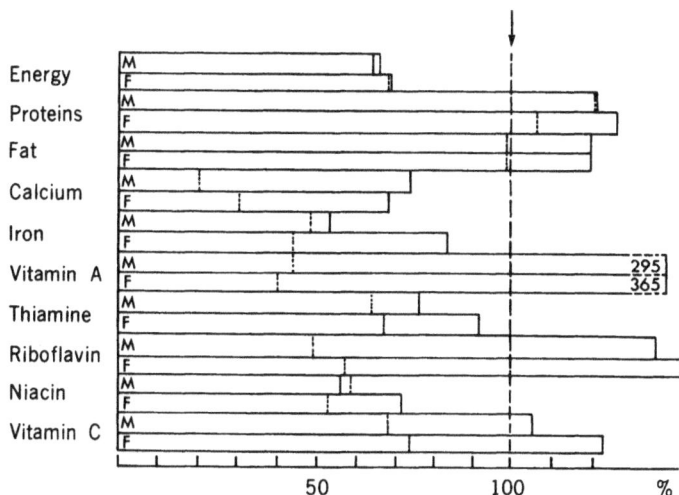

Figure 5   Mean energy and nutrient intake as a percentage
of recommended allowances, for Skolt Lapps aged 13 to 15
years (N = 20-8, winter, solid lines; N = 16-12, summer,
broken lines)

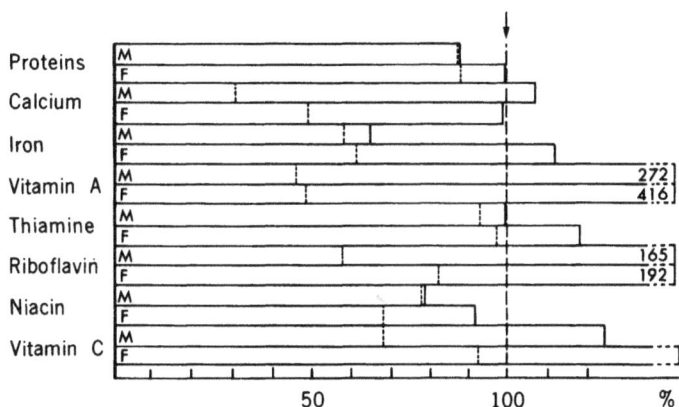

Figure 6   Mean intake of nutrients per 1,000 kcal as a percentage of recommended allowances, for Skolt Lapps aged 13
to 15 years (N = 20-8, winter, solid lines; N = 16-12,
summer, broken lines)

to 1 mg niacin. According to studies performed earlier in
Finland (5) the intake of niacin equivalents is about 4 mg
per 1,000 calories. In this material, it makes a contribution of 7 mg to vitamin intake. The total intake of niacin
equivalents would then be 17 mg, which is well above the
recommended level (13 mg). The summer diet was very poor in
this age group, too.

With the exception of the low iron intake, the quality
of school feeding was satisfactory when evaluated per 1,000
kcal (Figure 4).

For boys (M) and girls (F) aged 13 to 15, the mean daily
intakes of energy were only 66 to 69 per cent of the recommended level (Figure 5). Because of the low intake of food
energy, the consumed quantities of calcium, iron, and thiamine were generally low, even in winter.

The boys had lower values than the girls, as can be
seen when comparing the figures per 1,000 kcal of food
energy (Figure 6). The school meals were well balanced and
for the most part filled nutritional requirements. In
summer, 34 to 36 per cent of energy was covered by white
bread and sugar, whereas the corresponding figures in
winter were 15 to 23 per cent. This indicates the poor
qualitative composition of the summer diet.

In the three age groups presented here, most of the figures for both calories and nutrients were below accepted
norms. Children living at home received an unsatisfactory
diet both in winter and in summer. The school feeding program gave satisfactory values for all nutrients except
iron. Proteins expressed as a percentage of energy were
within normal limits. The low values for vitamin intake indicate a need for wider use of multi-vitamin preparations.
Both children and their parents need much instruction, so
that the children's diet may be improved.

SUMMARY

A dietary survey by the exact weighing method was undertaken on Finnish Skolt Lapps in 1970. The survey included
about 120 children. The average energy intake varied in
winter from 870 to 2,188 kcal/day and in summer from 1,070
to 1,970 kcal/day in different age groups. Proteins contributed 11-16 per cent to the total energy, and fats 27-
36 per cent.

For the age groups 4-6, 7-9, and 13-15 years, the intakes of calories and most nutrients were lower than the
accepted norms. Children living at home were most un-

favourably situated. School meals were qualitatively well
balanced and filled requirements for all nutrients except
iron. The daily intake of calcium was 290-1,200 mg. The intake of vitamin C was 16-68 mg in winter and 17-34 mg in
summer. The intake of B-group vitamins was also low.

REFERENCES

1. FAO/WHO, "Requirements of vitamin A, thiamine, riboflavin and niacin," WHO Tech. Rep. Ser., 362 (Geneva,
   1967)
2. FAO/WHO, "Energy and protein requirements," WHO Tech.
   Rep. Ser., 522 (Geneva, 1973)
3. Food and Nutrition Board, Recommended dietary allowances,
   Seventh revised ed. (National Research Council, Publ.
   No 1694, Washington, D.C., 1968)
4. Hasunen, K. and Pekkarinen, M. "The dietary intake of
   the Finnish Skolt children," Third International Symposium on Circumpolar Health, Yellowknife, Canada, July
   1974, Abstracts of papers
5. Seppänen, R., Koskinen, E.H., Pekkarinen, M., and Roine,
   P. "Dietary surveys in connection with epidemiological
   studies in Finland," Kansaneläkelaitoksen julkaisuja,
   ML 2:1-62 (1973)
6. Statens institut för folkhälsan, Önskvärd halt av
   näringsämnen per 1,000 kcal., Vår föda, 21: 167 (1969)

Investigation of blood lipids and food composition
of Greenlandic Eskimos

H.O. BANG, J. DYERBERG, and N. HJØRNE

Ischaemic heart disease is rare in Greenland Eskimos, although their consumption of animal products containing a
good deal of fat is thought to be rather high. During the
summer of 1970, we studied serum lipids in 130 Eskimos (61
male and 69 female) aged 30 years or more, the men living
as hunters and/or fishermen in the district of Umanak, on
the west coast of Greenland, some 500 km north of the Polar
Circle. Total serum lipids, cholesterol, triglycerides,

TABLE 1
Serum lipid and lipoprotein concentrations in Greenlandic Eskimos and
Danes

	Eskimos	Danes
Total lipid (g/l)	6.18	7.15
Cholesterol (mmol/l)	5.91	7.27
Triglycerides (mmol/l)	0.57	1.23
Phospholipids (mmol/l)	3.07	2.96
Chylomicrons (g/l)	0.27	0.19
Pre-β-lipoprotein (g/l)	0.43	1.29
β-lipoprotein (g/l)	4.45	5.21
α-lipoprotein (g/l)	4.00	3.34

phospholipids, and lipoproteins (1) were compared with results for some 300 healthy Danes of the same age (Table 1).

As in earlier studies, we found lower serum cholesterol
in the Eskimos. A new finding was the much lower level of
serum triglycerides; β-lipoproteins and especially the pre-
β-lipoproteins were lower than in the Danish population. In
order to test whether these differences in serum lipids were
of genetic origin, we also examined some 30 Greenlandic
Eskimos living in Denmark, on Danish food. The serum lipid
and lipoprotein pattern of these Eskimos did not differ from
that of other Danes. Consequently, differences in serum
lipids between Greenlandic Eskimos and Danes must be considered of environmental origin, presumably caused by the
special nature of Eskimo food. The number of seals and
whales caught in the Umanak district in 1970 was essentially
similar to that of other years. It was calculated that on
average every Eskimo - from baby to old man - ate about
400 g of seal or whale meat per day.

As the pattern of ester-bound serum fatty acids is considered to reflect that of the food consumed, we carried out
gas-liquid chromatographic analyses of the serum fatty acids
bound as cholesterol esters, triglycerides, and phospholipids, comparing the results with those for Danish controls. There were considerable differences. The levels of
palmitic, palmitoleic, oleic, and timnodonic acids were
higher in Eskimos, whereas linoleic, linolenic, and arachidonic acid levels were lower. The total quantities of saturated and monounsaturated fatty acids (Table 2) were a
little higher in Eskimos than in Danes, whereas the total
of polyunsaturated acids was a little lower than in Danes.

TABLE 2
Distribution of esterified fatty acids in the plasma lipids of Greenlandic Eskimos (G) and Danes (D). Data expressed as a percentage of
total for saturated, monoenes, and polyunsaturated components

Fatty acids	Cholesterol esters		Triglycerides		Phospholipids		Total	
	G	D	G	D	G	D	G	D
Saturated	22	14	36	37	58	49	39	33
Monoenes	36	27	45	46	21	17	34	30
Polyunsaturated	42	59	19	17	21	34	27	37

Two years later, we visited the same district and collected
duplicate samples of Eskimo food for chemical analysis. The
technique of Ancel Keys was used, food samples being taken
from 7 Eskimos over 7 days, in all 49 specimens. The food
was weighed, homogenized, and aliquots frozen for later examination in Denmark.

Our results were compared with the average composition
of Danish food for the same year (1972). We found a much
higher intake of protein (26 versus 11 cal per cent), a
fat intake of the same magnitude as that of Danes (37 versus 42 cal per cent), and a smaller intake of carbohydrates
(37 versus 47 cal per cent).

The composition of the fat was determined by gas-liquid
chromatography (Table 3). It differed from that of Danish
food, the main differences being a higher content of palmitoleic, timnodonic, and eicosahexaenoic acid, and a low
content of stearic, linoleic, and linolenic acid.

The total quantity of saturated fatty acids in the Eskimo food was lower than in Danish food, as was the total of
polyunsaturated fatty acids (Table 4). The cholesterol intake was higher in the Eskimos than in the Danes (245 mg/
1,000 calories in Eskimos and 139 mg/1,000 calories in
Danes). The lower level of serum cholesterol in the Eskimos
cannot be explained simply by the proportions of saturated
and polyunsaturated fatty acid in Eskimo food as suggested
in the formula by Ancel Keys (2). If Keys's formula is
applied to our figures, the difference in serum cholesterol
level should average 0.39 mmol/ℓ less in the Eskimos. However, the observed difference was much greater (0.70 to
2.49 in different age groups, averaging 1.35 mmol/ℓ).

If the lower serum cholesterol in Eskimos is caused by
the fatty acids ingested, the special long-chained polyunsaturated acids of timnodonic acid (C20:5) and

TABLE 3
The average fatty acid composition of Eskimo food, expressed as a percentage of total fatty acids, with corresponding figures for average Danish food (1972), mean and standard deviation

	Eskimos	Danes
C 12:0	1.1 ± 1.0	5.9
C 14:0	5.7 ± 1.1	7.5
C 16:0	19.2 ± 4.7	25.5
C 16:1	13.5 ± 4.5	3.8
C 18:0	4.9 ± 2.5	9.5
C 18:1	29.7 ± 5.3	29.2
C 18:2	4.7 ± 2.7	10.0
C 18:3	0.4 ± 0.3	2.0
C 20:0	0.6 ± 0.8	4.3
C 20:1	6.9 ± 3.5	0.4
C 20:4	0.1 ± 0.4	0
C 20:5	2.3 ± 1.4	0.4
C 22:0	1.8 ± 2.3	0
C 22:1	4.6 ± 2.9	1.2
C 22:6	2.2 ± 2.2	0.3
C 24:0	0.4 ± 0.8	0
C 24:1	1.9 ± 2.1	0

TABLE 4
The sum of the saturated, monounsaturated, and polyunsaturated fatty acids in Eskimo and Danish food (1972), given as a percentage of total fatty acids

	Eskimos	Danes
Saturated fatty acids	33.7	52.7
Monounsaturated fatty acids	56.6	34.6
Polyunsaturated fatty acids	9.7	12.7

eicosahexaenoic acid (C22:6) may act in a qualitatively different way than the C18 polyunsaturated fatty acids in Danish food.

The explanation of the very low level of serum triglycerides and pre-β-lipoprotein is obscure but may be of major importance - together with the lower serum cholesterol level - in explaining the low incidence of ischaemic heart disease, and the almost total absence of diabetes mellitus.

SUMMARY

Serum lipid and lipoprotein concentrations were measured in 130 Eskimos (61 males and 69 females) aged 30 years and over, living in northwest Greenland. The serum cholesterol

was lower than in Danes and triglyceride concentrations
were much lower. Serum β-lipoprotein and pre-β-lipoprotein
concentrations showed a parallel reduction. However, Greenland Eskimos living in Denmark had similar serum lipid and
lipoprotein levels to Danes. Environmental factors must
thus be responsible for the differences in serum lipids between Greenland Eskimos and Danes. The ester-bound fatty
acids in the serum lipids differed between Eskimos and
Danes, the levels of palmitic, palmitoleic, oleic, and
timnodonic acids being higher, and those of linoleic, linolenic, and arachidonic acids being lower in Eskimos. Eskimos had a lower intake of carbohydrates and a much higher
protein intake than Danes. The intake of both saturated
and polyunsaturated fatty acids was lower in Eskimos.

REFERENCES

1. Bang, H.O. and Dyerberg, J., "Plasma lipids and lipoproteins in Greenlandic Westcoast Eskimos," Acta med.
   scand., 192: 85-94 (1972)
2. Keys, A., Anderson, J.T., and Grande, F., "Prediction
   of serum-cholesterol responses of man to changes in fats
   in the diet," Lancet, II: 959-66 (1957)

Isolated adult-type lactose malabsorption in Finnish Lapps

T. SAHI, A.W. ERIKSSON, M. ISOKOSKI, and M. KIRJARINTA

Isolated adult-type lactose malabsorption (LM) due to a low
lactase activity in the jejunum is inherited. The inheritance is controlled by a single autosomal recessive gene
(8). The gene frequency and the prevalence of LM varies considerably around the world. In some populations, especially
in coloured people, the prevalence is 70-100 per cent and
the frequency of the lm gene 0.84-1.00. In other groups,
the prevalence is under 20 per cent (gene frequency under
0.45) (6); such people are generally descended from white

Europeans. In Finland the prevalence of LM among the Finnish-speaking population is 17 per cent and among the
Swedish-speaking population 8 per cent, the estimated frequencies of the Im gene being 0.41 and 0.28, respectively
(7).

The purpose of this study was to ascertain the prevalence of LM and to estimate the frequency of the lm gene in
Utsjoki Lapps. The hypothesis was that the gene frequency
would be distinctly higher among the Lapps than among the
Finns, because of the shorter history of milk consumption
in the former; the longer the time during which people have
consumed milk as adults, the lower is the gene frequency
(9).

MATERIAL AND METHODS

Utsjoki is the northernmost commune in Finland. Three-
quarters of its inhabitants are Lapps. The number of Lapps
over 15 years old with Lapp parents was 488. Of this group,
200 were selected by random sampling and invited to undergo
examination for lactose malabsorption and certain other
genetic disorders. One hundred and sixty people (80 per
cent) participated, but one of these had a Finnish mother
and was excluded and one person discontinued the examination. Forty-nine per cent (78/158) of the people examined
were men and 51 per cent (80/158) were women.

After overnight fasting, all subjects had a lactose
tolerance test with ethanol (LTTE) (4). They were given
0.3 g/kg of ethanol and 15 minutes later 50g of lactose.
Capillary blood samples for glucose and galactose determinations by the glucose-oxidase and galactose-oxidase methods were taken before and also 20 and 40 minutes after
the lactose load. The samples were refrigerated and sent by
air to Helsinki for analyses. The criteria for LM were a
maximum rise in blood glucose concentration of <20 mg/100
ml and a rise in galactose concentration of <5 mg/100 ml
(8).

General malabsorption was excluded in persons with LM
by a glucose-galactose tolerance test with ethanol (GGTTE)
(4). A quick method was needed for screening those subjects on whom the GGTTE had to be performed, because the
results of the determinations of blood glucose and galactose were available only later. Blood glucose concentrations were therefore determined immediately, using Dextrostix (Ames Co.) and a Dextrostix Reflectance colorimeter. People with a maximum rise in blood-glucose <25 mg/

100 ml were considered to have LM and were invited to take
the GGTTE.

RESULTS

Fifty-four persons (34 per cent) had a maximum glucose rise
<25 mg/100 ml as determined by the Dextrostix method. Seven
of the 54 persons refused the GGTTE. One subject vomited
during the LTTE and GGTTE and she was excluded.

Forty-nine people fulfilled the criteria of LM in the
LTTE, when the glucose and galactose concentrations were
determined by the glucose- and galactose-oxidase methods,
and 96 people had normal lactose absorption; 46 people
(93.9 per cent) in the former group and 92 people (95.8
per cent) in the latter had the same diagnosis as that obtained by the rapid Dextrostix method.

In 12 subjects, only one of the criteria of LM was fulfilled. In 7 of these lactose was considered to be absorbed
because of a high rise in glucose or galactose concentration. Four subjects were considered to have LM. They had a
maximum rise in glucose concentration of 21 to 29 mg/100 ml
and a rise in galactose concentration of only 0 to 1 mg/
100 ml, and all had diarrhoea or meteorism after the test.

In one subject, the result remained equivocal and he
also was excluded. No general malabsorption was found by
the GGTTE. Eleven of the 53 people who had LM had no GGTTE.
They were not, however, excluded because general malabsorption was not found in any other of the Lapps and in the
Finnish population general malabsorption is very rare (5,
7,8).

Thus the prevalence of isolated LM among the Utsjoki
Lapps was 34 per cent (53/156). The estimated frequency of
the lm gene was 0.583; this was significantly higher than
the frequency in the Finns (p < 0.001), so that the result
was in keeping with the hypothesis. The prevalence of LM
was 35 per cent in males and 33 per cent in females and it
was the same in all age groups.

Milk consumption was similar in the groups with LM and
with normal lactose absorption. Most people drank 2 to 3
glasses of milk per day.

DISCUSSION

It may be supposed that before man began to consume milk
as an adult, most adults had LM. When milk consumption began, subjects with normal lactose absorption were better

able to use all constituents of milk without diarrhoea
(6,9). This possibly constituted a selecting factor, where-
by the frequency of the lm gene decreased among milk-
consuming populations.

The Lapps have used cow's milk for about 100 to 150
years and reindeer's milk for about 300 years, although
consumption has been scanty (3). Based on this hypothesis,
one would thus suppose that the frequency of the lm gene
would be higher than 0.58 among the Lapps. On the other
hand, although the people examined were "pure" Lapps, it is
probable that the Utsjoki community has received a gene
flow from Finns and Norwegians, among whom LM is not so
frequent (7).

Among other Lapp populations the frequency of the lm
gene may be higher. Among Finnish Skolt Lapps in Sevettijärvi and Nellim the frequency was about 0.77 and the prevalence of LM about 60 per cent (Sahi, unpublished data).
This figure is significantly higher than that for Utsjoki
Lapps and indeed is the highest in Europe, if studies with
a small number of subjects are excluded. Skolt Lapps consume less milk than Utsjoki Lapps and the duration of milk
consumption is shorter, which might explain the difference
in gene frequencies.

The hypothesis has been criticized, because nowadays
diarrhoea in people with LM is not so severe that the absorption of other milk constituents is prejudiced (2).
However, it has been observed that lactose enhances calcium absorption, so that in persons with LM calcium absorption is probably decreased (1). In addition, vitamin D
enhances calcium absorption, and so especially in Northern
Europe, where production of vitamin D has been insufficient
because of restricted ultraviolet irradiation in winter,
normal lactose absorption has been a factor favouring calcium absorption (2) and thus preventing rickets and osteo-
malacia. This could be the selecting factor which has increased the gene frequency of normal lactose absorption
among the Lapps, although the hypothesis still demands further investigation.

ACKNOWLEDGMENT

This study was aided by grants from the Finnish Cultural
Association and the Nordic Council for Arctic Research.

SUMMARY

Isolated adult-type lactose malabsorption (LM) is inherited.
The inheritance is controlled by a single autosomal recessive gene. The frequency of the lm gene has been estimated
to be 0.41 among the Finns, with a 17 per cent prevalence
of LM. The Finns have been using milk for 3,000 years and
the Lapps for 300 years. The authors developed a hypothesis
that the frequency of the lm gene would be higher in the
Lapps than in the Finns; this was verified. The frequency
of the lm gene (0.58) was significantly higher for 158 of
the adult Lapp population at Utsjoki than among the Finns.
However, it was also significantly lower than the frequency
found in Skolt Lapps (about 0.77).

REFERENCES

1. Condon, J.R., Nassim, J.R., Millard, F.J.C., Hilbe, A.,
   and Stainthorpe, E.M., "Calcium and phosphorus metabolism in relation to lactose intolerance," Lancet, I:
   1027-9 (1970)
2. Flatz, G. and Rotthauwe, H.W., "Lactose nutrition and
   natural selection," Lancet, II: 76-7 (1973)
3. Itkonen, T.I., Suomen lappalaiset vuoteen 1945 (Porvoo,
   Finland: Werner Soderstrom Oy, 1948)
4. Jussila, J., "Diagnosis of lactose malabsorption by the
   lactose tolerance test with peroral ethanol administration," Scand. J. Gastroenterol., 4: 361-8 (1969)
5. Jussila, J., Isokoski, M., and Launiala, K., "Prevalence of lactose malabsorption in a Finnish rural population," Scand. J. Gastroenterol., 5: 49-56 (1970)
6. McCracken, R.D., "Lactase deficiency: an example of
   dietary evolution," Curr. Anthropol., 12: 479-517 (1971)
7. Sahi, T., "Lactose malabsorption in Finnish-speaking
   and Swedish-speaking populations in Finland," Scand.
   J. Gastroenterol., 9: 303-8 (1974)
8. Sahi, T., Isokoski, M., Jussila, J., Launiala, K., and
   Pyorala, K., "Recessive inheritance of adult-type lactose malabsorption," Lancet, II: 823-6 (1973)
9. Simoons, F.J., "Primary adult lactose intolerance and
   the milking habit: a problem in biologic and cultural
   interrelations," Am. J. dig. Dis., 15: 695-710 (1970)

Dietary habits of Greenland school children

LISBET BERG

GENERAL FEATURES OF GREENLAND DIET

Previous investigations of the diets and dietary habits of populations have shown dependence on both general and specific environmental factors. Topography and climate are among the most important general factors, influencing the fauna and flora available for direct dietary use and as trading objects. The preparation of food varies according to both traditions and the taste of the population. Some groups like their meat perfectly boiled, for example, while others prefer the meat dried or raw. Some throw away the bowels while in other groups this is a favourite dish - maybe because it provides some dietary requirement.

Specific factors show seasonal and more long-term trends - for instance, the extent of the permafrost, ambient temperature, precipitation, and the difference between midnight sun and midday darkness.

In the Greenlandic population, occupations change from the north to the south, from fishing via trading and service-functions to farming and sheep-breeding. Often several occupations are combined. Industrialization is increasing in the towns, but nevertheless workers go out hunting and fishing whenever they get the opportunity. In the summertime, they sometimes spend months at places that are good for fishing, taking the whole family with them. In the summer, it is not difficult to grow vegetables and fruits. Grain, however, does not ripen. Indirectly, it enters the chain of nourishment by serving as food for domestic animals - sheeps, cows, and horses. Vegetables are for many Greenlanders of real worth, particularly in the summer and autumn. The shepherds carry root vegetables such as beets and potatoes, cabbage and rhubarb for sale in bigger towns along the coast.

In Greenland as a whole, the "bread-winner" still provides a large part of the household food by hunting or by fishing. If he returns with a seal, this is prepared and the whole family eats from the pot at all meals (breakfast, lunch, afternoon and dinner) until the pot is empty. Nevertheless, store food makes up an increasing part of the Greenlander's diet, particularly in the towns.

The concentration of the population in towns makes it difficult to reach good fishing and hunting places and also leads to difficulties in storing provisions. More than two-thirds of Greenland's housing takes the form of flats, which have quite inadequate facilities for storing provisions. Store food consists mainly of bread and grain-products. Fruits and vegetables are expensive to transport across the Atlantic and in the winter it becomes almost impossible to reach harbours because of snow and ice. Natural milk is unavailable, but the stores sell dried milk, eggs, and cheese. Tinned food is making up an increasing part of the diet, especially fruits canned in syrup. Sweets, pop-corn, chocolate, and biscuits are also rising in consumption.

This paper describes a detailed survey of dietary habits among children in the south-Greenland town of Narssaq, conducted in the years 1966 and 1970-71.

THE NARSSAQ SURVEYS

The first investigation was conducted in 1966. It was not easy to construct a suitable questionnaire for the interviews. Our initial pattern was based on an investigation of a large number of Danish schoolchildren living in a rural district. However, the schoolchildren of Narssaq faced quite different conditions and we had to compile and reject many formats before we found a suitable one. Interviews took place in the classrooms and in all we interviewed 47 children in grades 4 and 5, 25 males and 22 females. It was not possible to interview younger grades because the children could not help answering in the same way and words as other pupils, especially those with whom they shared their desks. The children were very co-operative, but we had the impression that they gave answers which they thought we would like to hear. Each student was interviewed about his breakfast, lunch, and supper, and was also asked what he had to eat when returning from school and in the afternoon. A very large number of the children bought sweets, cakes, and biscuits in the shops every day - much like other school-children. In 1966, they got no milk and no school-meals.

In December 1970, all the Greenlandic school-children in grades 2, 3, and 4 of the Narssaq school were interviewed, a total of 106 children, 45 males and 61 females. In March '71 the same classes were re-interviewed (a total of 117 children, 49 males and 68 females). We interviewed

only children whose parents were both Greenlanders. Ages
ranged from 9 to 12 years. Some 61 per cent of the children
lived in households with 1 to 4 children and 39 per cent in
families with 5 or more children. In this survey, questions
concerned the meals on the chosen day and one day and two
days before the elected day. For breakfast, 4 per cent of
the children in Grade 2 got nothing to eat and 2 per cent
nothing to drink. In Grade 3, the corresponding numbers
were 13 and 3 per cent, while in Grade 4 they were 8 and 2
per cent.

Some 84 per cent of Grade 2 participated in school-meals
at mid-day. In Grades 3 and 4, 90 and 82 per cent participated. The fact that less than 100 per cent took school-
meals reflects the erratic nature of school attendance.
Concerning supper, 3 per cent of Grade 2, 9 per cent of
Grade 3, and 10 per cent of Grade 4 had nothing to eat,
with 5, 9, and 10 per cent having nothing to drink. By way
of comparison, the Danish investigation found that 6 per
cent of school-children had nothing to eat in the morning
and 5 per cent had nothing for lunch, but all had something
to eat for supper.

Details of the individual meals were as follows:

Breakfast
Most children had bread and butter or sandwich bread; 42
per cent had rye-bread only, 4 per cent white bread only,
and 41 per cent a combination; 33 per cent had porridge,
17 per cent oat meal or corn-flakes with milk and sugar;
63 per cent had coffee or tea. Only 10 per cent drank milk,
while 10 per cent drank juice, lemonade or water. From the
total of 106 children, 8 had nothing to eat and 2 nothing to
drink.

Mid-day Meal
Most children took the school-meal. Among the others, 19
per cent had a hot fish-dish and 25 per cent a hot meat
dish, often the special Greenlandic "suaussat," usually
taken with potatoes and soup, but sometimes with rice or
barley-corn; 14 per cent had bread and butter (rye-bread),
8 per cent had ryebread pure, and 12 per cent had white
bread. In all, 8 per cent said that they had nothing to eat
in the middle of the day; 31 per cent had coffee to drink,
9 per cent had milk, 8 per cent had juice, and 13 per cent
had pure water.

Supper

Most of the children told us that they had a hot supper. Seventeen per cent had fish, 20 per cent fowl, 2 per cent seal- or whale-meat, 6 per cent lamb; 19 per cent had potatoes and 20 per cent had soup with their meal; 18 per cent had bread and butter and 9 per cent dry bread, 14 per cent had white bread. For a beverage, 39 per cent had coffee or tea, 13 per cent got milk, 8 per cent juice or lemonade, and 9 per cent pure water; 8 per cent had nothing to drink.

Wide variations of response were encountered according to (1) the season, (2) the sort of food available in the home, (3) the sort of food that the "bread-winner" brought home, and (4) the age of the persons interviewed.

We conclude from the survey (1) that Narssaq is among the more prosperous of the towns along the coast, (2) the diet of the children is varied and quite good, (3) through various educational channels such as the women's assemblies, the evening-schools and consumer education groups the parents seem to have learned the nature of a good diet.

SOCIAL STRUCTURE OF THE FAMILIES

Some 71 per cent of the children investigated came from well-knit families, formally married and with both parents living at home. In 10 per cent, the supporter was single and unmarried, but frequently there was more than one child in the family and often several other persons lived in the same house, for example, the grandparents, brothers and sisters, or a "lodger." In 5 per cent, the "bread-winner" was a widow or a widower and in a further 5 per cent the parents were divorced or separated. The domestic situation was unknown in 7 per cent.

The traditional family is thus still the most common structure in Greenlandic society. However, many couples do not marry formally until they have several children, and the husband is not always the biological father of all the children.

With regard to occupation of the "bread-winner", in the towns hunting and fishing are no longer the main occupations. For 42.5 per cent of the children interviewed, the main supporter was employed in a factory, while 30 per cent were described as hunters, fishermen, or shepherds. Many workers still make a secondary occupation of fishing and hunting, but nevertheless their main employment is in the town. This is reflected in increasing purchases of common daily items of diet. Steadily rising trade in corn,

sugar, and flour is reported by the royal trading company.
Of the remaining providers, 5 per cent were independent
tradesmen or handworkers, while 11.5 per cent were public
workers, either in institutions or in shops. The occupation of 6.7 per cent of the "bread-winners" was unknown,
while 4 per cent were housewives.

We lived in a hamlet near Narssaq in order to examine
the results of hunting. As expected, seal-hunting was most
active in the second and third quarters of the year. At
this season, the seals came south with the ice floes. Fewest seals were caught in the final quarter of the year - 11
compared with 116 in the third quarter. The total kill of
the hamlet for the period 1970-71 was 472 seals, compared
with 273 seals in 1969-70. To this was added an unspecified
consumption of fish (cod, Greenland halibut, flounder,
salmon, and sea trout) and sea birds. Taking account of
the large number of seals shot and their high average
weight, it appears that the seals are the main source of
food followed by sea birds and fishes.

SUMMARY

General features of the Greenlandic diet are discussed, together with specific details of the food eaten by the
children of Narssaq (ages 9-12) during 1966 and 1970-71.
The children for the most part have a good diet, and it is
concluded that measures of dietary education are working
quite well. Information on family structure and the occupation of the "bread-winner" is discussed briefly.

Commentaries

"Nutritional status of Indians and Eskimos as revealed by
Nutrition Canada," by A.L. Forbes (Bureau of Nutritional
Health, Department of National Health and Welfare, Ottawa,
Canada). The survey encompassed clinical, biochemical, and
dietary studies on 1,865 Indians from six regions across
the country and 366 Eskimos from four major settlements. In
children and adolescents some weight deficits were observed,
particularly among Eskimos. Protein intakes were not fully
adequate among all children, but serum protein levels were

normal. Iron deficiency was common. Eskimos showed almost
universally low serum folate values, and Indians somewhat
less frequently. Intakes of vitamin D and calcium were low
in most diets, but serum calcium levels were normal and
rickets was not observed. Dietary deficits of vitamin A
were common. Vitamin C deficits were striking among Eskimos
and moderately prevalent among Indians. In adults onset of
obesity was early in Eskimos, although caloric intakes were
strikingly low. Iron deficiency was demonstrable in significant proportions of most age and sex groups. Eskimo men had
a higher prevalence of anaemia in the presence of good iron
intakes. The folate situation was the same as for children.
Vitamin A intakes were frequently low. Eskimos had the
highest prevalence of clinical signs suggestive of vitamin
C deficiency. Low serum vitamin C levels and low dietary
intakes were frequent among Indians and very common among
Eskimos. Goitre was rare among Eskimos and infrequent among
Indians. In general the nutritional status of the general
population was better than that of Indians, which in turn
was better than that of Eskimos.

"Metabolic disease in arctic populations," by Edward M.
Scott (Alaska Activities, Center for Disease Control,
Anchorage, Alaska, USA). Small populations, inadequate
methodology, and lack of a base for comparison have made
the prevalence of metabolic disease difficult to determine
in the arctic. Diabetes mellitus has been shown to be rare
in Eskimos and northern Indians, but is more common in
Aleuts. Eskimos have become less tolerant of glucose in the
past ten years. Analysis of discharge diagnoses from
Alaskan hospitals suggests unusual distributions and occurrence of certain diseases. Although goitre, presumably due
to iodine deficiency, was demonstrated earlier, it is not
found now. Both thyrotoxicosis and myxoedema in Athabaskan
Indians occur with only one-third the frequency that is
found in Eskimos and in Tlingit Indians. Cholelithiasis is
only half as frequent in northern Eskimos and Athabaskans
as in southern Eskimos and Tlingits. Rheumatoid arthritis
is much more frequent in Tlingits but in Eskimos and
Indians it is as common in men as in women. A small number
of cases of gout were reported in southern Eskimos.

"Glucose tolerance among Aleuts on the Pribilof Islands,"
by S.E. Dippe, P.H. Bennett, D.W. Dippe, T. Humphry, J.
Burks, and M. Miller (Southwestern Field Studies Section,
NIAMDD, NIH, Phoenix, Ariz., USA). An oral glucose tolerance test using a 75 g carbohydrate load was performed on
335 Aleuts (175 male and 160 female) aged 10 to 78 years.
Twenty-four Aleuts (9M, 15F) had a 2-hour plasma glucose
(2hPG) $\geq$ 200 mg/100 ml. Over 39 years of age, 8 of 79 males
(10 per cent) and 13 of 49 females (27 per cent) were
found to have a 2hPG $\geq$ 200 mg/100 ml. The frequencies of
occurrence of a 2hPG $\geq$ 160 mg/100 ml and $\geq$ 140 mg/100 ml
were 22 per cent and 25 per cent for males and 35 per cent
and 45 per cent for females, respectively. Eleven of the
24 Aleuts (46 per cent) who had a 2hPG $\geq$ 200 mg/100 ml
said they had diabetes and 9 were taking some hypoglycaemic
agent. The mean duration was 5 years. Three persons with a
2hPG < 200 mg/100 ml (68, 188, 167) said they had diabetes.

Females were heavier than males and diabetics were
heavier than non-diabetics. Using the mean percentage desirable weight (MPDW), the following results were obtained:

2hPG		< 140	140-199	> 200
MPDW	M	116	137	133
	F	134	150	154

Thirty-one per cent of all Aleuts had a serum triglyceride level greater than 150 mg/100 ml, whereas 88 per
cent of diabetics (2h$\geq$200 mg/100 ml) had triglyceride
levels above 150 mg/100 ml. Six of the 10 Aleuts with a
triglyceride level $\geq$ 500 mg/100 ml were diabetic. Cholesterol levels did not differ between diabetics and non-
diabetics. The frequency of occurrence of diabetes on the
islands of St Paul and St George which make up the Pribilof
Islands was the same.

Diabetes mellitus is very prevalent among Aleuts of the
Pribilof Islands and is considerably more prevalent than
among Eskimos and Alaskan Indians. The frequency of occurrence of diabetes is lower but more closely related to
that of the Pima Indians of Arizona, who have the highest
reported prevalence in the world.

"Biochemical mechanisms of human adaptation to the extreme
factors of the north," by L. Panin (Institute of Clinical
and Experimental Medicine of the Siberian Branch of the
Academy of Medical Sciences of the USSR, Novosibirsk, USSR).
Adaptation of aboriginal and alien populations in the polar
regions is an extremely complicated process, the study of

which requires an assessment of such factors as sex, age,
nutritional status, and the duration of residence in the
north. We have found an increase in the II-oxysteroid level
in the alien population of Norilsk after 1 to 2 months of
living in the north. In Nganasans the II-oxysteroid content
was the same as in the corresponding group in Novosibirsk.
We have established 12-hour rhythms in the sugar content of
blood, and 24-hour rhythms in the free fatty acid content,
lipoprotein, and II-oxysteroid content. We have also found
marked seasonal fluctuations in the indices of carbohydrate-
lipid metabolism. They are characterized by an increase in
the content of sugar, pyruvic and lactic acids, and phospholipids with a simultaneous decrease in the content of
free fatty acid and total lipids during the polar day, and
a decrease in the content of sugar, pyruvic and lactic
acids, and phospholipids with a simultaneous increase in
the content of free fatty acid and total lipids during the
polar night. The ascorbic acid content of plasma and its
excretion with urine are within the normal limits during
the polar night and sharply decrease during the polar day.
We believe that seasonal fluctuations in some indices of
carbohydrate-lipid metabolism (sugar, pyruvic and lactic
acids, free fatty acid) are determined by fluctuations in
the vitamin balance of the organisms and reflect disadapta-
tive changes.

"Bone mineral content of north Alaskan Eskimos," by Richard
B. Mazess and Warren Mather (Department of Radiology/
Medical Physics, University of Wisconsin Hospitals,
Madison, Wis., USA). Direct photon absorptiometry was used
to measure the bone mineral content of forearm bones in
Eskimo natives of the north coast of Alaska. The sample consisted of 217 children, 89 adults, and 107 elderly (over 50
years). Eskimo children had a lower bone mineral content
than United States whites by 5 to 10 per cent, but this was
consistent with their smaller body and bone size. Young
Eskimo adults (20 to 39 years) of both sexes were similar
to whites, but after age 40 the Eskimos of both sexes had a
deficit of from 10 to 15 per cent relative to white standards. Aging bone loss, which occurs in many populations,
has an earlier onset and greater intensity in the Eskimos.
Nutritional factors of high protein, high nitrogen, high
phosphorus, and low calcium intakes may be implicated. The
results are summarized in Tables 1 - 6. (Note that the
complete paper will appear in American Journal of Clinical
Nutrition, Vol. 27, 1974.)

TABLE 1
Morphology of Alaskan Eskimo children and adults and Eskimo values as a percentage of white values

Age (years)	No.	Height (cm)				Weight (kg)			
		X̄	SD	CV	%	X̄	SD	CV	%
Males									
5-7	23	116.9	5.3	4.6	93.2*	23.3	2.8	12.1	94.0
8-9	19	129.8	7.5	5.8	94.1*	30.4	5.1	16.8	97.4
10-11	22	140.1	7.4	5.3	95.6*	35.2	5.4	15.4	95.4
12-14	20	151.0	8.9	5.9	94.0*	47.5	10.8	22.7	94.8
15-16	9	162.9	5.6	3.5	92.6*	55.1	6.5	11.8	81.6*
17-19	15	171.0	8.5	5.0	94.9*	69.7	7.0	10.0	91.3**
20-29	16	168.6	4.7	2.8	94.2*	70.0	6.5	9.3	91.7**
30-39	17	167.7	7.1	4.2	93.4*	67.4	10.1	15.0	84.5**
40-49	7	166.9	6.8	4.1	94.3*	67.9	8.9	13.0	86.2*
50-59	13	166.1	4.0	2.4	93.6*	74.5	11.6	15.5	93.7
60-69	27	163.2	4.8	2.9	93.2*	67.7	12.9	19.0	89.2**
70-82	13	163.0	4.8	2.9	93.2*	69.8	12.6	18.1	94.2
Females									
5-7	26	119.5	7.5	6.3	94.4*	24.8	5.8	23.4	102.5
8-9	22	123.0	5.9	4.6	90.2*	28.9	3.9	13.7	97.6
10-11	17	139.7	7.7	5.5	95.5*	37.3	8.2	21.9	100.3
12-14	22	151.8	6.5	4.3	93.3*	53.1	11.1	21.6	107.9
15-16	10	157.4	3.8	2.4	94.6*	58.7	6.6	11.3	104.6
17-19	12	157.6	4.6	2.9	95.3*	59.8	5.3	8.8	102.4
20-29	14	157.1	5.6	3.5	96.0*	60.8	12.7	20.9	104.6
30-39	19	155.1	6.0	3.9	94.1*	63.6	14.2	22.3	97.5
40-49	16	152.3	7.6	5.0	95.0*	65.5	15.9	24.2	102.7
50-59	23	153.3	7.7	5.0	95.2*	62.4	11.5	18.5	97.8
60-69	20	152.8	5.6	3.7	96.0*	65.5	15.4	23.6	104.3
70-81	11	141.3	10.2	7.2	89.3*	48.6	10.7	22.0	77.6*

* Significance of difference by t test: $p < 0.01$.
** Significance of difference by t test: $p < 0.05$.

TABLE 2

Bone mineral measurements of the shaft of the radius of Alaskan Eskimo children and adults and Eskimo values as a percentage of white values

Age (years)	No.	Mineral (mg/cm)				Width (m × 10⁻⁵)				BMC/W			
		$\bar{X}$	SD	CV	%	$\bar{X}$	SD	CV	%	$\bar{X}$	SD	CD	%
Males													
5-7	23	462	73	15.9	93.3	1,006	203	20.2	102.3	0.466	0.061	13.0	92.6*
8-9	19	536	71	13.3	92.6**	1,005	117	11.6	96.0	0.533	0.045	8.6	96.4
10-11	22	626	90	14.4	93.7	1,086	93	8.5	96.4	0.574	0.060	10.5	96.8
12-14	20	760	138	18.1	92.9	1,189	137	11.5	94.7**	0.636	0.060	9.4	98.0
15-16	9	926	87	9.4	84.5*	1,293	87	6.7	89.7*	0.715	0.050	7.0	94.1
17-19	15	1,163	130	11.8	94.2	1,411	95	6.7	95.4	0.823	0.059	7.1	98.4
20-29	16	1,273	155	12.2	97.4	1,497	157	10.5	101.4	0.852	0.088	10.4	96.3
30-39	17	1,200	117	9.7	90.8*	1,458	110	7.6	98.6	0.823	0.066	8.0	92.0*
40-49	7	1,171	91	7.8	89.8*	1,514	128	8.4	102.0	0.774	0.061	7.8	88.0*
50-59	13	1,125	96	8.5	87.7*	1,508	119	7.9	101.3	0.748	0.072	9.6	85.0*
60-69	27	1,017	160	15.7	83.0*	1,499	160	10.6	95.5	0.680	0.100	14.7	86.1*
70-82	13	1,058	103	9.7	84.2*	1,530	148	9.6	98.5	0.693	0.063	9.1	85.5*
Females													
5-7	26	437	72	16.4	98.2	922	151	16.4	101.2	0.475	0.056	11.9	97.3
8-9	22	483	53	11.0	92.4**	929	121	12.4	97.3	0.497	0.054	11.0	90.7*
10-11	17	558	70	12.6	91.9	958	104	10.9	92.6*	0.582	0.040	6.9	99.7
12-14	22	762	129	16.9	96.7	1,115	135	12.1	95.9	0.681	0.078	11.4	100.6
15-16	10	848	50	5.8	97.0	1,184	103	8.7	98.7	0.718	0.045	6.3	98.5
17-19	12	878	100	11.4	95.7	1,192	154	12.9	97.5	0.738	0.049	6.6	98.4
20-29	14	889	108	12.1	93.4**	1,116	144	12.3	94.8**	0.764	0.055	7.2	98.7
30-39	19	928	127	13.7	92.8	1,262	168	13.3	96.8	0.736	0.059	8.0	95.7
40-49	16	883	124	14.1	90.4*	1,273	125	10.0	98.1	0.693	0.066	9.5	90.8*
50-59	23	782	140	17.8	88.4*	1,282	118	9.2	102.4	0.609	0.081	13.4	86.3*
60-69	20	685	112	16.4	89.1**	1,278	144	11.3	101.5	0.536	0.072	13.5	87.9*
70-81	11	507	131	25.9	70.2*	1,264	78	6.2	100.7	0.399	0.090	-22.5	69.4*

* Significance of difference by t test: p < 0.01.
** Significance of difference by t test: p < 0.05.

TABLE 3
Bone mineral measurements of the shaft of the ulna of Alaskan Eskimo children and adults and Eskimo values as a percentage of white values

Age (years)	No.	Mineral (mg/cm)				Width (m × 10^{-5})				BMC/w			
		X̄	SD	CV	%	X̄	SD	CV	%	X̄	SD	CV	%
Males													
5-7	23	402	71	17.5	99.5	906	129	14.3	105.8	0.443	0.041	9.4	93.7**
8-9	19	456	84	18.4	95.6	928	149	16.1	99.8	0.490	0.050	10.2	95.5
10-11	22	543	94	17.3	98.0	1,012	107	10.6	105.2**	0.535	0.064	12.0	92.7*
12-14	20	661	111	16.7	100.5	1,062	114	10.7	102.7	0.618	0.058	9.3	97.3
15-16	9	817	62	7.6	89.0**	1,162	95	8.2	96.8	0.706	0.073	10.4	92.4
17-19	15	1,005	126	12.6	97.2	1,167	70	6.0	92.6**	0.859	0.085	9.8	103.9
20-29	16	1,060	119	11.3		1,205	90	7.4		0.877	0.069	7.8	
30-39	17	1,067	135	12.7		1,189	81	6.8		0.895	0.083	9.3	
40-49	7	1,032	85	8.2		1,223	84	6.9		0.844	0.053	6.3	
50-59	13	1,066	132	12.4		1,308	102	7.8		0.815	0.072	8.8	
60-69	27	930	181	19.5		1,235	136	11.0		0.751	0.111	14.7	
70-82	13	946	125	13.2		1,251	82	6.6		0.755	0.075	9.9	
Females													
5-7	26	371	63	16.7	100.8	826	80	9.7	103.1	0.455	0.055	12.0	98.9
8-9	22	412	58	14.0	892.0	865	94	10.9	100.6	0.477	0.053	11.2	90.9**
10-11	17	480	60	12.6	95.4	862	117	13.6	94.8	0.558	0.046	8.2	101.5
12-14	22	642	117	18.2		958	107	11.1		0.669	0.093	13.9	
15-16	10	752	45	6.0		1,043	69	6.6		0.721	0.045	6.3	
17-19	12	767	98	12.8		1,011	95	9.4		0.759	0.070	9.2	
20-29	14	793	65	8.2	94.1	980	87	8.9	91.2	0.810	0.057	7.1	102.4
30-39	19	815	88	10.7	93.7	1,024	102	9.9	95.8	0.797	0.076	9.5	96.7
40-49	16	811	90	11.2		1,106	118	10.6		0.734	0.058	8.0	
50-59	23	712	148	20.8	88.6**	1,096	112	10.2	99.2	0.646	0.093	14.4	88.7*
60-69	20	647	105	16.3	92.2	1,110	129	11.6	100.1	0.585	0.093	15.9	93.6
70-81	11	462	133	28.9	75.1*	1,037	109	16.5	94.0	0.442	0.106	23.9	78.6*

See Table 2 for explanation of * and **.

TABLE 4

Bone mineral measurements of the midshaft of the humerus of Alaskan Eskimo children and adults and Eskimo values as a percentage of white values

Age (years)	No.	Mineral (mg/cm)				Width (m x 10^{-5})				M/W			
		X̄	SD	CV	%	X̄	SD	CV	%	X̄	SD	CV	%
Males													
5–7	9	974	147	15.1	90.4	1,384	115	8.3	95.2	0.701	0.082	11.8	94.6
8–9	10	1,138	153	13.4	89.7*	1,535	125	8.1	97.0	0.737	0.056	7.6	91.8*
10–11	8	1,432	168	11.7	97.6	1,699	117	6.9	98.1	0.840	0.059	7.0	99.2
12–14	7	1,773	256	14.4	101.5	1,883	90	4.8	98.5	0.937	0.116	12.4	102.6
15–16	3	1,982	276	13.9	84.4	1,987	46	2.3	91.2**	0.995	0.122	12.3	92.5
17–19	8	2,518	316	12.5	91.4**	2,110	81	3.8	93.2**	1.191	0.133	11.1	97.7
20–29	12	2,760	327	11.8	99.8	2,157	160	7.4	93.6***	1.279	0.122	9.5	106.6*
30–39	10	2,840	393	13.8	103.9	2,256	140	6.2	98.1	1.254	0.125	10.0	105.6
40–49	4	2,748	349	12.7	104.0	2,145	126	5.9	92.7	1.279	0.143	11.1	108.3
50–59	3	2,763	233	8.4	99.4	2,213	193	8.7	94.5	1.259	0.196	15.6	105.9
60–69	9	2,336	472	20.2	90.6	2,228	92	4.1	96.9	1.047	0.201	19.2	93.3
70–82													
Females													
5–7	12	917	146	16.0	93.4	1,309	112	8.5	92.4**	0.696	0.069	10.0	100.3
8–9	9	1,015	137	13.5	86.6*	1,433	92	6.4	93.1**	0.706	0.090	12.8	92.9**
10–11	9	1,106	154	13.9	87.5	1,519	63	4.2	95.1	0.727	0.099	13.6	92.5
12–14	14	1,635	278	17.0	97.2	1,771	169	9.6	97.0	0.920	0.116	12.6	100.1
15–16	5	1,898	167	8.8	100.1	1,812	151	8.3	96.6	1.045	0.054	5.2	103.2
17–19	4	1,724	226	13.1	86.5	1,852	123	6.6	98.3	0.929	0.099	10.7	87.9**
20–29	6	1,820	215	11.8	86.7**	1,817	93	5.1	91.4**	0.988	0.067	6.8	93.6
30–39	9	2,001	257	12.9	94.5	1,902	191	10.0	96.6	1.052	0.104	9.8	98.0
40–49	4	1,911	206	10.8	91.8	1,917	67	3.5	95.2	0.993	0.075	7.6	96.1
50–59	4	1,570	184	11.7	86.7	1,845	130	7.1	95.1	0.855	0.137	16.1	90.7
60–69													
70–81													

See Table 1 or 2 for explanation of * and **.

TABLE 5

Bone mineral measurements of the distal radius of Alaskan Eskimo children and adults; Eskimo values as a percentage of white values are given

Age (years)	No.	Mineral (mg/cm)				Width (m × 10⁻⁵)				BMC/W			
		X̄	SD	CV	%	X̄	SD	CV	%	X̄	SD	CV	%
Males													
5-7	14	478	86	18.0		1,464	194	13.2		0.326	0.043	13.1	
8-9	9	554	80	14.5		1,592	269	16.9		0.349	0.019	15.4	
10-11	14	608	80	13.2		1,740	164	9.4		0.349	0.039	11.1	
12-14	13	769	207	26.9		1,917	489	25.5		0.407	0.072	17.6	
15-16	6	1,007	225	22.3		2,459	501	20.4		0.409	0.033	8.0	
17-19	7	1,397	248	17.7		2,701	391	14.5		0.517	0.068	13.1	
20-29	4	1,568	179	11.4	113.1	3,020	391	13.0	128.9*	0.523	0.069	13.2	87.2
30-39	7	1,433	185	12.9	108.8	2,702	221	8.2	118.4*	0.530	0.058	11.0	90.1
40-49	3	1,308	238	18.2	100.8	3,300	171	5.2	152.6*	0.395	0.062	15.7	65.0*
50-59	19	1,213	255	21.0	912.0	2,847	348	12.2	129.3*	0.428	0.090	21.0	69.7*
60-69	18	1,052	209	19.9	88.3	2,712	335	12.3	114.8**	0.394	0.098	24.8	76.4*
70-82	10	1,029	190	18.4	86.7	2,535	396	15.6	108.8	0.410	0.075	18.2	76.5**
Females													
5-7	14	423	67	15.8		1,305	180	13.8		0.326	0.048	14.8	
8-9	13	438	80	18.2		1,442	271	18.8		0.307	0.044	14.5	
10-11	8	539	83	15.4		1,561	297	19.1		0.357	0.087	24.3	
12-14	8	712	185	25.9		2,014	346	17.2		0.352	0.058	16.5	
15-16	5	881	182	20.6		2,352	90	3.8		0.373	0.066	17.7	
17-19	8	969	153	15.8		2,121	513	24.2		0.473	0.092	19.5	
20-29	8	1,080	191	17.7	109.8	2,435	480	19.7	131.1*	0.449	0.060	13.4	83.3*
30-39	10	964	163	16.9	100.9	2,404	423	17.6	147.0*	0.468	0.079	16.9	83.0**
40-49	12	1,042	162	15.6	111.7	2,364	256	10.8	121.0**	0.444	0.069	15.6	89.9
50-59	10	935	218	23.3	105.4	2,382	362	15.2	128.3*	0.397	0.097	24.4	82.4*
60-69	18	696	161	23.2	93.8	2,256	368	16.3	118.6*	0.315	0.088	27.9	78.4*
70-81	11	472	146	30.9	65.7*	1,830	457	24.9	100.5*	0.263	0.084	31.9	65.9*

See Table 1 or 2 for explanation of * and **.

TABLE 6

Bone mineral measurements of the distal ulna of Eskimo children and adults; Eskimo values as a percentage of white values are given

Age (years)	No.	Mineral (mg/cm)				Width (m × 10^-5)				BMC/W			
		X̄	SD	CV	%	X̄	SD	CV	%	X̄	SD	CV	%
Males													
5-7	14	271	54	19.9		876	103	11.8		0.311	0.055	17.6	
8-9	9	305	57	18.7		915	181	19.7		0.336	0.033	9.9	
10-11	14	330	49	14.9		945	108	11.5		0.351	0.050	14.5	
12-14	13	415	87	21.1		1,045	220	21.1		0.400	0.066	16.6	
15-16	6	520	82	15.8		1,191	147	12.3		0.436	0.044	10.2	
17-19	7	712	142	20.0		1,319	273	20.7		0.544	0.078	14.3	
20-29	4	847	103	12.1		1,423	241	17.0		0.598	0.034	5.7	
30-39	7	721	103	14.3		1,140	116	10.2		0.630	0.046	7.3	
40-49	4	699	54	7.7		1,285	110	8.5		0.545	0.038	6.9	
50-59	10	656	125	19.1		1,242	126	10.2		0.532	0.110	20.6	
60-69	18	563	118	20.9		1,196	136	11.4		0.472	0.086	18.3	
70-82	10	514	81	15.7		1,133	159	14.1		0.455	0.053	11.6	
Females													
5-7	14	234	35	15.0		776	88	11.4		0.303	0.048	15.8	
8-9	13	236	35	14.7		831	114	13.7		0.287	0.046	16.2	
10-11	8	307	64	20.9		876	87	10.0		0.355	0.092	26.1	
12-14	8	368	71	19.4		1,057	149	14.1		0.348	0.052	14.9	
15-16	5	465	91	19.6		1,171	211	18.1		0.406	0.098	24.2	
17-19	8	503	76	15.1		1,091	251	23.0		0.476	0.095	20.0	
20-29	8	528	98	18.7	103.3	1,089	207	19.0	109.0	0.494	0.099	20.0	96.7
30-39	10	483	70	14.6	96.9	1,042	125	12.0	103.4	0.468	0.079	16.9	92.4
40-49	12	503	118	23.4		1,052	118	11.2		0.479	0.099	20.6	
50-59	19	470	102	21.7	104.0	1,098	129	11.8	113.1*	0.427	0.071	16.6	91.0
60-69	18	333	75	22.6	91.5	1,012	130	12.9	101.2	0.332	0.079	23.9	90.7
70-81	11	220	74	33.8	66.7*	889	259	29.1	85.6**	0.254	0.066	26.3	79.9**

See Table 1 or 2 for explanation of * and **.

"Bone mineral content in Canadian Eskimos," by Richard B.
Mazess and Warren E. Mather (Department of Radiology/
Medical Physics, University of Wisconsin Hospitals,
Madison, Wis., USA). Bone mineral content was measured
using direct photon absorptiometry in the forearm bones of
Canadian Eskimos in the northern Foxe Basin. The sample
consisted of 177 children, 92 young adults, and 66 older
adults. Canadian Eskimo children had a slightly lower bone
mineral content, 4 to 5 per cent, than Alaskan Eskimo
children, and a much lower bone mineral content, 10 to 13
per cent, than US Whites, but these group differences were
commensurate with the lower weights of the Canadian children. Throughout adulthood, the Canadian Eskimo bone mineral content was almost identical with average values for
Alaskan Eskimos; the major differences were lower mineral-
width ratios in the Canadian Eskimo males over 50 years of
age. Thus the Canadian Eskimo-White differences paralleled
the relative deficit demonstrated for Alaskan Eskimos, with
the exception that relative bone loss in elderly males
seemed even greater in the Canadian than in the Alaskan
group. Eskimo males had a bone loss of about 10 per cent a
decade, and Eskimo females about 15 per cent a decade, beginning in the forties; in both sexes, this was about 5 per
cent per decade greater than the aging bone loss seen in
the US Whites; the onset of the bone loss was also a decade
sooner in Eskimo males. (Note that the complete paper will
appear in Human Biology, 1974.)

GENETIC CONSIDERATIONS

Current genetic trends in the Greenlandic population

B.J. HARVALD

During the last decade, most genetic polymorphisms (i.e. gene loci where the frequencies of at least two alleles are higher than 0.01) have been examined in the Greenlandic population. The population is composed of three distinct groups: West-Greenlanders, East-Greenlanders, and Thule Eskimos. Among the two latter groups, there are subgroups with very little or no admixture of European blood.

Table 1 surveys the most consistent results. In all four groups of polymorphisms, erythrocyte enzymes (1), erthrocyte antigens (2), immunoglobulins (6,7) and transplantation antigens (3), there is a characteristic absence of alleles that attain considerable frequencies in Caucasian populations. There is a special "shortage" of alleles with regard to immunoglobulins (where apparently only two different chromosome types are found in Eskimos against at least 11 types in Caucasians), and HL-A antigens (where only 9 are found in Eskimos against at least 33 in Caucasians).

On assumption that the different alleles listed in Table 1 were missing in the original Eskimo population of West-Greenland, their current presence must be due to admixture of European alleles with the original gene pool. On the basis of the frequencies observed in West-Greenland and in Northern Europe, from where most immigrants are derived, it is possible to estimate the ratio between Eskimo and European genes in the West-Greenlandic population. From independent studies, this averages 3:1 in people born in Greenland of Greenlandic mothers. Of course, the ratio is not fixed; since 1950, the number of Danes working in Greenland has increased, and this has accelerated the cross-breeding process.

Some alleles missing in Eskimos occur with modest frequencies among East-Asians but in other cases the same alleles are also missing in Indian and in East-Asian gene

TABLE 1
Polymorphisms in "pure" Eskimos from Thule and Angmassalik

Locus	Characteristics
Erythrocyte enzymes	
Adenylate kinase (AK)	no AK^2-allele
6-phosphogluconate dehydrogenase (PGD)	no PGD^b-allele
Adenosine deaminase (ADA)	no ADA^2-allele
Acid phosphatase	no P^c-allele
Erythrocyte antigens	
ABO-system	no A_2-allele
Rhesus-system	no cde-allele
Kell-system	no K-allele
Immunoglobulins	
Heavy chain subgroups	only two types of chromosomes: az; $g_3 5$ az; $b^2 b^5$ - st b^0 (Caucasians 11 types)
Transplantation antigens	
LA series + Four series	9 antigens (Caucasians 33 antigens)

pools (8). This is the case with regard to the listed erythrocyte antigens, to most of the heavy chain subgroups,
and to the transplantation antigens. Thus the "shortage".of
alleles seems a common trait of East-Asians, Indians, and
Eskimos, who are thought to descend from the same ancestors.

It cannot be totally excluded that the apparent "shortage" of alleles in East Asians is due to the fact that polymorphisms in Caucasians have been studied much more intensively, leaving special East-Asian polymorphisms to be described in the future. If the shortage of alleles is real,
one explanation could be that the East-Asians have descended from a small original population that has lived a rather
isolated existence without admixture of foreign genes. This
may hold true in East-Asia, in contrast to Europe, which
has been overrun by intruding conquerors time after time.
Conquests by Asians, together with a considerable importa-
tion of African slaves, have probably contributed to an en-
richment of the European gene pool.

It looks as if the original Eskimo and Indian gene pools
are even poorer than the East-Asian, probably a result of
small numbers in the original population ("founder effect")
combined with a dropping out of low frequency alleles by
mere chance ("genetic drift"). Selective forces may, of
course, have been active in this process.

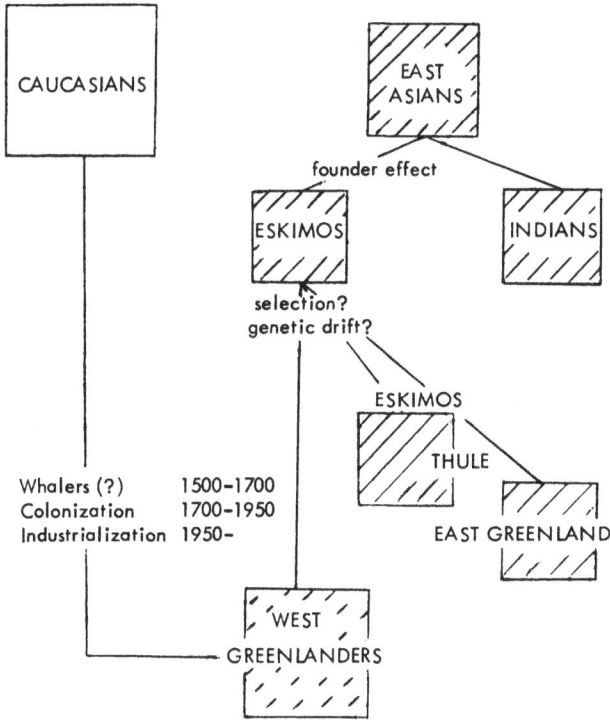

Figure 1   Estimate of gene pools, on the basis of the number of alleles in polymorphic systems

Figure 1 gives a rough estimate of the gene pools in these different populations. A high number of alleles and high frequencies of several alleles in the same locus mean a higher chance of heterozygotism, so the areas of the squares are thought to express the average relative chance of heterozygotism. With the massive influx of Caucasian genes into West-Greenland, the gene pool of West-Greenlanders must be expected to increase.

The practical implications of the described differences in polymorphic systems are not totally clear. Heterozygotism may mean a higher degree of adaptability and in this way an increased probability of survival. The connection between erythrocyte type and disease has been known for 20 years, and more recently even stronger correlations between transplantation antigens and diseases have been described. In this context it is of interest that the Hl-A antigen 27 is correlated with morbus Bechterew, morbus Reiter,

gonorrhoeaic, Yersinia and Salmonella arthritis, and anterior uveitis (9). These disorders are very frequent in
Greenland and at the same time the HL-A antigen 27 is four
times as frequent in pure Eskimos as in the Danish population. Multiple sclerosis is correlated with HL-A 3, HL-A 7,
and W 18, which all occur with low frequencies in pure Eskimos, in whom also multiple sclerosis seem to be rare.
Juvenile diabetes is correlated with HL-A 1 and 8 (5);
these antigens do not occur in Eskimos, offering a possible
explanation of the non-occurrence of juvenile diabetes in
Greenlanders. The high frequency of choriocarcinoma in
Greenland may be a consequence of the low number of transplantation antigens, giving a higher chance of mother-child
compatibility, which may in turn mean a higher chance for
the chorion cells to survive in the maternal organism (4).

SUMMARY

In several polymorphic systems, alleles that have considerable frequencies in Caucasians do not occur in Eskimos.
The relative "shortage" of alleles means a lower average
heterozygotism of which the origin and genetic implications
are not totally clear. Considering the well-known associations between erythrocyte- and HL-A-antigens and different
diseases, differences in the polymorphic systems may explain in part the different occurrences of many disorders
in Caucasian and Eskimo populations. Thus, the non-
occurrence of juvenile diabetes in Eskimos may be due to
low frequencies of HL-A antigen 1 and 8.

REFERENCES

1. Dissing, J., "Erythrocyte enzyme polymorphism in Greenland," Second International Symposium on Circumpolar
   Health, Oulu, 1971
2. Gürtler, H., Gilberg, Aa., and Tingsgaard, P., "Blodtypefordelingen i Grønland," Dansk Medicinsk Selskab,
   1: 21 (1973)
3. Kissmeyer-Nielsen, F., Andersen, H., Hauge, M., Karen
   E. Kjerbye, Mogensen, B., and Svejgaard, A., "HL-A-
   types in Danish Eskimos from Greenland," Tissue Antigens, 1: 74-80 (1971)
4. Mogensen, B., and Kissmeyer-Nielsen, F., "The prognostic
   application of HL-A and ABO typing in placental choriocarcinoma," Dan. med. Bull., 16: 243 (1969)

5. Neerup, J., "HL-A and diabetes mellitus," Paper read at
   the 34th Nordic Congress of Internal Medicine, Aalborg
   (Denmark), 27-29 June 1974
6. Nielsen, J.C., Martensson, L., Gürtler, H., Gilberg, Aa.,
   and Tingsgård, P., "Gm types of Greenlandic Eskimos,"
   Human Hered., 21: 405-9 (1971)
7. Persson, I., Rivat, L., Rousseau, P.Y., and Ropartz,
   C., "Ten Gm factors and the Inv system in Eskimos in
   Greenland," Human Hered., 22: 519-28 (1972)
8. Scott, E.M., Duncan, I.W., Ekstrand, V., and Wright,
   R.C., "Frequency of polymorphic types of red cell enzymes and serum factors in Alaskan Eskimos and Indians,"
   Am. J. hum. Genet., 18: 408-12 (1966)
9. Svejgaard, A., "HL-A and disease," Paper read at the
   34th Nordic Congress of Internal Medicine, Aalborg
   (Denmark), 27-29 June 1974

The origin of the Lapps in the light of
recent genetic studies

A.W. ERIKSSON, J. FELLMAN, H. FORSIUS, W. LEHMANN,
T. LEWIN, and P. LUUKKA

The Lapps deviate in many genetic and external characters
from other peoples of the Finno-Ugrian language group, such
as Finns and Estonians. The relation between Lappish and
other Finno-Ugrian languages (including Finnish) is still
controversial (7). A considerable proportion of the ancestors of the present-day Lapps are supposed to have been
spread over almost the whole of Finland and the northern
parts of Fennoscandia. Five hundred years ago considerable
areas of northern and eastern Finland were inhabited mainly
by Lapps (Figure 1). Today there are about 35,000 Lapps in
the whole of Fennoscandia: 20,000 in Norway, 10,000 in
Sweden, 3,500 in Finland, and 1,500 on the Kola peninsula
in the Soviet Union.

One of the reasons why the commune of Inari was selected
for International Biological Program Human Adaptability
studies (9) was that this region is inhabited by three

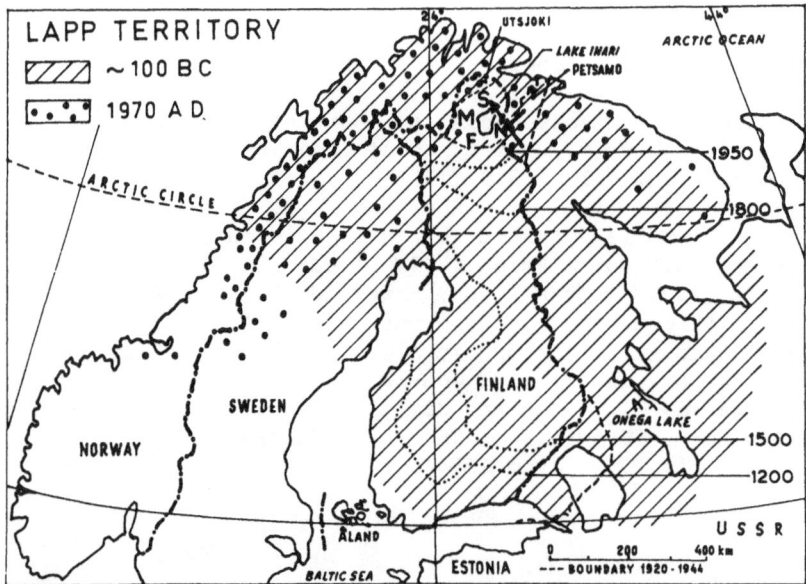

Figure 1   A comparison of Lapp territory, around 100 BC and 1970 AD

rather different Lapp populations: the Skolt Lapps in the eastern parts, the Fisher Lapps around Lake Inari, and the Mountain Lapps in the western parts of the commune. After World War II the Sevettijärvi Skolt Lapps were evacuated from the village of Suenjel and the Nellim Skolt Lapps from the regions south of the River Pasvik (Figure 1). Since World War II, the proportion of Lapps in Inari has declined markedly, although their absolute number has not decreased.

For the calculations of gene frequencies, the four groups of Sevettijärvi Skolt, Nellim Skolt, Fisher, and Mountain Lapps have been used as representatives of pure, unmixed Lapps, with only those whose ancestors over the last three generations are at least 75 per cent aboriginal Lapps being accepted. More than 95 per cent of the Skolts, 60 per cent of the Fisher Lapps, and more than 50 per cent of the Mountain Lapps have been studied. The Utsjoki series is a random sample investigated in 1973.

PHYSICAL ANTHROPOLOGY OF LAPPS

In external characteristics, the majority of the Lapps deviate from the surrounding populations. In contrast with

other Scandinavian peoples, who are among the tallest in the
world, the Lapps are short, with legs that are short both
relatively and absolutely. The Lapps are also among the most
brachycephalic (round-headed) peoples in the world, with a
cephalic index of up to 85. They have rather prominent cheekbones and a low facial height (11). The flattening of the
face, the prominence of the cheekbones, and the reduction of
the nasal prominence are not nearly so marked in Lapps as in
Mongolian populations. The inner eyefold, covering the inner
margin of the eye and responsible for the half-moon slant-
eye of many Asiatic and Amerindian peoples, is rare in Lapps.

Pigmentation

Some Lapps may have a light complexion in childhood with
quite fair hair. However, the darkening of the hair during
adolescence is much more intense than in other Nordic
peoples. A screening of hair pigmentation with "Fisher-
Saller's Haarfarbentafel," using 30 different hair colour
shades (Figure 2), shows that the Lapps, particularly the
Finnish Mountain Lapps, have considerably darker hair than
the Finns, who are one of the blondest peoples in the world
(6).
    Eye colours have been determined using Martin-Saller's
scale (Figure 3). The pigmentation of the irises and the eye
grounds (fundi) is much stronger than among the other Nordic
populations. Almost 30 per cent of the Fisher Lapps but
hardly 5 per cent of the Skolt Lapps have deep brown eyes
(7 and 8). On average, no less than 40-60 per cent of Finnish Lapps have blue eyes.
    Reflectance spectrophotometry has shown that among Fin-
nish Lapps skin colour is not yellow, as in Mongolians (unpublished observations). The Mongol spot can be found in
most children of the Mongolian race but is rare among those
of Lappish and other European populations.

Hirsute Traits of Lapps

The Lapps have soft and not uncommonly wavy hair, in contrast to the coarse, straight hair of the Mongolian race.
Microscopic studies show that the hair texture and hair pigmentation of the Skolt Lapps should be classified as European (Caucasian), not as Mongoloid (14).
    In its ample growth of hair, the white race resembles
monkeys more than any other human race. Among Lapps, beard
growth is rather sparse, and sideburns on the cheeks are
often missing. Among the Lapps, body and axillary hair

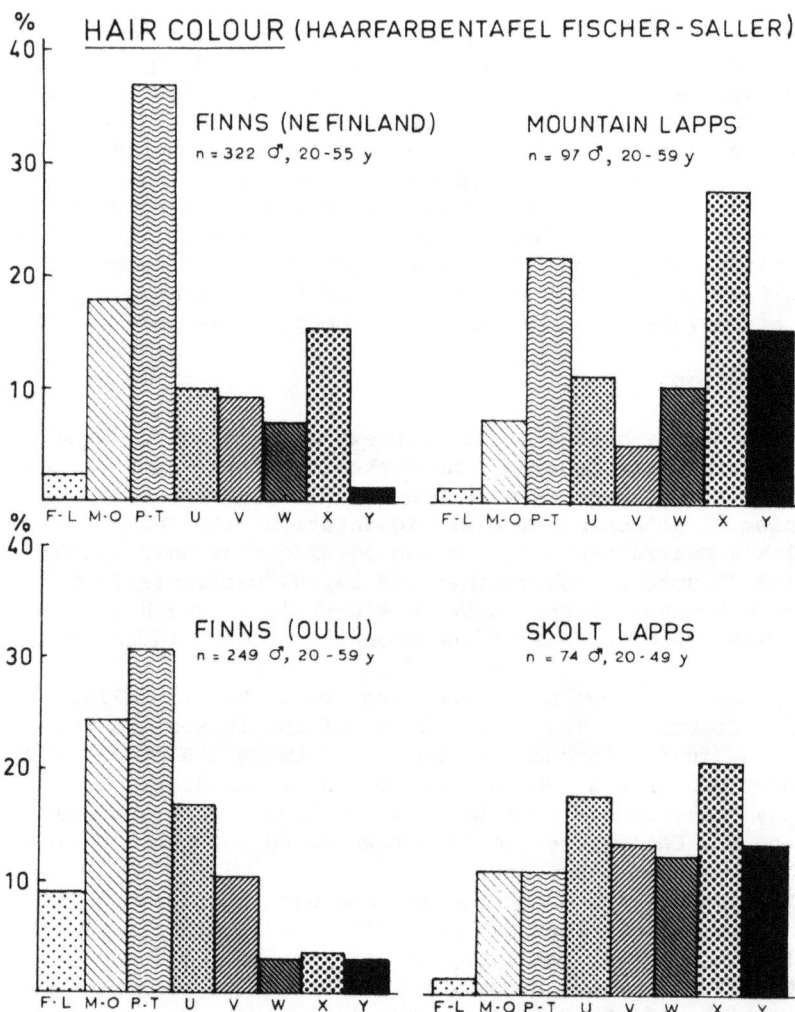

Figure 2   A comparison of hair coloration in Finns and Lapps (F-L, blond; M-O, fair; P-T, brown; U-Y, brown to black)

growth too is commonly sparse, as among the Mongoloid race.

The occurrence of middle-phalangeal hair, at least among Lapps in Finland, is as high as among other Fennoscandian populations (Swedes 70 per cent, NE Finns 80 per cent, Skolt females 75 per cent, Skolt males 95 per cent, Utsjoki Lapp females 69 per cent, Utsjoki Lapp males 74 per cent (unpublished observations). The majority of the populations

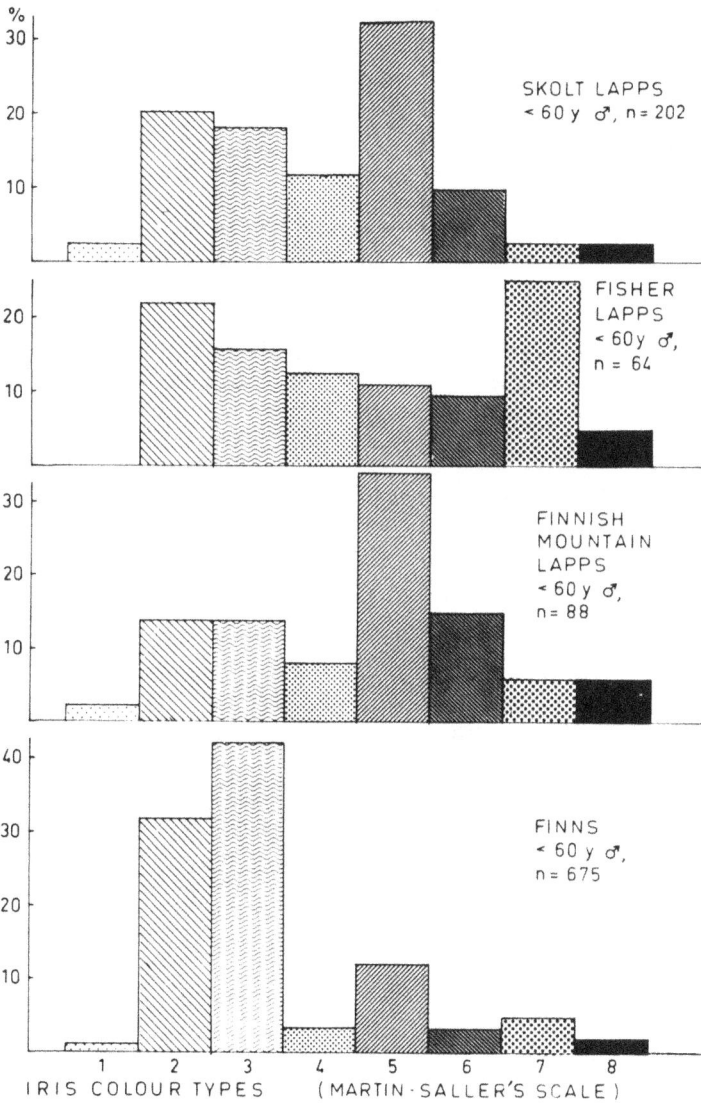

Figure 3 A comparison of iris colour types (Martin Saller's scale) for Lapps and Finns

of Mongoloid affinity so far studied seem to have considerably lower frequencies of individuals with middle-phalangeal hair.

Dermatoglyphics

The patterns of skin ridges of Skolt Lapps are mainly of
European type (8).
   The frequency of congenital dislocation of the hip among
Lapps is 20-30 times as high as among other North-European
populations.

MONOGENIC TRAITS

High Gene Frequency in Lapps

The majority of the Lapp populations so far studied in
Fennoscandia have some genetic traits in common. In comparison with the Scandinavians, the Lapps have very high frequencies of some markers. The most striking is the gene A_2,
which is about 2 to 5 times as high as in the surrounding
populations (Table 1). The Lapps have the highest frequency
of the A_2 gene in the world. The rather high frequency of
this gene in other Scandinavian populations has been interpreted as a sign of Lappish gene flow to the surrounding
populations (4).

TABLE 1
High and low gene frequencies in Lapps; the arrows indicate that the
gene frequencies resemble eastern (→) and western (←) traits

	Lapps	Other Scandinavians
High frequency in Lapps		
A_2	25 (14-37)	5
$NS_{1,13}$	15 (5-22)	8
Gm^1	2 (0-4)	1?
Inv^x	18 (13-26)	7
Ag^2	50 (40-61)	25
PGM_1^c	40 (21-55)	20
P^2	10 (2-19)	8
ADA	12 (10-16)	7
lm	60 (58-80)	30
w (dry cerumen)	30 (18-37)	17
Low frequency in Lapps		
B	6 (0-32)	11
r_2	17 (6-29)	38
Gc^2	14 (2-33)	24
se	16 (12-21)	48
AK_2^{3F}	1 (0-2)	5
C	6 (2-9)	19
t (PTC)	35 (26-55)	50

Until now, it has been believed that the A_2 gene had a
very low frequency among Siberian North-Asiatic populations.
However, a high frequency of the A_2 gene has been found recently in a north-Altayan group (Sukernik, personal communication). It will be very interesting to see what continued
subtyping of the blood group A will show in the north-
Siberian populations. A high frequency of A_2 in the northern
USSR could be interpreted in two ways, either as an indication of a relationship with the Lapps, or as evidence that
the A_2 gene is of selective advantage in arctic and subarctic regions. However, the A_2 gene seems to be completely
missing among the Ainu and the pure Eskimos.

The Mongolian gammaglobulin haplotype $Gm^{1,13}$ has been
found in all Finnish Lapp populations except Fisher Lapps.
This Mongoloid trait has, however, also been found in other
European populations, e.g. in Åland Islanders, Finns, and
Maris (13).

Figure 4 shows that among Europeans there is a distinct
increase of the Gm(1) allotype frequency in the northern
direction (south-north cline). Mediterranean populations,
e.g. Yugoslavs and Greeks, have frequencies of 30 to 40 per
cent, but in north-European populations frequencies are
60 to 70 per cent. The Lapps living in the Far North, the

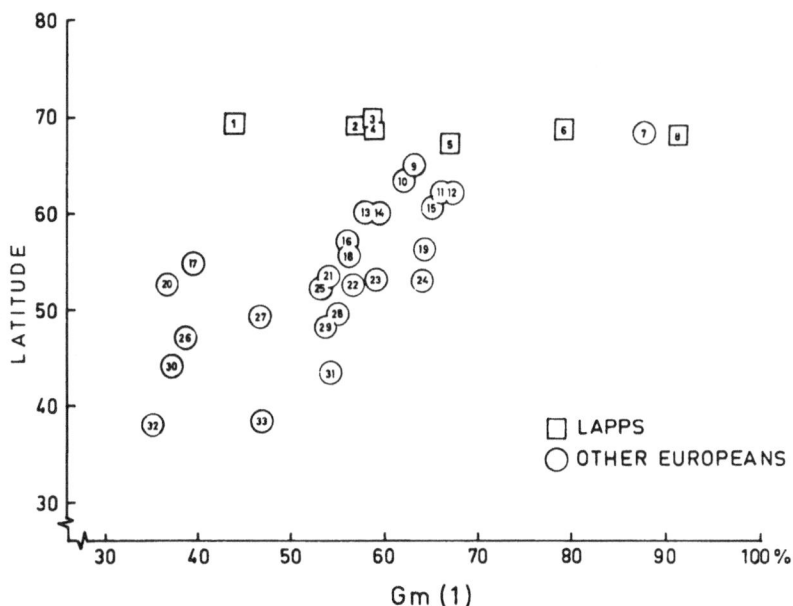

Figure 4   The relationship between latitude and frequency
of occurrence of Gm(1) gene

Inari Fisher Lapps and the Swedish Lapps have frequencies in good agreement with an increasing frequency of the Gm(1) allotype with latitude. The other Lapp populations, however, deviate from this rule, especially the Nellim Skolt Lapps, who have frequencies similar to those of Central Europeans. The advantage of having a Gm(1) constitution does not seem to be important, and in small isolated populations the effect of genetic drift, including founder effect, may be more important than any selective factors.

Among the Lapps the frequency of the gammaglobulin allele Inv[1] is 13 to 28 per cent, i.e. 2 to 4 times as high as among other Europeans. In other Finno-Ugrian populations, such as Finns and Maris, the frequency is the lowest in Europe, only 2 to 5 per cent (13).

Among Finnish Lapps the inherited lipoprotein antigen allele Ag^x is about twice as high as in other Scandinavian populations (3). Mongoloid peoples seem to have a higher frequency of Ag^x than Caucasians.

The PGM_1^2 allele seems to be another Lappish characteristic. It has an average frequency about twice as high as among other Scandinavians and the highest among Europeans. The frequency of the PGM_1^2 allele increases toward the north, both in Norway and in Finland (4). More studies are needed to elucidate whether this increasing PGM_1^2 frequency in the northern direction should be interpreted as a Lapp influence or as an effect of selection.

The red cell acid phosphatase gene P^c has a high frequency among Finnish Lapps. Among Skolt Lapps and Fisher Lapps the P^c frequency is the highest so far reported (13-19 per cent). The P^c allele is completely missing among all Asiatic populations so far studied. This trait may therefore be interpreted as a western gene.

It has been suggested that the acid phosphatase allele P^b is of selective advantage in a tropical environment (1). Recent studies have shown, however, that at least some circumpolar populations have high P^b frequencies (4).

The frequency of the adenosine deaminase gene ADA^2 among the Finnish Lapps is the highest so far reported.

Like other Europeans, the Lapps have a rather low frequency of the dry ear wax type (Figure 5).

The frequency of lactose malabsorption among adult Finnish Lapps is the highest so far reported among Europeans (see Sahi et al., this volume).

```
1.0 ─── N.CHINESE
        ─── KOREANS
        ─── MONGOLS
 .9     ─── JAPANESE

 .8

 .7     ─── NAVAJO,SIOUX
MONGOLOIDS
        ─── AINU
 .6

 .5     ─── ESKIMOS
            (N.W.Greenland)
 .4     ─── UTSJOKI LAPPS
        ─── NELLIM SKOLT LAPPS
        ─── SEVETTIJÄRVI SKOLT LAPPS
 .3     ─── MARI

        ─── FISHER LAPPS
CAUCASOIDS
 .2     ─── MOUNTAIN LAPPS
        ─── WHITES
 .1     ─── NE FINNS
        ─── U.S. NEGROES
NEGROES
 0
```

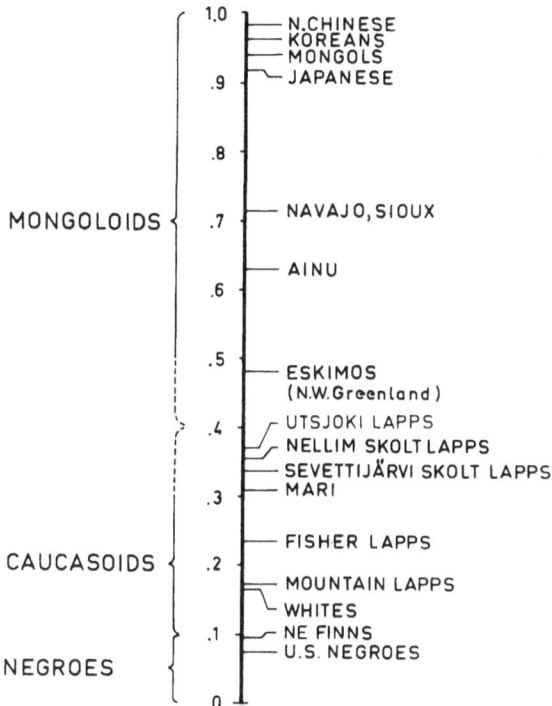

Figure 5 Frequencies of the allele for dry cerumen (w) in selected races

Low Gene Frequencies in Lapps

Except for the marginal population, known as Skolts, the Lapps have a frequency of the B gene that is about a half of that found in surrounding populations.

The frequency of Rhesus-negative individuals among western Europeans is about 15 per cent, but among Lapps is only between 2 and 9 per cent.

ABH non-secretors and Lewis (a+) subjects are only about one-third as frequent as among other Scandinavians (see Eskola et al., this volume).

To exemplify what contrasting gene frequencies can be found in small neighbouring isolates, we may mention that the Gc^2 gene frequency is extremely high in Nellim Skolt Lapps (33 per cent) with the lowest reported among Europeans in their neighbours, the Fisher Lapps (2 per cent). As far as we know, there has not been any gene exchange between these Lapp populations in recent generations.

Among all the Lapp populations studied so far, the adenylate kinase gene AK^2 is so extremely low that it may be supposed to have been extinct among the aboriginal Lapps. If genealogical studies can show that subjects with a rare allele are not pure Lapps and that the presence of this allele depends entirely on gene flow from surrounding populations, this gene frequency may be used as an indicator of gene flow from surrounding populations. Estimates based on the frequency of AK^2 and other rare genes, such as B or r, among Lapps suggest that the gene flow from the Finns to the Lapps in Inari has been between 20 and 40 per cent.

Studies of the genetic polymorphism of the third component of complement (C^l3) in serum have shown that the gene C^{3F} ($C'3^l$) is considerably lower among Lapps than among other Scandinavians (2).

The frequency of PTC non-tasters is low among Lapps in the central Lapp region, while the proportion of PTC tasters among the Skolt Lapps is the same as among other Europeans (5).

CONCLUSIONS

In some morphological characteristics, the Lapps are different from other Nordic populations. However, Swedes, Norwegians, Finns, and Russians are among the tallest and least pigmented peoples in the world. The Lapps are not more pigmented than many Central-European populations and have a considerably lighter complexion than other long-resident circumpolar populations.

Some monogenic traits of the Lapps suggest a trace of the Mongolian race. However, the Diego factor, Di(a+), restricted to the Mongolian race, has not been found in the Lapps studied so far. The transferrin alleles Tf^B0-1 and Tf^DChi are characteristic of Mongoloids and occur in fairly high frequencies in Finns and Estonians, but are rare among Lapps (4).

The Skolt Lapps deviate in many hereditary characteristics from other Lapp populations. In contrast to other Lapps, the Skolts have high frequencies of the genes B, M, r, Gc^2, and t (PTC non-tasters). There is evidence to show that the majority of the ancestors (founders) of the Skolt Lapps descended from only a few families in the sixteenth century (10).

The Lapps have always been a small ethnic group, probably never larger than today. The founder effect and randomness must have had a great influence on the gene pool.

However, this, in combination with inbreeding (16) and
selection, can hardly explain all the peculiar genetic
characteristics common to the majority of the Lapp populations so far investigated.

It is surprising that so many of the Lapp populations
have such a unique "Lappish" gene pattern, for according
to history and verbal tradition there has been a considerable gene flow from the nearby majority populations (see
von Bonsdorff et al., this volume). The fact that the Lapps
differ to such a high degree from other Nordic peoples in
both monogenic markers and external characteristics suggests
that in their ancestry they differed markedly from the
present Finns, Swedes, and Norwegians.

Certainly some of the morphological traits, such as
stature and craniofacial dimensions, have been influenced
by the hard conditions of the subarctic areas. The younger
generations of Lapps have not such extreme somatometric
characteristics (11).

For the linguist it has been a problem why the Lapps
speak a Finno-Ugrian language in spite of the fact that
they deviate so markedly from Finns and Estonians. However,
Baltic Finnish, spoken by Finns and Estonians, lacks the
dual which is typical of Lappish, Samoyedish, and Obugrish
(7). The culture of the Lapps as a whole also differs
sharply from that of the surrounding peoples, e.g. the
troll-drum used to evoke ecstasy, skin-covered skis, and
reindeer breeding. These factors indicate contact with
peoples of the northern USSR. Certain physical features and
osteological traits have been established as similar in
Lapps and Samoyeds (12).

It remains uncertain whether the ancestors of the Lapps
may have comprised relics of one or more proto-European
populations (15) and whether they may have had any contact
with peoples of the cultures of the Mesolithic periods,
about 8000 to 4500 BC, the cultures of Kunda, Suomusjärvi,
and Komsa (Ruija).

Recent studies have confirmed that the majority of the
Lapp populations still have a distinct distribution of
many genetic traits and deviate from the surrounding majority populations in some external characteristics. One is inclined to consider the Lapps, if not as a separate race,
then at least as a population descended from an original
stock. Some of the ancestral populations of the Lapps may
have had some extreme gene frequencies, which today are
still reflected in the majority of Lapp populations.

To reach more definite conclusions about the origin of the Lapps, more Lapps and neighbouring populations will have to be studied. Of particular interest are the circumpolar populations in the USSR.

ACKNOWLEDGMENTS

This work was aided by grants from the Nordiska Kulturfonden, the Finnish National Man and Biosphere Committee, and the Deutsche Forschungsgemeinschaft.

SUMMARY

In contrast to the tall, blond, and doliocephalic Nordic people, the Lapps are relatively short and dark, and among the most brachycephalic people in the world. The majority of the Lapp populations deviate from Finnish and other populations in northwestern Europe in having the highest noted frequencies of the blood group gene A_2, high frequencies of the alleles Fy^a, PGM^2, P^c, ADA^2, and low frequencies of the alleles B, r, P_1, Jk^a, Le^a, se, Gc^2, AK^2, t (PTC non-tasters). Of the gammaglobulin allotypes, Lapps have essentially Caucasoid haplotypes, with a small portion of the $Gm^{1,13}$ haplotype characteristic of Mongoloid populations. The frequency of the gene Inv^1 in Finnish Lapps is the highest known among Europeans, and w (dry cerumen) is rare. The frequency of congenital dislocation of the hip is 20 to 30 times as high among Lapps as in other North-European populations. In spite of gene flow from the surrounding majority populations and genetic drift and inbreeding in the rather small and isolated groups, most Lapp populations show similarities in several distinct gene frequencies. The inference is that the Lapps originated from different ancient peoples inhabiting northwestern Europe and at least some of these seem to have had some extreme gene frequencies that are still reflected in the present-day Lapps.

REFERENCES

1. Ananthakrishnan, R. and Walter, H., "Some notes on the geographical distribution of the human red cell acid phosphatase phenotypes," Hum. Genet., 15: 177-81 (1972)
2. Arvilommi, H., Berg, K., and Eriksson, A.W., "C3 types and their inheritance in Finnish Lapps, Maris (Cheremisses) and Greenland Eskimos," Hum. Genet., 18: 253-9 (1973)

3. Berg, K. and Eriksson, A.W., "Genetic marker systems in Arctic populations, V. The inherited Ag(x) serum lipo-protein antigen in Finnish Lapps," Human Hered., 23: 241-6 (1973)

4. Eriksson, A.W., "Genetic polymorphisms in Finno-Ugrian populations: Finns, Lapps and Maris," Israel J. med. Sci., 9: 1156-70 (1973)

5. Eriksson, A.W., Fellman, J., Forsius, H., and Lehmann, W., "Phenylthiocarbamide tasting ability among Lapps and Finns," Human Hered., 20: 623-30 (1970)

6. Forsius, H., Luukka, H., Lehmann, W., Fellman, J., and Eriksson, A.W., "Ophthalmogenetical studies on Skolt Lapps and Finns: corneal thickness, corneal refraction and iris pigmentation," Nord. Med., 84: 1559-61 (1970)

7. Itkonen, E., "Die Herkunft und Vorgeschichte der Lappen im Lichte der Sprachwissenschaft," Ural-Altaische Jb., 27: 32-44 (1955)

8. Lehmann, W., Jürgens, H.w., Forsius, H., Eriksson, A.W., Haack, M., Junkelmann, B., Bahlmann, E., and Pape, G., "Über das Hautleistensystem der Skoltlappen," Z. Morph. Anthrop., 62: 61-99 (1970)

9. Lewin, T. and Eriksson, A.W., "The Scandinavian International Biological Program, Section for Human Adaptability, IBP/HA, Scandinavian IBP/HA Investigations in 1967-1969," Arct. Anthrop. 7: 63-9 (1970)

10. Lewin, T., Rundgren, Å., Forsius, H., and Eriksson, A.W., "Demography of the Skolt Lapps in Northern Finland," Finska TandläkSällsk.Förhandl., 67: Suppl. 1: 24-38 (1971)

11. Lewin, T., Skrobak-Kaczynski, J., and Sigholm, G., "Secular changes in craniofacial dimensions in a homogeneous population," Acta morph. neerl.-scand., 11: 289-319 (1973)

12. Schreiner, K.E., Zur Osteologie der Lappen (Oslo: A.W. Brøgger, 1935)

13. Steinberg, A.G., Tiilikainen, A., Eskola, M.-R., and Erikson, A.W., "Gammaglobulin allotypes in Finnish Lapps, Finns, Åland Islanders, Maris (Cheremis), and Greenland Eskimos," Am. J. hum. Genet., 26: 223-43 (1974)

14. Stybalkowski, M., "Mikroskopische Untersuchungen an Querschnitten von Kopfhaaren der Sevettijärvi-Skolt-Lappen," Anthrop. Anz., 33: 219-32 (1972)

15. Torgersen, J., Getz, B., and Simonsen, P., "Varanger-funnene. I. Funn av menniskeskjeletter," Tromsø Mus. Skr., 7: 1-28 (1959)

16. Vollenbruck, S., Lewin, T., and Lehmann, W., "On the inbreeding of Skolts," Nord. Coun. Arct. med. res. Rept. 1974 (in press)

Demographic studies on the Inari Lapps in Finland

C. VON BONSDORFF, J. FELLMAN, and T. LEWIN

The genetic background of the inhabitants of Inari (northern Finland) in the eighteenth and nineteenth centuries has already been studied by genealogical and population-statistical methods (1). The Lapps are represented by two main groups, Skolt Lapps comprising about 600 individuals, and Inari Lapps, about 1,500 individuals. The great majority of the Inari Lapps belong to the subgroup Fisher Lapps and a minority to the subgroup Mountain Lapps. Since the demography of the Skolt Lapps has been investigated earlier (3), we study here only the Inari Lapps and their subgroups.

MATERIAL AND METHODS

This study is based partly on the official census of 1970 (4), in which Lapps were counted as a separate group for the first time. Here, the Lapps are defined by linguistic criteria. Secondly, we have studied a genealogical sample based on individuals included in the Scandinavian IBP/HA investigations of the Inari Lapps in 1969 and 1970. In the latter case, the sampling method aimed at finding Lapps as "pure" as possible for the investigations. The selection was based on church registers and earlier studies made by official committees working on socio-economic problems in northern Finland. Questionnaires completed during interviews of persons summoned to the IBP examinations included the following items: birth place, maternal age, birth interval, birth rank, number of siblings, age at and date of marriage, age at first menstruation and climacterium, use of contraceptives, and number of pregnancies. The information obtained at the interviews was supplemented by data from church registers and other official compilations to

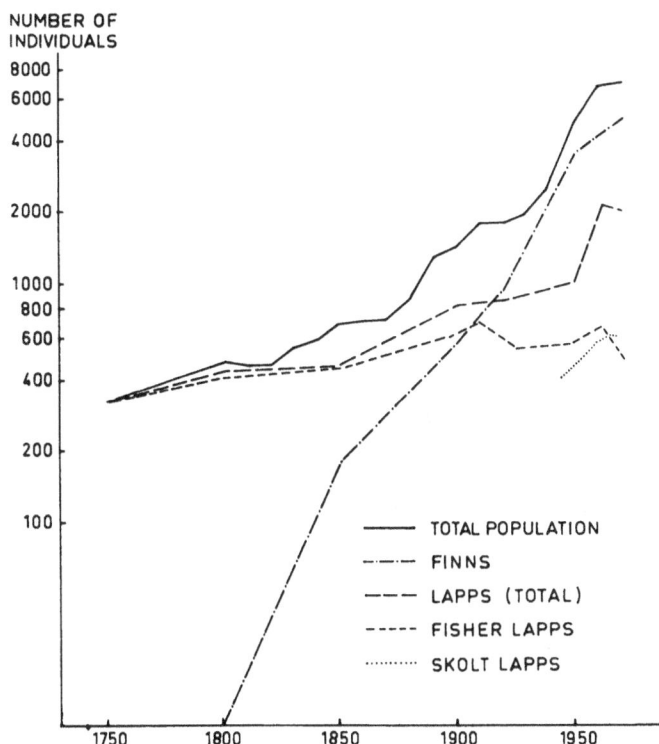

Figure 1 The development of the total population and the
subpopulations in Inari, 1750-1970

TABLE 1
Frequency distribution of individuals composing the genealogic sample
of Inari Lapps relative to the frequency of Mountain Lapp, Fisher Lapp,
and Finnish genes

Gene frequency classes	Individuals with Mountain Lapp genes		Individuals with Fisher Lapp genes		Individuals with Finnish genes	
%	n	%	n	%	n	%
100	26	2.8	150	16.3	51	5.5
99-75	139	15.1	254	27.5	110	11.9
74-50	101	10.9	227	24.6	236	25.6
49-25	152	16.5	190	20.6	81	8.8
24-1	108	11.7	98	10.6	135	14.6
0	423	45.8	154	16.7	361	39.1
100-0	923	100.0	923	100.0	923	100.0

yield a final four-generation genealogical sample of 923
individuals.

RESULTS

Figure 1 shows the growth of the population of Inari from
1750 to 1970, both as a whole and in the subpopulations:
Lapps, Finns, and the Fisher Lapps from 1750 to 1970, and
the Skolt Lapps from 1945 to 1967. From 1750 to 1970 the
total population of Inari increased from about 400 inhabitants to almost 7,000. The great increase was caused mainly
by immigration of Finns; this started about 1750, when two
Finnish women married Lappish men living in Inari. The increasing number of Finns has forced the Lapps into a minority position. At the end of the last century, the Lapps comprised about 60 per cent of the total population, but today they make up only 30 per cent. Of the four communes in
northern Finland in 1970, only Utsjoki had a Lapp majority;
nevertheless, more than 50 per cent of the total number of
Lapps in Finland lived in Inari.

In the sample examined, only 3 per cent were "pure"
Mountain Lapps, 16 per cent were "pure" Fisher Lapps, and
6 per cent were "pure" Finns. Mountain Lapp genes were
lacking in 46 per cent, Fisher Lapp genes in 17 per cent,
and Finnish genes in 39 per cent of the individuals. Of the
total gene pool in the sample, there were 46 per cent
Fisher Lapp genes, 25 per cent Mountain Lapp genes, 1 per
cent Skolt Lapp genes, and 28 per cent Finn genes (Table 1).

The age and sex distribution of the total population and
its subgroups is shown in Figure 2. The population pyramids
of Finns and Lapps have the same configuration from age
0-4 years up to age 10-14 years. After the age group 10-14
years there is a steady reduction of population up to the
age group 25-29 years, which comprises 5-6 per cent of the
total for Finns and Lapps. This age group size is then
maintained to age 50 in the Finns and to age 70 in the
Lapps, with successive reductions thereafter.

Males are in the majority up to 55 years. In the total
population of Inari this is also the case in the age group
55-64 and in the Finnish subpopulation even at ages above
64 years. Among the Lapps, male predominance is most pronounced at ages up to 35 years, but among the Finns the
peak occurs at a higher age.

♂   ♀

—— TOTAL POPULATION

— LAPPS (CENSUS)

········ LAPPS (GENEALOGIC SAMPLE)

----- FINNS

85
80
75
70
65 69
60 64
55 59
50 54
45 49
40 44
35 39
30 34
25 29
20 24
15 19
10 14
5   9
0   4

84
79
74

450 400 350 300 250 200 150 100 50 | 50 100 150 200 250 300 350 400 450

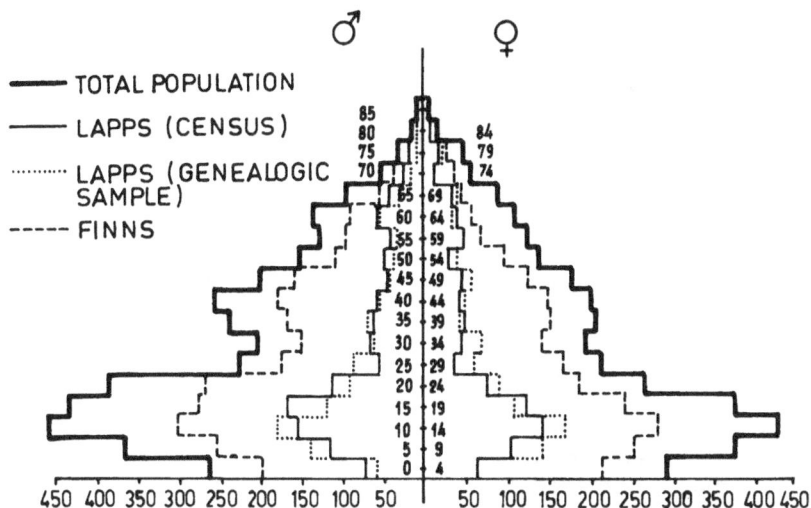

Figure 2 Population pyramids for the total population, the Finns, and the Lapps

TABLE 2
Trends in the crude birth rate and crude death rate in Inari and in Finland, 1841–1970

Year	Crude birth rate		Crude death rate	
	Inari	Finland	Inari	Finland
1841–1850	24.7	35.5*	13.5	22.2*
1851–1860	29.2	36.3*	19.0	28.2*
1861–1870	29.1	37.0*	15.5	25.8*
1871–1880	31.1	37.0	17.5	22.2
1881–1890	32.2	35.0	18.6	21.3
1891–1900	31.4	32.0	12.7	19.9
1901–1910	34.9	32.4	14.7	18.7
1911–1920	21.6	27.0	28.2	18.9
1921–1930	21.3	23.6	11.5	14.9
1931–1940	22.4	19.7	13.0	14.0
1941–1950	19.8	24.3	12.8	13.6
1951–1960	31.3	20.7	7.1	9.3
1961–1970	21.0	16.7	6.5	9.5

* First 5-year period

Natality and Reproductivity

The crude birth rate (Table 2) of the total population in
Inari was fairly steady at about 30 per 1,000 from 1840 to
1910; it then fell to about 20 up to the fifties, when it
became rather high for several years, finally declining
again to 13.3 in 1970. That year the Finns at Inari had a
birth rate of 16.9 and the Lapps only 12.9.

The age distribution of the female population shows a
pre-reproductive part of about 33 per cent. The reproductive part for the total and for the Finnish female population was about 50 per cent, but for the Lappish female
population it was somewhat below 45 per cent. These facts
naturally influence the birth rates and reproductivity.

Data on family size are available only for Lapps. In
Lappish families completed during the last 50 years, the
average number of children was 5.9. The most frequent number of children was 7 or 8 per family, with rather less
than half of the families giving birth to somewhat more
than two-thirds of the total children. The high mean size
of the sibships in comparison with the low crude birth rate
is explained partly by the small number of reproductive
females and partly by the fact that the Lappish women have
a lower marriage frequency than the Finnish women in Inari.

Sexual maturity tends to be reached at a lower age in
the later cohorts. For the total sample, the mean age at
the climacterium was again rather high, 49.4 years. The
average age at marriage was 24.6 for women and 29.3 for
men.

Mortality

The crude death rate (Table 2) of the population of Inari
fluctuated between 1850 and 1970. It reached a peak of 28
during the second decade of this century because of the
great increase in deaths during the civil war of 1918 and
the influenza pandemic (Spanish flu) at the end of World
War I. Since 1950, the mortality rate has been rather low.
The same trend is seen in the infant mortality rate, which
fell from 106 for the decade 1931-40 to a little over 20
after 1950.

In the genealogical sample going back to about 1870, all
deaths were registered. Calculations based on these deaths
gave mean ages at death of 46.7 years for females and 44.4
years for males.

Migration

Only limited studies of migration have been carried out so
far. For marriages contracted between 1954 and 1964, only
55 per cent of the partners had their residence at Inari.
Husband and wife originated from the same village in only
30 per cent of marriages. The situation was very much the
same a hundred years earlier. In the nineteenth century,
the endogamy rate was somewhat higher, 41 per cent. The
migratory activity is greater among Finns. Migration from
Inari is observable especially in the highest reproductive
age groups and in females, influencing both the sex ratio
and fertility.

CONCLUSIONS

Data relating to the genealogical sample are not representative of the whole population of Inari. In spite of this,
the data presented indicate that genes of Fisher Lapps make
up something between one-third and one-half of the Lappish
gene pool of Inari, and Mountain Lappish genes make up
about one-fourth, as do Finnish genes. The genealogical investigations indicate that division of individuals into
Lapps and Finns on a linguistic basis is very crude. In a
population consisting of several subpopulations, the majority of the individuals cannot be classified as "pure" representatives of a certain subpopulation. The contributions
of the different subpopulations to the genetic composition
of the individuals range from 0 to 100 per cent on a virtually continuous scale. This intermixture adds interest
to the study of the gene frequencies of the population of
Inari (2).

ACKNOWLEDGMENT

This work was aided by grants from the Nordiska Kulturfonden and Oskar Öflunds Foundation.

SUMMARY

Investigations of the genetic structure of the population
of Inari have been based on the 1970 census and on a
sample. In the census data, the individuals are classified
according to linguistic criteria. In the sample, the
classification is based on genealogical studies. The census data and the sample are analysed demographically and
discrepancies in the results are discussed. The genealo-

gical investigations indicate that linguistic division of
the individuals into Lapps and Finns is very crude. In a
population consisting of several subpopulations, the majority of individuals cannot be classified as pure representatives of any given subpopulation. The contributions of
different subpopulations to the genetic composition of individuals range from 0 to 100 per cent on a virtually continuous scale.

REFERENCES

1. Bonsdorff, C. von, "Gene flow from Finns to Lapps," 2nd
   Int. Symp. Circumpolar Health, Oulu, Finland, 21-24 June
   1971
2. Fellman, J., "Using a regression model to estimate the
   gene frequencies in aboriginal populations from observations in hybrid individuals," 3rd Congr. Bulg. Math.,
   IFIP TC-4 Working Conference on "Mathematical Models in
   Biology and Medicine," Varna, 6-11 Sept. 1972
3. Lewin, T., Rundgren, Å., Forsius, H., and Eriksson,
   A.W., "Demography of the Skolt Lapps in Northern Finland," Finska TandläkSällsk.Förhandl., 67: Suppl. I:
   24-38 (1971)
4. Official statistics of Finland: 1970 Population Census

Genetic polymorphisms in Utsjoki Lapps

M.-R. ESKOLA, M. KIRJARINTA, L.E. NIJENHUIS,
E. VAN DEN BERG-LOONEN, E. VAN LOGHEM, M. ISOKOSKI,
T. SAHI, and A.W. ERIKSSON

The blood groups of 172 Utsjoki Lapps were investigated in
June 1973. Utsjoki is the northernmost commune in Finland
and about 85 per cent of the population is still composed
of Lapps, the so-called Mountain Lapps.

Figures 1-4 show the percentages of some polymorphic
blood groups, serum proteins, and red cell enzymes in
different Fennoscandian populations. The Utsjoki Lapps are
denoted with black. The next four populations are other
Finnish Lapp populations in the commune of Inari, the next

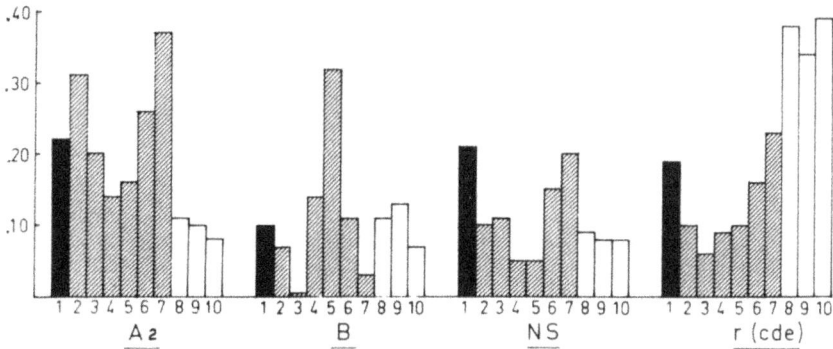

Figure 1   Approximate blood group gene frequencies in some
Fennoscandian populations (1, Utsjoki Lapps; 2, Inari
Mountain Lapps, 3, Inari Fisher Lapps; 4, Sevettijärvi
Skolt Lapps; 5, Nellim Skolt Lapps; 6, Norwegian Lapps;
7, Swedish Lapps, 8, Finns, northeastern Finland; 9, Finns,
whole country; 10, Norwegians and Swedes)

two are Norwegian and Swedish Lapps, and the last three are
Finns, Norwegians, and Swedes, in other words non-Lappish
populations. In the ABO blood group system (Figure 1) the
gene A^2 can be considered typical of Lapps. The frequency
of this gene is considerably higher in Lapp populations
than in non-Lapps. There is no definite distribution pattern for the gene B. The Nellim Skolt Lapps have a very
high frequency, while in the Fisher Lapps the gene B is almost absent. The estimated frequency of the gene complex NS
is around 7 per cent for Caucasians. Here, the Utsjoki Lapps
differ markedly from other Finnish Lapps, and resemble the
Norwegian and Swedish Lapps in having a much higher frequency.

The frequency of Rhesus-negative subjects is clearly
much lower in all Lapp populations than in non-Lapps.

For the gene P$_1$, the approximate value for Europeans is
50 per cent; the Lapps, with the exception of the Utsjoki
Lapps (51 per cent), all have lower frequencies.

The frequency of the Fy^a (Duffy) is well above the European average, which is about 40 per cent; in all the Lapp
populations it is over 50 per cent, and among the Finnish
Skolt Lapps it is as high as 70 per cent.

In the Kell system there are no marked differences between the different populations, the frequency of the gene
K being rather low.

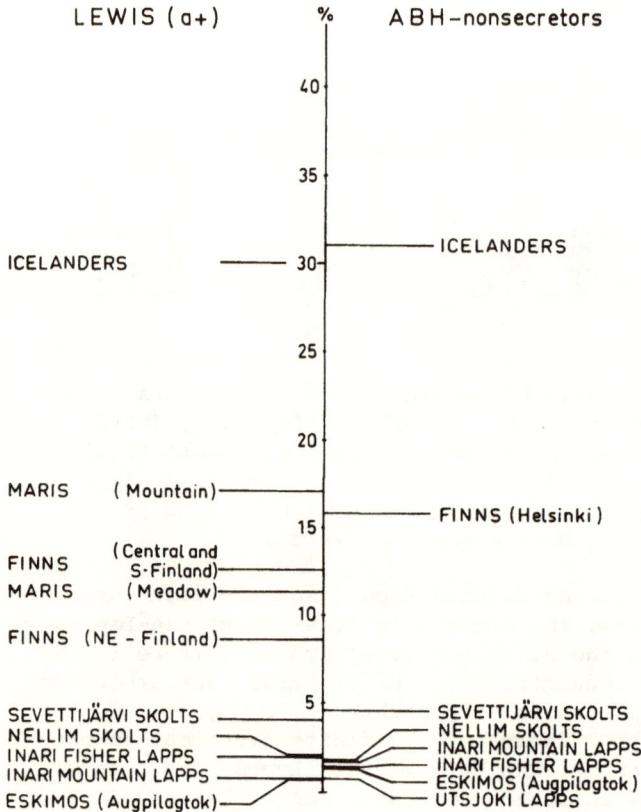

Figure 2   The frequency of Lewis (a+) and ABH non-secretors in selected populations

Almost all subjects with the Lewis antigen Le (a+) are also ABH non-secretors (Figure 2). About 25 per cent of western Europeans (e.g. Icelanders) have the antigen Le (a+). However, the Finno-Ugrian populations, Finns and Maris living on the Volga bend in the USSR, have much lower frequencies. All the Finnish Lapps, and especially the Ut-sjoki Lapps, have extremely low frequencies of these traits (<5 per cent). This could be considered an eastern influence, since the Mongoloid populations studied so far have almost zero frequencies of the genes se and Le[a]. Three different samples of Finns have been typed either for Le (a) or ABH. The Finns from NE Finland, who live closest to the Lapps, have the lowest frequencies.

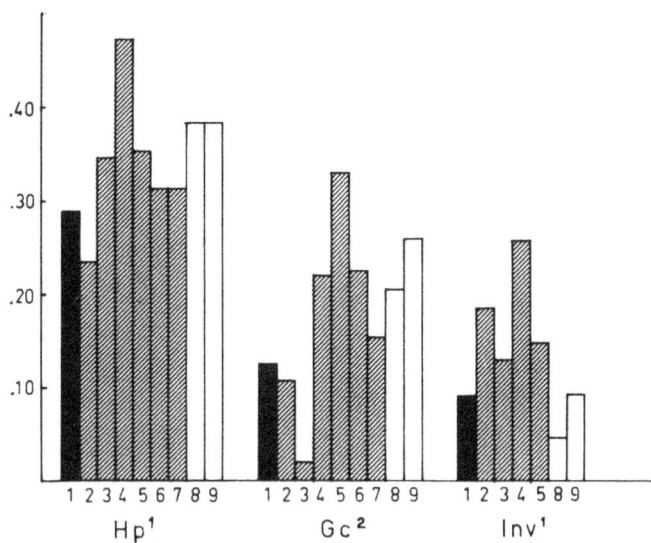

Figure 3 Approximate gene frequencies of serum groups in some Fennoscandian populations (1, Utsjoki Lapps, 2, Inari Mountain Lapps; 3, Inari Fisher Lapps; 4, Sevettijärvi Skolt Lapps; 5, Nellim Skolt Lapps; 6, Norwegian Lapps, 7, Swedish Lapps; 8, Finns; 9, Norwegians and Swedes)

The frequency of the haptoglobin gene Hp^1 (Figure 3) is roughly the same throughout most of the European continent, ranging from 35 to 43 per cent. The Utsjoki Lapps and Inari Mountain Lapps have frequencies well below 30 per cent.

The group-specific component gene Gc^2 shows a very heterogeneous pattern, only 3 per cent among the Inari Fisher Lapps and as high as 33 per cent among the Nellim Skolt Lapps.

The only variants of the transferrin system in the Lapp populations are the phenotypes B_{0-1} and CD_{Chi}, but their frequencies are much lower than among other Finno-Ugrian populations (1). Of the 168 Utsjoki sera, only three were of the slow-moving variant type CD_{Chi}.

The frequency of the Inv^1 (Km^1) gene among the Lapps is two- to five-fold that of other Nordic populations. For the Sevettijärvi Skolt Lapps the frequency is more than twice as high as any previously reported in European populations (3).

In the Gm system the haplotype zag is more frequent than in other Europeans, whereas fnb is much rarer. The frequency of zag is 26 per cent and of fnb 35 per cent.

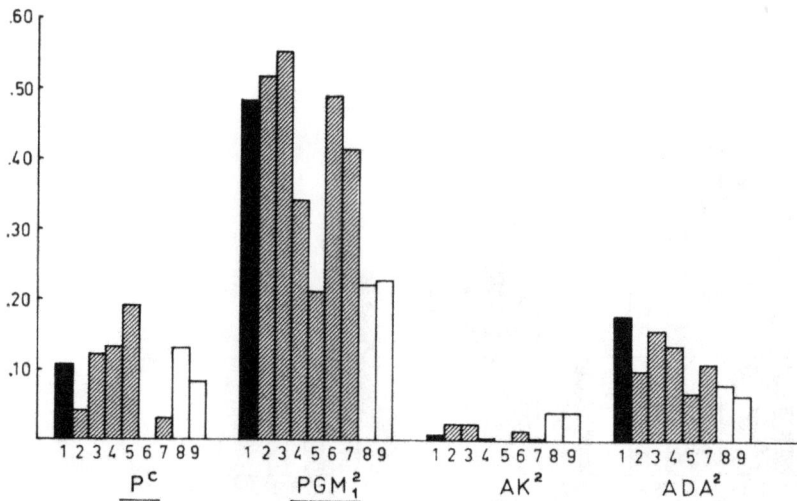

Figure 4   Approximate gene frequencies for red cell enzymes in some Fennoscandian populations (1, Utsjoki Lapps;
2, Inari Mountain Lapps, 3, Inari Fisher Lapps; 4, Sevettijärvi Skolt Lapps; 5, Nellim Skolt Lapps; 6, Norwegian
Lapps; 7, Swedish Lapps; 8, Finns; 9, Norwegians and Swedes)

As for the HL-A frequencies of the Utsjoki Lapps, the
most striking differences, in comparison with other European populations, are the high frequencies of HL-A, 3, 9,
27, W 15 and W 20, and the low frequencies of HL-A 1, 8,
and 12. As compared with the other Caucasian populations,
the Lapps show higher frequencies of HL-A 3 and W 15, and
low frequencies of HL-A 12 (4).

As in other Europeans, no polymorphism was found for the
A_2m markers, the sample being 100 per cent A_2m (1+2-).
In this respect these Lapps differ from Eskimos, in whom
polymorphism for the A_2m marker has been found. The degree
of polymorphism in the red cell enzymes is rather high
(Figure 4), e.g. the acid phosphatase gene p^C has a frequency in all Finnish Lapp populations that ranks among the
highest in the world.

Of the Caucasian populations only the Habbanite Jews
have a phosphoglucomutase gene PGM_1^2 frequency higher than
50 per cent. With the exception of the Finnish Skolt Lapps,
all the Lapp populations have high frequencies of this
gene.

The frequency of the adenylate kinase gene AK^2 in Lapp
populations is very low; among the Skolt Lapps it is almost
absent (2). The only cases with the phenotype AK 1-2 could

be traced to Finnish ancestry.

The adenosine deaminase gene ADA^2 has very high frequencies, especially in the Utsjoki Lapp population.

The results confirm that in so far as genetic markers are concerned the Utsjoki Lapps, like other Lapp populations, have several characteristics distinguishing them from the neighbouring non-Lappish populations. Which of these differing characteristics are due to isolation, genetic drift, or the founder effect is difficult to say.

ACKNOWLEDGMENT

This study was aided by grants from the Nordic Council for Arctic Medical Research and the Free University, Amsterdam.

SUMMARY

A genetic survey of 172 Utsjoki Lapps from Finnish Lapland included tests of red cell antigens, serum groups, red cell enzymes, and secretion of ABH antigens. The Utsjoki Lapps had high frequencies of the genes A_2, NS, Fy^a, R_1, R_2, and PGM_1^2, and low frequencies of the genes A_1, MS, r, and Gc^2. The frequency of ABH non-secretors was also very low. The frequencies found fit well into the range reported for neighbouring Lapp populations of Fennoscandia.

REFERENCES

1. Eriksson, A.W., "Genetic polymorphisms in Finno-Ugrian populations: Finns, Lapps and Maris," Israel J. med. Sci., 9: 1156-70 (1973)
2. Eriksson, A.W., Fellman, J., Kirjarinta, M., Eskola, M.-R., Singh, S., Benkmann, H.-G., Goedde, H.W., Mourant, A.E., Tills, D., and Lehmann, W., "Adenylate kinase polymorphism in populations in Finland (Swedes, Finns, Lapps), in Maris, and in Greenland Eskimos," Hum. Genet., 12: 123-30 (1971)
3. Steinberg, A.G., Tiilikainen, A., Eskola, M.-R., and Eriksson, A.W., "Gammaglobulin allotypes in Finnish Lapps, Åland Islanders, Maris (Cheremis), and Greenland Eskimos," Am. J. hum. Genet., 26: 223-43 (1974)
4. Tiilikainen, A., Eriksson, A.W., McQueen, J.M., and Amos, D.B., "The Hl-A system in the Skolt Lapp population," Monogr. Histocompatibility Testing (Copenhagen: Munksgaard, 1972), pp. 85-92

Correlation between glutathione reductase activity and acid phosphatase phenotypes: a biochemical population genetic study in Skolts and other Lapps

MIKKO KIRJARINTA

Glutathione reductase (GSSG-R) activity is significantly lower in Skolts than in other Lapp populations (7). Riboflavin deficiency has been discussed as a cause of the low activity of this enzyme among the Skolts (5). GSSG-R is a flavin enzyme. Its prosthetic group is flavin adenine dinucleotide (FAD), which is formed from riboflavin-5-phosphate (FMN) (Figure 1). FMN is the best natural substrate of acid phosphatase (8). The ratio of the enzyme activities corresponding to the genes P^a:P^b:P^c is roughly 2:3:4, and the effects of these three alleles are additive (6). The frequency of the gene P^c is extremely high among Lapps, and several homozygous CC subjects were found (3). The significance of human acid phosphatases has been discussed in a review (9).

The dependence between GSSG-R activity and acid phosphatase phenotypes has been studied. The activity of GSSG-R is correlated with socio-economic status (4), apparently due to inequalities in the dietary supply of riboflavin. In isolated homogeneous populations such as the Lapps the exogenous bias can be minimized. It has been possible to demonstrate a negative correlation between GSSG-R activities and acid phosphatase phenotypes with different activities (Table 1).

In Figure 2 the same results are shown schematically. Bottini and Modiano (2) have noticed that low reduced glutathione levels or high oxidized glutathione levels are associated with a decrease in acid phosphatase activity. Bottini et al. (1) have also studied the effect of acetyl-phenylhydrazine on red cell acid phosphatases.

Differences in the average values of GSSG-R activity between populations may be explained at least partly by the distribution of acid phosphatase phenotypes.

NUTRITION

INTESTINAL FLORA

RIBOFLAVIN

ACID PHOSPHATASES | FLAVOKINASE
MG++, ATP

FMN

FAD PYROPHOSPHORYLASE
MG++, ATP

ALLELE I → POLYPEPTIDE I
LOCUS   APO-E + FAD ⇌ APO-E-FAD + FAD ⇌ APO-E-FAD
                                         DIMERE   HOLOENZYME   HOLOENZYME
ALLELE II → POLYPEPTIDE II   GSSG-R   GSSG-R

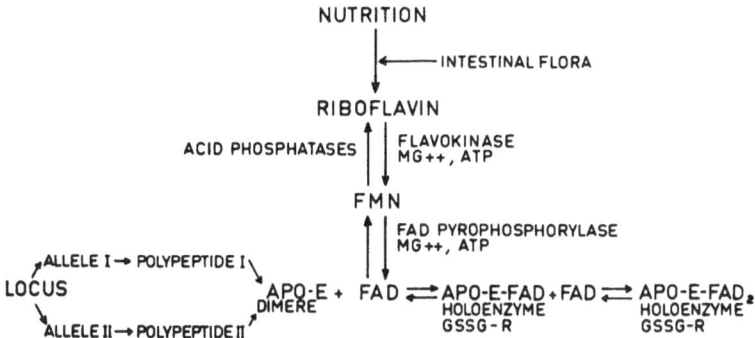

Figure 1 Factors in the formation of active glutathione
reductase (GSSG-R)

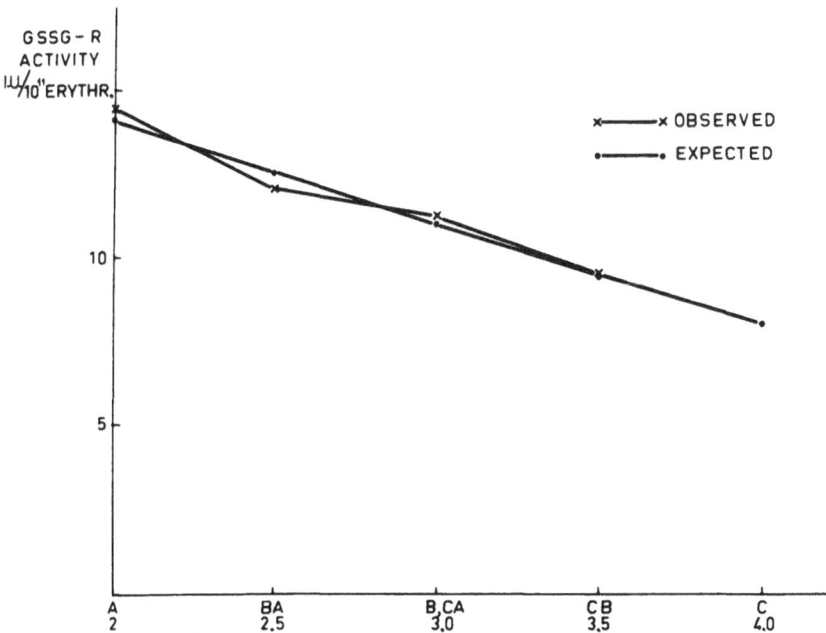

Figure 2 Acid phosphatase phenotypes and their relative
activities

TABLE 1
Influence of acid phosphatase phenotypes on glutathione reductase
activity, preliminary test of additivity

Acid phosphatase phenotypes				Observed GSSG-R activity, average	Expected activity
A $\quad a_0$ + $2a_1$			=	14.45	14.14
BA $\quad a_0$ + a_1 + a_2			=	12.10	12.54
B $\quad a_0$ + $2a_2$			=	11.15	10.94
CA $\quad a_0$ + a_1			=	10.95	11.07
CB $\quad a_0$ + a_2			=	9.60	9.47
C $\quad a_0$			=	–	8.00

$a_0 = 8.00; \quad a_1 = 3.07; \quad a_2 = 1.47.$

ACKNOWLEDGMENT

This work has been aided by grants from the Nordiska
Kulturfonden and Deutsche Forschungsgemeinschaft.

SUMMARY

It has proved possible to demonstrate a negative correlation between GSSG-R activities and acid phosphatase phenotypes with different activities.

REFERENCES

1. Bottini, E., Lucarelli, P., Tucciarone, L., Carapella,
   E., and Palmarino, R., "In vitro effect of acetylphenyl-
   hydrazine on acid phosphatases of fetal red blood cells,"
   Biol. Neonatale, 15: 57-60 (1970)
2. Bottini, E. and Modiano, G., "Effect of oxidized glutathione on human red cell acid phosphatases," Biochem.
   biophys. Res. Commun., 17: 260-4 (1964)
3. Eriksson, A.W., Kirjarinta, M., Gustafsson, B.,
   Bustavsson, B., Damsten, R., and Kajanoja, P., "Red cell
   enzyme polymorphisms in populations in Finland and in
   Greenland Eskimos," Scand. J. clin. Lab. Invest., 23,
   Suppl. 108: 45 (1969)

4. Flatz, G., "Population study of erythrocyte glutathione reductase activity. I. Stimulation of the enzyme by flavin adenine dinucleotide and by riboflavin supplementation," Hum. Genet., 11: 269-77 (1971)
5. Gustafsson, B., Gustafsson, C., Kirjarinta, M., Eriksson, A.W., Sjöblom, L., and Lehmann, W., "Some aspects on the red cell glutathione reductase deficiency among Skolt Lapps," 2nd Int. Symp. Circumpolar Health, Oulu, 21-24 June 1971
6. Hopkinson, D.A., Spencer, N., and Harris, H., "Genetical studies on human red cell acid phosphatase," Am. J. hum. Genet., 16: 141-54 (1964)
7. Kirjarinta, M., Lehtosalo, T., Eskola, M.-R., Eriksson, A.W., Gustafsson, B., and Lehmann, W., "Population genetical studies on glutathione reductase activity of red cells," Scand. J. clin. Lab. Invest., 25, Suppl. 113: 63 (1970)
8. Luffman, J.E. and Harris, H., "A comparison of some properties of human red cell acid phosphatase in different phenotypes," Ann. hum. Genet., 30: 387-401 (1967)
9. Yam, L.T., "Clinical significance of the human acid phosphatases," Am. J. Med., 56: 604-16 (1974)

Erythrocyte alanine amino transferase polymorphism in a Lappish population

K. VIRTARANTA, M. KIRJARINTA, A.W. ERIKSSON,
T. SAHI, and M. ISOKOSKI

The red cell enzyme alanine amino transferase (A*l*AT, E.C: 2.6.1.2), also called glutamate pyruvate transaminase (GPT), has recently attracted much attention from population geneticists because of its high degree of polymorphism and its wide variation in the populations so far studied. The polymorphism was first described in 1971 in a study of three different ethnic groups in America (1). Since then, 38 further populations have been studied, all showing a high degree of polymorphism at this locus.

The transferase exists in two molecular forms, the soluble form present in the cytoplasm and the mitochondrial form. The enzyme has an important function in the interconversion of carbohydrate and amino acid metabolites (2).

It has a requirement for vitamin B_6, or more exactly pyri-
doxal phosphate (5).

The polymorphism involves one autosomal locus with two
common codominant alleles, 1 and 2, which give rise to the
three expected phenotypes. The enzyme is a dimer, and in
heterozygotes a hybrid band is found in addition to the
two parental bands (2). Five rare alleles have also been
found (2, 7), and there is some evidence for the occurrence
of a silent allele (8).

The observed activities of the three most common phenotypes, 1-1, 2-1, and 2-2, differ markedly, and are normally
in the ratio of 4:3:2 (2). The role played by selection in
maintaining this high level of polymorphism in the populations studied is obscure, and the physiological consequences of the different phenotypes are still under investigation.

We have studied the amino transferase allele frequencies
in a Lapp population in the Utsjoki area of Finland. Blood
samples from individuals were typed by starch gel electro-
phoresis followed by substrate solution staining (6). Enzyme activity was detected by the following reactions:

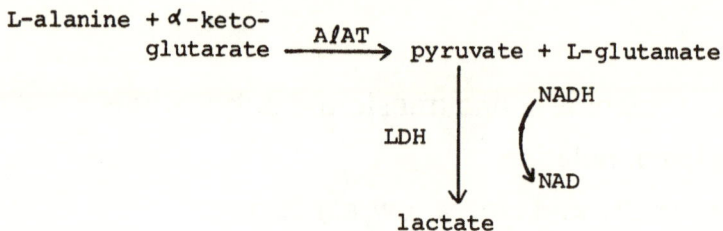

$$\text{L-alanine} + \alpha\text{-keto-glutarate} \xrightarrow{\text{A}l\text{AT}} \text{pyruvate} + \text{L-glutamate}$$

pyruvate $\xrightarrow[\text{LDH}]{\text{NADH} \rightarrow \text{NAD}}$ lactate

Each homozygote shows one band of activity, 1-1 giving a
"slow," intensely staining band, and 2-2 a "fast," weakly
staining band. The heterozygote shows both parental bands
and an extra intermediate hybrid band.

In an attempt to increase the intensity of staining, we
incubated samples with the co-enzyme vitamin B_6. This procedure was effective in increasing enzyme activity and made
typing easier. Certain Lapp populations have a low intake
of many vitamins (4). Possibly some of the individuals
studied here had a low intake of vitamin B_6, and this might
account for the low levels of enzyme activity observed initially, especially because AlAT activity is very sensitive
to the presence of vitamin B_6 (5).

The frequency of allele 1 in our population of Finnish Lapps was 0.503. The lowest frequencies for the allele 1 have been found among the Philippinos, 0.295; the highest, from 0.8 to 0.9, are found in African populations (2). In Caucasians the two alleles are almost equally common, their frequencies ranging from 0.48 to 0.55. Norwegian Lapps 0.610 (9), Canadian Eskimos 0.596 (2), and a group of Orientals 0.598 (1) have higher frequencies of allele 1 than any Caucasian population yet examined.

The frequency of allele 1 found for the Finnish Lapps in this study, 0.503, is well within the range reported for other European populations. A Norwegian study showed that Norwegian Lapps have a significantly higher allele 1 frequency than do other European populations (9). These Norwegian and Finnish Lapp populations are separated by only a few kilometres, but their allele 1 frequencies differ significantly. There are several possible explanations for this surprising situation. The most likely is some founder effect during the history of these populations; a second cause might be a slight difference in breeding structure between the two populations; thirdly, differences in the action of selection cannot be excluded.

As mentioned before, some Oriental populations have rather high allele 1 frequencies compared with Caucasian populations. The origin of the Lapps has been much discussed (3). The high frequency of allele 1 in Norwegian Lapps is not inconsistent with the hypothesis of a partly eastern origin of the Lapps. In contrast, the much lower frequency now found in the Utsjoki Lapps is very close to the frequencies found in several Caucasian populations.

ACKNOWLEDGMENT

This study was aided by grants from the Nordic Council for Arctic Medical Research and the Nordiska Kulturfonden.

SUMMARY

The soluble red cell enzyme alanine amino transferase (AℓAT) polymorphism was studied in a Lapp population of 171 individuals. The gene frequencies found were AℓAT^1 0.503 and AℓAT^2 0.497. These figures agree with other results obtained for Caucasians. The enzyme activity was enhanced by incubating the samples with the co-enzyme vitamin B_6.

REFERENCES

1. Chen, S.-H., and Giblett, E.R., "Polymorphism of soluble glutamic-pyruvic transaminase: a new genetic marker in man," Science, 173: 148-9 (1971)

2. Chen, S.-H., Giblett, E.R., Anderson, J.E., and Fossum, B.L.G., "Genetics of glutamic-pyruvic transaminase: its inheritance, common and rare variants, population distribution, and differences in catalytic activity," Ann. hum. Genet., 35: 401-9 (1972)

3. Eriksson, A.W., Fellman, J., Forsius, H., Lehmann, W., Lewin, T., and Luukka, P., "The origin of the Lapps in the light of recent genetic studies," This volume.

4. Hasunen, K., and Pekkarinen, M., "The food intake of the Finnish Lapps estimated by one-day recall," 2nd Int. Symp. Circumpolar Health, Oulu, Finland, 21-24 June 1971

5. Jacobs, A., Cavill, A.J., and Hughes, J.N.P., "Erythrocyte transaminase activity. Effect of age, sex and vitamin B_6 supplementation," Am. J. clin. Nutr., 21: 502-7 (1968)

6. Kömpf, J., "Zytoplasmatische glutamat-pyruvat-transaminase (E.C. 2.6.1.2): Bestimmungstechnik," Ärztl. Lab., 18: 25-6 (1972)

7. Olaisen, B., "Two rare GPT phenotypes in a Norwegian family. Evidence of a seventh allele," Hum. Genet., 19: 289-91 (1973)

8. Olaisen, B., "Atypical segregation of erythrocyte glutamic-pyruvic transaminase in a Norwegian family. Evidence of a silent allele," Hum. Hered., 23: 595-602 (1973)

9. Olaisen, B., and Teisberg, P., "Erythrocyte alanine aminotransferase polymorphism in Norwegian Lapps," Hum. Hered., 22: 380-6 (1972)

Unusual hereditary diseases in northern Sweden: a review, with particular reference to primary familial amyloidosis with polyneuropathy, Urbach-Wiethe disease, and Huntington's chorea

B. WINBLAD, R. ANDERSSON, P.-Å. HOFER,
B. MATTSSON, and S. FALKMER

For purposes of health care, Sweden is subdivided into seven regions, each with 1-2 million inhabitants, several large, medium-sized, or smaller hospitals, and one large regional hospital - usually a university hospital - equipped with facilities for clinical and experimental medical research. The University Hospital in Umeå serves the northernmost of these regions. Its disease panorama is in many respects unusual. Apart from the well-known higher frequency of some infectious diseases, particularly tuberculosis (see Winblad and Duchek's report in this volume), there is also a high frequency of unusual hereditary diseases (3,4). Families with fructose intolerance, malabsorption of glucose and galactose, Gaucher's disease, juvenile nephronophthisis, pseudoxanthoma elasticum, keratosis follicularis Darier, Ehlers-Danlos' syndrome, homocysteinuria, and oxalosis have all been described. Most known cases of some other rare diseases, such as Sjögren-Larsson's syndrome, infantile hereditary agranulocytosis, and keratodermia palmaris et plantaris, have been reported from this region. The families of northern Sweden used to be few but large, living in isolated regions (4); such a background favours the origin of both recessive and dominant hereditary diseases.

The present report is a brief review of three rare inheritable diseases recently studied at the University of Umeå, viz. primary familial amyloidosis with polyneuropathy, where more than 60 cases are known (1, 2, 7), Urbach-Wiethe disease (UWD) with 27 cases distributed among 14 families (5, 6, 8), and Huntington's chorea (HC) where 43 families with 162 cases are known (9).

PRIMARY FAMILIAL AMYLOIDOSIS WITH NEUROPATHY (1, 2, 7)

Familial occurrence of amyloidosis with polyneuropathy was
first described in Portugal more than 20 years ago. Since
then, similar diseases have been found in other countries,
and subtypes of the disorder have been described. Our own
material contains both familial and possibly non-familial
cases and conforms essentially to that from Portugal. The
sporadic cases show the same clinical pattern and histopathological lesions as the familial ones. The symptoms of
polyneuropathy start and become most severe in the lower
limbs. Biopsy of the peripheral nerves shows extensive
deposits of amyloid (1). In addition, amyloid is deposited
in the nerves of the autonomous system (7), in the vessel
walls of a multitude of tissues including the glomerular
tufts of the kidneys (2), and in collagenous connective
tissue and various kinds of musculature (7). As a consequence, signs of both sensory and motor nerve affection

Figure 1   Geographic distribution and mode of inheritance
of primary familial amyloidosis with polyneuropathy
A. Schematic map of Sweden and surrounding countries
showing the seven health care regions in Sweden and the
places of birth for 65 cases of primary amyloidosis with
polyneuropathy found (● 5 cases; ● 2 cases)
B. Part of the pedigree of a family with amyloidotic polyneuropathy (□ , male; 0, female; ◇ and 0, siblings of both
sexes;■ and ●, members with advanced polyneuropathy; ◘ and
◐, members showing slight signs and symptoms of neuropathy;
X, amyloidosis proved by histological examination; ↗, proband). The autosomal dominant mode of inheritance is seen

A

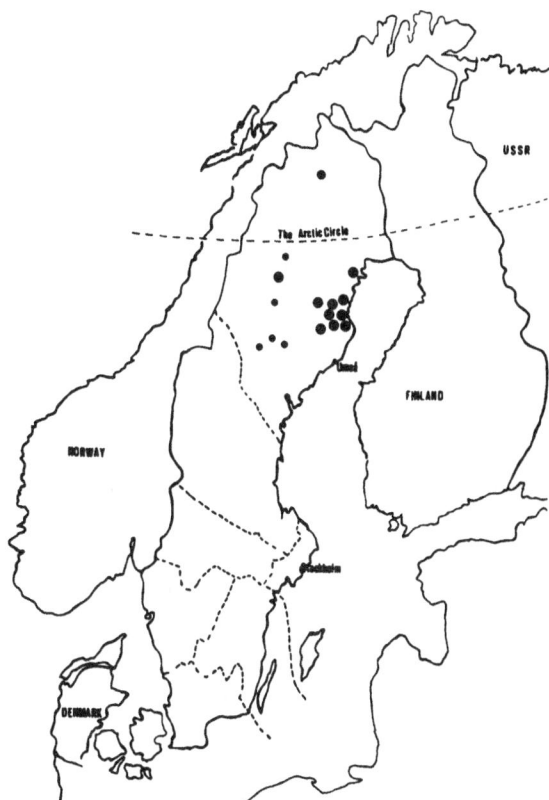

B

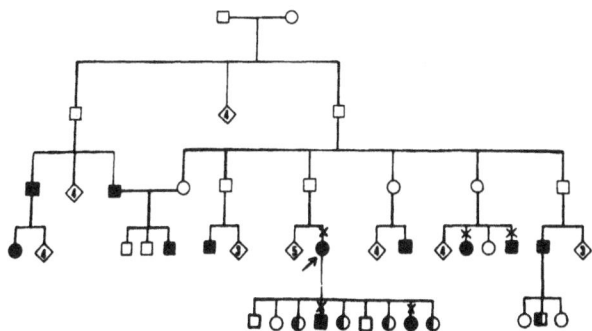

are observed, with ultimate flaccid paresis and muscular
atrophy. We have found that genito-urinary disturbances
with urinary bladder dysfunction and - in male patients -
impotence are early and common manifestations (2). Gastrointestinal dysfunction, including even malabsorption, has
also been observed, as well as cardiac insufficiency, postu-
ral hypotension, hoarseness, and characteristic opacities
of the vitreous body of the eyes (1). The mode of inheritance in the Portuguese cases is autosomal dominant. Our
preliminary genetic studies are in conformity with these
observations (Figure 1).

URBACH-WIETHE DISEASE (LIPOGLYCOPROTEINOSIS, HYALINOSIS
CUTIS ET MUCOSE) (5, 6, 8)

This disease was first described 45 years ago, but only
about 200 cases have been reported until now, usually as
conventional case reports (5). It is reasonable to assume
that the disease may be less rare than would appear from
the literature. The clinical manifestations can easily
lead to a wrong diagnosis and the morphological lesions are
often misinterpreted by the pathologist (5). Only exceptionally have any large number of patients been analysed.
Consequently, our material, consisting of 27 patients from
3 to 72 years of age, some observed for 7-10 years, should
be of particular interest (8).

Figure 2 Geographic distribution and mode of inheritance
in Urbach-Wiethe disease (UWD)
A. The symbol ● is used to indicate the birth places of
parents of UWD patients from northern Sweden. If not
immediately adjacent, the birth places of a pair of parents
are connected with a line. One parent's birth place was in
northernmost Sweden (outside the map)
B. Pedigree of UWD family with many intermarriages (□ and
○, examined, not affected by UWD; ■ and ●, UWD patient;
■ and ●, proband; ⊘ and ⊘, not examined; ⊠ and ⊗, deceased, not examined; ▩ and ⊛, deceased individual, presumably with UWD, as anamnesis indicated chronic hoarseness;
⊡ and ⊙, Heterozygous for the UWD gene, considering diagnosed cases of UWD; ⊠ and ⊗, deceased, presumed heterozygous for the UWD gene, considering presumed cases of UWD:
⊡⊡, monozygotic twins). The recessive mode of inheritance
is seen (Hofer, ref. 6; by courtesy of the editor of
Hereditas)

A

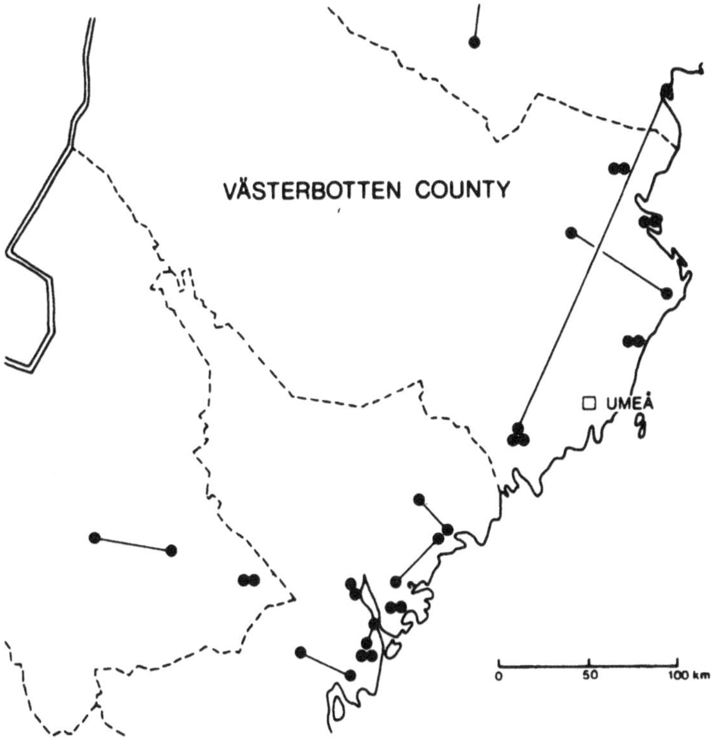

VÄSTERBOTTEN COUNTY

□ UMEÅ

0   50   100 km

B

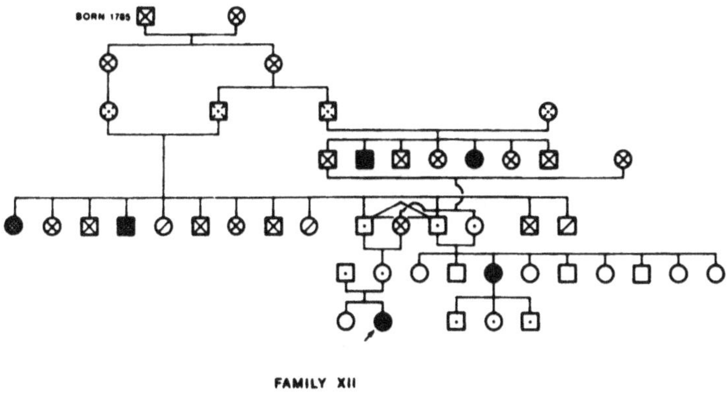

BORN 1785

FAMILY XII

The disease is characterized by lesions in the skin and
the mucous membranes of the mouth, pharynx, and larynx, due
to extracellular deposits of an amorphous substance. The
lesions are often discrete. They appear as acne-like scars,
but occur also outside typical acne locations; they may also
present as infiltrates, often in the skin over knees, el-
bows and fingers, in the axillae, on the scrotum, and as a
row of small papules along the free edge of the eyelids.
The laryngeal lesions cause hoarseness from early childhood.
Oral manifestations occur in the lips, the frenulum of the
tongue, the palate, and the back wall of the pharynx, and
there may be associated dental anomalies. Microscopic deposits accumulate particularly in vessel walls and connective tissue. Histochemically, they seem to contain glyco-
proteins and lipids since they are usually both PAS-positive
and sudanophil (8).

Carriers of the gene seem diffusely spread along the
coast of northern Sweden (Figure 2A). As shown in the pedigree in Figure 2B, many intermarriages have occurred among
relatives of UWD patients. Some presumptive gene carriers
had discrete lesions that could represent micro-manifesta-
tions of the disease (8). The genetic data indicate an
autosomal recessive mode of inheritance (6).

HUNTINGTON'S CHOREA (9, 10)

Huntington's chorea (HC) is transmitted by a dominant autosomal gene. The onset is usually between 35 and 40 years of
age. The possibility of reducing the incidence of HC depends
on early identification of gene carriers and the early establishment of a correct diagnosis.

Almost half of our patients first displayed psychiatric
symptoms, such as personality changes, loss of judgment,
alcoholism, criminality, and attempts at suicide. In some
cases, schizophrenic syndromes had persisted for years before neurologic symptoms appeared. Almost all the patients
who presented with neurologic symptoms were hyperkinetic
from the beginning. There was a smaller variation of age
of onset within than between families (9).

As it is still impossible to detect clinically healthy
carriers of the HC allele, a search for association and
linkage between HC and 15 various genetic marker systems
was made in 37 families. The only phenotypic association
found was with the Duffy blood group phenotype Fy(a$^+$); the
significance of this observation is still unclear.

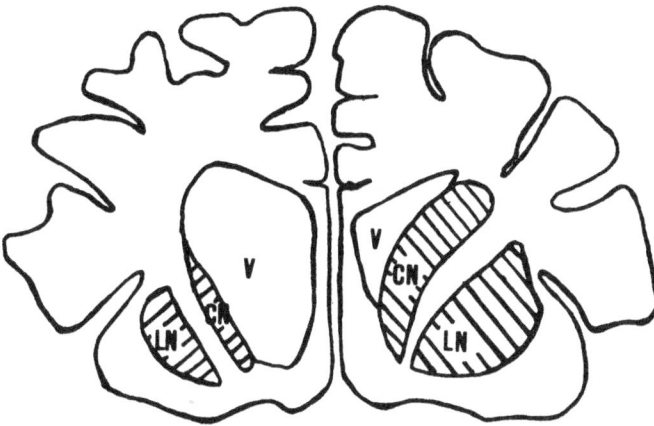

Figure 3   Schematic drawing where the hemisphere to the
left is from a case of Huntington's chorea and that on the
right is from a normal man. Note the shrunken lenticular
nucleus (LN) with the shrunken caudate nucleus (CN) as a
thin ribbon at the bottom of the dilated ventricle (V)

TABLE 1
Dopamine (DA) and homovanillic acid (HVA) in the caudate nucleus and
putamen in deceased patients with Huntington's chorea (HC) compared
to controls.   Concentration in μg/g tissue; means (M); standard
deviations (SD); number of subjects (N).   The significance of the
difference between the means is tested with Student's t-test (T)

	Amine/meta-bolite	HC patients			Controls				
		M	SD	N	M	SD	N	T	p
Caudate	DA	1.06	0.74	5	1.16	0.06	15	0.29	
nucleus	HVA	1.75	0.42	5	3.32	1.62	35	4.73	<0.001
Putamen	DA	2.03	1.92	5	1.08	0.53	15	-0.87	
	HVA	5.53	1.89	5	7.01	2.56	35	1.81	

Autopsies of five fatal cases of HC (10) showed a marked
atrophy of the basal ganglia of the brain, particularly
the putamen and the caudate nucleus (Figure 3), with severe
loss of nerve cells and a spongy condition of the paraven-
tricular region. Significantly lower concentrations of the
dopamine metabolite homovanillic acid were observed in the
caudate nucleus of the five HC cases when compared with an
age-matched control group (Table 1). This supports the
view that a disturbed dopaminergic balance of the basal

ganglia of the brain plays a major role in the pathogenesis of HC.

CONCLUSION

This review illustrates how it is possible to get an insight into the aetiology and pathogenesis of poorly known, rare, inheritable diseases by studying circumpolar populations where the living conditions favour the origin of such diseases. New features of more frequently encountered inherited diseases such as diabetic microangiopathy (5) and diseases of the central nervous system with abnormal dopamine metabolism (9) may also be brought to light through the investigation of such populations.

ACKNOWLEDGMENTS

This work was supported in part by grants from the Swedish Medical Research Council, the Nordic Insulin fund, the Swedish diabetes association, the Anna Cederbergs foundation, the Karl Oskar Hansson Foundation, the Edward Welander Foundation, the Board for Medical Research of the Swedish Life Insurance Companies, and the Medical Faculty of the University of Umeå.

SUMMARY

Isolation, large families, and frequent in-breeding have probably favoured the origin of rare inheritable diseases in northern Sweden. A large number of unusual familial diseases are described from this area. Recently, our clinical, histopathological, and genetical studies have been concentrated upon primary familial amyloidosis with polyneuropathy, Urbach-Wiethe disease, and Huntington's chorea. The number of cases of these three diseases is at least 60, 27, and 102, respectively, and several patients have been examined repeatedly over more than 10 years. The prolonged observation time and the large number of patients provide an excellent opportunity to follow the evolution of these rare diseases and to get an insight into their pathogenesis and mode of inheritance. Huntington's chorea and apparently also the polyneuropathic amyloidosis are transmitted by a dominant autosomal gene, whereas Urbach-Wiethe disease is probably inherited in an autosomal recessive manner.

REFERENCES

1. Andersson, R., "Hereditary amyloidosis with polyneuropathy," Acta Med. Scand., 188: 85-94 (1970)
2. Andersson, R., and Hofer, P.-Å., "Genitourinary disturbances in familial and sporadic cases of primary amyloidosis with polyneuropathy," Acta Med. Scand., 195:
49-58 (1974)
3. Falkmer, S., "Some rare diseases of morphological interest in the public medical service region of Umeå:
Keratosis follicularis Darier, Ehlers-Danlos' syndrome,
and lipoglycoproteinosis Urbach-Wiethe," Acta Path.
Microbiol. Scand., 66: 267 (1966)
4. Falkmer, S., Hofer, P.-Å., and Hollström, E., "Lipoglycoproteinosis (Urbach-Wiethe). A preliminary report,"
Acta Derm-Venereol. Sven Hellerström 65 years (Suppl.):
47-54 (1966)
5. Hofer, P.-Å., "Urbach-Wiethe disease (lipoglycoproteinosis; lipoid proteinosis; hyalinosis cutis et mucosae).
A review," Acta Derm-Venereol. (Suppl. 71): 1-52 (1973)
6. Hofer, P.-Å., "Urbach-Wiethe disease (lipoglycoproteinosis; lipoid proteinosis; hyalinosis cutis et mucosae). A clinico-genetic study of 14 families from northern Sweden," Hereditas, 77 (1974)
7. Hofer, P.-Å., and Andersson, R., "Postmortem findings
in primary familial amyloidosis with polyneuropathy.
A study based on six cases from Northern Sweden," Acta
Neuropath. (in press, 1975)
8. Hofer, P.-Å., Larsson, P.-Å., Ek, B., Göller, H.,
Laurell, H., and Lorentzon, R., "A clinical and histopathological study of twenty-seven cases of Urbach-
Wiethe disease. Dermatologic, gastroenterologic, neuro-
physiologic, ophthalmologic, and roentgendiagnostic
aspects, as well as the results of some clinico-chemi-
cal and histochemical examinations," Acta Path.
Microbiol. Scand., 82A, Suppl. 245: 1-87 (1974)
9. Mattsson, B., "Clinical, genetic and pharmacological
studies in Huntington's chorea," Umeå Univ. Med. Diss.,
No. 7: 1-120 (1974)
10. Mattsson, B., Gottfries, C.-G., Roos, B.-E., and Winblad, B., "Huntington's chorea: Pathology and brain
amines," Acta Psychiat. Scand., Suppl. (in press, 1974)

Immunological homeostasis in a population migrated to polar regions

V.P. LOZOVOY

Studies on infectious and non-infectious immunology in man living at high latitudes require a complex approach. Human adaptation to adverse environments involves immunological mechanisms not only as a system of defence against infection, but also as a means of regulating the antigenic composition of organs and tissues, the pool of hemopoietic cells and their transformation into macrophagic and stromal cell populations (Fridenstein et al.). These functions are evidenced by data on the "trophocyte" properties of lymphocytes which serve as suppliers of material (Khrushchov, Skurskaya et al., 1961) as well as sources of morphogenetic information, regulating the proliferation and differentiation of different tissues (Svet-Moldavski, 1964; Petrov et al., 1972). Lymphocytes are involved in the regeneration process (Babaeva, 1972) and control the pathways and regeneration rate of stem hemopoietic cells. Antibody production and the regulation of humoral and cellular immune responses are also functions of special organs and lymphoid cells. Based on the classical studies of Mechnikov, Maksimov, and Bogomolts and in agreement with modern immunological concepts (Burnet, 1972), a concept of the physiological system of antigenic structural homeostasis may be formulated. This physiological system has many components which defend the organism from everything alien, controlling the constancy and adequacy of the antigenic structure of all organs and tissues; the same system provides appropriate interaction between cells, tissues, and organs through cellular and humoral complementary factors (Figure 1).

The antigenic structural (immune-structural) homeostasis system comprises the following elements (Figure 2):

(1) The control element (central organs of immunity - thymus, analogue of bursus Fabricii).

(2) The element accepting antigenic information - antigen-responsive T-lymphocytes.

(3) The effector elements - concerned with the synthesis of cellular and humoral antibodies, co-operation, differentiation, and proliferation of lymphoid T and B cells, production of lymphokins and so on.

(4) A system of direct and feedback control, with appropriate temporal and spatial relations.

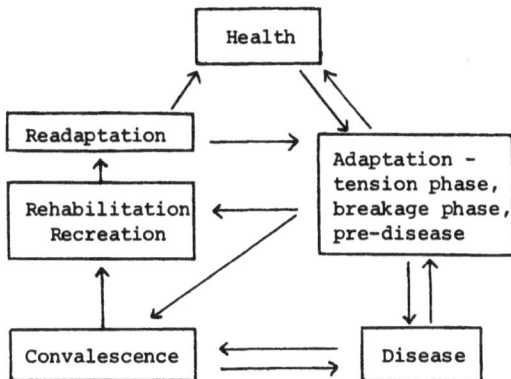

Figure 1   The system of immunological homeostasis (note that the following must be taken into account: specificity of the participating factors, biorhythms, phases of onto-genesis, genetic peculiarities of the individual)

(5) Cells that serve as stores of immunological memory.

(6) Non-specific factors concerned in the induction and development of immune responses, such as complement, inter-feron.

It is necessary to assess the magnitude of the response of tissues and target cells to the antigen-antibody res-ponse. An immunologically competent lymphoid cell is a discrete unit of immunological homeostasis and has the capacity to accept, transform, transmit, and store anti-genic information; it is capable of specific interaction and of synthesizing complementary structures. This complex system responds as a single unit, although the over-all effect is to a large extent due to the function of the separate components and each individual is distinguished by characteristic geno- and pheno-typic features of these components.

Immune homeostasis is subject to the influence of other physiological and pathological systems. It is always under the control of the neuroendocrine apparatus and must be supplied with adequate material and energy; it also has to be replenished periodically with cells from the pool of polypotent bone marrow stem cells.

A good idea of the functioning of immunostructural ho-meostasis and its component parts may be obtained under antigenic and non-antigenic loads. Transitional states are studied, when the system is first exposed to factors in the external or internal environment (including antigens);

```
                    ┌─────────────────────────┐
                    │  Neuroendocrine system  │
                    └─────────────────────────┘
                              ↑  │
┌─────────────────────┐       │  │       ┌─────────────────────┐
│ Plastic and energic │───────┼──┼──────→│ Polypotent stem cell│
│      provision      │       │  │       │        pool         │
└─────────────────────┘       │  ↓       └─────────────────────┘
         ↖  ↘                            ↖  ↗
          Antigen-structural homeostasis
```

```
┌──────────────────────────────────────────────────────────┐
│   ┌────────────────────────────────────────────────┐      │
│   │    Controlling link                             │      │
│ ┌─│ 1.  Thymus                                      │      │
│ │ └────────────────────────────────────────────────┘      │
│ │                    ↑ ↓                                   │
│ │ ┌────────────────────────────────────────────────┐      │
│ └→│ 2.  Link of perception of antigenic             │      │
│   │     information                                 │      │
│   │     macrophage, antigen-reactive cell           │      │
│   └────────────────────────────────────────────────┘      │
│                      ↑ ↓                                   │
│   ┌────────────────────────────────────────────────┐      │
│   │    Effectors link                               │      │
│   │ 3.  Co-operation, differentiation,              │      │
│   │     proliferation, antibody synthesis,          │      │
│   │     lymphocytes and other mediators             │      │
│   └────────────────────────────────────────────────┘      │
│              ↖  ↗   ↓ ↑                                     │
│              │   ┌────────────────┐                        │
│              │   │ Immunological  │                        │
│              │   │    memory      │                        │
│              ↓   └────────────────┘                        │
│   ┌────────────────────────────────────┐   ↓              │
│ ┌→│ Tissues, target-cells - realization │                  │
│ │ │ of immune responses by organs,      │                  │
│ │ │ anatomi-cal and physiological       │                  │
│ │ │ systems                             │                  │
│ │ └────────────────────────────────────┘                  │
└──────────────────────────────────────────────────────────┘
```

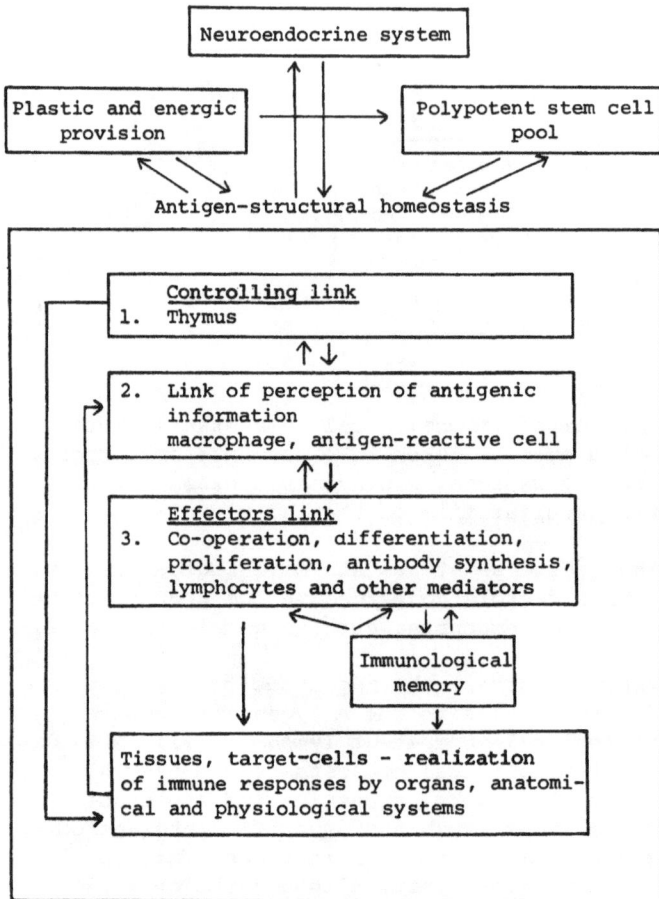

Figure 2   Elements of the system of immunological homeostasis

one may examine the triggering of adaptive mechanisms and
determine the subsequent state of antigenic-structural homeostasis - normalization and ultimate exhaustion (immunological deficiencies), along with such immunopathological
processes as allergy and autoimmune diseases (Figure 3).
   Studies on the role of immunological homeostasis in the
adaptation processes of man currently include exposure to
high altitudes and high latitudes, together with an examination of the role of immunity in pathological processes and
diseases developing under high latitude conditions. We are

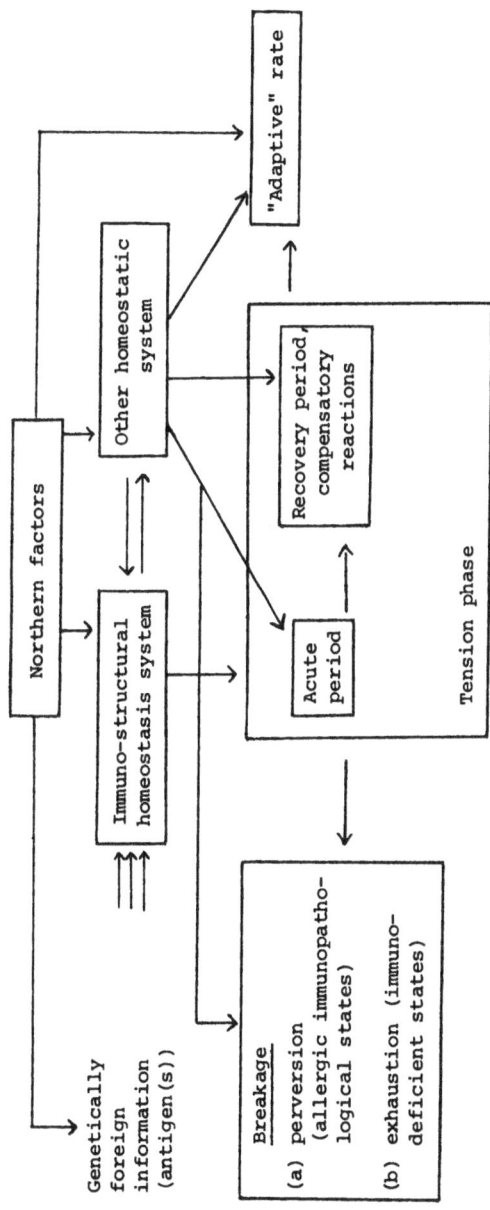

Figure 3   Phases of immuno-structural homeostasis during adaptation to a northern climate

concerned to develop methods and criteria to estimate the
functions of immunological homeostasis in normal subjects
at different phases of adaptive responses and under pathological conditions of homeostasis, at the levels of both organisms and populations. Our analysis seeks to take account
of the influence of the neuroendocrine apparatus, the supply
of materials and energy for immunological responses, the
registration of spatial and temporal characteristics, the
scanning of functions in time and space, and the measurements of rhythms and functional desynchronization.

By developing methods of predicting the behaviour of
systems of immunological homeostasis, and detecting impairments, it should be possible to determine the course of
some diseases and to work out a rationale for treatment.
It may also be useful to select men for work and permanent
residence in high latitude areas on the basis of immunological criteria. Applied aspects could include the development of scheduled inoculations and anti-epidemiological
measures.

RESULTS OF IMMUNOLOGICAL STUDIES IN THE NORTH

The specific studies performed to date include an examination of non-specific immunity factors in the North, a study
of lymphocyte properties using the phytophaemoagglutinin
test, the reaction of rosette-forming cells with autoery-
throcytes, antigen-conjugated connective tissue (the sedimentation reaction of erythrocytes with leucocytes), the
percentage of T-cells in the reaction of rosette-forming
cells with sheep erythrocytes, the cytopathic features of
blood lymphocytes, the number and relative content of im-
munoglobins A, G, M in residents of high and low latitudes
of Siberia. Determinations of the immunological status of
normal subjects and patients with autoimmune diseases included measurements of diurnal and seasonal fluctuations,
and metabolic assays of proteins, lipids, and carbohydrates. The groups analysed have comprised men living in
northern and southern latitudes of Siberia for different
periods of time. In assessing results, it is important to
take into account variations of immunological responses related to diurnal and seasonal dynamics.

Thus, the percentage of T-lymphocytes in the peripheral
blood varies from 29.2 to 65.2 per cent of the total number
of lymphocytes in the blood of normal youths (Figure 4).
This is significant in view of the fact that T-lymphocytes
are the most important elements of the immune system.

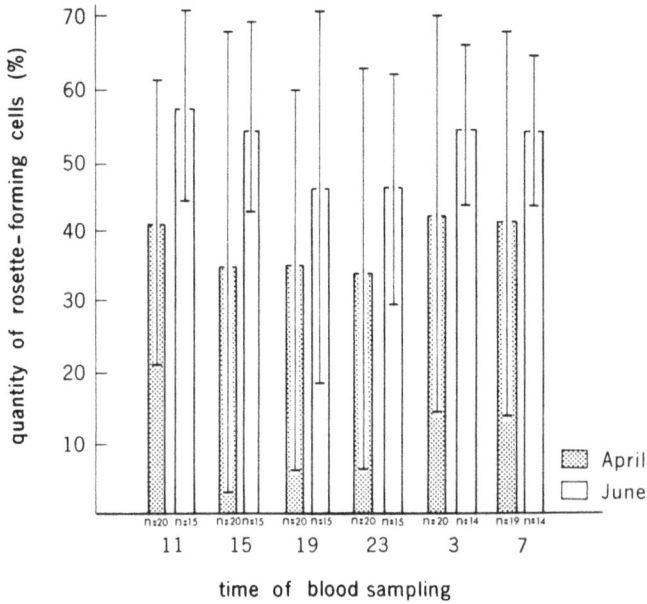

Figure 4   24-hour dynamics of T-cells in peripheral blood
of healthy subjects during spring (April) and summer (June)
at Novosibirsk

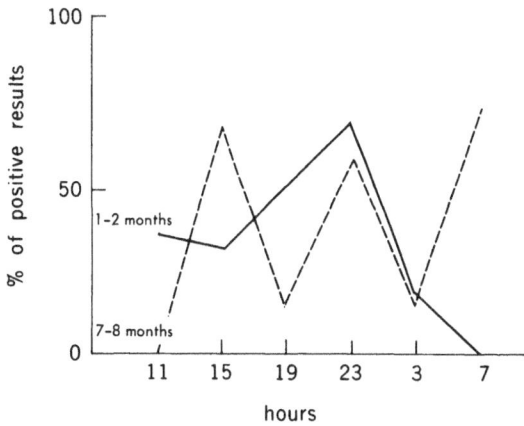

Figure 5   Daily rhythm of positive reactions of erythrocytes with leucocytes for men after 1-2 and 7-8 months of
residence in the arctic

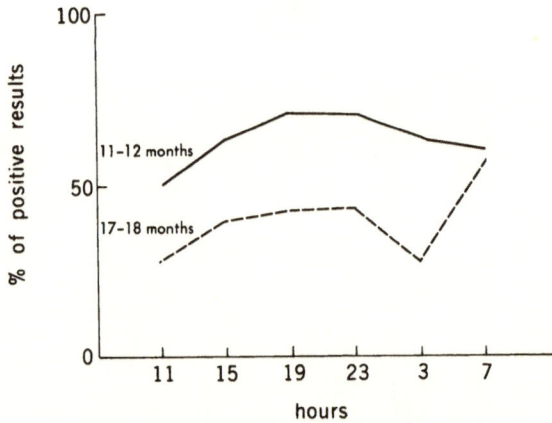

Figure 6 Daily rhythm of positive reactions of erythrocytes with leucocytes for men after 11-12 months and 17-18
months of residence in the arctic

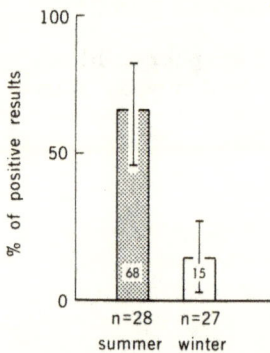

Figure 7 Histogram of positive reactions of erythrocytes with leucocytes in
newcomers to the arctic
during summer and winter (χ^2
= 12, p < 0.01)

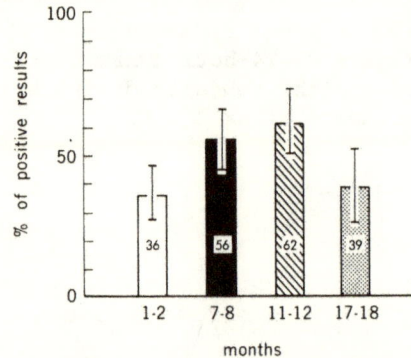

Figure 8 Average percentage
of positive reactions of erythrocytes with leucocytes for
men after varying periods of
residence in the arctic (χ^2
= 18.5, p < 0.001)

This heterogeneous cell subpopulation performs the function
of detecting and regulating the proliferation processes of
bone marrow cells participating in the immune response.
These cells are also involved in reactions associated with
transplantation and anti-tumour immunity.

According to our observations, functional detection (sedimentation test of erythrocytes with leucocytes) of T-cells varies at different times of the day and at different seasons of the year, both in North and South Siberia. Different types of curves have also been obtained in subjects living in transpolar areas for different periods of time. Subjects who had lived in the North for 6 to 12 months showed 15 to 20 per cent of positive reactions during the polar day, as compared with 5 to 9 per cent of positive reactions during the polar night. After 1.5 years of residence in the North interseasonal differences disappeared. (Figures 5-8 and Table 1). In summer, the total number of T-cells in the blood was increased in some normal subjects. The sedimentation test and the content of T-cells was directly correlated with plasma corticoid content (Figure 7).

The blast-transformation of lymphocytes in cultures stimulated with PHA did not detect any differences between groups of residents of high and low latitudes depending on the duration of their residence, time of day, or season of the year (Table 2). This test gives valuable data in cases of immunodeficient and autoimmune processes, chronic inflammation of the lungs and so on; such conditions lead to decrease of blast-transformation and a phase shift of the reaction.

Depending on the duration of residence in the north, significant changes were detected in seasonal and diurnal variations of the complement titres, heterophylic antibodies, and the phagocytic activities of leucocytes. After 2 to 12 months of residence, the activity of non-specific immunity factors was restored to normal levels, and by 1.5 to 2 years it often surpassed the initial level. Over 1.5 years of residence, there were also changes in the blood serum spectrum, with decrease of albumins, increase of haemaglobulins, and changes in the relative content of different classes of immunoglobulins. During the initial period of residence in the North, newcomers showed an activation of foci of chronic infection and an aggravation of allergic reactions.

Thus, in the first 1.5 to 2 years, newcomers to the North show changes of lymphocyte properties, decreased non-specific immunological resistance, and a tendency towards development of immunological processes. The second phase of immunostructural homeostasis is characterized by a normalization of the functions of immunological homeostasis, with clear-out diurnal and seasonal periodicity and often a breakdown of some type (allergy, chronic, microbic,

TABLE 1
Positive reactions of erythrocytes with leucocytes in newcomers to
the arctic during spring (April) and summer (June)

	7 a.m.	11 a.m.	3 p.m.	7 p.m.	11 p.m.	3 a.m.
April, 18 men						
Average No. with reaction	1	4	1	8	4	7
Mean and SD (%)	6 ± 6	22 ± 10	6 ± 6	44 ± 12	22 ± 10	39 ± 12
Range (%)	0–26	6–48	0–26	22–69	6–48	17–64
June, 20 men						
Average No. with reaction	2	1	1	1	1	0
Mean and SD (%)	10 ± 7	5 ± 5	5 ± 5	5 ± 5	5 ± 5	0 ± 5
Range (%)	1–32	0–24	0–24	0–24	0–24	0–17

TABLE 2
Correlations between plasma 11-oxycorticosteroids and
(a) erythrocyte/leucocyte reaction and (b) titre of
heterophyllic antibodies for first one to eight months
of residence in the arctic

	Time of day			
	3 p.m.	7 p.m.	11 p.m.	3 a.m.
RAEL	+0.724	+0.768	+0.890	+0.470
Titre of heterophyllic antibodies	+0.682	+0.796	+0.760	+0.048

TABLE 3
Correlations between plasma 11-oxycorticosteroids and
(a) erythrocyte/leucocyte reaction and (b) titre of
heterophyllic antibodies for first two years of residence
in the arctic

	Time of day			
	7 a.m.	3 p.m.	7 p.m.	11 p.m.
RAEL	−0.946	−0.006	+0.566	+0.768
Titre of heterophyllic antibodies	+0.742	+0.759	+0.212	+0.796

or viral infection, autoimmune disturbances, lymphoproli-
ferative processes, and so on). The detection of this critical period in immunological homeostasis requires early prophylactic measures.

SUMMARY

The central role of the lymphocytes in immuno-structural
homeostasis is stressed. The immune system is described,
and its importance in adaptation to the arctic environment
is discussed. Objective measurements of the reaction between leucocytes and sheep red cell erythrocytes show 24-
hour and summer/winter differences in antibody titres
which are modified as the subject becomes adapted to the
Arctic. The method used may have practical value in demonstrating a tension phase in the process of adjustment,
where the immunological system is under particular stress;
if such a stage can be demonstrated, appropriate prophylactic measures could then be instituted.

Commentaries

"A comparison of genetic markers in the blood of circumpolar populations," by Nancy E. Simpson and Phyllis J.
McAlpine (Departments of Paediatrics and Biology, Queen's
University, Kingston, Canada). Eleven out of 38 loci for
markers in blood which had alleles which were common
enough to be considered polymorphic in the Igloolik population were examined. The definition of polymorphism used
was an arbitrary one proposed by Harris, i.e. when there
is evidence for two or more alleles determining a variant
form of a marker and the frequency of the least common
allele appears to be no less than 0.01. The Igloolik markers reported here exclude the blood groups. The eleven
polymorphic loci were the six red cell enzymes 2, 3-DPGM,
sGOT, sGPT, PGM_1, PGD, and AcP; four serum markers E_2 cho-
linesterase, haptoglobin, Gm, and Inv; and the Hl-A lymphocyte antigens. When the allele frequencies of all of the
markers which were tested were compared, a few allele frequencies exhibited clines which may represent migratory

patterns; some were extremely variable for the different
populations and probably were the result of genetic drift;
there were some markers that were thought to be introduced
from Caucasian populations and some rare new variants found
which may represent alleles which are exclusive to that particular population.

"Histocompatibility studies on Canadian Inuit (Eskimos),"
by J.B. Dossetor, J.W. Schlaut, L. Olson, J.M. Alton, T.
Kovithavongs, P.R. McConnachie (Medical Research Council
Transplantation Group and Department of Clinical Pathology,
University of Alberta, Edmonton, Canada). Isolated populations are subject to the pressure of natural selection and
the phenomenon of genetic drift. Both these lead to restricted polymorphism and increased homozygosity. The
latter, for histocompatibility genes, might lead to increased graft survival. Two populations of Canadian Inuit
(Eskimos), 236 individuals in the MacKenzie Delta and 336
at Igloolik, were tissue typed for HL-A antigens. In Igloolik, lymphocytes were also obtained for selective mixed
leucocyte culture (MLC). Thus data on the serologically defined (SD) and lymphocyte defined (LD) antigens of the
major histocompatibility complex (MHC) were obtained. Then,
in Igloolik, 190 selected 6 mm punch skin grafts were observed for survival.
    The HL-A antigens (SD) of Inuit show marked polymorphic
restriction with very high frequencies for HL-A 9 (88 per
cent) and HL-W10 (80 per cent) and 30 per cent of cells
were homozygous for these two antigens. No evidence could
be obtained of Inuit specific antigens not marked by Caucasoid typing sera. Over all, skin grafts between Inuit survived longer (17 days) than between Caucasoids (11 days).
However, although grafts between HL-A identical family members lasted longest (27 days), those between HL-A identi-
cals of different families lasted only 18.5 days and there
was MLC stimulation between 9 of 11 in the latter group.
This established that SD factors of the MHC in this population are associated with more than one LD factor and that
SD identity, alone, does not favour graft survival. This
was confirmed in one unique family where both parents and
all siblings were SD identical and yet MLC showed that the
two parents were LD different, and there were several MLC
groups amongst the siblings; in this family the skin grafts
also did not survive more than 30 days. No conclusion can
be drawn, at present, on whether this homozygosity reflects

natural selection for survival in the north or is merely
genetic drift.(Supported by MRC and IBP (Canada).)

"Deficiency of secretory IgA in Eskimo saliva," by Hamdy
Sayed, J. Sayed, J.A. Hildes, and O. Schaefer (University
of Manitoba, Winnipeg, and Health and Welfare Canada,
Edmonton). Local immune mechanisms may be of greater importance in resistance to respiratory viral infections than
circulating mechanisms; and high levels of serum immunoglobulins may indicate failure of the local mechanisms to
prevent infection. Parotid saliva from 14 Igloolik Eskimos
and 4 Eskimos resident in Winnipeg were studied by electro-
immunodiffusion for secretory IgA and by a specific antibody test for secretory piece. Twelve of the 14 had serum
samples for immunoglobulin assays by radial immune diffu-
sion and immunoelectrophoresis. Three of the Iglooligmiuts
had absent salivary IIS-IgA and increased 7S-IgG. In two
others the salivary IIS-IgA was only detected in trace
amounts, and again the predominant salivary immunoglobulin
was 7S-IgG. All the other saliva samples had low normal values of IIS-IgA but again the 7S-IgG was predominant. The
salivary concentrations of secretory piece were in comfor-
mity: the three cases with absent IIS-IgA had absent secretory piece, the two cases had very low levels, and the
remainder had low normal levels. The sera of the 3 subjects with absent salivary IIS-IgA showed a broad bowed arc
with beta-electrophoretic mobility which failed to react
with anti-IgM, anti-IgD, or anti-IgE and also failed to
react with the γ chain components characteristic of IgG.
However reacting these sera with anti-L immune serum was
suggestive of a lambda A myeloma protein. In contrast
sera from the two subjects with trace amounts of secretory
IgA indicated striking increases of IgG, IgM, and IgA
polyclonal in nature. Quantitative testing also indicated
polyclonal hypergammaglobulinemia; in contrast to the ano-
malous protein demonstrated in the other 3 subjects. These
findings may have significance for understanding patterns
of disease prevalence in Eskimos. (Supported by the Canadian Committee for IBP.)

"Demographic aspects of the Canadian Eskimo communities of Igloolik and Hall Beach," by Phyllis J. McAlpine and Nancy E. Simpson (Department of Paediatrics and Biology, Queen's University, Kingston, Canada). Demographic data from the closely related Eskimo communities of Igloolik and Hall Beach in the eastern Canadian Arctic have been collected and analysed. Low median age groups, 10 to 14 years for males and females in Igloolik and females in Hall Beach and 15 to 19 years for males in Hall Beach, reflect the high proportion of young persons in both communities. Post-menopausal women in Hall Beach had larger families than their counterparts in Igloolik, but the mean family size of pre-menopausal women in the two communities were similar. The birth rate per thousand population was greater in Igloolik than in Hall Beach but no difference in the sex ratios of births was detected between communities. Multiple births were frequent. The high infant and childhood mortality in both communities indicated that as many as one-third of all liveborn children did not survive long enough to have off-spring. Of the present marriages in the two communities 8.2 per cent were known to be consanguineous relationships, and the coefficient of inbreeding among their offspring was es-timated to be 0.001 per cent. Caucasian admixture was esti-mated to be about 3 per cent from family history analysis and about 7 per cent from genetic marker data.

GROWTH AND DEVELOPMENT

Growth of Eskimo children in northwestern Alaska

P.L. JAMISON

MATERIALS

The growth data reported in this paper were collected as
part of the US/IBP research on Eskimos living in northwestern Alaska. Field trips to Alaska occurred during the
summers of 1968 through 1971 and children were measured in
five villages: Wainwright, Point Hope, Anaktuvik Pass, Kak-
tovik (Barter Island), and Barrow. The entire cross-
sectional sample numbers 488 children (253 males, 235 females) between the ages of 1 and 20 years. Growth rates
have also been estimated on a smaller longitudinal sample
of males from the village of Wainwright.

There is some apparent variation in the growth status
of children in different Eskimo villages, as well as variation between hybrids and non-hybrids. Based on the present
data, Barrow children are shorter and lighter than the
children in Point Hope or Wainwright. Hybrid versus non-
hybrid comparisons demonstrate smaller differences than
those between villages. White admixture predominates in
the hybrids although Eskimo/Black hybrids occur in Point
Hope. Since the primary purpose of this paper is to describe the growth of northwestern Alaskan Eskimo children
relative to a White standard and also relative to other
Eskimo series, both village of residence and admixture
status have been submerged in the analysis.

METHODS

All of the data on north Alaskan Eskimos reported here
were derived from measurements taken by the author himself.
The measurements were taken on subjects wearing light, indoor clothing - usually jeans and T-shirts for boys or
slacks and blouses for girls, plus undergarments. Subjects assumed an erect but not military attention posture

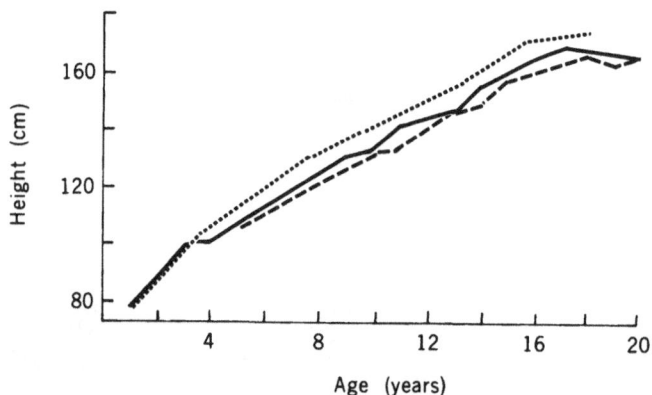

Figure 1   Male stature (—— Alaskan Eskimo; --- Canadian Eskimo; -·- US white)

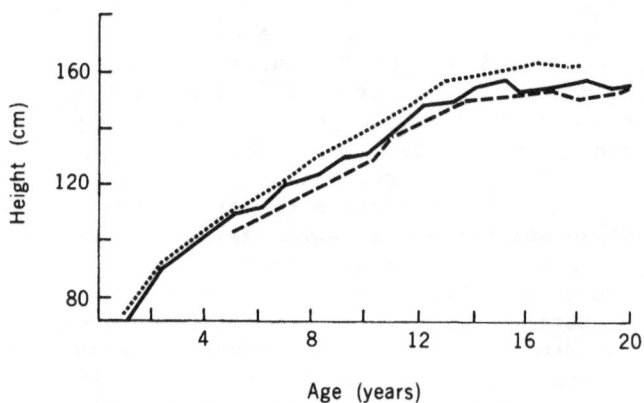

Figure 2   Female stature (—— Alaskan Eskimo; --- Canadian Eskimo; -·- US white)

for the measurement of stature. All weights were recorded on the same Health-O-Meter beam and balance scale. The decimal method of Weiner and Lourie (9) was used to record ages and the 6-year-old age group (for example) included children between the ages of 5.500 and 6.499 years.

RESULTS

Figures 1 and 2 (for males and females respectively) present the distance curves of growth in stature for Alaskan Eskimos as the solid lines between two broken ones. The

upper broken line in both figures represents the 50th percentile of a growth standard for US Whites, based on Stuart
and Meredith's data as reported in Watson and Lowry (8).
The stature of the Alaskan Eskimos generally falls between
the 10th and 25th percentiles of this standard. During
adolescence, both sexes approach the 25th percentile. At
age 18 there is a 6 cm difference for males and a 4.5 cm
difference for females between the Eskimos and the Whites.

The lower broken line in both figures represents growth
data on Canadian Eskimos from IBP research conducted in
Igloolik and Hall Beach, Northwest Territories. These data
reflect a mixed longitudinal series measured by Dr. Joan de
Peña (2). It is apparent that the Canadian Eskimos are
shorter than the Alaskans at all ages. In fact, the Canadians fall below the 10th percentile of the US White Standard until age 15 when they approximate this level. By age
18 the two Eskimo growth lines converge so that they reach
similar end points at the age limit of the present study.

Data from two other Alaskan Eskimo growth studies provide useful comparative material. The most recent study is
that of Heller, Scott, and Hammes (3), involving 286 boys
and 275 girls measured in nine villages in western Alaska
between 1957 and 1961. For stature, these data closely
approximate the Alaskan IBP data until the age of 11-12 in
both males and females. After this age, the earlier data
resemble those for the Canadian Eskimos.

A second body of Alaskan Eskimo growth data is that of
Hrdlicka (4) who analysed a mixed longitudinal series of
97 children who lived in Bethel (southwestern Alaska) between 1928 and 1931. At all ages, stature in these children is below that seen in the Alaskan IBP data. Hrdlicka's
data approximate the Canadian IBP data until age 11-12 and
then drop below the Canadian. In both sexes the discrepancy between the present Alaskan data and that from Bethel
(40 years earlier) gets progressively wider during adolescence.

Figures 3 and 4 show distance curves for weight, using
the same graphic representation of the populations as before. Alaskan Eskimo weights initially fall very close to
the 50th percentile of the White standard (until age 16
in males and 11 in females), but then they move up to the
75th percentile. At age 18, the Eskimo males are 16 pounds
heavier than the Whites and the females are 12 pounds
heavier. Canadian Eskimos lie just above the 25th percentile of the US standard until the early teens, when both
sexes also begin a trend upwards, in this case to the 50th

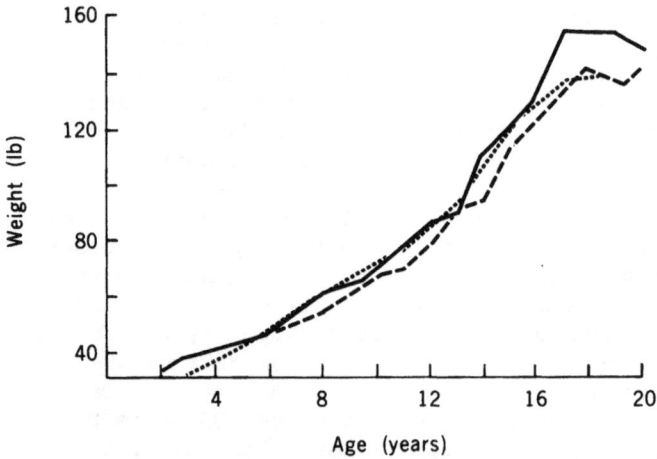

Figure 3   Male weight (—— Alaskan Eskimo; --- Canadian Eskimo; ••• US white)

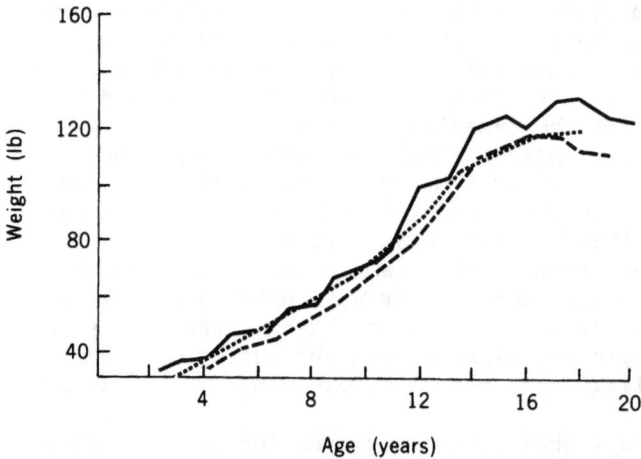

Figure 4   Female weight (—— Alaskan Eskimo; --- Canadian Eskimo; ••• US white)

percentile. At all ages the Canadian Eskimo weights are lower than that of their Alaskan counterparts; at age 20 the difference is 5-7 pounds.

The Alaskan Eskimo weight data from Heller et al. (3) show males to be between current north Alaskans and Canadians in weight until age 12, when the earlier data fall

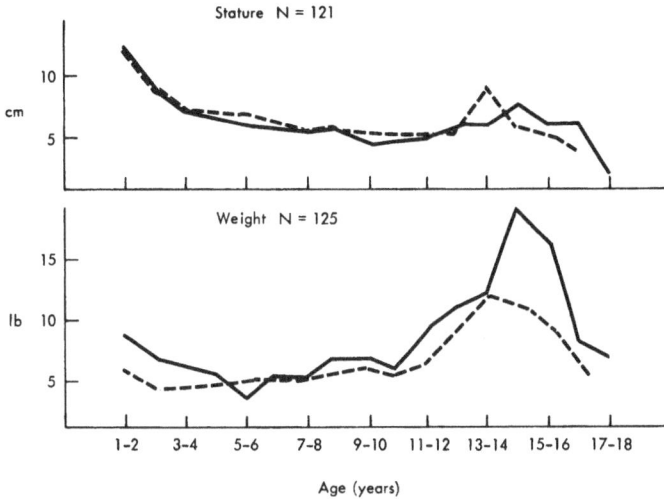

Figure 5   Mean annual increments for males (— Alaskan Eskimo; --- US white)

off to more closely resemble the Canadian data. Hrdlicka's
data on Bethel children lie just beneath the Canadian Eskimo data in Figures 3 and 4 until age 9-10. At this age
the Bethel weights continue in a linear fashion with no
apparent growth spurt.

   Figure 5 shows mean annual increments in male stature
and weight, calculated from a semilongitudinal series of
67 Wainwright Eskimos and graphed by chronological age.
The velocity curves are based on 121 replicate measurements
for stature and 125 replicates for weight. Eskimo mean
annual increments (solid lines) are again compared with US
White data from Watson and Lowry (8). For stature, the Eskimo growth rate is below the standard up to the adolescent
period. The peak velocity for the Eskimos occurs between
the ages of 14 and 15, or one year later than for Whites.
The adolescent growth spurt for stature reaches a lower
peak among the Eskimos, but the increased velocity lasts
longer. By age 17-18 the growth rate has fallen to 2 cm
per year, indicating that the point of effective growth
cessation is near.

   For weight, the rate curve for Wainwright Eskimos is
somewhat above the White standard at nearly all ages, an
again the peak velocity is one year later than that seen
for Whites. The magnitude of the Eskimo peak velocity is
surely a sampling error, but it is very likely that the
actual peak velocity is greater than that of the White

standard. This follows the results seen in the distance
curves as well.

DISCUSSION

The point frequently made concerning Eskimo growth is that
there is a higher weight per unit stature than is seen for
Whites. The Alaskan IBP data are no exception to this generalization. However, a shift is apparently occurring to
higher rates of growth of both stature and weight. When
compared with the White standard, stature moves from the
10th to the 25th percentile and for weight from the 50th
to the 75th percentile. Is this a feature of the traditional
Eskimo growth pattern or an aspect of relatively recent
change related to secular trends?

When present results are compared with the earlier Alaskan data, a tendency is seen for a greater disparity during
adolescence than before it. The increasing north Alaskan
Eskimo stature seen previously (5) can be described more
specifically as an increased rate of growth during adolescence.

The difference between the Alaskan and Canadian IBP data
must relate to the genetic-environment interaction taking
place in both populations. Central Canadian Eskimos are
generally shorter in stature than northwestern Alaskan
Eskimos as seen in the data of Jenness (6), Seltzer (7),
Birket-Smith (1), and de Peña (2), suggesting that a genetic predisposition for size may be involved. However,
different nutritional regimes, varying health conditions,
and perhaps a slightly different stage in the development
of secular trends in the two populations have likely entered into the situation. The national and international
syntheses of IBP data currently in preparation will allow
more definitive statements to be made about the specifics
of this interaction between genetics and environment.

SUMMARY

Stature and weight data on Eskimo children living in northwestern Alaska were collected as part of the US contribution to the International Biological Program (IBP). These
data are compared to a US White growth standard, Canadian
Eskimo IBP data, and data from two earlier Alaskan Eskimo
growth studies. The data indicate that north Alaskan Eskimos are taller and heavier at all ages than central Canadian Eskimos. In comparison with the US standard, Alaskan

Eskimo stature falls between the 10th and 25th percentiles
and their weight lies between the 50th and 75th percentiles.
During adolescence both variables approach higher percentiles of the White standard. A male, semilongitudinal
series indicates that peak growth velocity for stature and
weight occurs a year later among Alaskan Eskimos than among
Whites and the adolescent spurt appears to be of longer duration.

REFERENCES

1. Birket-Smith, K., "Anthropological observations on the
   Central Eskimos," Rept. of the Fifth Thule Exped. 1921-
   1924, 3(2): 1-126 (1940)
2. de Peña, J., "Growth and development," in D.R. Hughes
   (ed.), IBP Annual Report No. 4, Human Adaptability Proj-
   ject, Univ. of Toronto Anthrop.Series, No. 11, pp. 47-
   69, 1972
3. Heller, C.A., Scott, E.M., and Hammes, L.M., "Height,
   weight and growth of Alaskan Eskimos," Am. J. Dis.
   Child., 113: 338-44 (1967)
4. Hrdlicka, A. Height and weight in Eskimo children. Am.
   J. Phy. Anthropol., 28: 331-341 (1941)
5. Jamison, P.L., "Growth of Wainwright Eskimos: stature
   and weight," Arctic Anthropol. 7 (1): 86-94 (1970)
6. Jenness, D., "The Copper Eskimos. Part B: Physical
   characteristics of the Copper Eskimos," Rept. Canad.
   Arctic Exped. 1913-1918, 12 (B): 1-87 (1923)
7. Seltzer, C.C., "The anthropometry of the Western and
   Copper Eskimos, based on data of Vilhjalmur Stefansson,"
   Hum. Biol. 5 (3): 313-70 (1933)
8. Watson, E.H., and Lowry, G.H., Growth and Development
   of Children, 5th ed. (Chicago: Year Book Medical Publ.,
   1967)
9. Weiner, J.S., and Lourie, J.A., Human Biology, A Guide
   to Field Methods (Philadelphia: F.A. Davis CO., 1969)

Growth, development, and fitness of the Canadian Eskimo*

A. RODE and R.J. SHEPHARD

Eskimo residents in the Canadian Arctic settlement of Igloo-lik currently have an above average level of cardiorespiratory fitness (page 78). It is thus of interest to examine the growth and development of physiological variables related to cardiorespiratory performance within this population.

METHODOLOGY

A cross-sectional study of 58 boys and 52 girls aged 9-19 years was completed in the summer of 1970 and studies were repeated on 49 of the group 12-14 months later. Tests conformed to the protocol established by the International Biological Program (6). Anthropometric measures included standing height, body weight, and the thickness of three skinfolds - triceps, subscapular, and suprailiac. Cardiorespiratory performance was assessed by a progressive submaximal step-test and maximum oxygen intake was predicted by means of the Åstrand nomogram. Knee extension strength was assessed by cable tensiometer, and hand grip by Stoelting dynamometer.

STANDING HEIGHT

Cross-sectional data for standing height (Figure 1) showed that both sexes were substantially shorter than recent series studied in southern Canada, the US, and the UK; indeed, the Eskimo children were slightly shorter than Toronto children of 1939 (2). The period of greatest increase in average height occurred around the age of 14 in the boys and 11 in the girls - a few months later than in southern Ontario Whites.

Unlike White girls, the Eskimo girls were taller than the boys from the age of 11 to 14. As in southern communities, they grew little after the age of 14, and reached full adult stature at about 16 years. The boys continued

---

* This study forms part of the multidisciplinary Canadian International Biological Program, Human Adaptability Project.

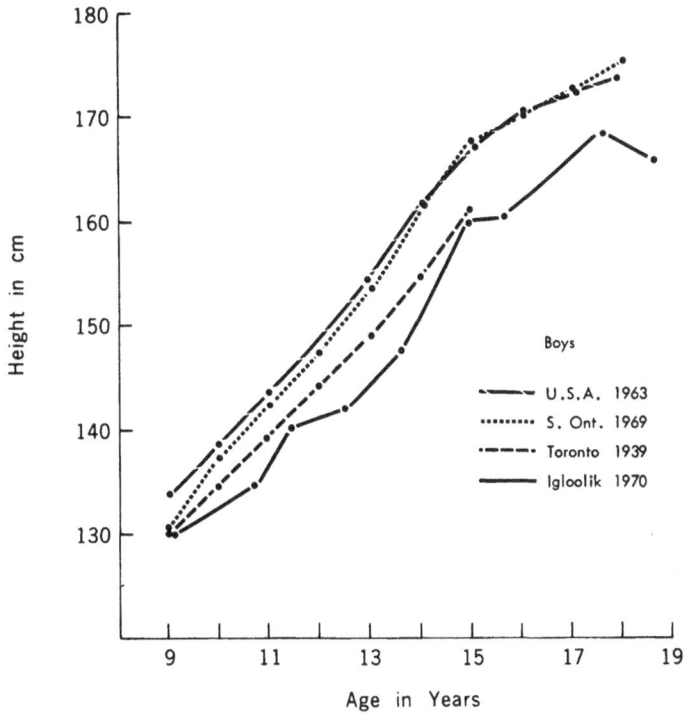

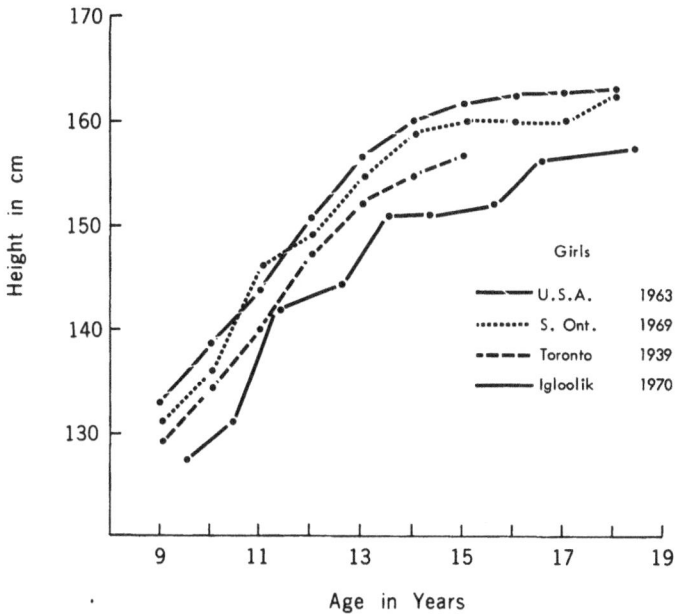

Figure 1   Comparison of height in boys and girls; data from cross-sectional studies

to grow to the age of 17, with a final advantage of some
10 cm relative to the girls.

The general form of the growth curve did not differ substantially from that anticipated in a White community, although in common with many primitive groups the average age
of peak growth was delayed by a few months relative to
current generations of city-dwellers.

Apparent Secular Trend

Younger adults were taller than older adults. Taken at
face value, the difference was equivalent to a secular
trend of 1.7 cm/decade in the male Eskimos and 1.9 cm/de-
cade in the females.

The fully grown Igloolik Eskimo is currently 6-7 cm
shorter than the average North American White, attaining a
maximum stature of 167-168 cm in the male and some 157 cm
in the female. Such values are comparable with recently reported standing heights of pure-bred Alaskan Eskimos (2)
and are substantially greater than the 1967 heights of
Skolt Lapps (4).

The short stature of the Eskimo must be remembered when
assessing various indices of fitness, whether simple performance tests or more precise measures of cardiorespiratory physiology. Some data such as lung volumes are related directly to standing height, and other variables such
as cardiac output are often related to body surface area.

BODY WEIGHT

Cross-sectional data indicate that in both sexes body
weights are less than current norms for the White population and are closely similar to published figures for
Toronto children of 1939 (Figure 2). In Eskimo boys, the
most rapid weight gain was apparently between the 14th and
15th years, while in girls the greatest gain was between
the 13th and 14th years. The longitudinal data placed the
period of rapid weight gain between 13.5 to 15.5 years in
the boys, and between 11 and 14.5 in the girls. Among individual girls, the rapid weight gain was initiated simul-
taneously with the height spurt, but in the boys the
weight spurt did not begin until almost one year after the
height spurt.

The girls had a greater weight than the boys between the
12th and the 14th years, and as with standing height the
sexual difference in body weight was more marked than in
the White population.

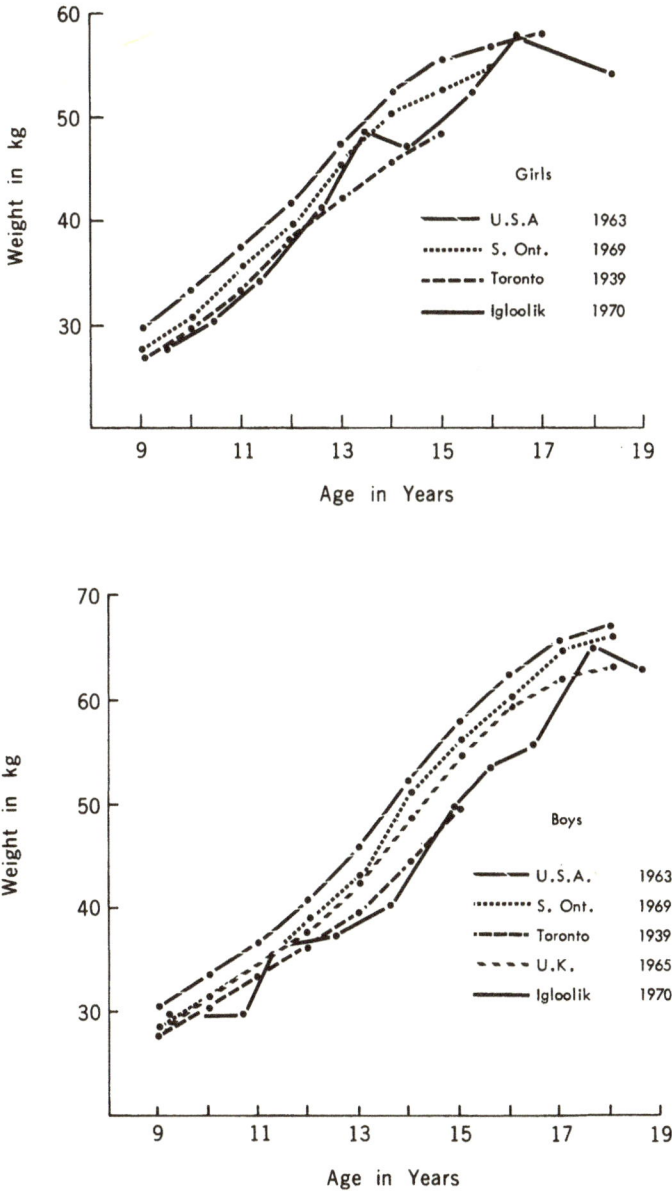

Figure 2   Comparison of weight in boys and girls; data from cross-sectional studies

SUBCUTANEOUS FAT

The boys showed a relatively uniform subcutaneous fat thickness between the 9th and 19th years. The final total of 18.2 mm for the sum of three folds was very modest by White standards and implies that the weight spurt initiated late in the 13th year was attributable almost entirely to lean tissue rather than fat.

At age 12, the girls had a summated fold thickness of approximately 18 mm, but this increased substantially with the onset of puberty. Cross-sectional and longitudinal data agree that the increase of thickness dated from the 13th year. Substantial quantities of subcutaneous fat were accumulated between the ages of 14 and 16, at a time when height was relatively static but body weight was still increasing.

Taking the sum of measurements for the three IBP skinfolds, recent figures for 9-13 year old boys are comparable in Toronto (22.7 mm) and Saskatoon (23.4 mm), but are little more than half as great in Igloolik (14.3 mm). Indeed, if we accept that in the Eskimo as in the white man each double fold of skin itself measures 4 mm, then there can be almost no subcutaneous fat in the young Eskimo boys. Even in late adolescence, the Eskimo boy remains thin, the average thickness at 17-18 years (18 mm) being much less than the comparable value for Torontonians (34 mm).

The figures for young Eskimo girls (with an average of 18.8 mm over the age span 9 to 13 years) are a little higher than for the boys, but are still much lower than in Toronto (average 30.6 mm). Eskimo girls accumulate a substantial quantity of fat in later adolescence, but the final readings (30-35 mm) remain below the 42 mm encountered in young Toronto adults.

MUSCLE STRENGTH

Cross-sectional data on the boys showed continuing development of handgrip strength to the 18th year (Figure 3) with particularly marked gains between 14 and 18. Leg extension strength showed a clearly defined spurt between 14 and 15 years of age. Longitudinal data suggested that both the grip and leg extension strengths of the boys began to increase rapidly in the 13th year, coincident with the initiations of rapid weight gain. Grip strength continued to increase throughout the period of observation, and gains of leg strength were also prolonged beyond the period of rapid weight gain.

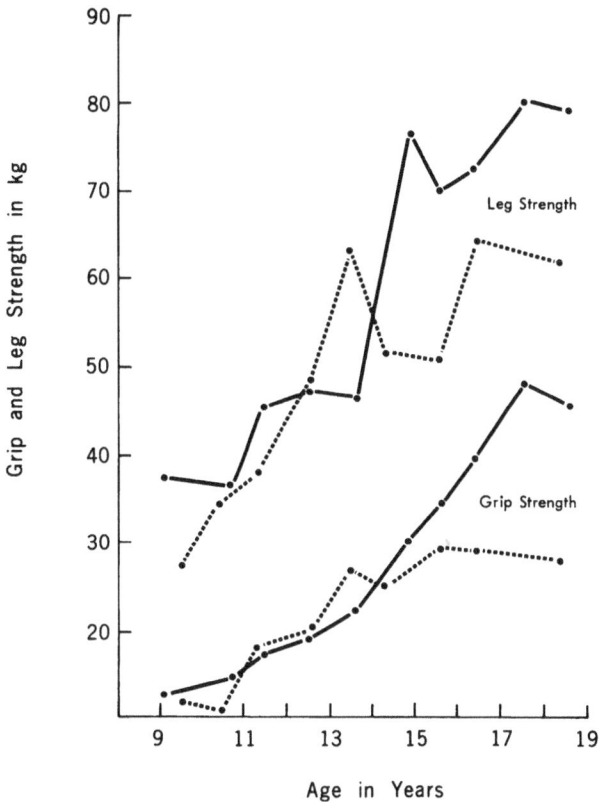

Figure 3 The increase of strength with age in Eskimo girls
(O) and boys (●); data from cross-sectional studies

Cross-sectional data for the girls indicated peak gains
in both grip and leg extension strength around the 13th
year, with little improvement of strength beyond 14 years
of age. An inspection of the longitudinal data indicated
rather earlier rapid gains of grip strength (from the 11th
to the 13th year) - with little improvement thereafter.
Leg extension strength developed vigorously from the 11th
to the 14th year.

In the boys, grip strength was consistently less than in
Toronto (5) and Edmonton (1). Leg extension strength was
similar in Igloolik and Toronto, but perhaps because of a
more complete immobilization of the trunk, was lower in
Edmonton. In the Eskimo girls the development of grip
strength ran closely parallel with that seen in Canadian

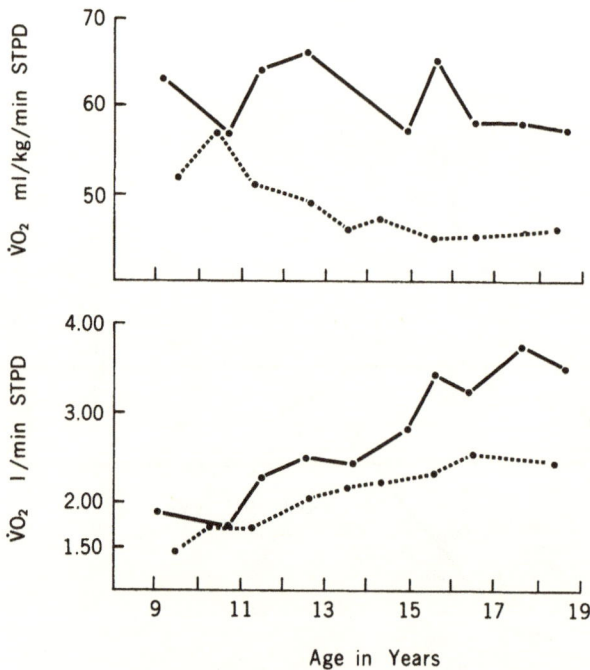

Figure 4   The predicted $\dot{V}_{O_2}$ max relative to age in Eskimo girls (O) and boys (●); data from cross-sectional studies

White communities. Leg extension strength in the younger girls was slightly greater than in Toronto and Edmonton; because development continued into late adolescence, final figures of 60 kg were 20 kg above those reported from Edmonton. A likely explanation for this continuing development of leg strength is the very common sight of a young girl carrying a 20-30 lb baby on her back in the traditional amauti as she goes about her chores and errands. At best, the terrain is uneven, and for most of the year snow makes walking with a load a good test of muscle power.

AEROBIC POWER

The boys showed a gradual development of absolute aerobic power throughout the period of observation (Figure 4). Inspection of this graph and our longitudinal data both suggest that the most marked increase (14-15 years) coincided with the period of maximum weight gain. The girls showed a rather slower development of absolute aerobic power; this reached a peak at the age of 16, with no clear sign of a growth spurt.

When the data were plotted relative to body weight, the boys maintained a rather constant ratio throughout the period of observation. The young girls had almost as large a relative aerobic power as the boys, but after the age of 10 there was a progressive decline, apparently related to the increase of body fat. The aerobic power of the late teenage girls was thus 20 per cent lower than at the age of 10.

If data are expressed relative to body weight, then the aerobic power of the Eskimo is at all ages substantially superior to that for White children. Part of the apparent fitness of the Eskimo child is attributable to a low percentage of body fat, and when data are expressed in absolute terms the discrepancy from previously reported material is less striking. Nevertheless, for most gross body movements, the per kilogram standard is the relevant measure of fitness.

The decline of aerobic power in the older Eskimo girls is at variance with their well-maintained leg strength. The final figure is still higher than in the White university entrant, but the deterioration through adolescence is at least as great as in the White group.

ON OUTGROWING ONE'S STRENGTH

Does the adolescent outgrow his strength at any stage of development? In the Eskimo boys, there is some evidence that increases of height precede increases of weight and absolute cardiorespiratory power, although the rapid increment of height is coincident with the development of grip and leg extension strength, and the aerobic power per unit of body weight remains remarkably constant throughout puberty. In the girls, the aerobic power per unit of body weight certainly decreases during adolescence, but there is no evidence that this is due to any limitations of potential growth.

ACKNOWLEDGMENT

This research was supported in part by a research grant from the National Research Council (Human Adaptability project).

SUMMARY

The growth, development, and fitness of Canadian Eskimo children living at Igloolik (69°40'N) has been evaluated by means of a semilongitudinal survey. Both height and weight growth curves have a similar form to those reported for southern Canadian and US cities, but the growth spurt is apparently delayed by a few months. At all ages, Canadian Eskimo children are shorter and lighter than their white counterparts, but the weight/height ratio is similar to that of the city-dweller. The secular trend to an increase of height (1.7 cm/decade in men, 1.9 cm/decade in women) suggests that the size differential between the White population and the Eskimos will disappear over the next few decades.

Skinfold thicknesses are extremely thin in Eskimo boys throughout development. The girls lay down a substantial quantity of subcutaneous fat during and following puberty, but remain thinner than city-dwellers. The boys are characterized by a rather poor grip strength and average leg strength. The girls have an average grip strength, but an unusual development of leg strength in late adolescence, perhaps caused by carrying small children on their backs over the rough terrain. The boys maintain a high level of relative aerobic power throughout the period of development. The girls show a progressive decline from the age of 12; this trend is thought to be socially conditioned.

REFERENCES

1. Howell, M.L., Loiselle, D.S., and Lucas, W.G., "Strength of Edmonton school-children," unpublished report, Fitness Research Unit, University of Alberta, Edmonton, 1966
2. Jamison, P.L., and Zigura, S.L., "An anthropometric study of the Eskimos of Wainwright, Alaska," Arctic Anthropol., 7: 125-43 (1970)
3. Keyfitz, N., A height and weight survey of Toronto elementary school-children, 1939 (Ottawa: Dominion Bureau of Statistics, 1942)
4. Lewin, T., Jurgens, H.W., and Louekari, L., "Secular trends in the adult height of Skolt Lapps," Arctic Anthropol., 7: 53-62 (1970)
5. Shephard, R.J., Allen, C., Bar-Or, O., Davies, C.T.M., Degré, S., Hedman, R., Ishii, K., Kaneko, M., La Cour, J.R., di Prampero, P.E., and Seliger, V., "The working

capacity of Toronto school-children." Canad. Med. Assoc.
J., 100: 500-66; 100: 705-14 (1968)
6. Weiner, J.S., and Lourie, J., Human Biology - a guide to
field methods (Oxford, UK: Blackwell Scientific Publications, 1969)

Secular changes in Lapps of northern Finland

J. SKROBAK-KACZYNSKI and T. LEWIN

The belief that the averages of body dimensions and proportions remain unchanged in human populations under conditions of genetical stability is fundamental to hominid taxonomy. Equally, in discussions of the origin and racial position of the Lapp people relative to other populations of
Europe and Asia, anthropometrical characteristics like stature, relative leg length, facial height and cephalic index
are considered important, conclusive issues.

The emphasis on body size for the racial classification
of Lapps is of rather recent origin. Earlier authors (e.g.
Schafferi (10), sic!) explained body particularities of
the Lapps - such as a short stature - on the basis of hard
living conditions, harsh climate, and poor nutrition. A
similar opinion was expressed by Virchow (13). Later investigators, however, rejected these opinions and started to
consider the body characteristics of Lapps as genetically
fixed racial marks. Bryn, for instance, wrote: "Ich glaube
dass es ganz richtig ist wenn man die Samen mit zu den
Pygmien rechnet"; he suggested that the lowest average ever
registered in any Lapp group should be considered the true
stature of Lapps, as any increase would be the effect of
Scandinavian admixture. The esimated stature of Lapps was
thus set around 150 cm - "ja vielleicht sogar bedeutende
unter diser Zahl" (10). Estimating the cephalic index of
Lapps in the same way, Bryn found values between 88 and 90.
The other morphological characteristics of Lapps were also
estimated in this manner, including only "rassenrein ausse-
hender Individen" - or "correcting" averages for possible
Scandinavian admixture, giving values which fitted the
author's ideas of what could be considered Lappish traits.

The conclusion was that "die Samen in einer Klasse für sich
selbst stehen, weit entfernt von allen anderen europeischen
Völksarten...". Any shortness of stature in Scandinavians
was explained by Lappish admixture, and any increase of stature in Lapps as a result of penetration by Scandinavian
genes.

More recent investigations of school age children of
Swedish and Norwegian Lapps (7,11) have pointed out strong
secular trends in these populations. A number of "Lappish
traits" now seem on the way out, these children achieving
a stature and some body proportions like other Scandinavians. The present study of northern Finnish Lapps was designed to allow not only a description of morphological
traits in the present generation of Lapps, but also to detect the existence, direction, and magnitude of any changes
in these traits over the last two to three generations,
with their possible causes. In the Lapp population, we can
determine the relationship between secular changes and environmental factors alone. In most other populations, however, the environmental changes are so closely interrelated
with increasing heterozygote that it is not possible to give
a final answer on the main cause of the secular trend.

MATERIAL AND METHODS

The Skolt Lapps are still genetically isolated both from the
Finns and from the Inari Lapps. Those of the latter included
in our sample also have none or very minor Finnish admixture. Altogether, 93 male and 83 female adult Skolts were
examined together with 133 male and 151 female adult Inari
Lapps. Anthropometric data on 48 male and 48 female Skolt
Lapps were taken from Nickul and Outakoski's study of 1934
(8). Data on 52 adult male and 50 adult female Inari Lapps
was taken from Näätänen's examinations of 1928 (9). These
data were pooled with the anthropometric studies of Lewin
and Skrobak-Kaczynski (1968-70), thereby providing figures
uninfluenced by age involution for individuals born in
1885-1905, 1905-20, 1920-40, and 1945-50 (Table 1). All
measurements included were taken according to the techniques
advised by Martin (6).

RESULTS AND DISCUSSION

From the many measurements collected, the following are
taken for comparison: stature, relative length of legs,
total arm length, facial height, bizygomatic and bigonial

TABLE 1
Number and sex of Skolt and Inari Lapps born in different periods

		Birth period				
		1885–1905	1905–20	1920–40	1945–50	Total
Skolt Lapps	♂	19	46	19	9	93
	♀	15	41	20	17	93
Inari Lapps	♂	15	58	42	18	133
	♀	18	60	41	32	151

TABLE 2
Differences in morphological characteristics of Skolt and Inari male Lapps born in 1885-1905 and 1945-50 (A, absolute difference; R, relative difference)

	Skolt Lapps		Inari Lapps	
Measurement	A	R (%)	A	R (%)
Stature	10.6 cm**	6.8	5.0 cm**	3.1
Symphysion height	5.7**	7.4	3.5	4.4
Total arm length	5.0**	6.0	3.0*	3.5
Femur cond. breadth	1.2 mm	1.3	-3.1 mm*	-3.3
Humerus epic. breadth	-0.6	-0.9	-4.7*	-6.7
Wrist breadth	-0.7	-1.2	-3.1*	-5.2
Indices, relative (% of stature)				
Symphysion height	0.5		0.4	
Total arm length	-0.9		-1.1	
Femur cond. breadth	-0.3**		-0.4**	
Humerus epic. breadth	-0.3**		-0.4**	

* Significant difference, $p < 0.05$
** Significant difference, $p < 0.01$

diameter, facial and cephalic index. The reason for such
selection is that these measurements are often considered
the best in discriminating Lapps from other European populations, indicating both their racial separateness and
their Mongolian affinity.

The stature of both Skolt and Inari Lapps shows a significant increase from those born in 1885-1905 to those born
in 1945-50 (Figure 1 and Table 2). The increase amounts to
10 cm in Skolt males, 6.7 cm in Skolt females, 5.0 cm in
Inari males, and 5.3 cm in Inari females. As the increase
has been greater in the Skolts, the difference between them
and the Inari Lapps - significant in the past - has diminished to 1 cm. The stature of Skolts in relation to Norwegians (12) has increased from 90.5 per cent for the generations born in 1885-1905 to 93 per cent for those born in
1945-50. Lapp children from Norway (11) have also increased
their stature to such a degree that they are currently of
the same body size as Norwegian children born only 50 years
earlier. At present, we cannot exclude the possibility that
over a shorter or longer period of time the difference in
stature will be completely eliminated.

The great relative arm length is another characteristic
referred to as a specific Lappish trait. This index has decreased over the last 60 to 70 years (Table 2), and Lapps
born between 1945 and 1950 have the same relative arm length
as Norwegians, when comparisons are made between groups with
similar stature. On the other hand, the relative length of
the legs (also considered a specific Lapp or Mongolian
trait) is at present the same as in previous generations
(Figure 2 and Table 2). But again, if we compare the Lapps
- not with the total Norwegian population - but with groups
of approximately the same stature as the Lapps, the relative length of the legs is the same in both populations.
From tables giving the relative length of the legs for every
5 cm class of stature (12), it appears that this index does
not increase linearly with stature. Up to 170 cm, almost no
change occurs, but there is a conspicuous rise above this
limit. As Lapps still have an average stature of less than
170 cm, we cannot yet expect any alteration of this proportion.

Breadth measurements of the wrist, femoral condyles, and
humerus epicondyles express the sturdiness of body build.
A comparison of relative values for the two generations of
Lapps shows a dramatic change towards gracilization (Table
2). The increase of length is accompanied by a less sturdy
body build, a typical phenomenon characterizing the secular

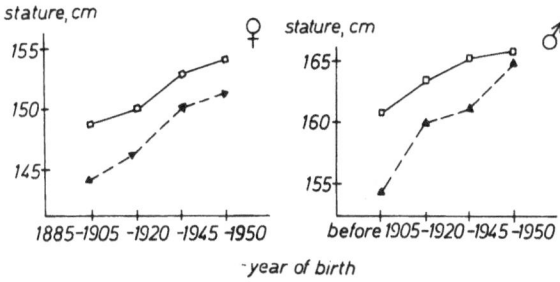

Figure 1   Changes of stature in Skolt and Inari Lapp men and women born in the period 1885-1950 (dashed line, Skolt Lapps; solid line, Inari Lapps)

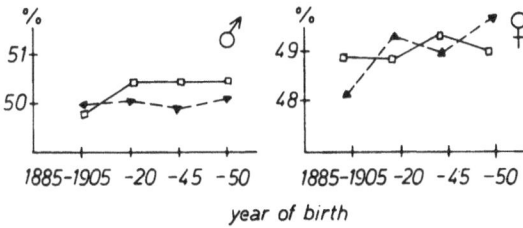

Figure 2   Relative symphysion height in Skolt and Inari Lapp men and women born in the period 1885-1950

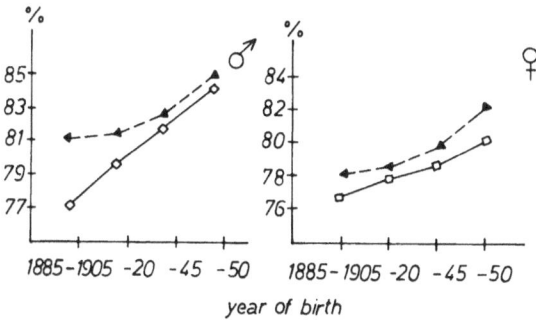

Figure 3   Changes of facial index in Skolt and Inari Lapp men and women born in the period 1885-1950

TABLE 3
Differences in craniofacial measurements of Skolt and Inari male
Lapps born in 1885-1905 and 1945-50 (A, absolute difference;
R, relative difference)

Measurement	Skolt Lapps		Inari Lapps	
	A	R (%)	A	R (%)
Head length	7.7**	4.2	3.2	1.7
Head breadth	0.1	0.0	0.4	0.2
Facial height	2.4	2.1	7.6**	6.8
Bizygomatic breadth	-2.5	-1.8	-4.3**	-3.1
Bigonial breadth	-1.9	-1.8	-5.2**	-4.5
Indices				
Relative head length	-0.29		-0.16	
Relative head breadth	-0.64**		-0.27	
Cephalic index	-3.6**		-1.6	
Relative face height	-0.33		0.25	
Relative bizyg. breadth	-0.73**		-0.53**	
Facial index	3.24**		7.71**	
Relative bigonial breadth	-0.56**		-0.53**	

** Significant change, $p < 0.01$.

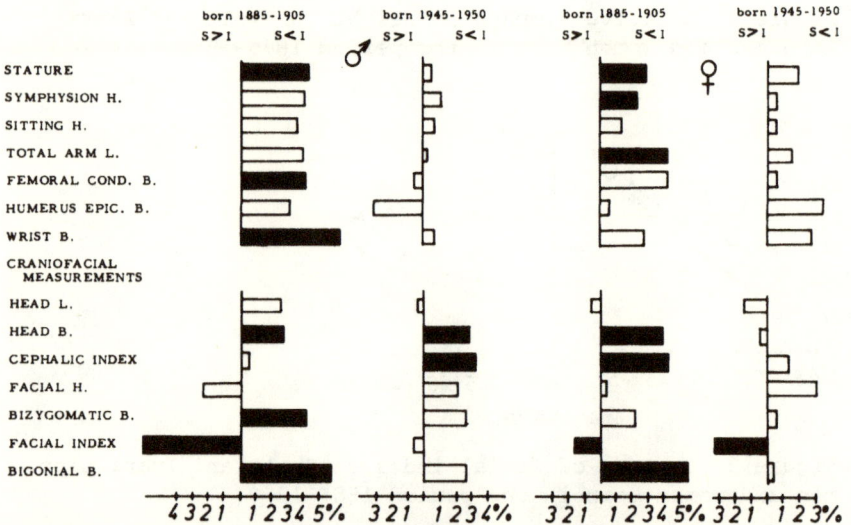

Figure 4   Comparison of morphological differences between
Skolts (S) and Inari (I) Lapps born 1885-1905 and 1945-50
(filled bars denote significant differences, $p < 0.05$)

trend. The craniofacial dimensions - particularly the low
facial height, great bizygomatical and bigonial breadth,
and high cephalic index - are considered specific Lappish
traits, or traits indicating a Mongolian origin (1,2,3).
However, increases of facial height and decreases of facial
breadth have reduced the difference between Lapps and the
Norwegians to one-half (Figure 3). Even the cephalic index
- considered the most important single racial mark in anthropology - appears less stable than is generally believed.
Both in Skolt and Inari Lapp males a decrease can be observed. Inari Lapp women also show a decrease of this index, but in the Skolt women the increase of head breadth
has been so marked that in spite of an increase of head
length, the cephalic index has increased slightly (by 0.5
index points, Table 3).

Differences between Skolt and Inari Lapps, conspicuous
and often significant in the 1885-1905 generation, have decreased in those born in 1945-50, and none are significant
in the later generation (Figure 4).

GENERAL DISCUSSION

The pace of changes in Lappish morphology is too rapid to
have a genetic origin. Changes by way of selection, mutation, or drift, all need a considerably longer period for
manifestation. We thus conclude the observed alterations
are of plastic character, expressions of an adaptation of
the human body to a changing environment.

Observations from India show that low caste Hindus are
shorter and more darkly pigmented than those of higher
caste. Similarly, comparisons of lower and higher social
classes in a number of European countries suggest that poor
living conditions are responsible for morphological characteristics that may give an impression of racial distinct-
ness, or admixture of some strange genes (such as the Mongolian origin long postulated for the Lapps).

If further studies on Lapps and other genetically isolated populations confirm our findings, it may have an important implication for hominid taxonomy; most of the sophisticated statistical methods used in such studies are based
on a belief in the stability of morphological traits with
a constant genetic pool. Measurements of anthropological
distances based on stature, cephalic index, etc. of populations living in different times and climates, with different nutritional standards, do not have much relevance as
tools for describing the origin of populations or their re-

lationship to one another. Such statistics should rather be used for measuring how far environment can change body characteristics.

The observation that Lapps born in 1945-50 are in some respects morphologically closer to Scandinavians than to their own ancestors (4,5) shows how dangerous mechanical acceptance of statistical results can be. One could now draw strange conclusions about the origin of the present generations of Lapps!

The possibility of fast changes in morphological characteristics can explain some puzzles in anthropology (e.g. the dominance of a Lapponoid "race" in Europe in Mesolithikum) by environmental changes rather than by speculations on possible migrations or warfare.

SUMMARY

Comparisons of morphological data on Skolt and Inari Lapps born between 1885 and 1905 and between 1945 and 1950 show that a secular trend is taking place in both populations. The main morphological changes in Lapps are an increase in stature and gracilization of body build, changes similar to those observed in other populations where a secular trend has been registered. The secular trend in Lapps can be wholly explained by amelioration of living conditions. Only subjects with known Lappish ancestors for the last four to five generations have been considered and increasing heterosis can be ruled out. A number of morphological characteristics considered as specific inherited Lappish traits are changing fast, revealing their dependence on environmental factors. Some, like relative shortness of the legs, have been erroneously considered as Lappish, since Scandinavians with no Lappish admixture but of comparably short stature share this and other so-called Lappish body proportions. The differences between Skolt and Inari Lapps have now disappeared almost completely, and were most probably caused in earlier generations by environmental rather than genetic factors. None of the characteristics investigated give any hint of a Mongolian admixture or origin of the Lapps. Further, it can be questioned in the light of the secular trend in Japan whether short stature is a Mongolian trait. Since metrical characteristics are dependent on environment, their usability for hominid taxonomy can be seriously questioned.

REFERENCES

1. Bryn, H., "Norwegische Samen. Mitt.," Anthrop. Ges., 62: Wien (1932)
2. Comas, J., Manual of Physical Anthropology (Springfield, Ill.: C.C. Thomas, 1960)
3. Coon, C.S., The Races of Europe (New York, MacMillan Company, 1954)
4. Lewin, T., and Hedegård, B., "Anthropometry among Skolts, other Lapps and other ethnic groups in northern Fennoscandia," Proc. Finnish Dent. Soc., 67: 71-98 (1971)
5. Lewin, T., Skrobak-Kaczynski, J., and Sigholm, G., "Secular changes in craniofacial dimensions in a homo-geneous population," Acta Morphol. Neerl.-Scand., 11: 289-319 (1973)
6. Martin, R., Lehrbuch der Anthropologie in systema-tischer Darstellung, 2. Aufl. Bd. 2 (Jena: Fischer Verlag, 1928)
7. Melbin, T., "The children of Swedish nomad Lapps," Acta Pedriatica, 51: Suppl. 131 (1962)
8. Nickul, K., "The Skolt Lapp Community Suenjelsijd during the Year 1938," Acta Lapponica, V. Gebers Förl., Stock-holm (1943)
9. Näätänen, E.K., "Ueber die Anthropologie der Lappen in Suomi," Ann. Acad. Sci. Fenn., A 47, No. 2 (1936)
10. Schafferi, J., Lapponia. Id est regionis Lapponium gen-tis, nova et verissima descriptio (Francofurti, 1673)
11. Skrobak-Kaczynski, J., Torp, K., Vandbakk, Ø, and Lange Andersen, K., "Growth pattern of Lappish children in Kautokeino, University of Oslo: IBP/HA, Report No. 11, 1971
12. Udjus, L., Anthropometrical changes in Norwegian men in the twentieth century (Oslo: Universitetsförlaget, 1964)
13. Virchow, R., Mitteilungen über die physischen Eigen-schaften der Lappen," Verh. Berl. Ges. Anthrop. Ethnol. u. Urgesch., 7: 31-6 (1875)

Skeletal maturation of the hand and wrist in
Finnish Lapps*

J. EDGREN, C. BRYNGELSSON, T. LEWIN, J. FELLMAN,
and J. SKROBAK-KACZYNSKI

Two of the most widely used methods of assessing skeletal
maturation are the "skeletal age" method of Greulich and
Pyle (5) and the "maturity score" method of Tanner, Whitehouse, and Healy (10). The present paper reports previously
published data (4) on the skeletal maturation of 215 Lapps
from the Inari district, studied according to the Greulich-
Pyle method (5) and skeletal maturation scores for 216
Skolt Lapps from Sevettijärvi and Nellim studied by the
method of Tanner et al. (10).

INARI LAPPS

Measurements were made during field expeditions to Inari
commune in the years 1968-70. The series comprised 112
males aged 3 to 21 years and 103 females aged $3\frac{1}{2}$ to 23
years. Two determinations of skeletal age, separated by a
time interval of one or two years, were made on 51 males and
40 females. The population consisted of Skolt Lapps and
Fisher and Mountain Lapps, but as no difference could be detected between the two populations, the information is presented here as a single unit.

Results

The rate of maturation was the same for male Lapps as indicated by the Greulich-Pyle standards (Figure 1). However,
the linear regression on chronological age (y = 0.978 x -
8.11) shows that skeletal maturation relative to the
Greulich and Pyle children was delayed by 11.1 ± 1.4 months
throughout the period of growth. In females aged 4 to 7
years, the skeletal age corresponded with that of the standards, but final maturation was delayed by about one year
(Figure 2).
    We estimated the age-dependent variation in the matura-
tion rate from data on individuals who were investigated

* This study forms part of an anthropological investigation
of Finnish Lapps, carried out by the Scandinavian section
of the International Biological Program, HA project.

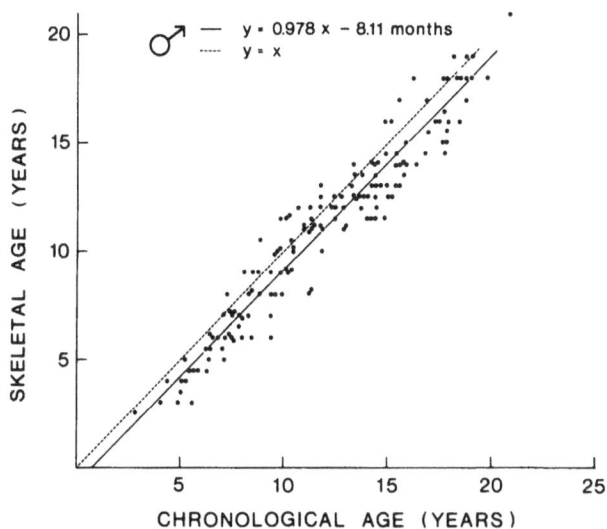

Figure 1   Data on 112 male Lapps showing relationship between chronological age and skeletal age according to Greulich and Pyle

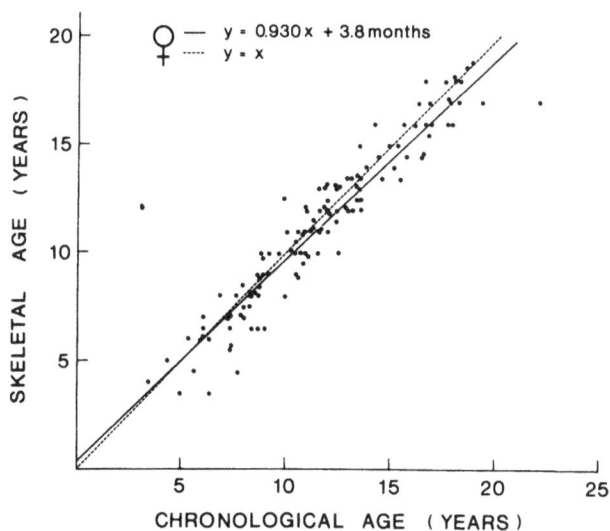

Figure 2   Data on 103 female Lapps showing relationship between chronological age and skeletal age according to Greulich and Pyle

twice. No correlation could be detected between the maturation rate and the chronological age, although maturation seemed to accelerate slightly after 17 years of age in the males and after 15 years in the females.

Conclusions

Our results suggest that the Greulich-Pyle method is sufficiently accurate for both population studies and longitudinal studies repeated at intervals of 1 to 2 years.

In the present study we found an over-all lag in skeletal maturation of 11.1 months in the males and a delayed maturation of nearly one year in the females, as compared with the Greulich-Pyle standards. Differences in growth pattern between populations of different racial origin have been reported previously (6,8). Studies of twins (2) have shown that genetic constitution plays an important role in determining the rate of bone maturation. The influence of social and nutritional status on skeletal development has also been pointed out (1,3). The children of the Greulich-Pyle series represented an American population of far above the average economic level; compared with this favoured group, children of a Finnish urban population showed a lag of skeletal maturation of 7.8 months for boys and 5.9 months for girls (7), while Danish children (1) showed a retardation of 5.9 months for boys and 5.2 months for girls. It seems likely that the retardation of skeletal maturation observed in the present group of Lapps is due mainly to environmental differences. The results also indicate that minor differences in skeletal maturation of genetic origin could only be detected if studies of this type were performed on populations living under comparable environmental conditions.

SKOLT LAPPS

The series consisted of girls aged 6 to 17 years and boys aged 6 to 19 years; 65 boys and 46 girls were from Sevettijärvi (S) and 54 boys and 51 girls were from Nellim (N). The children were observed in July, once to three times between 1968 and 1970. Altogether 350 observations were made; of these, 198 refer to S children and 152 to N children.

Results

The skeletal maturity scores of the Skolt children deviated from the chronological age throughout the period studied, as shown in Figures 3 and 4.

SA-CA
in years

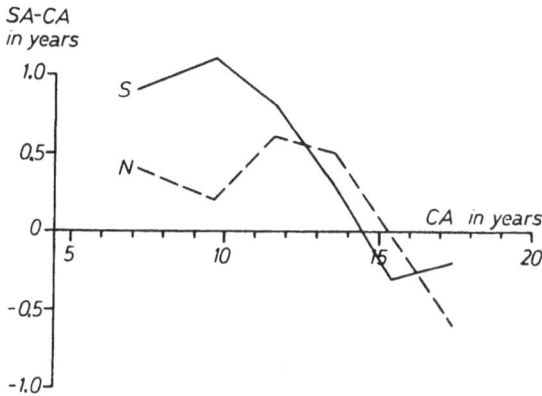

Figure 3   Deviations of skeletal age (SA) from chronological
age (CA) in males from Sevettijärvi (S) and Nellim (N)

SA-CA
in years

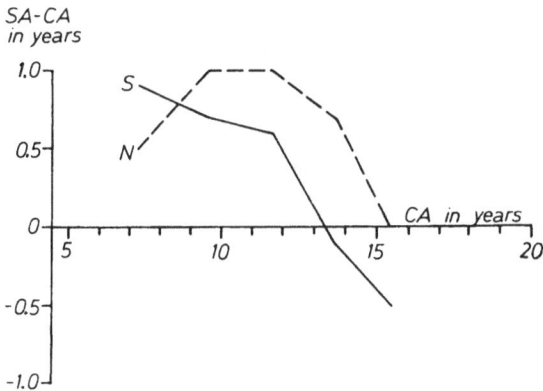

Figure 4   Deviations of skeletal age (SA) from chronological
age (CA) in females from Sevettijärvi (S) and Nellim (N)

In none of the chronological age intervals tested was
there any significant difference of mean scores between the
two groups of boys (S and N), although the boys in the S
group tended to be ahead of the boys in the N group at 9-
11 years. The girls of the N groups aged 13-15 years had a
tendency to earlier skeletal maturation than girls of the S
group, and at 15-17 years this difference was significant.

The "maturity score" has two components, the score for
the long bones of the hand, including the distal epiphyses
of radius and ulna, and the score for the short or round
bones in the wrist, viz. carpal bones. When the scores for

the long and the round bones were considered separately,
the total score of the S boys aged 9-11 years was found to
depend on a significantly higher round bone score in the
boys of the S group. On the other hand, the lagging of the
girls in the S group in relation to the girls from Nellim
depended on slower maturation of the long bones.

Conclusions

Others have shown that the skeletal age determined by the
"maturity score" method (10) anticipates chronological age.
Thus in Melbourne children (9), the boys successively increased the advance of skeletal age over chronological age
from about one month at the chronological age of 6-9 years.
After that, the advance decreased, reaching a value of one
month at age 13. Girls also showed an increase in the advance of skeletal over chronological age from 2 to 7 years·,
when the skeletal age was 12 months higher. The subsequent
decrease reduced this advance to about 6 months at the
chronological age of 10 years, after which it remained at
the level of 6 months.
    The present study of Skolt children from age 6 shows the
same decreasing advance of skeletal age as in the Melbourne
children. However, the average advance of the Skolt children was 2 to 4 months less than in the Melbourne children.
Furthermore, after age 15 in boys and 14 in girls the skeletal age of the Skolt children lagged behind their chronological age. When skeletal age in the Melbourne children was
assessed according to the standard of Greulich and Pyle (5),
it coincided with their chronological age. In the Skolt
children, on the other hand, it lagged behind the chronological age. Discrepancies between the methods of Greulich and
Pyle and Tanner et al. seem the same in the Skolt children
as in the Melbourne children, and reflect differences in the
populations on which the two scales were based (9).
    Despite the discrepancies shown above, the "maturity
score" provides a reliable method of analysing differences
in skeletal maturation between the boys and girls in the
two groups of Skolt children. The tendency of the boys at
Sevettijärvi to be significantly above the boys at Nellim
in the age group 9-11 years, because of higher scores for
their carpal bones, suggests a genetically determined advance in the former group, since they have a nutritional
level considerably below that of the Nellim boys. In the
girls the better nutritional level at Nellim than at
Sevettijärvi favours skeletal maturation, as shown by the

significant advance of the Nellim girls in relation to the
Sevettijärvi girls at ages over 13 years. The difference
in score depends on slower maturation of the long bones of
the girls at Sevettijärvi. Taken with the findings on the
boys, one may hypothesize that the genetically determined
advance of the Sevettijärvi children is mostly due to the
carpal bones. This view is supported by previous findings
(3) that in a group of undernourished children the carpal
bones were the least retarded in maturation.

SUMMARY

The skeletal maturation of 112 male and 103 female Lapps was
studied according to the Greulich-Pyle method. The skeletal
maturation of the boys lagged by an average of 11.1 ± 1.4
months throughout the period of growth. The girls showed a
retardation of skeletal maturation beginning at 7 years of
age, resulting in completion of skeletal maturation one
year after the standards. The lag in skeletal maturation of
the Lappish children was considered due mainly to environmental differences. The skeletal maturation of 216 Skolt
Lapp children was estimated according to the "maturity
score" method of Tanner, Whitehouse, and Healy. The findings
showed a discrepancy between this maturity score and the
skeletal age determined according to Greulich and Pyle. The
Skolt children had an advanced score until puberty, with
a lag after this period. Comparisons between two groups of
children showed that the advancement was due to genetic
factors influencing maturation of the carpal bones.

REFERENCES

1. Andersen, E., "Skeletal maturation of Danish school-
   children in relation to height, sexual development and
   social conditions." Acta paediatr. Scand., Suppl. 185
   (1968)
2. Bohacova, J., Fiserova, J., Hajnisova, M., and Kubic-
   kova, Z., "Bone age in twins," In Hrdlicka (ed.),
   Anthropological congress, proceedings 1969 (Prague:
   Czechoslovak Academy of Sciences, 1971), pp. 135-40
3. Driezen, S., Snodgrasse, R.M., Parker, G.S., Currie,
   C., and Spies, T.D., "Maturation of bone centers in
   hand and wrist of children with chronic nutritive
   failure," Am. J. Dis. Child. 87: 429-39 (1954)

4. Edgren, J., Fellman, J., and Lewin, T., "Skeletal maturation of the hand and wrist, a longitudinal study
   covering two years, among children of Finnish Lapps,"
   Acta Morphol. Neerl.-Scand., 12: 1-7 (1974)
5. Greulich, W.W., and Pyle, S.J., Radiographic atlas of
   skeletal development of the hand and wrist. 2nd Ed.
   (Stanford Univ. Press, Stanford, Calif., 1959)
6. Kimura, K., "On the skeletal maturation of the Japanese-
   American hybrids. A preliminary report," J. Anthrop.
   Soc. (Nippon), 79: 21-9 (1971)
7. Koski, K.J., Haataja, J., and Lappalainen, M., "Skeletal
   development of hand and wrist in Finnish children," Am.
   J. phys. Anthrop., 19: 379-82 (1961)
8. Malina, M.R., "Skeletal maturation studied longitudi-
   nally over one year in American whites and negroes six
   through thirteen years of age," Human Biol., 42: 377-
   90 (1970)
9. Roche, A.F., Davila, G.H., and Eyman, S.L., "A comparison between Greulich-Pyle and Tanner-Whitehouse assessments of skeletal maturity," Radiology, 98: 273-80 (1971)
10. Tanner, J.M., Whitehouse, R.H., and Healy, M.R.J., A
    new system for estimating skeletal maturity from the
    hand and wrist, with standards derived from a study of
    2600 healthy British children. Part II: The scoring
    system (Paris: International Children's Centre, 1962)

Feeding practices and growth of Igloolik infants

JUDITH E. SAYED, J.A. HILDES, and O. SCHAEFER

Among the first effects of acculturation, the Eskimos
change their sources of food. One of the results of dietary
change appears to be an increase of stature (8). It is well
established that nutrition is a major determinant of human
growth from the foetal period through adolescence. Thus,
infant feeding practices were examined and their effect
upon growth of Iglooligmiut children evaluated as part of
the Canadian IBP project.

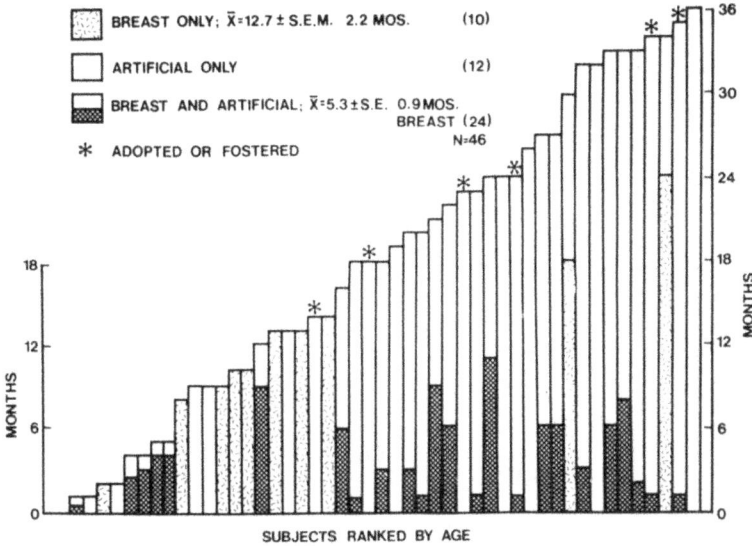

Figure 1   Patterns of infant feeding at Igloolik, 1972

FEEDING PRACTICES

During the 1972 field trip to Igloolik, NWT, mothers with
infants up to 36 months were interviewed about infant
feeding practices. About 80 per cent of the 50 infants were
breast fed for at least part of their infancy (Figure 1);
22 per cent were fed by breast only for a mean of 12.7
months; 52 per cent by breast for an average of 5.3 months,
followed by artifical feeding; and the remaining 26 per
cent, including three adopted or foster children, were
breast fed one month or less. The age at which solid foods
were introduced ranged from one to fourteen months of age,
most infants receiving solid foods at 6 months of age. For
41 per cent of the infants the first solid foods were native (seal, caribou, fish). Whole cereals and strained
foods were among the first for 35 per cent. The remainder
of the infants received biscuits, cookies, and candies as
first solid foods.

PHYSICAL GROWTH

The lengths and weights of children up to 60 months of age
were measured in 1969, 1971, and 1972. These data were compared with the Harvard standards (7), because the growth
of well-nourished children of different ethnic origins and

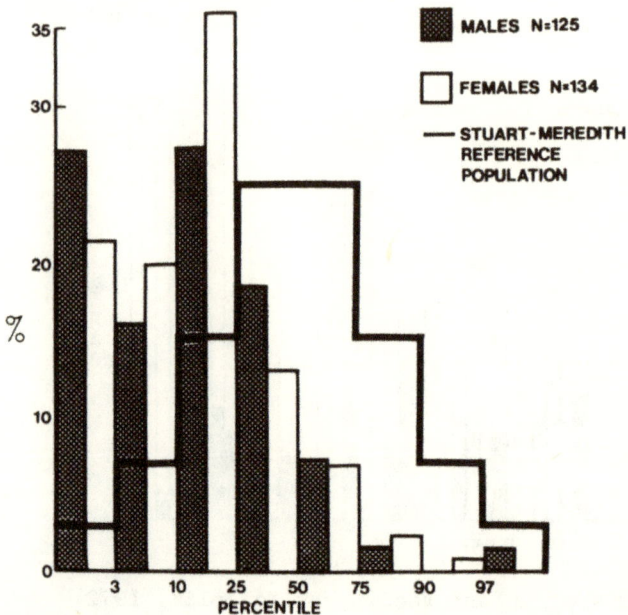

Figure 2   Distribution of length in Igloolik infants 0-60 months in age, 1969-72, relative to Stuart-Meredith reference population

geographic locations conforms to these standards (3).

However, the lengths of 70 per cent of the Igloolik boys and of 77 per cent of the girls fell below the 25th percentile of the standard (Figure 2). On the other hand, the distribution of weights of the Igloolik children conformed more closely to the reference population (Figure 3). The lengths and the weights of adopted and foster children did not differ from the rest.

MODE OF FEEDING AND GROWTH

The growth of bottle-fed infants was compared with that of infants fed wholly or partially by breast (Table 1). Weights and lengths have been calculated as a percentage of expected values. The lengths of infants in all feeding groups were independent of the mode of feeding and were significantly lower than the 50th percentile of the reference population. Infants who were fed by bottle were significantly lighter than those who were breast fed. The general impression that breast-fed infants tend to weigh less

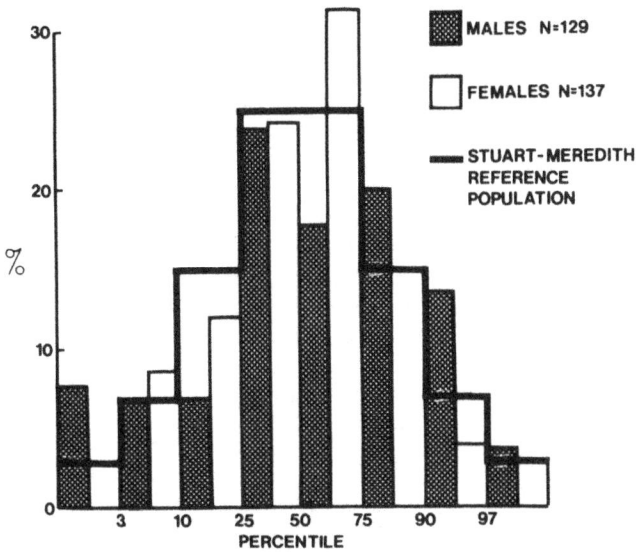

Figure 3   Distribution of weight in Igloolik infants 0-60 months of age, 1969-72, relative to Stuart-Meredith reference population

TABLE 1
Mode of feeding and infant growth

Mode	% weight			% length		
	N	Mean	SE	N	Mean	SE
Breast	76	102	1.2	74	96	0.5
Breast and artificial	106	102	1.1	104	95	0.4
Artificial	75	97*	1.5	70	95	0.6

* p < 0.01.

than those fed artificially is not supported. Other factors, biological, environmental, or social, perhaps create a negative influence for the artificially fed Iglooligmiut infant. The age at which solid foods were introduced did not influence the growth achievements of the 24 infants on whom data were available.

The Igloolik children are similar to the Alaskan Eskimo children (4), US Indians (6), and Peruvian children (1) in that they are short in stature and heavy for length as

compared to Caucasian standards. The postulation of Adrianzen et al. (1) regarding the body build of the Peruvian
children may also apply to Eskimo children. The lives of
these children may represent a series of attempts to re-
cover from intermittent malnutrition, with the periods of
nutritional rehabilitation of insufficient duration for linear growth to return to normal, but sufficiently long to
permit weight gain. This concept has support from human and
animal studies (2,5).

Seasonal variations in diet may be a significant factor
in the growth of Eskimo children (8). Synergism between infection and nutrition must also be considered; indeed, this
relationship may have been involved in the significantly
lower weights of the artificially fed infants as compared
to the breast-fed infants in this study.

SUMMARY

Of 50 Iglooligmiut infants aged 0 to 36 months available
for study, 84 per cent had been breast-fed wholly (22 per
cent) or partially (52 per cent for a mean of 5.3 months),
while 26 per cent had been bottle-fed from birth. Solid food
was introduced at a mean age of six months. It was of native sources (fish, caribou, seal) for 41 per cent of the
infants and comprised imported strained foods and cereals
for 35 per cent of the infants; the remainder first received
biscuits, candies, etc.

Seventy-five per cent of the Iglooligmiut children were
below the 25th percentile of the Harvard standard for
length, whereas the distribution of their weights conformed
more closely to these standards. Bottle-fed infants weighed
significantly less than those who were breast-fed wholly or
partially, but the mode of feeding did not influence linear
growth. Similar growth patterns in Peru and in US Indians
and Eskimos have been ascribed to chronic or intermittent
malnutrition.

REFERENCES

1. Adrianzen, T.B., Baertl, J.M., and Graham, G.G., "Growth
   of children from extremely poor families," Am. J. clin.
   Nutr., 26: 926 (1973)
2. Graham, G.G., Cordano, A., Blizzard, R.M., and Cheek,
   D.B., "Infantile malnutrition: changes in body composition during rehabilitation," Pediat. Res., 3: 579 (1969)

3. Habicht, J.P., Harbrough, C., Martorell, R., Malina, R.M.,
   and Klein, R.E., "Height and weight standards for preschool children. How relevant are ethnic differences in
   growth potential?" Lancet, 2: 611 (1974)
4. Heller, C.A., Scott, E.M., and Hammes, L.M., "Height,
   weight, and growth of Alaskan Eskimos," Am. J. Dis.
   Child., 113: 338 (1967)
5. Kerr, G.R., Allen, J.R., Scheffler, G., and Waisman,
   H.A., "Malnutrition studies in the rhesus monkey. 1.
   Effect on physical growth," Am. J. clin. Nutr., 23: 739
   (1970)
6. Moore, W.M., "Physical growth of North American Indian
   and Alaskan native children," in Moore, W.M., Silverberg,
   M.M., and Read, M.S. (eds), Nutrition, growth and
   development of North American Indian children (Washington, D.C.: US Government Printing Office, 1972), pp. 35-
   46
7. Nelson, W.E., Vaughan III, V.C., and McKay, R.J.,
   Textbook of Pediatrics, Ninth Ed. (Philadelphia: W.B.
   Saunders, 1969), pp. 15-54
8. Schaefer, O., "Pre and post natal growth acceleration
   and increased sugar consumption in Canadian Eskimos,"
   Canad. Med. Assoc. J., 103: 1059 (1970)

Trends in fertility in a northern Alaska community

G.S. MASNICK and S.H. KATZ

For the anthropologist, sociologist, and demographer, the
north slope Alaskan community of Barrow provides a setting
for gaining a deeper appreciation of the social and demographic interrelationships that characterize the process
we call "modernization." Over a period of a mere 50 years,
Barrow has grown from a small distant outpost of mostly Eskimo families banded together as hunters in a life-style
inherited from generations past, to become a city of over
2,000 with a movie theatre, several stores, a bank, a hospital, large public school, and many other amenities.
This transformation has been rapid, but it has not been
smooth. From the introduction of a cash economy with

reindeer herding in the beginning of the century to the
current activities surrounding the development of the northern oil fields, the sweeping economic changes can best be
described as "boom or bust." The reindeer industry in Barrow
started collapsing during the mid 1920s when the price per
carcass dropped from $5.00 to $2.00. The reindeer economy
was succeeded by a lively trade in Arctic fox fur, but when
pelts selling from $50.00 to $100.00 a piece in 1929 declined to $5.00 in 1932, the only sources of cash in the
village disappeared until World War II. During the war, the
active exploration for oil reserves brought a huge boom in
employment until about 1952 when the initial exploration
was completed, whereupon another period of economic depression followed. By 1958, another boom atmosphere was begun with the construction of the "Dew Line" early warning
defensive radar sites and the location of the Naval Arctic
Research Laboratories. Throughout the 1960s the economy
remained relatively stable, with employment related to the
Alaska pipeline gradually replacing those activities associated earlier with the Cold War. Finally, the Native Land
Claim Settlement, signed into law in 1971, provided Alaska
Eskimos and Indians with 40 million acres of land, a
$462.5 million cash settlement, and $500 million in mineral
rights on lands no longer owned by the natives. Economic
and social change will thus continue at a rapid pace in the
near future (Figure 1 and Table 1). This report presents a
preliminary analysis of fertility changes over the period
1940-1970, a first step in the analysis of population
changes in Barrow.

THE DATA BASE

Eleven censuses were conducted in Barrow between 1940 and
1970, in the years 1940, 1944, 1946, 1950, 1951, 1954,
1957, 1958, 1962, 1966, and 1970. Families were reconstituted for each date by linking children with mothers, and
fertility rates computed by noting additions to the family
between consecutive censuses. Births not entering into the
figures are children born and dying between censuses. Although this measure of fertility understates the true level
by a small fraction, it undoubtedly reflects trends and
differentials in age patterns and temporal swings accurate-
ly.

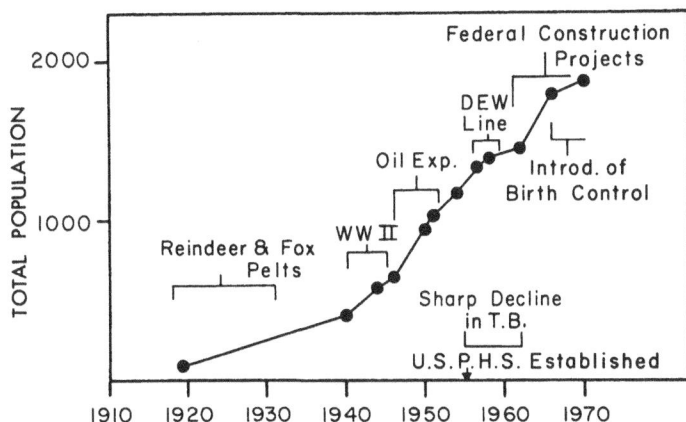

Figure 1   Schematic diagram showing factors influencing population of Barrow

TABLE 1
Rates of growth in Barrow, 1940-70

Period	Population at beginning of period	Population at end of period	Population change	Average annual rate of growth over period (%)
1940-44	406	566	160	8.7
1944-46	566	663	97	8.5
1946-50	663	956	293	11.0
1950-51	956	1,026	70	7.3
1951-54	1,026	1,157	131	4.3
1954-57	1,157	1,349	192	5.5
1957-58	1,349	1,383	34	2.5
1958-62	1,383	1,485	102	1.8
1962-66	1,485	1,782	297	5.0
1966-70	1,782	1,827	45	0.6

PERIOD FERTILITY

For all practical purposes childbearing does not begin in this population until after age 20 (Table 2). If reports of widespread teenage sexual activity among Eskimos are correct, the slow start of childbearing deserves closer examination.

The 20-24 age group begins to demonstrate a fertility swing over this thirty-year period that is strikingly similar to the fertility pattern in the "lower 48" of the United States. However, the absolute level of childbearing

262 Growth and development

TABLE 2
Period of fertility, number of births for women during each age
interval recorded in censuses between 1940 and 1970 (net of children
born and dying in the intercensal interval)

Age of mother	1941-45	1946-50	1951-55	1956-60	1961-65	1966-70
15-19	0.07	0.11	0.22	0.06	0.09	0.01
20-24	0.67	0.88	0.99	1.02	1.05	0.36
25-29	0.80	1.14	1.69	1.65	1.80	0.87
30-34	1.32	2.21	1.96	1.49	2.25	0.87
35-39	1.49	0.90	1.07	1.64	1.85	0.26
40-44	1.37	0.80	1.92	0.16	0.37	0.94
Total	5.72	6.04	7.85	6.02	7.41	3.31

in this age group is still far below what might be expected
in a high fertility population. Those who entered the 20-
24 age group in the earlier censuses were presumably affected by the depression and war years. Each succeeding cohort entering the 20-24 age group stepped up the pace of
childbearing, so that those entering this age group in the
early 1960s demonstrated the quickest start at family
building. The dramatic drop in fertility in the last half
of the 1960 decade coincides with the introduction to
Barrow of modern forms of contraception (especially the
IUD).

Women in the 25-29 and 30-34 age groups follow the pattern established in the previous age group with two important differences. First, the level of fertility is substantially higher. Secondly, a dip in fertility occurs in the
mid and late 1950s, probably in response to the adverse
economic circumstances at that time.

The pattern exhibited by women in the 35-39 age group
differs markedly from that for the younger age groups. By
this age, however, we would expect not only the economic,
social, and demographic events of the period to be influencing the rate of childbearing, but we would also anticipate that a women's previous fertility experience would
play a role. Thus, we have analysed the childbearing experience of Barrow mothers by following birth cohorts of
women through as much of their reproductive history as
covered by our census series.

TABLE 3

Cohort fertility, number of births per woman during five-year age intervals for women born between 1901 and 1950 (figures are net of children born and dying in the intercensal interval)

Cohort born in years	Age specific fertility and date cohort entered age group (in parentheses)						Cumulative total through age 44
	15-19	20-24	25-29	30-34	35-39	40-44	
1901-05	-	-	-	-	-	1.37 (1941-45)	8.68
1906-10	-	-	-	-	1.49 (1941-45)	0.80 (1946-50)	7.19
1911-15	-	-	-	1.32 (1941-45)	0.09 (1946-50)	1.92 (1951-55)	6.32
1916-20	-	-	0.80 (1941-45)	2.21 (1946-50)	1.07 (1951-55)	0.16 (1956-60)	5.52
1921-25	-	0.67 (1941-45)	2.17 (1946-50)	1.96 (1951-55)	1.64 (1956-60)	0.37 (1961-65)	6.81
1926-30	0.07 (1941-45)	0.88 (1946-50)	1.69 (1951-55)	1.49 (1956-60)	1.85 (1961-65)	0.94 (1966-70)	6.92
1931-35	0.11 (1946-50)	0.99 (1951-55)	1.65 (1956-60)	2.25 (1961-65)	0.26 (1966-70)	-	-
1936-40	0.22 (1951-55)	1.02 (1956-60)	1.80 (1961-65)	0.87 (1966-70)	-	-	-
1941-45	0.06 (1956-60)	1.05 (1961-65)	0.87 (1966-70)	-	-	-	-
1946-50	0.09 (1961-65)	0.36 (1966-70)	-	-	-	-	-

COHORT FERTILITY

Cohort analysis (Table 3) proceeds on the assumption that
rates at various stages in the reproductive period are not
measures of isolated events, but, in reality, strongly influence one another. Dashes in the table indicate age
groups for the various cohorts in which reproduction did or
will take place outside the 1940-70 limits set by our data.

The basic swing in fertility observed in the period data
of Table 2 is replicated in the cohort figures, with a few
minor variations. However, some important adaptive trends
are revealed by the cohort analysis. The initial downward
trend of cumulative totals extended through the cohorts born
from 1916 to 1920. Even though a major part of their reproductive ages came after 1946, when conditions were more favourable to childbearing, fertility was not "made up" by
this group, who got off to a slow start at childbearing.
They seemed to be unusually responsive in lowering their
fertility in response to the 1941-45 and 1956-60 recessions
(while they were age 25-29 and 40-44), and all told, their
completed fertility was reduced.

The rapid early childbearing of the post World War II
period resulted in a "baby boom" for the 1921-30 cohorts.
These cohorts showed little evidence of controlling their
later fertility during the 1956-60 and 1966-70 periods
(when they entered the 35-39 and 40-44 age groups). Their
high level of childbearing during years of recession might
well be attributed to their lack of an early experience in
controlling fertility. It is hypothesized that the 1921-30
birth cohorts of Barrow mothers shared the motivation to
control fertility during the later recessions, but, in contrast with the 1916-20 cohorts, were unable to learn the behaviour necessary to do so.

The decline in age-specific fertility of all cohorts has
been dramatic in the years 1966-70 for all cohorts except
those born in 1926-30. Even the 1931-35 cohort, who began
childbearing at an extremely fast pace, controlled their
fertility dramatically as they entered the age groups 35-
39. This pattern suggests that the modern contraceptive
technology introduced to this population by the Public
Health Service (an "outside" agency) can reduce fertility
in cohorts that might ordinarily not be expected to use
the traditional fertility regulating mechanisms effectively.
The 1931-35 birth cohort was still young enough in 1966-70
to adopt the innovation in contraceptive technology, but
probably would have been too old to control fertility

effectively by traditional methods requiring sustained motivation and a disruption of patterned sexual and childbearing behaviour because of fifteen prior years of regular
pregnancy and childbearing.

SUMMARY

A preliminary analysis of data for Barrow, Alaska, supports
the premise that Eskimo populations have in the past been
able to adjust fertility to changes in social and economic
conditions. Those cohorts who began childbearing under ad-
versity, and who had an early experience in controlling fertility, were better able to adjust their level of natality
when economic conditions were bad during later stages of
their life cycle. Those cohorts who began their reproductive years under a climate of prosperity had rapid early
childbearing, and were less able to control fertility at
later ages, even when the economy was depressed. These conclusions should be tested by examining birth intervals and
family composition directly. Such analyses of a community
undergoing rapid change can help us to understand the limits
of adaptability and health in the evolution that man is
undergoing in the late twentieth century.

Commentaries

"Correspondence of selected demographic and cultural factors to growth and development," by J.F. de Pena (Department of Anthropology, University of Manitoba, Winnipeg,
Canada). Body size attainments and rates of development in
human populations are known to have strong genetic components which interact variably to changing cultural features.
A short series of cultural-demographic factors were studied
for their separate and combined association with selected
variables of growth and development in a mixed longitudinal
sample of Igloolik and Hall Beach youth from 6 through 22
years of age. Stature, weight, biiliocristal diameter, and
skeletal age were assessed with respect to season of birth,
birth order, length of time of residence in settlements,
length of time in attendance at residential schools, religious affiliation, residence with biological birth unit,

and both the separate and composite features of a proposed
Igloolik Project "acculturation index." The data suggest
that, of the factors studied, the association of religious
affiliation and length of time in residential schools have
the strongest relationships to both body size achievements
and developmental rates.

"Growth patterns of Fort Chimo and Spotted Island Eskimos,"
by F. Auger (Département d'Anthropologie, Université de
Montréal, Canada). The Eskimo village of Fort Chimo is located at 58° 7'N, 68° 24'W on the west shore of the Koksoak
River, 35 miles south of Ungava Bay. Traditional cultural
and social values have remained relatively unchanged there
until fairly recently. However, as a consequence of closer
contact with more technically advanced societies, this
community is now rapidly undergoing substantial socio-
cultural changes. Along with these changes, the people of
Fort Chimo have also undergone genetic changes due to intermarriages with Whites and, to a lesser extent, with Indians.
This cross-sectional study was undertaken during the summer
of 1969. A total of 114 (87.69 per cent) Eskimos 5 to 25
years old were examined for body measurements. Using a portion of the growth curves (5 to 14.99 years old) we can
show some differences in size and shape between hybrids and
non-hybrids. For an interpopulational comparison, we used
data collected on mixed children of Spotted Island Eskimos
(Labrador). Differences in size and shape are well established between children of both communities.

"Associations of anaemia and illness in infancy with subsequent intellectual development of children," by J.M. Burks,
C. Baum, J.K. Fleshman, T.R. Bender, and T.A. Vieira
(Alaska Activities, Bureau of Epidemiology-CDC, USPHS, USA).
We have studied a cohort of 503 Eskimo children, in order
to determine whether anaemia and illness in infancy may play
a role in their intellectual development. A child whose mean
haemoglobin level between 6 and 17 months of age was less
than 11.0 grams was considered anaemic. Serious illnesses
occurring before age two were classified under the heading
of "significant illness" (SI). A separate illness category
was the occurrence of otitis media before age two, with subsequent hearing defect (OM). WISC intelligence tests and
standard school achievement tests were administered to
children at about age eight. Children who had either

anaemia, SI, or OM in infancy had significantly lower IQ and achievement test scores than children who had none of these conditions in infancy. The occurrence of two or all three of these conditions in infancy resulted in still lower scores. The presence of anaemia at the time of intelligence testing was not a factor in these results. Our data indicate that the intellectual development of children may be impaired by milder nutritional and illness insults than has been previously realized.

"Growth assessment through hand-wrist x-rays of some Fort Chimo males," by C. Eyman and E. Salter (Department of Archaeology, University of Calgary, Calgary, Canada). A sample of 83 males from Fort Chimo, ranging from 4 to 24 years of age, has been assessed for skeletal hand-wrist maturity by both the Greulich-Pyle and the Tanner-Whitehouse-Healy II standards. There appear to be practically no bony anomalies. These males show slightly accelerated bone maturation from their chronological ages when compared with the standards composing both of the maturational assessments. The Fort Chimo sample is heterogenous in that there are three subgroups: Eskimo, Eskimo-Indian, and Eskimo-Indian-Caucasian. There may be some skeletal hand-wrist maturational differences between these subgroups.

"Associations of nutrition and illness in infancy with subsequent growth of a cohort of children," by J.M. Burks, C. Baum, J.K. Fleshman, T.R. Bender, and T. Vieira (Alaska Activities, Bureau of Epidemiology-CDC, USPHS, USA). We have studied a cohort of 503 Eskimo children, in order to determine whether undernutrition in infancy may play a role in determining their ultimate stature. Severe malnutrition was not present in our cohort. Therefore, anaemia was used as a measure of undernutrition. Severe illness of whatever cause was categorized under the heading of "significant illness" (SI). Children were followed closely for the first two years of life, and were examined again at age eight. Growth of the cohort at the time of follow-up agreed closely with previously published findings for Eskimo children. Those children who acquired both anaemia and SI during infancy were essentially no different in stature at follow-up than children who acquire neither of these conditions. Children with retarded skeletal maturation at follow-up were smaller than those with normal skeletal maturation. However, even those with normal bone age reached only the

25th percentile in height. We conclude that anaemia and illness in infancy have not played a major role in the growth
of this cohort of children, and suggest that the genetically
determined height potential for Eskimos is equivalent to the
25th percentile of Caucasian standards.

"Social health and environmental factors associated with
variations in early growth and development of Eskimo children," by S.H. Katz, J. Hesser, G. Masnick, and E. Foulks.
Paper not submitted.

ARCTIC EPIDEMIOLOGY

Epidemiology of some non-infectious diseases in eastern Siberia

K.R. SEDOV

During recent years, the epidemiology and pathology of various chronic diseases has been studied in such towns of eastern Siberia as Irkutsk, Norilsk, Sludyanka, Kirensk, Yakutsk, Yerbogachen, Kachug, Mama, Tofalaria, and island Olhon (Lake Baikal).

Though the total incidence of myocardial infarction is comparatively low (0.5 per 1,000), in some settlements the annual rate exceeds 1.0. The inhabitants of Norilsk, Irkutsk, and other big cities suffer from various clinical forms of atherosclerosis, diabetes, bronchitis, rheumatic arthritis and rheumatic fever, while rural inhabitants suffer from gastric and duodenal ulcer, and leucocytosis. The wide range of morbidity in some settlements does not necessarily exclude an influence of environmental factors on morbidity.

The age distribution of chronic non-infectious diseases is not uniform. Many conditions such as myocardial infarction, atherosclerotic cardiosclerosis, hypertension, cholecystitis, rheumatic arthritis, diabetes, and chronic lymphocytosis increase in frequency with age. The atherosclerotic index of the aorta, the coronary vessels, and the circumflex branch of the left coronary artery, the incidence of myocardial infarction and of atherosclerotic cardiosclerosis all follow this pattern. On the other hand, anaemia and problems of the biliary ducts have a relatively uniform age distribution while the highest incidence of rheumatic fever and chronic leucocytosis is found in young people.

In general, diseases accompanied by exudative reactions are characteristic of young people and those accompanied by proliferative sclerotic reactions are typical of old age. Some diseases increase in incidence to the fourth and fifth decades and then decline in frequency. Gastric and duodenal

ulcer, chronic bronchitis, and effort angina are examples.
The first two of these diseases occur in people under the
age of 40, and the subsequent sharp decrease in number of
cases is due to natural losses. The decrease in number of
patients suffering from effort angina is accompanied by a
marked increase in painless forms of ischaemic heart disease in older age groups.

Sex has a definite influence on the incidence of many diseases. Women more often suffer from rheumatic fever, rheumatic arthritis, cholecystitis, problems of the bile passages, anaemia, diabetes, and chronic myeloid leukaemia. Men
suffer from gastric and duodenal ulcer, chronic bronchitis,
acute leucocytosis, chronic lymphocytosis. Coronary atherosclerosis occurs more often in men under the age of 50, but
in the elderly, women are commonly affected. The characteristic sex incidence of the various diseases is conditioned not only by differences in hormone profile, but also
by peculiarities of their daily work.

People primarily engaged in mental activities often suffer from myocardial infarction, effort angina, and chronic
bile disease; manual workers, on the other hand, suffer
from ulceration of the stomach and duodenum, and from chronic bronchitis. The nature of work does not seem to modify
the incidence of rheumatic fever, rheumatic arthritis, or
anaemia.

The climate of eastern Siberia is continental. A prolonged, cold winter and a short but hot summer are characteristic of most of this region, except for the Polar
circle, where summer air temperatures remain comparatively
low. Of all settlements examined, the highest contrasts of
air temperatures were recorded in Yerbogachen, Mama, and
Kirensk, where annual temperature fluctuated by 93.9° F
(Table 1). Much lower contrasts of air temperature are observed in the region of Lake Baikal (island Olhon, t.
Sludyanka), because of the vast area of water. Despite similar average indices of relative humidity, precipitation also differs considerably in the several regions (Table 1).
Weather factors did not have a clear impact on the distribution of chronic diseases among the population. In the regions with the most continental climate, the incidence was
no greater than in the other settlements. However, meteorological factors did seem to influence the timing in the
exacerbation of some diseases. Chronic bronchitis, rheumatic fever, ulcer of the duodenum, and infarction apparently
tend to occur in the period when fluctuations of daily
temperature, air humidity, and wind velocity are large.

TABLE 1
Meteorological features in the regions of Eastern Siberia that were examined

Settlement	Air temperature (°C)				Av. atm. press. (mb)	Rel. humidity (%)	Total precip. (mm)
	Av. ann.	Abs. max.	Abs. min.	Ann. range			
Norilsk	-9.9	29.4	-48.3	77.8	1,005.1	76.8	470.8
Yerbogachen	-8.5	32.9	-61.0	93.9	985.0	71.1	367.2
Mama	-4.6	36.5	-48.7	85.2	990.5	71.3	512.6
Kirensk	-4.7	33.7	-52.7	86.4	987.4	71.2	360.0
Kachug	-3.6	33.2	-49.5	82.7	952.2	68.0	334.0
Olhon	-1.1	28.3	-37.6	65.9	959.3	66.8	195.7
Sludyanka	-0.2	32.1	-34.4	56.5	962.8	71.6	422.5
Irkutsk	-0.4	32.3	-41.1	71.0	962.3	72.3	412.2
Tofalaria	2.6	30.4	-47.1	77.5	904.4	68.9	486.5

Serious cardiovascular diseases show a correlation with
heliogeophysical data such as oscillations in the magnetic
field of the earth and the sunshine hours of the region.

Nutritional study of the populations was based on
questioning and the weighing method (Table 2). The diet was
varied, with respect to composition, preparation, and ener-
getic value. Fats constituted 26.0-36.5 per cent, proteins
12.6-19.3 per cent and carbohydrates 45.1-61.2 per cent.
There was no obvious dependence of morbidity on diet. Indeed, some paradoxical phenomena were observed including a
very low incidence of clinical forms of coronary atherosclerosis in aborigines using plenty of fat. Coronary

TABLE 2
Percentage of calories provided by main foodstuffs
in populations of Eastern Siberia

Region	Protein (%)	Fat (%)	Carbohydrate (%)
Norilsk	14.3	32.5	53.2
Yerbogachen	18.4	36.4	45.2
Mama	14.6	98.0	57.4
Kirensk	17.8	32.2	50.0
Katchug	19.3	31.4	55.3
Olhon	16.8	31.2	52.0
Slyudyanka	12.5	26.3	61.2
Irkutsk	12.6	26.2	61.2
Tofalaria	18.4	36.5	45.1

artherosclerosis is rare among rural inhabitants and especially among aborigines although meat with a high fat content prevails in the rations of the latter group. We studied
4,060 sets of coronary vessels and aorta in Irkutsk and more
than 600 in Yakutsk using WHO methodology. The affected area
of the aorta and coronary vessels was smaller in Irkutsk
than in Moscow and Riga and higher than Yakutiya. The index
appeared to be considerably lower among the aboriginal population than among recent immigrants. Constant manual labour
and nutrition no more than adequate to meet energy losses
seem important preconditions for reduction of morbidity from
this disease.

Smoking aggravates some forms of chronic disease including chronic bronchitis, gastric and duodenal ulcer, angina
of effort, and atherosclerotic cardiosclerosis (Table 3).

TABLE 3
Incidence of some chronic diseases among smokers and nonsmokers (per 1,000 people)

Pathology	Smokers	Non-smokers
Effort angina	26.8 ± 2.1	16.3 ± 3.5
Atherosclerotic cardiosclerosis	127.1 ± 4.7	90.2 ± 8.0
Chronic bronchitis	42.8 ± 3.8	8.8 ± 1.0
Gastric and duodenal ulcer	68.0 ± 5.1	20.0 ± 1.7

The leading aetiological factor in the occurrence and distribution of rheumatic fever is a reservoir of streptococci
and immunologic reactivity of the local population (Table 4).

TABLE 4
Incidence of rheumatic fever, manifest positive cultures of
beta-haemolytic streptococci and titre of ASL-O in specific
regions of USSR

Region	Incidence of rheumatic fever	Positive cultures of beta-haemolytic streptococci	Average titre of ASL-O
Olhon	1.40 ± 0.41	7.38 ± 1.44	317.3 ± 6.16
Kichugski	1.60 ± 0.40	7.27 ± 6.50	344.0 ± 4.37
Katanski	3.40 ± 0.51	26.9 ± 1.82	388.3 ± 6.75
Irkutsk	3.70 ± 0.19	27.1 ± 1.79	434.1 ± 3.80
Tafalariya	4.95 ± 0.90	32.9 ± 3.52	494.7 ± 9.10

Frequent isolation of beta-haemolytic streptococci from the pharynx and high titre of ASL-O were observed in inhabitants of the regions with a high incidence of rheumatic fever. There was also a direct and close connection between the geographic distribution of rheumatic fever and the population incidence of positive beta-haemolytic streptococcal cultures (τ = ± 0.95 ± 0.022), average titre of ASL-O (τ = 0.98 ± 0.003), and distribution of chronic tonsillitis (τ = 0.95 ± 0.012), or correlation between common immunological reactivity and an allergic response to streptococcal toxins (τ = 0.92 ±-0.004), an inverse correlation with common immunologic reactivity (r = 0.94 ± 0.009), and moderate positive correlations with average readings of streptococcal sensitization (r = 0.56 ± 0.002) and sensitization to heart antigen (r = 0.69 ± 0.0014). Weak immunologic reactivity (respective values 20.1-27.0 per cent and 5.6-6.8 per cent) and more rarely good or average reactivity (respective values 54.8-69.4 per cent and 74.8-86.5 per cent) was observed more often in regions with a high incidence of rheumatic fever in regions where this disease was uncommon. Lingering and lethal diseases occurred rather frequently in the people suffering from rheumatic fever (group 12-WHO).

Infection and common immunologic reactivity of the organism plays a major role in the incidence of chronic bronchitis. Chronic bronchitis occurs in the population of great cities (Irkutsk, Norilsk) more often than in small rural settlements. Staphylococci (50.2 per cent), more rarely streptococci (19.9 per cent), protei (11.9 per cent), and much rarer Candida ablicans (6.7 per cent), intestinal bacillus (4.2 per cent), blue-green pus (2.9 per cent), and pneumococci (1.7 per cent) can be cultured from the sputum of patients suffering from chronic bronchitis. Pathogenic staphylococci are cultured 1.5 times more often from bronchitic patients living in the town than from those living in the country. The disease is generally mild in character and 89.7 per cent of patients are able to work.

Irregular and insufficiently balanced nutrition and harmful dietary habits are the most probable reasons for the high incidence of ulcer in some northern regions. Irregular meals, the use of hot and cold food, and a high consumption of alcohol were noted more often in the country, especially among aborigines. Reflex influences on the abdominal organs (20.1 per cent) and previous psychic trauma (4.1 per cent) were the most common causes of ulcer. Our material makes us doubt the viewpoint of some authors who have considered the disease as a "disease of civilization."

There is a direct relationship between the incidence of cholecystitis, disorders of the bile ducts and the mineral content of drinking water. The major incidence of chronic bile disease is observed in settlements that use hard water with too great a content of chlorides and sulphates. Alimentary disturbances and infections are also factors promoting the development of these diseases.

There is one area where iron deficiency anaemia is endemic (t. Kirensk). The diet lacks iron, copper, and manganese, and there are correspondingly low levels of these ions in the blood. Blood losses and achlorhydria are other factors leading directly to development of anaemia. However, of all patients with anaemia, iron deficiency was revealed in 98.9 per cent, chronic haemolytic anaemia in 0.7 per cent, and haemolytic anaemia in 0.1 per cent. B_{12} deficiency anaemia was not found.

A rise in the well-being of the population and an improvement of preventive medical care has led to a significant reduction in the incidence of and mortality from tuberculosis. From 1964 to 1973, the incidence of tuberculosis decreased to almost a third in Yakut Autonomous Soviet Socialist Republic, while morbidity and mortality were halved.

SUMMARY

Differences in the incidence of disease between urban and rural areas of eastern Siberia are discussed in relation to age, sex, and climate. The extreme range of temperatures encountered appeared to influence the timing of chronic bronchitis, rheumatic fever, ulcer, and myocardial infarction. The latter was also related to heliogeophysical data such as hours of sunshine. Nutrition was generally good, and aboriginal groups showed a low incidence of atherosclerosis despite a high fat diet. Coronary atherosclerosis was shown by post-mortem analysis to be rarer in rural than in urban areas. Rheumatic fever was correlated with the frequency of the β haemolytic streptococcus in the population. Chronic bronchitis was more common in the cities. Predominant microorganisms are described. Biliary diseases were related to an excessive mineral content of the water. Anaemia was usually due to iron deficiency. Over the past 10 years, the incidence of tuberculosis has fallen to one-third of its initial figure.

Leukaemia in northern Finland

I.P. PALVA, H.L.A. PALVA, and S.J. SALOKANNEL

During the years 1970-73, a centrally supervised but de-centralized system provided diagnosis and treatment of haematological diseases for adults living in northern Finland. Bone marrow smears from all hospitals and health centres were examined for adults (over 15 years) totalling 410,000 in 1970, and the large sample size has allowed a more precise study of morbidity in various haematological diseases than is normally possible.

All diagnoses were based on the morphological findings of the same team, and the diagnostic criteria thus remained the same for the whole series. Solid lymphatic tumours without leukaemic involvement were not included.

Preliminary data covers the period 1970-72, corresponding to 1,230,000 man-years of observation. The annual incidence of neoplastic blood diseases detected is shown in Table 1.

In 1970, the Finnish Cancer Register reported that in adults the total incidence was 4.5 per 100,000 for all types of leukaemia and 2.3 for multiple myeloma. According to our observations, the incidence of neoplastic blood diseases in northern Finland is about double that reported by the Finnish Cancer Register. What is the reason for this discrepancy?

1. The Cancer Registry figures are based on the number of deaths, whereas our figures indicate the number of new cases diagnosed. During the period of observation, the median survival period was about six months for adults with acute leukaemia and about two years for those with chronic leukaemia or multiple myeloma. As these diseases are fatal,

TABLE 1
Neoplastic blood diseases detected in adults in north Finland in 1970-72 annually per 100,000 inhabitants

Acute leukaemia	3.8
Chronic granulocytic leukaemia	1.3
Myelofibrosis (myeloid metaplasia)	0.5
Polycythemia vera	2.4
Chronic lymphatic leukaemia	5.0
Multiple myeloma	5.3
Waldenström's disease	0.2

the annual number of deaths should be practically identical
with the number of new cases. The different source of the
data thus should not lead to any difference in incidence figures.

2. Is there really a higher incidence of neoplastic blood
diseases in northern Finland as compared with other parts of
the country? We cannot exlude this possibility. However, the
population of northern Finland is mainly a mixed Finnish
population, with a similar age distribution to that found in
the south. Any real difference, therefore, seems unlikely.

3. Different diagnostic criteria may be the main source
of the difference. Most patients with chronic leukaemias and
multiple myeloma and many with acute leukaemia are elderly
people. As the final cause of death is often an infection
(in leukaemia) or uremia (in myeloma), the basic disease may
remain undisclosed in many cases, with pneumonia or chronic
pyelonephritis being indicated as the cause of death. This
would be especially true of the large group of patients
whose blood disease runs a course with few symptoms until
the fulminant terminal phase. We cannot exclude a certain
underdiagnosis of this type even in our series. According to
our data, however, it seems likely that the physicians of
northern Finland have been more aware of the possibility of
neoplastic blood diseases than has been the case in the
country as a whole. The incidence figures for leukaemias
and myeloma reported by the Finnish Cancer Register are
lower than those in many western countries, while our data
are close to the highest incidences reported. In our opinion, the latter data represent the real situation.

In conclusion, we can state that a centrally supervised,
but decentralized system has been effective in diagnosing
new cases of neoplastic blood diseases in the most remote
areas of Finland. Indeed, it seems that it has been even
more effective in this respect than the medical system in
the country as a whole.

SUMMARY

All bone marrow smears from hospitals and health centres in
northern Finland were examined by a single team during the
years 1970-72. Preliminary figures give the following incidences for various types of leukaemia and myeloma: acute
leukaemia 3.8/100,000/year, chronic myeloid leukaemia 1.3,
myelofibrosis 0.5, polycythaemia vera 2.4, chronic lymphatic leukaemia 5.0, multiple myeloma 5.3, and Waldenström's
disease 0.2. The incidence of leukaemias and myeloma re-

ported by the Finnish Cancer Register is lower than those in
many western countries, though our data are close to the
highest incidences reported. The main source of this discrepancy could be the number of cases not reported to the
Cancer Register and perhaps not diagnosed at all. According
to our data, haematological diagnosis has been at least as
effective in the remote areas of northern Finland as in the
country as a whole.

The changing pattern of neoplastic disease in
Canadian Eskimos

O. SCHAEFER, J.A. HILDES, L.M. MEDD, and D.G. CAMERON

Review of hospital files at three main referral centres revealed 164 histologically proven cases of neoplastic disease in Canadian Eskimos over observation periods varying
from 6 years in eastern to 26 years in central and western
Arctic Eskimos.

Table 1 summarizes and lists in order of prevalence of
primary organ site or histological type all cases found in
these centres, while Table 2 records similarly the 64 cancer deaths reported on death certificates of Eskimos from
the Northwest Territories from 1967 to 1972 inclusive.
Table 3 demonstrates a very significant increase in both
cancer morbidity and mortality when comparing earlier and
more recent survey periods. This cannot be explained by
aging of population structure, as, indeed, the relative proportion of NWT Eskimos over 40 years of age decreased from
8.59 to 7.48 per cent for men and from 7.13 to 6.26 per
cent for women between the 1961 and the 1971 census.

Of even greater interest is the unusual prevalence of
certain tumour types in traditional Canadian Eskimos
(Table 4), and a highly significant change in the order of
prevalence of "traditional" tumours such as salivary gland
and renal neoplasms, and "modern" tumours such as lung and
cervical cancer when comparing an earlier (1947-66) and a
more recent period (1967-73). Between 1947 and 1966, 59
Eskimos were diagnosed as having neoplastic disease - 13

TABLE 1
Summary of 164 cases of neoplastic disease in Eskimos from the Northwest Territories proven histologically in Edmonton, Winnipeg, Montreal,
and Toronto, 1950-74

Organ of primary or histological diagnosis	Number (and mean age) of cases		
	Total	Males	Females
Lung			
Bronchial carcinoma	26 (57.4)	11 (60.7)	15 (55.1)
Carcinoid adenoma	1 (46)	1 (46)	
Salivary gland tumours			
(19 carcinoma, 5 "mixed tumours")	24 (38.8)	11 (40.4)	13 (37.4)
Cervix			
Invasive	10 (39.4)		10 (39.4)
"In situ"	8 (34.0)		8 (34.0)
Nasopharynx	17 (54.8)	15 (56.7)	2 (40.0)
Blood and reticulo-endothelial system	12 (23.5)	7 (28.3)	5 (16.7)
Renal (9 carcinoma, 1 fibrosarcoma, 1 Wilm's)	11 (56.0)	8 (53.9)	3 (61.7)
Colon and rectum	11 (59.4)	4 (54.5)	7 (62.2)
CNS and retina (blastoma and melanoma)	6 (2.9)	2 (3.7)	4 (2.5)
Biliary tract (4 ampulla, 2 gall-bladder)	6 (56.3)	4 (56.0)	2 (54.0)
Oesophagus	5 (65.6)	3 (65.0)	2 (66.5)
Urinary bladder	4 (58.25)	1 (91)	3 (47.1)
Osteogenic sarcoma	3 (61.3)		3 (61.3)
Prostate	3 (65.0)	3 (65.0)	
Breast			
Invasive	2 (41.5)		2 (41.5)
"In situ"	1 (36.0)		1 (36.0)
Liver (hepatoma)	2 (73.5)	1 (74)	1 (73)
Stomach and duodenum	2 (55.5)	2 (55.5)	
Skin	1 (36)		1 (36)
Lip	1 (39)		1 (39)
Vulva	1 (52)		1 (52)
Choriocarcinoma	1 (47)		1 (47)
Ovary	1 (35)		1 (35)
Pancreas	1 (61)	1 (61)	
Thyroid adenoma	1 (36)		1 (36)
General carcinomatosis, primary site unknown	3 (50.0)	3 (50.0)	
All forms of cancer	164 (47.0)	77 (50.9)	87 (43.2)

TABLE 2
Primary site or type of cancer reported in death certificates for Eskimos from the Northwest Territories, 1967-72, and cancer death rates for various groups

Primary site or histological type of neoplasm	No.	Mean age	M	F	Origin of patients*				
					D	C	N	K	B
Lung (bronch.)	19	58.3	10	9	2	1	3	6	7
Nasopharynx	8	52.3	7	1	2	2	-	3	1
Colon and rectum	5	61.2	1	4	1	2	-	-	2
Blood and RES	5	25.0	-	3	-	-	-	3	2
Parotid gland	4	38.8	3	1	-	1	-	1	2
CNS									
Medulloblastomas	3	5.7	2	1	1	-	-	1	1
Astrocytoma	1	51.0	1	-	-	-	-	-	1
Cervix	3	45.7	-	3	1	1	-	1	-
Renal (hypernephroma)	2	60.5	2	-	1	-	-	-	1
Liver (hepatoma)	2	73.5	1	1	-	-	2	-	-
Pancreas	2	53.0	2	-	-	1	-	-	1
Oesophagus	2	68.0	-	2	-	-	-	2	-
Stomach and duodenum	2	55.5	2	-	2	-	-	-	-
Biliary (ampulla of Vater)	1	51.0	1	-	-	-	-	1	-
Testes	1	66.0	1	-	-	1	-	-	-
Prostate	1	57.0	1	-	-	-	-	1	-
General carcinomatosis, primary site not known	3	70.1	1	2	-	-	1	-	2
All cancer cases	64	51.9	37	27	10	9	6	19	20

	Total	M	F	D	C	N	K	B
Population estimates (January 1970)	11,175	5,643	5,532	1,772	1,492	780	2,375	4,756
Cancer rates per 100,000 per annum	95.5	109.3	81.3	94.1	100.5	128.2	133.3	70.1

* D = Mackenzie Delta, C = Coppermine, N = Netchiligmiut, K = Keewatin Zone, B = Baffin Zone.

with salivary gland, 7 with renal, and 6 with nasopharyngeal tumours. In contrast, only 4 had lung and one a cervical cancer. Of the 84 Eskimos diagnosed with malignant disease in the same centres between 1967 and 1973, lung cancer accounted for by far the largest group (20 cases, 23.8 per cent, compared with 6.35 per cent of all cancer cases registered in Alberta during 1969 and 1970), followed by cervical cancer; on the other hand, salivary gland tumours

TABLE 3
Increase of cancer morbidity and mortality of Eskimos as reflected by
(a) number of newly diagnosed cases, 1950-73, in Edmonton and Winnipeg,
and, (b) number of cancer deaths reported for Eskimos from the Northwest Territories, 1960-72

Year	(a)	(b)
1950	1	
51	4	
52	4	
53	1	
54	2	
55	2	
56	2	
57	6	
58	4	
59	3	
60	2	2
61	4	3
62	4	6
63	0	3
64	6	3
65	3	5
66	11	8
67	13	9
68	6	7
69	12	10
70	13	13
71	14	11
72	12	14
73	9	
Totals	80	94

(a) column annotations:
19 cancer cases in 6 years (3.167 annually) in population of 4,250 (Jan. 1958), 74.5 per 100,000 annually

Difference significant at p< 0.001

70 cancer cases in 6 years in population of 6,300 (Jan. 1969), 185.2 per 100,000 annually*

(b) column annotations:
22 cases in 6 years (3.7 annually) in population of 8,565 (Jan. 1963), 42.8 per 100,000

Difference significant at p<0.001

64 or 10.7 annually in a population of 11,175 (mid-1970), 99.5 per 100,000

* Six "in situ" cervical cancers were all found in the later period,
perhaps due to more screening with IUD's and birth control medication.
If these six cases were omitted, the figures would decrease to 64
cases or 169.3 per 100,000 and the significance level of the difference would drop to p< 0.002.

(9) had fallen to the fourth and renal neoplasms (3) to the
seventh place. Nasopharyngeal carcinoma remained in third
place, and was the leading form of cancer for males (15 of
74 with identified site of origin, 20.3 per cent of the
total series).

In recent years, morbidity and mortality rates from
bronchogenic carcinoma appear to have been higher in Eskimos of both sexes than in other Canadians, particularly
when age-adjusted rates are taken into consideration.

TABLE 4
Significance of changing order of incidence of cancer
observed in western and central arctic Eskimos in
early (1947-66) and recent (1967-73) periods

Type of neoplasm	1947-66	1967-73
Two leading "traditional" Eskimo neoplasms (salivary and renal)	20	12 $p < 0.01$
Two leading "modern" Eskimo cancers (lung and cervix)	5	34 $p < 0.001$
Total no. of all types of neoplasms	59	84

Note: There was a significant decrease in the relative prevalence of "traditional" tumours and a highly
significant increase in "modern" Eskimo tumours in
the last versus the first 20 years of the survey.
The significance of the over-all change of order ($x^2 <$
19) is even higher.

For NWT Eskimo males over 40 years of age we calculated for
the period 1967-72 inclusive an annual lung cancer mortality
rate of 204 per 100,000 compared with 96 per 100,000 in all
Canadian men of the same age groups in 1965. Corresponding
rates for Eskimo and Canadian women were 220 and 15 per
100,000. Eskimo women over the age of 40 years had 15 times
more chance to die of lung cancer than their southern Canadian counterparts if they lived in the NWT, and more than
30 times more risk of a lung cancer death if they lived in
the central Arctic.

Practically all Eskimos smoke from puberty onwards, the
amount and intensity of smoke exposure (number of cigarettes smoked, depth of inhalation, use of non-filter
brands, length of discarded stub) being quite high but about
equal in both sexes during the last two decades (specific
data for one settlement is given on page 320).

The unique predominance of females in this cancer form,
striking in the earlier observation period, when all four
recorded lung cancer cases were found in women, must be explained by additional Eskimo specific factor(s). Greater
affliction of females in areas where until a few years ago
seal oil lamps were used and cared for day and night by
women make us inclined to hypothesize that inhalation of
smoke from these open lamps played a role, particularly

when bronchial cleansing mechanisms were impaired by primary or secondary inhalation of cigarette smoke.

Salivary gland tumours were particularly prevalent in the least acculturated Eskimos of the Barren Lands and their Northern neighbours the Netchiligmiut. We are at a loss to explain either the extraordinary propensity of traditional Eskimos of both sexes for salivary gland tumours or the liability to cancer of the nasopharynx and to a lesser degree of the kidneys among Eskimo men. Changes of relative prevalence with time and geographical area suggest that environmental factors related to life-style may be responsible. Possibly, nutritional habits and climatic factors faciliate viral invasion.

Cancer of the cervix was diagnosed only once in the first 20 years of our survey, but has now jumped to second place if we count only invasive cases or to first place in females if 6 *in situ* cases are included. In either instance, the rate increase is highly significant. Almost all cases came from the larger and more promiscuous settlements, where there has been a manyfold increase of specific and unspecific vaginal infections; this supports recent claims of a relationship between cervical cancer and vaginal infections.

Breast cancer is still extremely rare in Eskimos (3.5 per cent of female cancer cases compared with 21.6 per cent in Alberta). In more than 25 years, only one Eskimo woman in the Northwest Territories died of breast carcinoma, that is an annual rate of approximately 5 per 100,000 females 35 years and older, whereas the breast cancer mortality for all Canadian women over 35 years of age was 63.7 in 1965. All our three cases had their first children before 19 years of age; gestation did not differ significantly from that of their unaffected cohorts, but lactation history was very different. The two cases with invasive breast carcinoma had a history of 10 and 6 births respectively, but did not nurse more than a total of one and three months respectively with the breast that was later affected. The third woman was diagnosed incidentally while in a Tuberculosis Sanatorium; she had an *in situ* lobular breast carcinoma, and reported a total of 60 months lactation with three births. The traditional practice, pretty widespread until moving into settlements in the mid 1960s, was to lactate each child until the next one was born – usually 3½ years later. This gave practically all women age 35 and older a lactation experience in excess of 200 months (1,2,3).

SUMMARY

The three main referral centres encountered 164 histologically proven cases of neoplastic disease over observation
periods of 6 years (eastern Arctic) to 26 years (central
and western Arctic). An unusual prevalence of tumours of
the salivary glands (14.9 per cent) and nasopharynx (20.3
per cent of neoplasms in males) was found. Differences in
geographic distribution and significant changes in the
relative prevalence of certain cancer types when compared
to an earlier period (1947-66) suggest that environmental
factors associated with acculturation are related to (a)
the absolute and relative increase of cancer morbidity and
mortality of Canadian Eskimos, and (b) the relative decrease
of traditional Eskimo tumours such as salivary gland and
renal neoplasms, with the dramatic increase of cancer of
the lung and of the cervix. More women than men had lung
cancer, perhaps caused by tending the traditional seal oil
lamps. Breast cancer is still a rarity, perhaps because of
lactation practices of the Eskimo.

REFERENCES

1. Schaefer, O., "Medical observations and problems in
   Canadian Arctic; Part II," Canad. Med. Assoc. J., 81:
   386-93 (1959)
2. Schaefer, O., "Cancer of the breast and lactation"
   (Letter to the Editor), Canad. Med. Assoc. J., 100:
   625-6 (1969)
3. Hildes, J.A. and Schaefer, O., "Health of Igloolik Eskimos and changes with urbanization," J. hum. Evol., 2:
   241-6 (1973)

Cancer in native populations in Labrador

G.W. THOMAS and J.H. WILLIAMS

In the past, it was thought that there was little or no carcinoma among the native populations of the North. Around
1960, some doubt was cast upon this generalization, and
over the past decade numerous authors have reported carcinoma in native populations of this area (1,2). The present

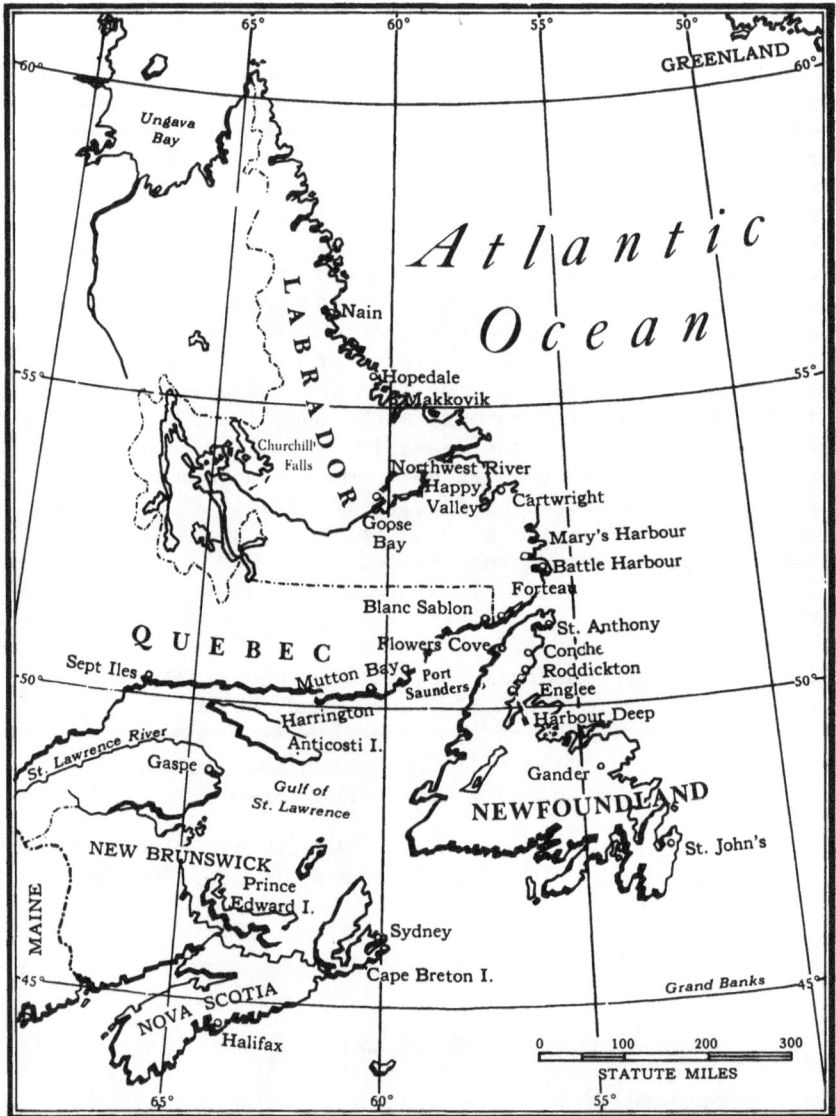

Figure 1 Geographical area of study

communication describes our experience of cancer among the
Eskimo and Indian populations of northern Labrador over the
period 1950-70. The only medical agency working in this
area is the International Grenfell Association and, because
of this, the native peoples are under the close medical
supervision of a single integrated medical service. It

would seem logical to assume that there is little likelihood
of a carcinoma occurring in an Eskimo or Indian person in
the area and escaping detection. The geographical area
served is shown in Figure 1. Nain, Davis Inlet, Hopedale,
Makkovik, and North West River are the principal areas where
native populations reside. Over the period of study, the Eskimo population averaged about 1,000, and the Indian population about 500.

The systemic incidence of the 25 histologically proven
carcinomas among the Eskimo population is shown in Table 1.
The commonest site was the gastrointestinal tract, with
primary growths in the stomach (3), common bile duct (1),
caecum (2), descending colon (2), and rectum (1). The next
commonest group of carcinomas occurred in the cervix (7).
The clinical details of the cervical tumours are summarized
in Table 2. The young age and the late stage of presentation are noteworthy. Three of the stage IV carcinomas were
seen in patients 25, 26, and 32 years old; the remaining
four were aged 38, 42, 44, and 51 years respectively. At
the time of diagnosis, four of the seven carcinomas had
reached stage IV and all patients died within two years
despite surgery and radiotherapy. The three carcinomas
in situ were treated surgically; the patients have survived
for over five years and remain well.

Three tumours of the parotid gland were seen over the 20-
year period. The incidence, 0.15 cases per thousand population per annum, is similar to that reported by Wallace et
al. (4); they found 14 salivary gland tumours over a 9-year
period in an Eskimo population of approximately 11,500
drawn from throughout the Canadian North, but excluding
Labrador (annual incidence 0.13 per thousand population per
year). In the series of Wallace et al., only 3 of their 14
tumours were of typical "mixed parotid" type; the remainder
were carcinomas, 9 being poorly differentiated with local
invasion and involvement of the regional lymph nodes. Histologically, this latter group resembled malignant lympho-
epitheliomas, but the authors suggested that they were pure
carcinomas of an unusual type.

Two of the three tumours in the present series were of
the typical "mixed parotid" type. The third case was a
further example of the variant described by Wallace et al.
(4); a 50-year-old Eskimo from Hopedale presented in July
1969 with a left parotid tumour measuring 4.5 X 3 X 3 cm,
which had grown rapidly in one year. Biopsy confirmed the
clinical diagnosis of a malignant tumour and a radical excision of the parotid gland with extensive dissection of

TABLE 1
Systemic incidence of cancer in Eskimos (number of
cases in a population of about 1,000 over 20 years)

Gl tract	9	Skin	1
Cervix	7	Bladder	1
Parotid	3	Bone	1
ENT	2	Breast	1

TABLE 2
Carcinoma of the cervix in an Eskimo population (clinical details
for seven patients)

Age	Year	Diagnostic stage	Treatment	Result
26	1951	IV	Radium implant	Died 1951
25	1951	IV	Radium implant	Died 1953
38	1959	0	Hysterectomy	Alive and well 1974
51	1961	IV	Radiotherapy	Died 1962
32	1961	IV	Radiotherapy	Died 1962
42	1967	0	Cone biopsy	Alive and well 1974
44	1968	la	Total hysterectomy Salpingo-oophorectomy	Alive and well 1974

the regional lymph nodes was carried out. Histologically,
the tumour had two distinct cellular patterns. The main tumour mass consisted of adenoid cyst exciting a moderate
round cell reaction in the adjacent fibrous stroma; closely
associated with this lesion were undifferentiated foci of
epithelial carcinoma with considerable lymphoid infiltra-
tion. The carcinomatous area showed highly cellular tumour
nests; the cells were large with pale cytoplasm and the
nuclei showed considerable variation in size with prominent
nucleoli. Similar tumour masses were seen in the adjacent
lymph nodes. No immediate postoperative radiation was
given, but a local recurrence in December 1971, eighteen
months after the primary excision, was treated with a course
of cobalt 60 to a total dosage of 4,500 Rads over a three-
week period. The patient died from extensive disease in
1973. An autopsy was not performed.

Of the other tumours, two arose in the nasopharynx;
these were an epidermoid carcinoma of the tonsils and a
secondary epidermoid carcinoma of the cervical lymph nodes
of indeterminate origin. An osteosarcoma of the right leg
was seen in a young man of 15; this was treated with a high

amputation and he remains well 23 years after the event - a remarkable survival. A tumour of the head of the pancreas and a sarcomatous lesion of the face were also seen. Only a single case of carcinoma of the breast was recorded. Carcinoma of the breast is certainly uncommon; the 53-year-old Eskimo lady, who had scirrhous carcinoma of the right breast, treated by a radical mastectomy and radio therapy, has been described previously (2). This lady remained well for 17 years following the initial diagnosis and treatment. In May 1974 she complained of gastric discomfort and was found to have extensive carcinoma of the stomach. A total gastrectomy was performed in July 1974, and metastases to the regional lymph nodes only were found. She died of cardio-respiratory complications on the 16th postoperative day. At autopsy, it was confirmed that the spread of the gastric neoplasm was confined to the regional lymph nodes; no evidence of any neoplastic disease of mammary origin was detected. This woman represents the first case in our experience of a double primary growth occurring in a native person.

During a similar period, only five patients with carcinoma were seen among the Indian population. The problem of keeping this population under close medical supervision is made more difficult because of their nomadic way of life and many of them still are somewhat reticent about seeking medical care. It is possible, therefore, that some cases of carcinoma among the Indians may not have been detected.

TABLE 3
Systemic incidence of cancer in Indians
(number of cases in a population of about
500 over a 20 year period)

Gl tract	2
Skin	2
Parotid	1

Table 3 shows the systemic incidence of cancer in the Indian population. Two cases of gastrointestinal carcinoma were seen, one of the rectum, and one of the head of the pancreas. Although carcinoma of the lip represents one of the types with the highest incidence in the white population of Labrador (5), no cases were observed in the Eskimo population; one case was seen in a 68-year-old Indian man from North West River who had a squamous cell carcinoma of his lower lip. A solitary carcinoma of the salivary gland was seen during this period and was of the common "mixed parotid" type.

Carcinoma of the breast was not encountered in any Indian person during the twenty-year period of review. In 1971, a 42-year-old Indian woman presented with a mass in the breast which consisted of a soft tumour 4 cm in diameter in the subareolar region. Histological examination showed moderately well-differentiated cellular carcinoma, with extensive lymph node involvement. This lady survived two years following radical mastectomy and radiotherapy.

Twenty-five proven cases of carcinoma were seen in a small group of Labrador Eskimos over the twenty-year period 1950-70. The over-all incidence of carcinoma (1.25 new cases per thousand population per annum) is similar (Newfoundland Tumour Registry - personal communication) to the incidence seen in the general population of Newfoundland and Labrador (1.5 per 1,000 of population). The incidence of carcinoma in the Indian population, 0.5 per 1,000 per year, is considerably lower than that seen in either the population as a whole or in the native Eskimos. However, the Indian figure may be artificially low because of social and environmental factors, and it may not represent the true incidence of carcinoma in that particular population.

An educational program to promote screening procedures for the early detection of carcinoma in native populations is likely to be the most effective way to reduce mortality and morbidity. However, such programs are difficult to carry out because of problems of environment and language. An active gynaecological cytology service appears to have reduced the number of advanced cancers of the cervix seen over the past 10 years. Extension of the service to include early detection of mammary and gastrointestinal neoplasms would appear to be indicated.

ACKNOWLEDGMENT

We are grateful to Dr W.A. Paddon and the staff of North West River Hospital for referring these patients and for assistance with the follow-up reports.

SUMMARY

The occurrence of carcinoma in the Eskimo and Indian population of Labrador from 150 to 1970 is reviewed. The incidence of carcinoma in the Eskimo group, 1.25 new cases per thousand population per annum, is similar to that recorded for the entire population of Newfoundland; however, the incidence of carcinoma in the Indian population is only 0.5

new cases per thousand population per annum. The importance of an active cancer detection program is stressed.

REFERENCES

1. Hildes, J.A., "Health Problems in the Arctic," Canad. Med. Assoc. J., 83: 1255 (1960)
2. Thomas, G.W., "Carcinoma among Labrador Eskimos and Indians," Canad. J. Surg., 4: 465 (1961)
3. Kraus, F.T., Gynaecologic Pathology (St. Louis: C.V. Mosby Co.), 1967
4. Wallace, A.C., Macdougall, J.T., Hildes, J.A., and Lederman, J.M., "Salivary gland tumours in Canadian Eskimos," Cancer 16: 1338 (1963)
5. Spitzer, W.O., Hill, G.B., Chambers, L.W., and Murphy, H.B., "Clinical epidemiology of cancer of the lip in Newfoundland," Ann. Roy. Coll. Phys. & Surg. Canada, p. 44, Jan. 1974

Allergy in the Yukon Territories: a review of
fifty-six patients, with a botanical study of allergenic flora

J.D. MARTIN and R. PORSILD

Between 1 January 1971 and 5 December 1973, 56 residents of the Yukon (14 per cent of them born in the Territory) were seen with symptoms (Table 1) suggesting an allergy; 37.5 per cent were male and 62.5 per cent female, the age distribution being as shown in Table 2. The patients received a full allergy work-up including skin testing.

Among the 16 persons who presented with wheezing, skin testing revealed a high incidence of positive reactions to house dust and animal allergens which correlated well with the history (Table 3). All 16 showed at least one positive reaction to dog or cat, and nine reacted positively to house dust.

Among the 25 persons who presented with chronic rhinitis, there was a high incidence of positive reactions to house dust and moulds (Table 4).

TABLE 1
Presenting symptoms suggestive of allergy

	Number of cases
1. Nasal discharge and/or obstruction	25
2. Post-nasal drip	5
3. Chronic conjunctivitis	8
4. Wheezing	16
5. Loss of hearing	1
6. Sinusitis	2
7. Chronic cough	2
8. Chronic headache	2
9. Eczema	4
10. Urticaria	3
11. Angioneurotic edema	4
12. Recurrent nose bleeds	1
13. Sneezing	3

TABLE 2
Age distribution of subjects with
symptoms suggesting an allergy

Age (years)	Number
0-9	7
10-19	11
20-29	13
30-39	16
40-49	8
50-59	1
60+	0

TABLE 3
Positive skin reactions among patients
presenting with wheezing

House dust	9
Moulds	2
Animals	
Dog	7
Cat	9
Grasses	1

Of the 56 patients, 12 received allergy desensitization
solutions. Unfortunately many of these people are not
available for follow-up, so that the effectiveness of this
treatment cannot be analysed. The majority of patients
responded to a program of avoidance of the allergen, e.g.
animals, and to a house dust eradication program in the
home.

TABLE 4
Positive skin reactions among 25
patients presenting with rhinitis

House dust	11
Moulds	7
Cat	4
Feathers	2
No reaction	6

Three patients with chronic rhinitis and no evidence of allergy were thought to have symptoms precipitated by oral contraceptives. One woman with nasal obstruction was found to have used a nasal spray for several months and responded well when she stopped using the spray. Four patients referred to the Ear, Nose and Throat Consultant required surgery. One woman being desensitized to pollens collapsed in the office following an injection and required adrenaline.

BOTANICAL SURVEY OF ALLERGENIC FLORA

The Yukon Territory lies in Canada's north-western corner. Approximately 20,000 people live in an area of 207,076 square miles, over half of them in Whitehorse, the Yukon's capital city. High elevation and a semi-arid climate produce warm summer weather, varying from cool evenings to 80° F and higher during the long daylight hours from June to September. Average winter temperatures compare with those of Regina and Winnipeg. The southern interior is a great plateau, drained by the Yukon and its tributary rivers. The St Elias Range in the west is an extension of the Coast Range of British Columbia. Here are the highest peaks in Canada, including Mount Logan at 19,850 feet.

There are many potentially allergenic plants in the Yukon (Table 5), but allergy does not appear to be a problem clinically. Some of the fifty-six patients had manifestations of pollen allergy elsewhere in Canada, but most were relieved of symptoms in the Yukon. Ragweed is not seen in this area.

DISCUSSION

From this limited survey, it would seem that seasonal allergy is uncommon; most patients present with perennial allergic manifestations. House dust and dog and cat allergens are frequently the cause of rhinitis and asthma. Although there are many pollen producing plants in the Yukon, the paucity

TABLE 5
Hay fever inducing plants, Yukon species, common with Alaska and
northern British Columbia

Tree or plant	Popular names	Latin names	More populated areas
Alder	Mountain alder	*Alnus incana*	Common near damp ground
		Alnus crispa	Common near damp ground
Poplar	Aspen	*Populus tremuloides*	Common
	Black cottonwood	*Populus trichocarpa*	Local near southern borders
Birch	Balsam poplar	*Populus tricacakocca*	Common
	Shrub birch 1	*Betula glandielosa*	Fairly common
	Shrub birch 2	*Betula occidentalis*	Fairly common
	Paper birch	*Betula papyrifera*	Fairly common
Willow		32 *Salix* species	Some common
Pine	Lodgepole pine	*Pinus contorta*	Common, but local, Whitehorse area
Spruce	White spruce	*Picea glauca*	Common, but local, Whitehorse area
	Black spruce	*Picea mariana*	Common, but local, Whitehorse area
Fir	Alpine fir	*Abies lasciocarpa*	Only on high ground, Elsa Mine
Larch	Tamarack	*Larix laricina*	Local, common in Watson Lake area
Grass	Annual June	*Poa annua*	Common, introduced
	Kentucky blue	*Poa pratensis*	Common, introduced
	Bent	*Agrostis* species	Common
	Wild rye	*Elymus glaucus*	Local
	Fescue	*Festica* species	Scarce
	Quack	*Agropyron* species	Common
	Brome	*Bromus* species	Common
	Timothy	*Phleum pratense*	Common, introduced
Weed	Dock or sorrel	*Rumex* species	Common near wet ground
	English plantain	*Plantago lanceolata*	Local, common, Mayo
	Plantain	*Plantago major*	Common
	Lamb's quarters	*Chenopodium* species	Common
	Sage	*Artemesia* species	*A. frigida*, very common
	Dandelion	*Taraxacum taraxacum*	Very common

of symptoms suggests that pollen counts are low; counts to
verify this point are planned for 1975. Factors that likely
hold down the pollen count are the mountainous terrain and
a low rainfall (as little as eleven inches annually in
Whitehorse).

SUMMARY

Fifty-six residents of the Yukon Territories seen between
1 January 1971 and 5 December 1973 had symptoms suggesting
an allergy. The majority of patients presented with nasal
discharge and/or obstruction, chronic conjunctivitis, and
wheezing. In the sixteen persons who presented with
wheezing, skin testing revealed a high incidence of positive reactions to house dust and animal allergens, particularly dog and cat. In twenty-five persons presenting with
chronic rhinitis, skin testing revealed a high incidence of
positive reactions to house dust and moulds, with fewer
reactions to dog and cat allergens. Of the fifty-six patients, twelve received allergy desensitization injections.
A list of common "hay fever" producing plants of the Yukon
Territories has been compiled. Although there are many potentially allergenic plants, pollen allergy does not appear
to be a problem clinically. Some of the fifty-six patients
had developed allergy to pollens elsewhere in Canada, but
most were relieved of these symptoms in the Yukon. Ragweed
is not seen in this area.

REFERENCES

1. Samter, Max, and Durham, Oren C., Regional Allergy of
   the United States, Canada, Mexico and Cuba, A Symposium
   of Thirty-nine Contributors (Springfield, Ill.: C.C.
   Thomas, 1955)

Commentaries

"Differences in coronary heart disease incidence and risk
factors between northern and southern Sweden," by C. Fur-
berg, L. Wilhelmsen, and G. Tibblin (Central Hospital,
Boden and Sahlgrenska Hospital, Gothenburg, Sweden). A myocardial infarction (MI) register, covering the total populations between the ages of 20 and 64 years (totalling 23,372
and 274,870 persons, respectively), was operating in the
city of Boden and its rural surroundings in northern Sweden
and in the city of Gothenberg in the southwest from January

1 to December 31, 1971. The combined incidence of non-fatal
and fatal MI was 4.8 in Boden and 2.8 in Gothenburg per
1,000 men and 1.6 and 0.7 respectively per 1,000 women. Angina pectoris, previous MI, and diabetes prior to the
present MI were equally common in both areas, but intermittent claudication, cerebrovascular accidents, and hypertension were slightly more common in the Boden area. The
average delay between onset of symptoms and admission to
the hospital was 240 minutes in the north as compared to
150 minutes in Gothenburg. A population survey among middle-
aged men was running in the two areas at the same period as
the register. Data on the composition of the risk factors
for coronary heart disease (CHD) revealed that middle-aged
men on Boden had somewhat higher plasma cholesterol,
higher physical activity at work and during leisure time,
and smoked less than men in Gothenburg. There were no
differences in systolic or diastolic blood pressures or
body weight. The difference in the incidence of MI was essentially not explained by any of the factors studied.

"Coronary heart disease risk factors in relation to urbanization in Alaskan Eskimo men," by J.E. Maynard (Center for
Disease Control, US Public Health Service, Anchorage,
Alaska, USA). During an epidemiologic study to provide new
descriptive information on blood pressure, coronary heart
disease, and associated risk factors in relation to the
rural-urban gradient, 2,356 Alaskan Eskimo males over the
age of 14 were examined. Prevalences of systolic and diastolic hypertension were lower in Eskimos than in the general US population, and Eskimos residing in towns and
cities had higher frequencies of systolic and diastolic
hypertension than did those living in villages. Serum
cholesterol levels in Eskimos were found to be among the
highest reported to date. Although the association of
cholesterol level with the Eskimo rural-urban gradient was
inconstant, its persistent negative association with educational level suggested a possible relationship to dietary
pattern associated with the educational aspects of acculturation. The Eskimo demonstrated higher levels of serum
uric acid and lower levels of triglycerides than those
found in North American population comparisons. The positive association of serum triglycerides and the negative
association of uric acid with the Eskimo rural-urban gradient suggested differences in relative intakes of fat, protein, and carbohydrate between the rural and urban environ-

ments. Electrocardiographic abnormalities indicative of
prior mycardial infarction were absent in Eskimo men under
50 years of age. However, prevalence of these abnormalities
in the older age groups was only slightly lower than in
other US population comparisons, with no discernible relationship to the Eskimo rural-urban gradient. Although
there were no significant associations between frequency of
infarction-related abnormalities and levels of serum triglycerides, cholesterol, uric acid, or with smoking history, the data did not support the assertion of an unusually low prevalence of coronary heart disease in the Eskimo
men. The data are, however, at variance with the assumption
of a uniform positive relationship between serum cholesterol level and coronary heart disease prevalence in populations where both attributes are measured.

"Cholelithiasis in Alaskan Indians and Eskimos," by I.W.
Duncan (Arctic Health Research Center, Center for Disease
Control, USPHS, Fairbanks, Alaska, USA). Alaska's large
size, wide variation in environmental conditions, and the
geographic distribution of ethnic groups within the state
make the study of geographic clustering of disease of unusual interest. Inpatient records from Alaska Native
Health Service Hospitals for the fiscal years 1966-70 were
searched by computer for the diagnosis of cholelithiasis.
Cholelithiasis was found to be more prevalent in older individuals in females and in southeastern Alaska Indians,
and an association with urbanization and obesity was suggested. Utilization of hospitals by Aleuts, Eskimos, and
Indians was in direct proportion to their respective populations. The over-all rate of hospitalization of persons
(per 1,000 populations at risk) because of cholelithiasis
was not grossly different from rates found in studies of
non-Indian populations. The high prevalence of cholelithiasis reported in previous studies of North American Indians
was not indicated.

ZOONOTIC AND INFECTIOUS DISEASES

Mosquito vectors of California encephalitis virus in a Canadian subarctic region

D.M. MCLEAN

Isolation of the snowshoe hare subtype of California encephalitis (CE) virus from several species of *Aedes* mosquitoes and the blood of snowshoe hares (*Lepus americanus*) near Tok (63° N, 143° W) in east-central Alaska during the summer of 1970 (2) has stimulated investigations of the prevalence of CE virus throughout the Yukon Territory during successive summers since 1971 (6). Serological evidence of human infections with CE virus was also found in Alaska (2). Previously recorded northern foci of prevalence of the CE virus include the snowshoe hare subtype near Rochester, Alberta (54° N, 113° W) (3) and the Inkoo subtype near Helsinki, Finland (60° N, 20° E) (1).

During the summers of 1971, 1972, and 1973, strains of CE virus were isolated from 22 of 176 pools comprising four species of unengorged wild-caught female mosquitoes (*Aedes canadensis, A. cinereus, A. communis,* and *Culiseta inornata*), collected at five sites throughout the Yukon Territory, from Marsh Lake (61° N, 134° W) near Whitehorse, to mile 123 on the Dempster Highway (66° N, 138° W) in the north (5). Minimum field infection rates ranged from 1:160 to 1:2854 (Table 1). During the summer of 1974, CE virus was isolated from one pool of *A. canadensis* mosquitoes collected near Carmacks (62° N, 135° W).

Sera were collected from 4,133 small forest rodents at seven principal locations throughout the Yukon Territory during the summers of 1971 to 1973 (Table 2). A Yukon mosquito isolate of the snowshoe hare subtype of CE virus (Marsh Lake 23 strain) was neutralized by 661 (16 per cent) sera including 426 of 1,070 (41 per cent) snowshoe hares (*Lepus americanus*), 237 of 2,854 (8 per cent) ground squirrels (*Citellus undulatus*), and 8 of 209 (4 per cent)

TABLE 1
California encephalitis virus isolations from Yukon
mosquitoes, 1971-73

Location	Year	Week no.	Species	Ratio	MFIR
Marsh Lake	1971	26-29	A.canadensis	6/34	1:282
(61°N, 134°W)	1972	27-31	A.communis	4/40	1:668
	1973	28	A.canadensis	1/6	1:295
	1973	27	A.communis	1/20	1:1117
Lookout	1971	29	A.canadensis	5/16	1:160
(61°N, 135°W)	1973	23	Cs.inornata	1/9	1:179
Mayo Road					
(61½°N, 135°W)	1971	27	A.canadensis	1/6	1:650
Hunker Creek					
(64°N, 138°W)	1972	30	A.communis	1/21	1:1654
Dempster Hwy	1972	30	A.communis	1/19	1:2854
(66°N, 138°W)	1973	23	A.cinereus	1/5	1:370

red squirrels (*Tamiasciurus hudsonicus*). During the summer
of 1974, with the precipitous decline in the population of
snowshoe hares, the 44 of 780 (5.6 per cent) sera which
neutralized CE virus were derived almost exclusively from
39 of 756 (5.2 per cent) ground squirrels. Other reactions
included 4 of 6 snowshoe hares and 1 of 18 red squirrels.

Infectivity was detected at high titre in the salivary
glands of *Culiseta inornata* mosquitoes which were incubated
at 40° F for 76 days, and at 30° F thereafter for as long
as 194 days, following intrathoracic injection of 30 mouse
LD_{50} of the Marsh Lake 23 strain. Enveloped virions 45 nm
in diameter were observed by electron microscopy of thin
sections of salivary glands 59 days after intrathoracic injection with 300 mouse LD_{50}, following incubation at 55° F.
Transmission of virus by biting suckling mice was effected
by *Cs. inornata* after 17 days extrinsic incubation at 80° F
following intrathoracic injection with 30 mouse LD_{50} of
Marsh Lake 23 virus (5). When incubated at 55° F, both
Cs. inornata and *Aedes cinereus* became infected following
intrathoracic injection with as small a quantity of CE virus as 0.03 mouse LD_{50} (5). Transmission by biting mice was
also effected by *A. cinereus* which were incubated for 15
days at 55° F following intrathoracic injection with 30 and
3 mouse LD_{50} (5).

The immunoperoxidase test (4) was used successfully to
demonstrate the presence of CE antigen in the cytoplasm of
acinar cells of salivary glands of *Cs. inornata* mosquitoes

TABLE 2

California encephalitis neutralizing antibodies in small mammals, Yukon, 1971-73 (La = snowshoe hare, Cu = ground squirrel, Th = red squirrel)

Location	1971			1972			1973			Total			
	La	Cu	Th	La	Cu	Th	La	Cu	Th	La	Cu	Th	All
Lookout (61°N, 135°W)	22/105	0/13	0/3	33/88	13/112	0/1	21/75	13/77	0/6	76/268	26/202	0/10	102/480
Mayo Road (61¼°N, 135°W)	8/60	10/135	0/2	8/32	8/184	..	..	8/127	0/1	16/92	26/446	0/3	42/541
Carcross, etc. (60½°N, 135°W)	9/24	33/459	0/8	17/51	41/601	1/9	51/87	24/275	5/97	77/162	98/1,335	6/114	181/1,611
Marsh Lake (61°N, 134°W)	19/71	16/68	2/11	47/102	12/194	0/1	89/164	8/85	0/53	155/337	36/347	2/65	193/749
Haines Jn., etc. (61°N, 138°W)	3/9	16/203	0/3	0/2	6/138	0/1	51/112	6/85	0/7	54/123	28/426	0/11	82/560
Hunker Ck. (64°N, 138°W)	17/36	1/47	0/3	26/42	..	..	3/8	1/4	0/1	46/81	2/51	0/4	48/141
Dempster Hwy (66°N, 138°W)	..	..	..	2/2	4/14	..	..	7/33	0/2	2/2	11/47	0/2	13/51
Total no.	78/303	76/925	2/30	133/319	84/1,243	1/12	215/446	67/686	5/167	426/1,070	237/2,854	8/209	661/4,133
%	26	8	6	42	7	8	48	10	3	41	8	4	16
All no.		156/1,260			218/1,574			287/1,299			661/4,133		
%		12			14			22			16		

6 to 22 days after intrathoracic injection with 3,000 mouse LD_{50} of Marsh Lake 23 virus, and in the salivary glands of *A. canadensis* 4 to 22 days and *A. communis* 4 to 10 days after intrathoracic injection with 300 mouse LD_{50}, when mosquitoes were incubated both at 70° F and 55° F. Laboratory bred *A. aegypti* mosquitoes revealed immunoperoxidase staining in salivary glands removed one to 27 days after intrathoracic injection with 200 mouse LD_{50} CE virus after incubation at 70° F, but staining was also detected after 6 days incubation at 55° F.

These results indicate the prevalence of CE virus in natural foci throughout the Yukon Territory. The natural cycle for virus maintenance appears to involve small forest rodents, especially ground squirrels, as reservoirs, and various *Aedes* and *Culiseta* mosquitoes as vectors. In years of high prevalence of snowshoe hares, these lagomorphs also serve as extremely important natural reservoirs. The ability of mosquitoes to serve as arbovirus vectors at subarctic latitudes, where daytime temperatures rarely exceed 70° F and overnight temperatures may fall below 32° F even during summer, appears to arise from their ability to support CE virus replication at unusually low temperatures, from 55 to 30° F. It also seems likely that the adult *Culiseta* mosquito may provide a significant mechanism for overwintering, in view of the prolonged persistence of CE virus in salivary glands following incubation at 30° F.

Although human infections or illness due to CE virus have not been encountered in the Yukon to date, serological evidence of CE infection among human residents of a natural CE focus in east-central Alaska suggests that CE infections could become manifest among large groups of persons who were located suddenly but inadvertently in a natural focus where mosquito-abatement procedures were not pursued.

SUMMARY

California encephalitis (CE) virus (snowshoe hare subtype) has been isolated from wild-caught mosquitoes throughout the Yukon Territory during successive summers 1971 to 1974, as far north as 66° N. Principal natural mammalian reservoirs have been *Citellus undulatus* and *Lepus americanus*. *Culiseta inornata* and *Aedes cinereus* mosquitoes, collected in the Yukon, have transmitted virus by biting mice following intrathoracic injection and incubation for about two weeks at 80° F and 55° F respectively, and CE virus has persisted in *Cs. inornata* salivary glands up to 194 days

after holding at 40° F reducing to 30° F at 77 days. Immunoperoxidase techniques have revealed CE antigen in cytoplasm
of salivary glands of Yukon mosquitoes 2 to 22 days after
intrathoracic injection following incubation at 70° F and
55° F. Although human infections with CE virus have not
been diagnosed in Yukon residents, several cases were recognized among residents of east-central Alaska. CE infection
could become manifest among large groups of persons who
were located suddenly but inadvertently in a natural focus
where mosquito-abatement procedures were not pursued.

REFERENCES

1. Brummer-Korvenkonitio, M., Saikku, P., Korhonen, P.,
   Ulmanen, J., Reunala, T., and Karvonen, J., "Arboviruses
   in Finland. IV. Isolation and characterization of Inkoo
   virus, a Finnish representative of the California group,"
   Am. J. trop. Med. Hyg., 22: 404-13 (1973)
2. Feltz, E.T., List-Young, B., Ritter, D.G., Holden, P.,
   Noble, G.R., and Clarke, P.S., "California encephalitis
   virus: serological evidence of human infections in
   Alaska," Canad. J. Microbiol., 18: 757-62 (1972)
3. Iversen, J., Hanson, R.P., Papadopoulous, O., Morris,
   C.V., and De Foliart, G.R., "Isolation of viruses of the
   California encephalitis group from boreal Aedes mosquitoes," Am. J. trop. Med. Hy., 18: 735-42 (1969)
4. Kurstak, E., "The immunoperoxidase technique: localiza-
   tion of viral antigens in cells," in Methods in Virology,
   5 (New York: Academic Press, 1971), pp. 423-44
5. McLean, D.M., Bergman, S.K.A., Graham, E.A., Greenfield,
   G.P., Olsen, J.A., and Patterson, R.D., "California encephalitis virus prevalence in Yukon mosquitoes during
   1973," Canad. J. Pub. Health, 65: 23-8 (1974)
6. McLean, D.M., Goddard, E.J., Graham, E.A., Hardy, G.J.,
   and Purvin-Good, K.W., "California encephalitis virus
   isolations from Yukon mosquitoes, 1971," Am. J. Epidemiol., 95: 347-55 (1972)

Epizootiology of rabies in Canada

K.M. CHARLTON and H. TABEL

Two human cases of rabies were reported in Canada during the 19th century (3, 6). One case occurred near Ottawa, following the bite of a dog or a fox, and one occurred in Quebec City, following a dog bite. In the first half of the 20th century, there were sporadic epizootics near the Canadian-American border (8), outbreaks occurring in southern Saskatchewan (1905), southern Manitoba (1907), southern Ontario (1907-17), Red Deer, Alberta (1909), Victoria, (1914), Ottawa Valley, Ontario and Quebec (1917-26), Calgary, (1927), and southwestern Ontario (1942-45). These outbreaks involved domestic animals, especially dogs, and the disease did not become established in wildlife. Frequently, infection was traced to animals imported into Canada from the United States.

There are no reports of rabies in the Canadian Arctic (Northwest Territories and Yukon) in the 19th century. During the 1920s and 1930s, there were several reports from the NWT of a neurologic disease in sleigh dogs and wild animals (8). A disease resembling rabies was seen in dogs from Somerset Island in 1945, and in 1946, there were similar reports from Baffin Island and Baker Lake. The first laboratory diagnosis of rabies in the Canadian Arctic was made by Plummer at Baker Lake, NWT, in 1947 (7). This diagnosis, in a fox, was based on demonstration of Negri bodies and confirmed by animal inoculation. In the same year, the disease was diagnosed in a wolf at Aklavik in the Mackenzie Delta and in a sleigh dog at Frobisher Bay on Baffin Island. Since 1947, rabies has been diagnosed in the NWT and/or Yukon every year except four - 1949, 1950, 1957, and 1960. The distribution of accumulated cases is illustrated in Figure 1. During the period from 1961 to 1973, rabies has been diagnosed 9 years in the Mackenzie Delta, 5 years in the Yellowknife area, 7 years along the north shore, 8 years along the west shore of Hudson Bay, and 9 years in the northern islands. Rabies has thus been widespread and continuously present in the Canadian Arctic, at least since 1947. Because of the difficulties in transportation of suitable specimens for diagnosis and because of the known presence of rabies in Alaska, it is conceivable that rabies was also present, but undiagnosed, in the NWT prior to the first definite diagnoses in 1947. The

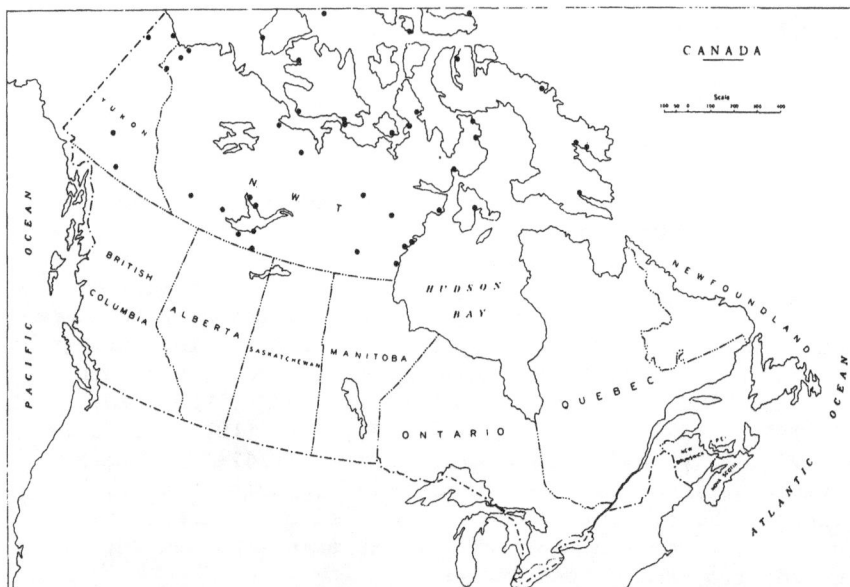

Figure 1   Location of rabies in the Northwest Territories
and the Yukon. Other parts of Canada not included. Each
site indicates diagnosis of rabies in one or more years
from 1947 to 1973

species currently affected include Arctic and red foxes,
wolves, dogs, cats, and caribou. The fox is the most frequently affected, with most diagnosis being made during the
winter months. The number of positive cases per year is
fairly small, with only slight fluctuations, and there is
insufficient evidence to suggest cyclic occurrence of rabies in the NWT.

Rabies in the Yukon and NWT has had a profound effect
on other parts of Canada, since outbreaks of rabies in
several provinces in the 1950s were caused by a southward
spread of the disease (8). The red fox was the predominant
wildlife vector concerned. In 1952, an epizootic began in
the vicinity of Fort Smith, NWT; it spread south throughout Alberta (Figure 2), and to a lesser extent into Saskatchewan and northeastern British Columbia, to subside in
the late 1950s. Rabies in northern Manitoba in the 1950s
probably originated in the NWT. Rabies was not diagnosed in
southern Ontario between 1945 and 1956, although the disease was present in New York state. The distribution and
sequence of diagnoses made in the eastern NWT and northern

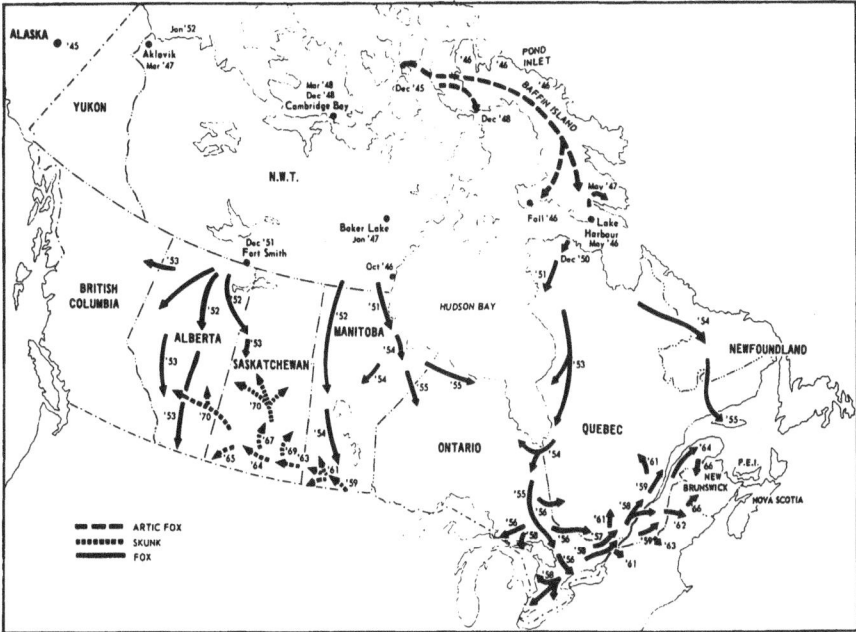

Figure 2   Arrows indicate the direction and extent of major epizootics of rabies in Canada from 1945 to 1972 (courtesy of *The Canadian Veterinary Journal*)

Quebec in the late 1940s and early 1950s suggest that rabies travelled south through the northern tip of Quebec in 1951, reaching Moosonee in 1954, and southern Ontario in 1956. In 1957, rabies was found in the striped skunks of Ontario and, since then, the skunk has become the second most important wildlife vector in Ontario and Quebec (4). In addition to remaining enzootic in Ontario and Quebec, the disease probably spread to adjacent areas of the northeastern United States (Figure 2). Rabies in Manitoba, Saskatchewan, and Alberta now occurs mainly in skunks, while in British Columbia it is almost entirely restricted to bats. The distribution of rabies across Canada in 1973 is depicted in Figure 3. The fox and skunk have been and continue to be the most important wildlife vectors in Canada (Table 1).

The climate of the Canadian Arctic allows the rabies virus to survive for prolonged periods in frozen carcasses. This may be an important factor in the epizootiology of rabies in Canada, maintaining a source of viable virus between

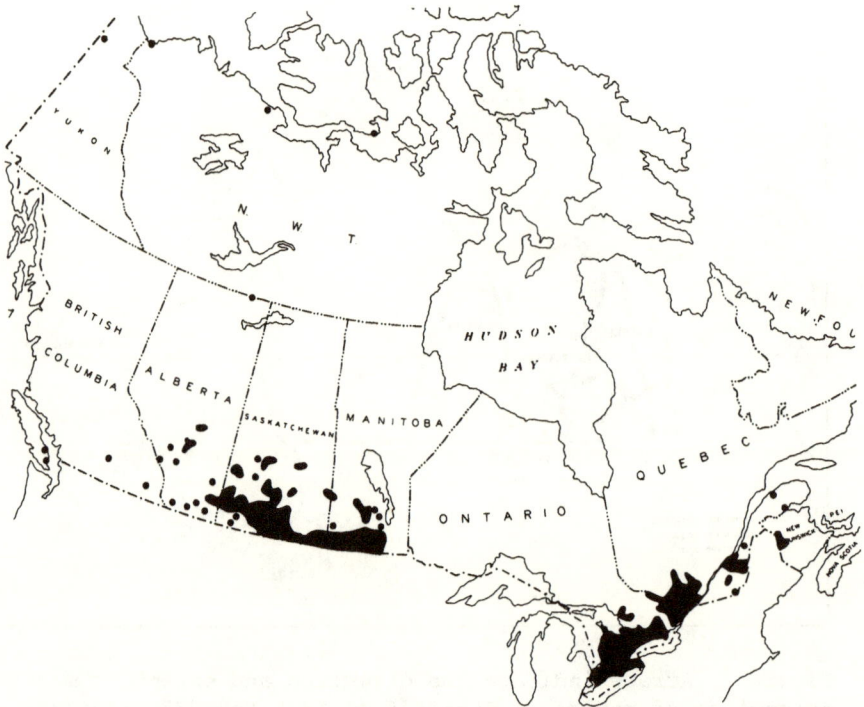

Figure 3   Distribution of rabies during 1973 (all species)

TABLE 1
Rabies in wildlife species in Canada, 1947-73

Species	Total
Fox *(Vulpes vulpes/Alopex lagopus)*	9,856
Striped skunk *(Mephitis mephitis)*	4,319
Bat *(Vespertilionidae)*	203
Raccoon *(Procyon lotor)*	124
Wolf *(Canis lupus)*	111
Coyote *(Canis latrans)*	86
Groundhog *(Marmota monax)*	18
Black bear *(Ursus americanus)*	9
Lynx *(Lynx canadensis)*	5
Muskrat *(Ondatra zibethica)*	4
Badger *(Taxidea taxus)*	2
Beaver *(Castor canadensis)*	2
Buffalo *(Bison bison)*	2
Caribou *(Rangifer tarandus)*	2
White-tailed deer *(Odocoileus virginianus)*	2
Rat *(Rattus norvegicus)*	2
Others	14

epizootics. Although rabies is usually transmitted by biting, experimental animals have been infected via the oral and respiratory routes (2, 5) and in one instance, dogs apparently acquired the infection after being fed frozen fox carcasses (8). Providing that such mechanisms could initiate an outbreak, the subsequent spread of the disease by the more usual mode of transmission would then depend on the many geographic and biological factors influencing the distribution and density of the species concerned.

SUMMARY

The history of rabies in Canada is traced from the first sporadic outbreaks of the disease initiated by imported dogs along the US border. The first confirmed diagnosis of rabies in the NWT was in 1947, and since this time the disease has become widespread, spreading southward into Ontario and Quebec. At the present time, rabies is found in domestic animals or wildlife in all Canadian provinces except Newfoundland, Prince Edward Island, and Nova Scotia. Climatic conditions of the Arctic help preserve the virus between epizootics, and maintain a source of infection for other areas of Canada. The arctic fox and the red fox are the main vectors in the NWT.

REFERENCES

1. Ballantyne, E.E. and O'Donoghue, J.G., "Rabies control in Alberta," J. Am. vet. med. Assoc., 125: 316-26 (1954)
2. Fischman, H.R., and Ward, F.E. III., "Oral transmission of rabies virus in experimental animals," Am. J. Epidemiol., 88: 132-8 (1968)
3. Historical Atlas of the county of Carleton, Ontario (Toronto: H. Belden & Co., 1879), p. XXXIII
4. Johnston, D.H., and Beauregard, M., "Rabies epidemiology in Ontario," Bull. Wildl. Dis. Assoc., 5: 357-70 (1969)
5. Johnson, R.T., "Pathogenesis of experimental rabies," in Y. Nagano and F.M. Davenport (eds.) Rabies (Baltimore: University Park Press, 1971), pp. 59-75
6. Mitchell, C.A., "Rabies in Quebec City. Case Report 1839," Med. Serv. J. Can., 23: 809-12 (1967)
7. Plummer, P.J.G., "Rabies in Canada, with special reference to wildlife reservoirs," Bull. Wld. Hlth. Org., 10: 767-74 (1954)
8. Tabel, H., Corner, A.H., Webster, W.A., and Casey, G.A., "History and epizootiology of rabies in Canada," Can. vet. J., in press

Parasites of Eskimos at Igloolik and Hall Beach, Northwest Territories

R.S. FREEMAN and J. JAMIESON

There are relatively few reports that discuss the incidence of human intestinal parasites in the people of the near-Arctic. There have been a few surveys along the coast of Alaska, others from Canada, mainly below the Arctic Circle (3,4,10) and at least one survey from the west coast of Greenland (2). All describe relatively high, albeit variable, incidences of intestinal parasites, including protozoans and usually some metazoan eggs. As Babbott et al. stated for Greenland (2), the level of parasitism "... was comparable to many tropical regions." There are a few studies on the biology of metazoan parasites of natives, mostly from Alaska (11, 12). The present report adds to scanty knowledge of the incidence of human intestinal parasites in the far north of eastern Canada (4,5,9) particularly Igloolik and Hall Beach, NWT (3). Particular objectives of the study were to establish the identity and shed light on the biology of *Diphyllobothrium* sp. (3), and to determine whether *D. latum* occurs in the eastern Canadian Arctic (1,5,9,11,16).

MATERIALS AND METHODS

The senior author collected faecal specimens on two short trips in May–June 1970 and August 1971. Local workers also collected faecal specimens at Hall Beach and Igloolik in September–October 1970; these were treated with formalin and sent to Toronto for examination. A total of 352 faecal samples, from more than 300 Eskimos out of a total native population of just over 700, were examined. In May–June 1970, 171 pinworm swabs were also collected.

A modified Ritchie-Formalin-Ether centrifugation concentration technique (RFE) (13) was used on all specimens. Some specimens were also stained with Scholton's modified iron haematoxylin (SIH) procedure (15).

One of us (J.J.) spent May–September 1971 collecting helminth parasites from Arctic char and a few other species of fish from nine areas of the upper Foxe Basin, as well as observing the biology of Eskimos in summer camp. Two types of tapeworm plerocercoids were removed from

Arctic char (*Salvelinus alpinus* (L.)) and a second worm
tentatively identified as *Diphyllobothrium* sp.; these were
fed to five Caucasian volunteers and two dogs. Two humans
and one dog became infected with one type.

Four adult worms were purged from the human volunteers
using magnesium sulphate, atabrine, sodium bicarbonate, and
phenobarbital as recommended by Rausch et al. (12). The
worms were fixed in hot or cold 10 per cent formalin,
stained, and either shaved, sectioned, or mounted in toto
for study.

RESULTS

Results are summarized in Table 1. Because of the low incidence of pinworms in May–June 1970, this aspect of the study
was not continued in the autumn of 1970 or in 1971. The data
for May–June 1970 and August 1971 are comparatively consistent, and are based on field study of RFE concentrates and
additional SIH specimens prepared on return to the laboratory in 1971. The apparent discrepancies between these samples and those collected in September–October 1970 may result from both smaller sample sizes and from the use of for-
malin-treated samples. The latter provide less consistent
information than results obtained with unfixed faecal samples. The higher incidence of parasites found in August
1971 undoubtedly reflects both a true increase in the incidence of helminth ova, and the fact that several protozoal
infections, overlooked in RFE procedures, were detected
with the SIH technique.

Two types of plerocercoids of *Diphyllobothrium* spp., the
stage infective to the homiothermic vertebrate host, were
commonly found on and within various viscera from Arctic
char. One type was large, characteristically wrinkled, or
even segmented (Figure 1), and was subsequently identified
as *Diphyllobothrium dendriticum* (Nitsch); this type was
less ubiquitous and less common in absolute numbers than
the second type. The latter was small, characteristically
"smooth" (Figure 2) and found in all areas where Arctic
char were collected, being at least four times more common
than *D. dendriticum*. The results of limited feedings of
both types of plerocercoids to Caucasian volunteers and
dogs (Table 2) were monitored with the RFE technique, beginning seven days after ingestion of plerocercoids and
continuing weekly for seven weeks if eggs were not found.
Four *Diphyllobothrium dendriticum* were purged from the
two infected humans (8), but one dog, although passing eggs

TABLE 1
Intestinal parasites of Eskimos in Hall Beach and Igloolik, NWT

	1949* August Igloolik	1970 May-June Igloolik	Hall Beach	1970 Sept.-Oct. Igloolik	Hall Beach	1971 August Igloolik
Pinworm swabs (examined/% infected)	60/33	77/5	94/2	-	-	-
Faecal samples (examined/% infected)	97/47	78/47**	73/48**	46/33**	32/59**	123/53**
Entamoeba coli (% infected)	8	30	38	17	38	29
Entamoeba histolytica (% infected)	0	0	0	0	3	0
Endolimax nana (% infected)	4	12	6	9	22	24
Giardia lamblia (% infected)	2	17	29	9	28	11
Other flagellates (% infected)	0	0	0	0	0	2
Diphyllobothrium sp. (% infected)	33	0	0	9	0	2
Diphyllobothrioid eggs (% infected)	0	0	0	0	0	6
Fluke (?) eggs (% infected)	0	0	0	0	0	2
Enterobius vermicularis (% infected)	?	0	0	0	0	2
Unidentified eggs (?) (% infected)	0	0	0	0	0	2

* From M. Brown, et al., *Can. J. Public Health* 41: 508-12 (1950).
** Some multiple infections.

TABLE 2
Results of feeding plerocercoids of *Diphyllobothrium* spp. to humans and dogs

	Number of plerocercoids fed	Days until eggs seen	Days until purge (p) or autopsy (a)	Worms obtained
Diphyllobothrium dendriticum				
Caucasian No. 1	3	11	72? (p)	3*
(second feeding)	6	?	14? (p)	
Caucasian No. 1	8	None seen	not done	0
Caucasian No. 2	6	10	32 (p)	1
Dog No. 1	6	None seen	24 (a)	0
Dog No. 2	6	7	24 (a)	0
Diphyllobothrium sp. (smooth)				
Caucasian No. 3	6	None seen	Not done	0
Caucasian No. 4	2	None seen	Not done	0
Caucasian No. 5	3	None seen	Not done	0

* Not known if adult worms 14 or 72 days old.

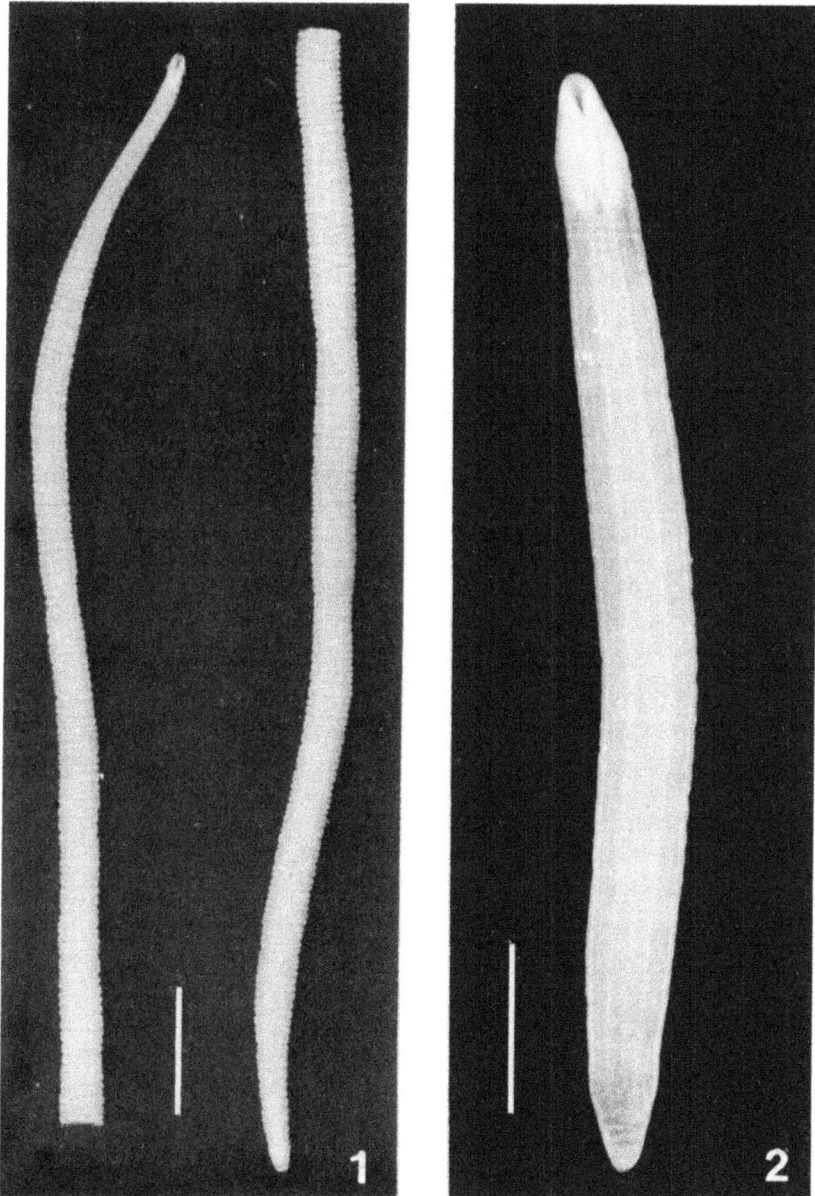

Figure 1   Plerocercoid of *Diphyllobothrium dendriticum*, anterior half on the left; notice distinct segmentation (scale = 5 mm)
Figure 2   Plerocercoid of *Diphyllobothrium* sp.; notice much smaller size, smooth outline of body, and lack of segmentation (scale = 1 mm)

within seven days, showed no parasites when autopsied 17
days later. The smaller plerocercoids did not establish
themselves in man (Table 2).

DISCUSSION

Changes in the incidence of parasites in 1970-71 compared
with 1949 (3) are presumably conservative estimates, since
in most instances the more recent data are based on single
samples. Pinworms (*E. vermicularis*) are down markedly, as
are head lice according to the nurses, although we did not
examine for them. Interestingly, the over-all incidence of
intestinal parasitism has not changed – nearly half the Eskimos still harbour one or more types of parasites – but the
relative incidence of various species of parasites has
changed. Protozoans have increased at least fourfold, while
worm infections have declined to a slightly smaller extent.
Giardia lamblia, a mild pathogen, is much more abundant
than formerly. The single infection with *Entamoeba histolytica* probably was acquired when this individual was receiving treatment for another condition in southern Canada.
Conceivably, *Dientamoeba fragilis* were overlooked in the
SIH preparations made in 1971.

The identity of the cestodes is intriguing. Towards the
end of the last collecting trip, an iodine-stained slide
dried by accident, and it was then discovered that at least
two types of eggs were present in the stools. One, with a
typical smooth shell, can be associated with *Diphyllobothrium* spp. of fresh-water origin (7). The other, with a
deeply pitted scrobiculate shell, is typically associated
with various diphyllobothrioid cestodes of marine origin
(7). Whether the latter were present in 1949 is unknown. A
single attempt to purge a patient passing scrobiculate eggs
was unsuccessful. Successfully infecting man and dog with
plerocercoids from Arctic char (Table 2) and producing non-
scrobiculate eggs (N = 350, range 48-72μ, $\bar{x}$ = 63.3μ)(8)
suggests that the smooth-shelled eggs of the same size
range obtained from the Eskimos are *Diphyllobothrium dendriticum*. This is almost certainly a zoonosis, maintained
elsewhere in the world by gulls. The species becomes patent in less than two weeks in man and is relatively small
and short-lived; in contrast, *D. latum* requires four weeks
or more to become patent, may live for several years, and
is quite large (8, 11). Since no eggs were found in the
stools in the spring, this further supports the assumption
that the smooth-shelled eggs found later in the summer are

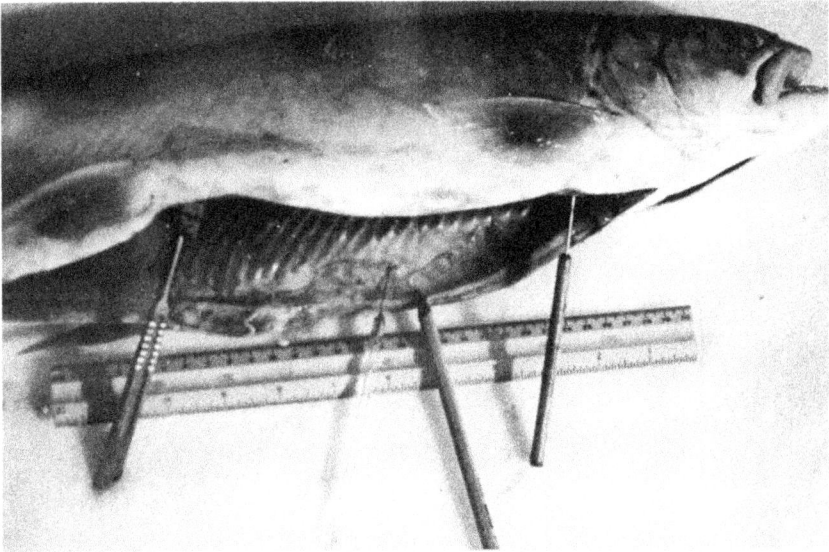

Figure 3 Photograph of eviscerated Arctic char with plerocercoids, indicated by pencil, encysted on lateral peritoneum.

the short-lived *D. dendriticum*. This species is probably of
little consequence to health.

The Eskimos continue to eat uncooked, unfrozen Arctic
char, although probably less than was formerly the case.
They eat only the flesh and occasionally a ripe roe. From
conversation and observation it is apparent that the Eskimos are unaware of the presence of the plerocercoids. How
are plerocercoids of *Diphyllobothrium* sp. ingested, since
they are relatively rare in the roe (<4 per cent) and do
not occur in the flesh, being mainly on and in other viscera (∼ 25 per cent) or attached to the lateral peritoneum
(∼ 10 per cent) (8)? Quite likely, a few plerocercoids from
roe are ingested, but probably most come from those
attached to the lateral peritoneum (Figure 3). Often the
fish are filleted and the flesh separated from the skeleton.
Most peritoneal plerocercoids are left behind with the
skeletal carcass. However, some remain on the peritoneum
of the abdominal wall when the fillet is removed from the
skeleton (Figure 4). Some people also have a habit of
using their teeth to comb off the flesh remaining on the
carcass after filleting. Quite likely, plerocercoids attached to the dorso-lateral peritoneum are ingested in

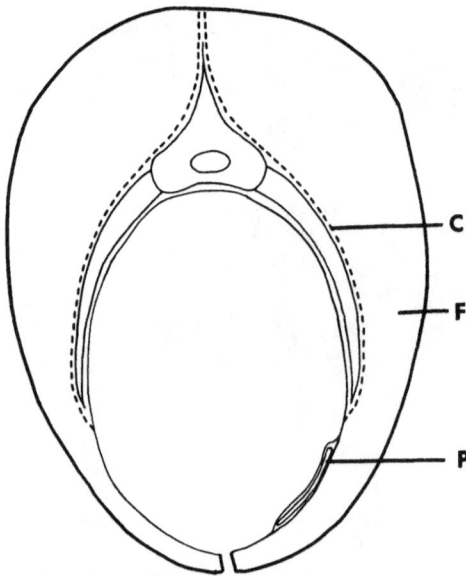

Figure 4   Diagram of cross-section of eviscerated Arctic
char illustrating how fillet is cut (C) leaving plerocercoid (P) on the ventral abdominal flap attached to the
fillet (F)

this way. Adequate energy for the cookstove in the village
and the portable camp stove permit more food to be cooked
now than in the past. This will probably result in a further decline of *Diphyllobothrium* sp. infections. However,
the complete elimination of uncooked fish from the diet
might do more harm than good, since it serves as an important source of vitamin C (14).

What the fluke (?) eggs are, and where they come from,
is a mystery. They are too small to be *Metorchis* sp. and
Crypotocotyle sp., as reported in other natives of North
America (5, 12). They may be of marine origin, since
freshwater molluscs are scarce or absent in this area (8).
It seems unlikely that the source of infection is the Arctic char, since metacercariae were not found in any of
the several hundred fish examined (8).

Unlike the worms, transmission of intestinal protozoans
is almost entirely via faecally contaminated food or drink
(10), or person-to-person contact (6). In 1949, Igloolik
had relatively few permanent residents, nomadic family
groups going to various camps for hunting and fishing, but

visiting Igloolik to trade. Now the reverse is true with
most families occupying permanent wooden housing. Only in
late spring do some families establish fishing and hunting
camps for relatively short periods. It is doubtful if
crowding within the dwellings is any greater now than in
the past. However, there is a mounting problem of handling
the human waste accumulating in plastic disposal bags. The
crowded conditions of permanent housing also give opportunity for faecal contamination of the permanent central water
tank. Small wonder that the incidence of protozoan parasites is high. A prime danger is the introduction and establishment of a severe pathogen such as *Entamoeba histolytica* in this environment. Such introduction becomes increasingly likely as these people have more contacts with
the south. For the foreseeable future, it is likely that
the incidence of protozoans will continue high, whereas
the incidence of helminths may decline even further.

ACKNOWLEDGMENTS

We thank the Eskimos, nurses, and other government personnel at Igloolik and Hall Beach who made this study possible. We are also grateful to the scientists who voluntari-
ly ingested plerocercoids, and to Mrs. Maria Staszak for
able technical assistance. The study was supported in part
by the International Biological Program Human Adaptability
project of Canada, and NRCC grant A-1969.

SUMMARY

A total of 352 faecal samples and 171 pinworm swabs were
examined from Eskimos at Hall Beach and Igloolik, NWT in
May-June and September-October 1970 and August 1971.
Approximately 50 per cent of all faeces (51.4 per cent of
105 samples from Hall Beach and 47.4 per cent of 247 from
Igloolik) contained one or more of the following: protozoa
- *Entamoeba coli, Entamoeba histolytica, Endolimax nana,
Giardia lamblia,* and other flagellates; helminth ova - *Di-
phyllobothrium* sp., diphyllobothrium-like, *Enterobius
vermicularis,* fluke (?), and unidentified. Eggs of pinworm,
E. vermicularis, occurred on 3.5 per cent of the swabs.
Protozoa occurred in both villages, but all helminth eggs
in faeces were from Igloolik. Eggs of *Diphyllobothrium* sp.
(spp.?) and other cestode and fluke eggs were present only
in the faecal samples obtained in August through October.
Feeding experiments with plerocercoids from Arctic char, a

staple food of these people, indicate that *Diphyllobothrium dendriticum,* but not *D. latum,* is one cestode involved. A comparison of the present data with a study conducted at Igloolik in 1949 by Brown et al. indicates that the incidence of protozoans is rising, whereas the helminths are declining. The implications of these changes are discussed.

REFERENCES

1. Arh, I., "Fish tapeworm in Eskimos in the Port Harrison area, Canada," Canad. J. Public Health, 51: 268-71 (1960)
2. Babbott, F.L. Jr., Frye, W.W., and Gordon, J.E., "Intestinal parasites of man in Arctic Greenland," Am. J. trop. Med. Hyg., 10: 185-90 (1961)
3. Brown, M., Green, J.E., Boag, T.J., Kuitunen-Ekbaum, E., "Parasitic infections in the Eskimos at Igloolik, N.W.T.," Canad. J. Public Health, 41: 508-12 (1950)
4. Burrows, R.B., "Prevalence of amebiasis in the United States and Canada," Am. J. trop. Med. Hyg., 10: 172-84 (1961)
5. Cameron, T.W.M., and Choquette, L.P.E., "Parasitological problems in high northern latitudes, with particular reference to Canada," The Polar Record, 11: 567-77 (1963)
6. Eaton, R.D.P., "Amebiasis in northern Saskatchewan: Epidemiological considerations," Canad. Med. Assoc. J., 99: 706-11 (1968)
7. Hilliard, D.K., "Studies on the helminth fauna of Alaska. LI. Observations on eggshell formation in some diphyllobothriid cestodes," Canad. J. Zool., 50: 585-92 (1972)
8. Jamieson, J.L., "Parasites of *Salvelinus alpinus* (Salmonidae) in the northern Foxe Basin, Northwest Territories, with emphasis on those of medical importance," M.Sc. Thesis, University of Toronto, Toronto, Canada, 1972
9. Laird, M. and Meerovitch, E., "Parasites from northern Canada. I. Entozoa of Chimo Eskimos," Canad. J. Zool., 39: 63-7 (1961)
10. Meerovitch, E., and Eaton, R.D.P., "Outbreak of amebiasis among Indians in northwestern Saskatchewan, Canada," Am. J. trop. Med. Hyg., 14: 719-23 (1965)
11. Rausch, R.L., and Hilliard, D.K., "Studies on the helminth fauna of Alaska. XLIX. The occurrence of Diphyllobothrium latum (Linnaeus, 1758) (Cestoda: Diphyllobothriidae) in Alaska, with notes on other species," Canad. J. Zool., 48: 1201-19 (1970)

12. Rausch, R.L., Scott, E.M., and Rausch, V.R., "Helminths
    in Eskimos in western Alaska, with particular reference
    to Diphyllobothrium infection and anaemia," Trans. Roy.
    Soc. Trop. Med. Hyg., 61: 351-7 (1967)
13. Ritchie, L.S., "An ether sedimentation technique for
    routine stool examinations," Bull. US Army M. Dept. 8:
    326 (1948)
14. Schaefer, O., "When the Eskimo comes to town," Nutrition
    Today, 6: 8-16 (1971)
15. Scholton, T.L., "An improved technique for the recovery
    of intestinal protozoa," J. Parasitol., 58: 633-4 (1972)
16. Wolfgang, R.W., "Indian and Eskimo diphyllobothriasis,"
    Canad. Med. Assoc. J., 70: 536-9 (1954)

Commentaries

"Hepatitis B in western Alaska," by D.H. Barrett, J.M.
Burks, B. McMahon, K.R. Berquist, and J.E. Maynard (Alaska
Activities, Bureau of Epidemiology-CDC, USPHS, USA). In
1973, epidemiological data and sera were collected from the
residents of two remote Alaskan villages located in an area
of high hepatitis incidence. A total of 418 sera were
analysed by radioimmunoassay for HBAg and HBAb. Epidemiological and serological correlations implied that most symptomatic hepatitis cases were caused by hepatitis B infection. The over-all infection rate of 54.8 per cent in the
two villages includes a 13.9 per cent prevalence of HBAb.
The high HBAb rate in adults, and a 46 per cent HBAg prevalence in the 0-10 year age group of one village, suggested
infection occurring in childhood. Families containing an
individual with HBAg had significantly higher infection
rates than those without antigen. Larger households, used
as an approximate index of crowded living conditions, had
higher rates of infection than smaller households. The preponderance of hepatitis cases noted in the fall suggested
mosquito-induced transmission of hepatitis B in June or
July, months of high mosquito populations. No evidence for
a genetic susceptibility to infection was found.

"Botulism Type B outbreak in an Alaskan Eskimo village," by
D.H. Barrett, M.S. Eisenberg, and J.M. Burks (Alaska Activities, Bureau of Epidemiology, CDC, USPHS USA). An outbreak
of Type B botulism involving nine persons occurred in
November 1973 in Chefornak, Alaska. Investigation revealed
principal involvement of one family and implicated home-
prepared dried smoked whitefish. Type B toxin was demonstrated in serum or faeces from five persons, and four
additional cases were diagnosed on the basis of appropriate
symptomatology. Toxin could not be found in any of the variety of native foods used by the family. Commercially prepared food had not been consumed near the the time of onset
of the disease. Clinical symptoms of diplopia, blurred
vision, dysphagia, and dry mouth and eyes were found in
every case. Most demonstrated mydriasis and evidence of
dysarthria. The outbreak was unusual because there were no
fatalities; many cases had been symptomatic for over two
weeks before being discovered. Only one patient had evidence
of respiratory impairment but responded well to treatment
with trivalent antitoxin (ABE). This is the first reported
outbreak of Type B botulism in Alaska. All prior cases investigated have been due to Type E, the only type yet found
in environmental samples collected in areas similar to
Chefornak. The importance of initial treatment with poly-
valent antitoxin prior to determination of the specific
type involved cannot be overemphasized.

"Epidemiology of brucellosis in the north," by G.F. Byelov,
A.N. Gudoshnik, and G.D. Netsky (Siberian Branch of the
Academy of Medical Sciences, Novosibirsk Medical Institute,
USSR). Clinically and with the help of laboratory tests 963
inhabitants of Taimir were studied (693 aborigines, 271
immigrants). In aborigines, brucellosis has been found only
in primary latent form. No chronic forms of the disease and
its consequences have been discovered in aborigines. In immigrants, brucellosis had primary latent, acute, and chronic
forms. It is supposed that a milder course of brucellosis
in aborigines is explained by mutual adaptation of organisms of the host and parasite. The infection of people
with brucellosis occurs mainly through the alimentary tract
and contact. The main reservoir of brucellosis infection on
Taimir are domestic and wild reindeer. A high incidence of
brucellosis among representatives of wild fauna (basic and
additional hosts) makes it possible to state that on Taimir
there are natural foci of brucellosis.

"Infectious hepatitis in Greenland, 1970-2," by Flemming
Mikkelsen (Deputy Chief Medical Officer in Greenland).
During the period 1970-2 an epidemic of infectious hepatitis (IH) occurred in Greenland. A total of 4,183 cases
were registered, corresponding to 8.9 per cent of the population, although this must be considerably less than the
number of cases which actually occurred, as cases from
settlements and outposts were not registered and a number
of cases from the towns did not come to the notice of the
health authorities. Seventeen deaths occurred during the
epidemic as a result of IH or where IH was an important contributory factor (fatality:0.4 per cent). The most frequent
cause of death was hepatic coma and the next haemorrhagic
diathesis. It did not prove possible to register all the
complications which occurred during the epidemic, but the
most frequent appear to have been hepatic failure and
haemorrhage. The age distribution is of special interest.
Only a few cases were described in children below the age
of one year and in adults over the age of 45 years. The
majority of cases occurred in the age-group from 1 to 14
years, corresponding to 63.8 per cent of notified cases.
The previous epidemic of IH occurred in west Greenland in
1947, and judging from the age distribution of the most
recent epidemic, the previous epidemic appears to have resulted in massive immunity in the population. Crowded
housing and the prevailing poor hygiene were conditions of
considerable importance for the spread of the epidemic,
this being described throughout as a contact epidemic.

"Problem of zooanthroponoses in the arctic area of Siberia,"
by G.I. Netsky (Omsk Institute of Natural Foci Infections
of the Ministry of Health of RSFSR, Siberian Branch of the
Academy of Medical Sciences of USSR, USSR). The mechanism
of adaptation is the principal basis of geographic pathology in the arctic area (V.P. Kaznacheyev). The mechanism of
adaptation is studied on two levels: the evolution of foci
and the interadaptation of man with the agents of zooanthroponoses in arctic conditions. These two aspects supplement
each other. The foci of zooanthroponoses in contemporary
arctic Siberia are a relic of foci that existed there at
the commencement of the posglacial period, when the tundra
was covered with forests. This is the most probable basis
for preservation of foci of zooanthroponoses and their
northward limits of spread seen today. Assumption of the
activity of agents of tick-borne encephalitis, rabies,
Asian tick-borne rickettsiosis, Q-rickettsiosis, leptospi-

rosis, tularaemia, and brucellosis in the arctic area of
Siberia has been confirmed during mass inspection of the
population, and of northern deer and lemmings. The activity
of the West Nile virus, probably connected with the mass
concentration of migrating birds, has also been ascertained.
The circumpolar distribution of some zooanthroponoses serves
as the basis for doing a comparative and cooperative study
of the structure, spread, and evolution of their foci in
different countries.

"Streptococcal surveillance and control in remote arctic
populations," by T.R. Bender, J.S. Edelen, and J.M. Burks
(Alaska Activities, Bureau of Epidemiology-CDC, USPHS, USA).
Rheumatic heart disease is a major cause of morbidity among
Alaskan natives. Because of this, a surveillance program to
detect streptococcal pharyngitis and non-suppurative se-
quellae has been operative in nine remote Alaskan Eskimo
villages since September 1971. The village health aide cultured a 25 per cent sample of school-children in each village each week, such that each child received a throat culture once a month. In addition, persons of any age with
symptomatic pharyngitis were cultured. Persons with cultures positive for group A streptococci were treated regardless of symptoms. Despite an average delay of 10 days
between culturing and treatment, group A streptococcal
prevalence was reduced from 27 to 10 per cent during the
first study year, and to 5 per cent at the end of the
second study year. In contrast, point prevalence in nine
matched control villages averaged 19 per cent. No cases of
acute rheumatic fever were detected in any of the study
villages. A streptococcal surveillance program of this
type can result in a significant decrease in group A streptococcal prevalence, even if mail-in procedures necessitate
considerable delay. Such a program is a feasible method of
streptococcal control in high-risk areas.

"Rheumatic fever and rheumatic heart disease among Alaskan
natives, 1964-73," by J.S. Edelen, J.M. Burks, D.H. Barrett,
and P. Steer (Alaska Activities, Bureau of Epidemiology-CDC,
USPHS, USA). Acute rheumatic fever (ARF) and rheumatic
heart disease (RHD) are major health problems among Alaska
natives. We have reviewed the medical records of all Alaska
natives who acquired ARF from FY 1964 through FY 1973, and
all with the diagnosis of RHD. The average annual incidence

of ARF among children aged 5-19 was 44 cases per 100,000
population. There was considerable variation within the
state: the Yukon-Kuskokwim delta area had an incident rate
of 82, whereas the incidence in the North Slope area was
only 16. Carditis was present in 70 per cent of the cases.
RHD prevalence in 1973 was 605 cases per 100,000 population
of all ages. For the 5-19 year age group, RHD prevalence
was 377 per 100,000. Regional variations within the state
again showed highest rates in the Yukon-Kuskokwim delta,
and lowest prevalence in the far north. Mitral stenosis
was diagnosed at a young age in an unusually high percentage of patients, suggesting that carditis is severe in
this population. Vigorous efforts to control group A streptococcal infections are indicated in those areas where the
incidence of rheumatic fever is high.

PULMONARY FUNCTION AND CHEST DISEASES

Pulmonary function of Canadian Eskimos

A. RODE and R.J. SHEPHARD

Despite recent advances in the delivery of health care to
the northern communities, respiratory adenovirus infections
are still prevalent, and many older Eskimos show late sequelae of pulmonary tuberculosis. There is thus a continuing need to survey respiratory health. In small and isolated settlements, a portable spirometer might provide a more
practical diagnostic tool than mass radiography, given (1)
appropriate normal standards for the population and (2)
demonstration of functional loss with the disease of concern.

Canadian Eskimos are currently undergoing rapid acculturation to White patterns of living. There is thus scientific interest in documenting their current status, comparing data with previous surveys, and developing a firm
baseline against which subsequent functional changes can
be charted. It is also pertinent to explore the apparent
paradox that couples a high level of cardiorespiratory fitness with almost universal cigarette consumption and widely prevalent respiratory disease.

Beaudry (2) conducted the only previous systematic study
of respiratory function in Canadian Eskimos. He found poor
0.75 second forced expiratory volume relative to normal
White standards. More recently, Rennie et al. (6) reported
above normal values for static and dynamic lung volumes of
Alaskan Eskimos. The present paper reports current static
and dynamic lung volumes, pulmonary diffusing capacity,
and smoking habits of the eastern Arctic Eskimo community
of Igloolik.

POPULATION SAMPLING

Respiratory function tests were conducted on 196 villagers
(77 per cent of the boys and 65 per cent of the girls aged
11 to 19, 67 per cent of the men and 56 per cent of the women aged 20 to 39, and 41 per cent of the men and 48 per
cent of the women over the age of 40). Some of those not
tested were very active hunters and thus absent from the
village; others were unco-operative and some were affected
by disease of various types. The sample thus should be
reasonably representative of the average Eskimo living in
this particular settlement.

METHODOLOGY

The one-second forced expiratory volume ($FEV_{1.0}$) and the
forced vital capacity (FVC) were measured with a 13.5 litre
Stead-Wells spirometer fitted with a lightweight bell.
Seated subjects were allowed two practice attempts followed
by three definitive trials. Results reported are the mean
of three "good" records. The total lung capacity (TLC) was
estimated by the radiographic technique of Pratt and Klugh
(5), and a "steady state" procedure was used to determine
pulmonary diffusing capacity at rest and during bicycle
ergometer exercise.

STATIC AND DYNAMIC LUNG VOLUMES

Adults were subdivided into a healthy group and a group
with a history of previous chest disease, mainly TB. In
healthy men, the FVC was similar at ages 17-19 and 20-29,
but thereafter decreased with age (Table 1). In healthy
women, volumes diminished continuously from age 16, and in
both sexes the $FEV_{1.0}$ decreased throughout the age range
tabulated.

Males averaged 12 per cent higher FVC than predicted by
the formula of Cotes (3) and 8 per cent higher than predicted by the formula of Anderson et al. (1); excluding subjects with a history of previous chest disease, these discrepancies increased to 13 and 9 per cent respectively.
Discrepancies for the women amounted to 17 and 21 per cent,
or after exclusion of disease, 19 and 22 per cent respectively.

Forced expiratory volumes (Table 2) were close to predicted values in the men, where in the women the $FEV_{1.0}$ was

TABLE 1

Lung volumes of healthy Igloolik Eskimos (patients with history of chest disease excluded)

Age (yr)	Male			Female		
	N	$FEV_{1.0}$ (1 BTPS)	FVC (1 BTPS)	N	$FEV_{1.0}$ (1 BTPS)	FVC (1 BTPS)
16/17-19	9	4.28	5.15	6	3.47	4.06
20-29	26	4.01	5.14	16	3.00	3.79
30-39	20	3.74	4.95	11	2.75	3.49
40-49	6	3.37	4.53	3	2.19	3.01
50-59	3	3.42	4.40	2	2.65	3.26

TABLE 2

A comparison of measured $FEV_{1.0}$ (1 BTPS) with estimate based on age and height (1)

Age (yr)	Men			Women		
	Measured	Measured/Estimated	(%)	Measured	Measured/Estimated	(%)
16/17-19	4.26	100.6		3.28	116.5	
20-29	4.03	99.2		3.00	111.7	
30-39	3.68	98.6		2.70	112.9	
40-49	3.26	98.4		2.31	104.1	
50-59	3.41	115.5		2.34	117.8	

greater than anticipated. After exclusion of subjects with a history of chest disease, male values were still no more than 101 per cent of predictions compared with 115 per cent in the women.

The ratio of $FEV_{1.0}$ was thus somewhat below anticipated results, being essentially similar in both healthy subjects and those with a history of chest disease.

Multiple regression equations for the prediction to static and dynamic lung volumes of the Eskimo (Table 3) have a precision much as in the White population, the standard deviations for the first four equations being 0.72, 0.44, 0.68, and 0.42 litre BTPS respectively. As in previous studies, the data for children were best satisfied by log/log relationships. After allowance for differences of standing height, the present figures for static and dynamic lung volumes of Eskimo children showed no sex differences. This agrees with the data of Engström et al. (4), but is in contrast with most other studies of White children.

TABLE 3
Equations for the prediction of static and dynamic lung volumes
of Igloolik Eskimos

Men
$$FEV_{1.0} = 0.0584(H,cm, \pm 0.0141) -0.0193(A,yr, \pm 0.0081) - 5.28$$
$$FVC = 0.0788(H,cm, \pm 0.0148) -0.0083(A,yr, \pm 0.0085) - 7.90$$
Women
$$FEV_{1.0} = 0.0075(H,cm, \pm 0.0027) -0.0268(A,yr, \pm 0.0060) + 2.50$$
$$FVC = 0.0056(H,cm, \pm 0.0028) -0.0275(A,yr, \pm 0.0063) + 3.57$$
Boys
$$FEV_{1.0} = 1.76 \times 10^{-7} \times H^{3.31}$$
$$FVC = 2.55 \times 10^{-7} \times H^{3.28}$$
Girls
$$FEV_{1.0} = 1.07 \times 10^{-5} \times H^{2.50}$$
$$FVC = 9.72 \times 10^{-7} \times H^{3.01}$$

Absolute volumes were 0.2 to 0.4 litre in excess of reported values for preadolescent White children, the discrepancy increasing with age (Table 3). The height expo-
nent of the log/log plot was greater than 3 for the Eskimo
children, but only around 2.8 in the White. Whether the Eskimo children show a greater spurt of thoracic strength at
puberty or the White postadolescent children are more reluctant to develop maximum thoracic force remains to be
determined.

PULMONARY DIFFUSING CAPACITY

There were no statistically significant differences of pulmonary diffusing capacity between subjects with and those
without a history of respiratory disease (Table 4).

TABLE 4
Pulmonary diffusing capacity of Igloolik Eskimos ($D_{L,CO}$ ml STPD/
min/mm Hg)

	Men			Women		
Age	N	Resting D_L	Exercise D_L	N	Resting D_L	Exercise D_L
14-16	11	19.0	34.9	–	–	–
16/17-19	4	19.5	43.8	6	17.7	28.8
20-29	15	21.1	43.2	18	15.3	29.9
30-39	17	14.6	37.8	17	11.4	23.2
40-49	9	14.0	33.6	6	8.8	21.4
50-59	5	10.9	30.5	5	9.3	21.1

Between the third and sixth decades, the resting $D_{L,CO}$ decreased by 48 per cent in the men and 39 per cent in the women, a finding comparable with the 33 per cent decrease of resting single-breath $D_{L,CO}$ reported by Cotes.

The men were heavier smokers than the women, and showed a significant decline in cigarette consumption between the third and the sixth decade, changes of reported consumption being confirmed by differences of blood carboxyhaemoglobin levels. The half-times of carbon monoxide elimination, as estimated from the reported time since the last cigarette, were 2.7 and 1.4 hours for men and women respectively, compared with 3.7 and 2.5 hours in Toronto subjects (7). Nonsmokers were relatively few, and their carboxyhaemoglobin levels were lower than in Toronto.

DISCUSSION

Our figures for Igloolik confirm that the majority of adult Eskimos smoke some cigarettes, although personal estimates of consumption and the objective evidence of blood carboxyhaemoglobin hardly support previous reports of "intense" smoking. Nor is respiratory disease as rampant as some anecdotal reports would suggest. The most common finding in our Igloolik subjects was a history of tuberculous disease. Minor hilar calcifications and primary foci had little impact upon lung fuction, but secondary tuberculosis was sometimes associated with parallel impairment of $FEV_{1.0}$ and FVC.

Exposure to the soot of burning seal oil lamps is now uncommon and the Eskimo generally encounters less air polution than the white man. Nevertheless, he is exposed to the combustion products of oil-fired furnaces and stoves, the tobacco smoke of crowded public facilities, and the exhaust fumes of motorized toboggans. Eskimos who do not smoke thus show blood carboxyhaemoglobin figures above the theoretical 0.4-0.5 per cent for a pollution free environment.

Body build has previously been blamed for both small and large lung volumes; certainly, in view of the unusual body build, any predictions that are used should be based on Eskimo subjects. Nevertheless, the adult size of the Igloolik Eskimos is increasing rapidly, and within a few decades White standards may be relevant.

The Igloolik Eskimo has a high level of cardiorespiratory fitness and this may contribute to his large lung volumes. However, we have not found any marked differences

in $FEV_{1.0}$ and FVC between active hunters and men working in
the settlement.

How may we resolve the apparent discrepancy between our
findings and the data of Beaudry? The most likely explanation seems that the health and the nutritional status of
the Eskimo has improved to the point where advantages conferred by physical activity, body build, low levels of air
pollution, and a moderate cigarette habit are now apparent.
Other factors could include the lapse of five years and the
difference in the prevalence of respiratory disease between
different areas of the Arctic.

With regard to the spirometric screening of respiratory
health, this approach apparently lacks sensitivity, and in
many cases of early pulmonary disease the $FEV_{1.0}$ and the
FVC show no significant deterioration. It is thus likely
that communities such as Igloolik will continue to place
greater reliance upon periodic visits by a radiography
team.

The functional significance of respiratory volumes is
assessed too rarely. Large changes of static and dynamic
volumes must occur before there is a significant reduction
of maximum oxygen intake. This is because the transport of
oxygen from the atmosphere to the working muscles depends
more upon circulatory than upon respiratory function, and
the normal shape of the oxygen dissociation curve can compensate for a substantial decrease of alveolar oxygen pressure. Here we see the main explanation of our initially
formulated paradox - the coupling of cardiorespiratory
fitness with moderate to substantial cigarette consumption
and a high incidence of respiratory disease.

SUMMARY

Multiple regression equations for predicting the lung function of the Canadian Eskimo were developed through tests
conducted on 139 adults and 57 children living in Igloolik.
Both $FEV_{1.0}$ and FVC of healthy Eskimos exceeded predicted
values for White communities, but the ratio $FEV_{1.0}$/FVC per
cent was somewhat subnormal. The residual volume and total
lung capacity, estimated radiographically, were as predicted for White subjects. The pulmonary diffusing capacity
(steady state/assumed dead space technique) was normal
both at rest and at a given exercise load; however, because of a high VO_2 (max), the estimated maximum diffusing
capacity was also large. Possible explanations of the large
$FEV_{1.0}$ and FVC include a high level of habitual activity,

some unusual features of body build, a relatively low level
of air pollution, a moderate and recently acquired cigarette habit, and recent improvements in general health and
nutritional status. A history of chest disease leads to the
anticipated changes in static and dynamic lung volumes,
residual volume, and pulmonary diffusing capacity. However,
because of the form of the oxygen dissociation curve, the
impact on maximum oxygen intake is usually slight.

REFERENCES

1. Anderson, T.W., Brown, J.R., Hall, J.W., and Shephard,
   R.J., "The limitations of linear regressions for the
   prediction of vital capacity and forced expiratory volume," Respiration, 25: 140-58 (1968)
2. Beaudry, P.H., "Pulmonary function of the Canadian Eastern Arctic Eskimo," Arch. environ. Hlth., 17: 524-8
   (1968)
3. Cotes, J.E., Lung function. Assessment and application
   in medicine (Oxford: Blackwell Scientific Publications,
   1965)
4. Engström, I., Karlberg, P., and Kraepelien, S., "Respiratory studies in children. Lung volumes in healthy
   children 6-14 years of age," Acta. Paediat. (Uppsala)
   45: 277-94 (1956)
5. Pratt, C.P., and Klugh, G.S., "A method for the determination of total lung capacity from posterior-anterior
   and lateral chest roentgenograms," Am. Rev. resp. Dis.,
   96: 548-52 (1967)
6. Rennie, D.W., di Prampero, P.E., Fitts, R.W., and Sinclair, L., "Physical fitness and respiratory function of
   Eskimos of Wainwright, Alaska," Arctic Anthropol., 7:
   73-82 (1970)
7. Rode, A., "Some factors influencing the fitness of a
   small Eskimo community," Ph.D. Thesis, University of
   Toronto, 1972

Chronic lung disease and cardiovascular consequences in Iglooligmiut

J.A. HILDES, O. SCHAEFER, JUDITH E. SAYED,
E.J. FITZGERALD, and E.A. KOCH

It appears that many Canadian Eskimos, particularly of middle and older age, suffer from non-tuberculous chronic lung disease characterized by productive cough, wheezing, and voluminous lungs. From an eastern Arctic survey in 1967 Beaudry (1) reported extensive impairment of pulmonary function, and in 1971 Schaefer (5) indicated that the chronic lung condition was associated with certain electro-cardiographic (ECG) patterns.

These observations prompted us to examine how closely abnormalities of lung function correlated with ECG changes in the Eskimos of the Northern Foxe Basin in the central Canadian Arctic. This population was the subject of multidisciplinary studies carried out as an International Biological Program project. As part of the medical aspects of the study, most of the population had a standardized medical examination and a chest radiograph. Ventilatory tests and ECG examinations were limited to 66 adults; those omitted tended to be patients without signs or symptoms*.

METHODS

Chest radiographs were taken at a standard distance in the postero-anterior and lateral planes on all members of the population available as part of the regular annual survey for tuberculosis control. In addition to reading these films for evidence of tuberculous infection, 315 chest X-rays of adults were read independently by two experienced

---

* A more complete series of lung function tests using laboratory spirometers with lightweight bells was carried out by the physiology team (see page 320).

observers and graded for the presence and severity of chronic obstructive lung disease (COLD). Pulmonary artery size
was measured on 304 of the adult chest radiographs, using
the method of Chang (2), which records the diameter of the
descending branch of the right pulmonary artery. Ventilatory function was assessed using a McKesson portable bellows spirometer; 161 tracings were available for analysis.
From the tracing, the one and six second forced expiratory
volumes were measured and the maximal mid-expiratory flow
rates calculated. ECG - standard 12 lead tracings were taken with a portable machine. Additional right anterior chest
leads and, when indicated, posterior chest leads were also
recorded. ECG tracings were available from 77 males and 38
females.

RESULTS AND DISCUSSION

More than a quarter of the adults over 50 years of age had
severe changes of COLD as judged from the chest radiographs, but the young men and women aged 20 to 29 were mostly reported as normal.

A summary of the ventilatory function data, normalized
for height, age, and sex (3), is shown in Table 1. FEV_1 for
the men had a mean value that was only 81 per cent of the
predicted level, but the vital capacity was close to it.
The maximum mid-expiratory flow rates were much below that
predicted - this may be related partly to the type of
equipment used, but it does not prevent internal comparisons; thus the data show a marked decline with age in men.

The ECG abnormalities found were similar to those previously reported by Schaefer (5), namely complete and incomplete right bundle branch block, clockwise rotation of

TABLE 1
McKesson-Scott bellow spirometer readings for a group of
66 Eskimos living in the Foxe basin (% of predicted for
age and height)

	Males (54)		Females (12)	
	Mean	SD	Mean	SD
FEV $_{1.0}$	81.4	16.6	70.0	11.7
VC	97.9	14.1	82.3	12.0
FEV $_{1.0}$/VC	72.0	9.1	73.0	8.4
MMF	48.6	22.0	35.9	15.5

TABLE 2
Diameter of right pulmonary artery (mm) as measured from
chest radiographs

Age group	Males			Females		
	Mean	SD	n	Mean	SD	n
20-29	16.1	1.4	90	14.4	1.3	55
30-39	17.3	1.3	50	15.1	1.1	35
40-49	18.2	1.3	25	15.9	1.7	14
50+	19.4	2.0	20	15.6	1.2	15

the heart, and what Schaefer has described as the "pseudo-infarction" pattern.

The pulmonary artery diameters are summarized in Table 2. There is a progressive increase with age in both males and females and particularly in the older age groups the mean diameters are abnormally high as compared with Chang's findings (normal males 9-16 mm, females 9-15 mm).

The two main features of the ECG, the electrical axis of the heart and the presence and degree of RBBB were treated as dependent variables in a multivariate analysis in which chest X-ray grading, pulmonary artery size, ventilatory function, and age were independent variables. Analyses were carried out separately for 54 men and 12 women. Whether considered separately or together, the independent variables failed to be useful predictors of the ECG. Age in years showed some relationship to ECG abnormalities, and the various ventilatory functions correlated fairly well with each other, but otherwise the results of the statistical analysis were negative. This raises the question of whether the hypothesis relating COLD to the cardiovascular changes is indeed correct or whether the ECG changes are normal variants in Eskimos. There are striking differences (Table 3) between the Eskimo ECG abnormalities and those

TABLE 3
Resting ECG abnormalities in 115 adult Eskimos compared with findings at Tecumseh (4), as a percentage

	Males		Females	
	Caucasian	Eskimos	Caucasian	Eskimos
Ischaemic changes	28.3	7.7	25.6	2.6
LBBB	0.2	0.0	0.4	0.0
RBBB	2.6	30.0	0.9	13.0

found among an adult population in Michigan (4). The US urban population had predominantly ischaemic ECG changes and
a low percentage of RBBB, whereas the opposite pertains in
the Eskimos. An additional fact revealed from the adult
chest radiographs is that aortic calcification was visible
in only 9 subjects and in 7 of these it was recorded as
faint. This also is in striking contrast to what would be
expected in a Caucasian urban population.

In spite of the failure to demonstrate statistically
that the ECG abnormalities of Eskimos can be predicted from
the chest X-ray, the pulmonary artery diameter, and ventilatory functions, the striking changes in these indices of
chronic pulmonary disease are most likely linked to the
prevalent ECG abnormalities since these originate from the
right side of the heart in contradistinction to the ischaemic type changes seen in a Caucasian population.

ACKNOWLEDGMENTS

This study was carried out with funds from the Canadian
Committee for the International Biological Program. The
help of Dr T.E. Cuddy with the ECG interpretations is
gratefully acknowledged.

SUMMARY

A review of chest X-rays of adult Eskimos living in the
Northern Foxe Basin showed that more than a quarter of subjects over 50 years had changes suggestive of chronic obstructive lung disease. The diameter of the descending
branch of the right pulmonary artery was also abnormally
increased in older males and females. Ventilatory function
as measured with a McKesson-Scott bellows spirometer was
decreased and the electrocardiogram showed a preponderance
of changes arising from the right side of the heart. The
electrocardiographic abnormalities are believed secondary
to chronic obstructive lung disease, although multivariate
analysis failed to confirm that the X-ray and pulmonary
function tests were good predictors of the electrocardiographic changes.

REFERENCES

1. Beaudry, P.H., "Pulmonary function survey of the Canadian Eastern Arctic Eskimo, Arch. environ. Health, 17:
   524-8 (1968)

2. Chang, C.H., "The normal roentgenographic measurement of the right descending pulmonary artery in 1085 cases," Am. J. Roentgen., 87: 828-935 (1962)
3. Cherniack, R.M., and Raber, M.B., "Normal standards for ventilatory function using an automated wedge spirometer," Am. Rev. resp. Dis., 106: 38-46 (1972)
4. Ostrander, L.D., Brandt, R.L., Kjelsberg, M.O., and Epstein, F.H., "Electrocardiographic findings among the adult population of a total natural community, Tecumseh, Michigan," Circulation, 31: 888-97 (1965)
5. Schaefer, O., "Right bundle branch block and pseudo-infarction ECG patterns in Eskimo men," Paper presented at second International Symposium on Circumpolar Health, Oulu, Finland, 1971

Tuberculosis in Finnish Lapland

I.P. PALVA and B. FINELL

Since the eighteenth century, Ostrobotnia and Lapland have been the most unfavourable parts of Finland with respect to morbidity and mortality from tuberculosis. However, in 1951 a tuberculosis hospital was opened for Lapland; at the same time out-patient clinics were placed under the auspices of the same administration, the association of local authorities. During the past 20 years, the statistics for tuberculosis have improved substantially in the whole of Finland but especially in Lapland.

MORBIDITY

The number of new cases of tuberculosis in Lapland during 1953 was 709, 403 per 100,000 inhabitants, compared with 211 per 100,000 for the whole of Finland. A steady improvement has subsequently taken place, the number of new cases being 275 per 100,000 in 1955, 225 in 1960, 129 in 1965, 86 in 1970, and 70 in 1972; currently, the rate is comparable with that of Finland as a whole (Table 1).

TABLE 1
New cases of pulmonary tuberculosis in the whole of Finland and
in Lapland, the number of radiographic examinations carried out
in Lapland, and the population of Lapland

Variable	1953	1955	1960	1965	1970
New cases in Finland (per 100,000)	212	160	137	108	80
New cases in Lapland (per 100,000)	403	275	225	129	86
Radiographic examinations (thousands)	34	37	49	51	56
Population of Lapland (thousands)	176	183	204	219	215

Among children under 15 years of age, the improvement
has been even more marked: in the 1960s, 20 to 30 new cases
of tuberculosis were detected among Lapp children every
year, but in 1970-72 the number dropped to 4 or 5.

MORTALITY

Although tuberculosis morbidity in Lapland has been very
unfavourable compared with that for the rest of Finland,
there is no difference in the average mortality. There are
areas of Finland with a much higher tuberculosis mortality
than Lapland, and the average statistics for the whole
country are at the same level as figures for Lapland. The
mortality rate for tuberculosis in Finland has declined
from 290 per 100,000 inhabitants in 1930 to 93 in 1950, 26
in 1960, and 8 in 1970.

SEARCH FOR NEW CASES

A population of some 200,000 Lapps is served by tuberculosis out-patient clinics arranging 10,000 to 15,000 consultations every year. In addition, mass radiographic examinations are performed to detect new cases (Table 1); currently, about 25 per cent of the population is screened annually.

BCG VACCINATION

During the past 25 years, most children in Finland have received BCG vaccination. Nowadays, about 90 per cent of
children are vaccinated during their first year of life.
Hence, almost the entire population of Finland under 30

years of age is BCG vaccinated. Vaccination is the exception among people over 45 years, but practically all of this group have been exposed to tuberculous infection in their youth.

PROPHYLACTIC THERAPY

Prophylactic therapy with antituberculous drugs has been administered only in selected and rather rare cases. In Lapland, 405 patients received prophylactic antituberculosis therapy in 1972.

RESOURCES: TUBERCULOSIS HOSPITALS

The tuberculosis hospital at Muurola was opened with 355 beds in 1951 and was enlarged to 459 beds in 1956. Admissions for tuberculosis reached their peak, 734 cases, in 1966, while the highest number of hospital days, 176,000, had already occurred in 1961. The average time of hospitalization was practically a year (352 days) in 1957, 258 days in 1961, 150 in 1966, and 66 in 1972. Part of Muurola hospital was taken over for other patients in 1968, 366 beds remaining for tuberculosis.

MANPOWER AND FINANCES

In 1972, the medical staff consisted of 3 full-time physicians and 3 part-time consultants, 4 vacancies being unfilled. The nursing staff comprised 90 hospital nurses and 4 working in out-patient clinics. The annual operating costs of the tuberculosis program in Lapland were 1.0 mill. Fmk in 1952, 3.3 mill. in 1962, and 6.2 mill. in 1972.

CONCLUSION

An intensive preventive and therapeutic program has reduced the incidence of tuberculosis in Lapland to the same rather favourable level found in Finland as a whole. The annual number of new cases has decreased to a fifth of that seen 20 years ago.

SUMMARY

In 1953, 403 new cases of pulmonary tuberculosis were detected per 100,000 inhabitants in Finnish Lapland, about twice the average for the whole country. During recent years, the situation has improved, and at present some 70 new cases of tuberculosis per 100,000 inhabitants are detected both in Lapland and in the country as a whole. In spite of a high morbidity with respect to tuberculosis, mortality due to it has been at the same level in Lapland as in other parts of Finland. The total mortality from tuberculosis in Finland has declined from 290 per 100,000 inhabitants in 1930 to 93 in 1950 and 8 in 1970. An intensive preventive and therapeutic program has brought Lapland to the same level of tuberculosis as Finland as a whole, the number of new cases having decreased by as much as 80 per cent during the last 20 years.

REFERENCE

1. Annual reports of Muurola Hospital and the Finnish Anti-Tuberculosis Association 1951-72

The relevance of studies of tuberculosis in Eskimos to antituberculous program planning

S. GRZYBOWSKI and K. STYBLO

Studies of tuberculosis among the Eskimo populations of three countries (Greenland, Alaska, and Canada) have certain general implications for tuberculosis control. In this presentation, a comparison has been made of the problem in these three populations, and the likely impact of the different control programs has been discussed.

THE SITUATION BEFORE THE INTRODUCTION OF COMPREHENSIVE ANTITUBERCULOUS PROGRAMS

Figure 1 is taken from a study on tuberculosis in the native population of Alaska in the late 1920s (1). At that time, mortality was extremely high - the over-all rate being 655 per 100,000 population. Almost exactly the same tuberculosis mortality rate, 653 per 100,000, was recorded in Alaskan natives in 1950 (5); thus there was no decline

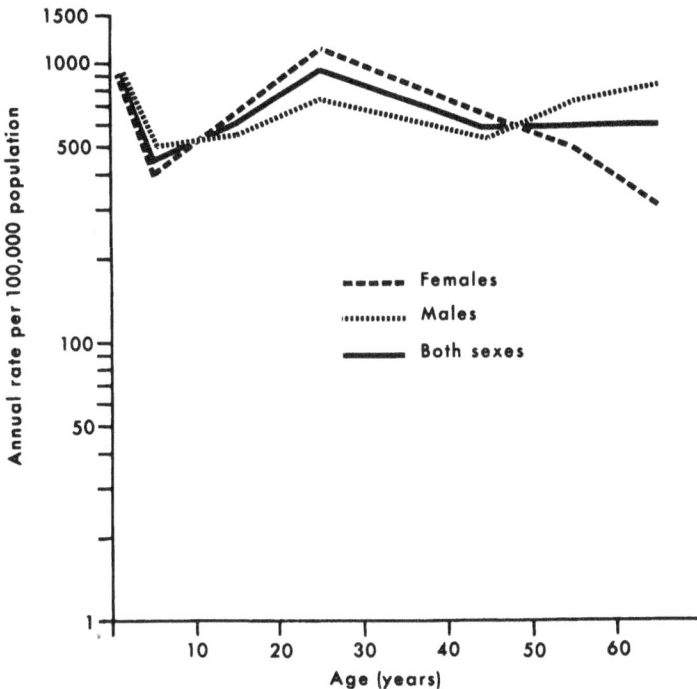

Figure 1   Mortality from tuberculosis, classified by age and sex, for Indian and Eskimo population of Alaska, 1926-30

between 1930 and 1950. The mortality rate in the 1920s did not differ substantially in different age groups. The lowest mortality was seen in females between 1 and 9 years of age, where the rate was 382 per 100,000, and the highest was 1,134 in women aged 20 to 29 years. When the present authors started their study, they also were struck by the fact that tuberculosis seemed almost equally frequent in all age groups. It was impossible to delineate the specific high and low risk groups so apparent among white North Americans.

Information on morbidity before the start of comprehensive control programs is scanty. Jensen (4) surveyed 3,400 inhabitants of the Julianehab District of Greenland and showed that 7 per cent of the population suffered from bacillary pulmonary tuberculosis. Johnson (5) found that the incidence of active tuberculosis in Alaska during the early 1950s was between 1.5 and 1.8 per cent. Wherrett (7) estimated the annual incidence rate in the Baffin Zone of the Northwest Territories was 2.9 per cent during the period 1955 to 1957.

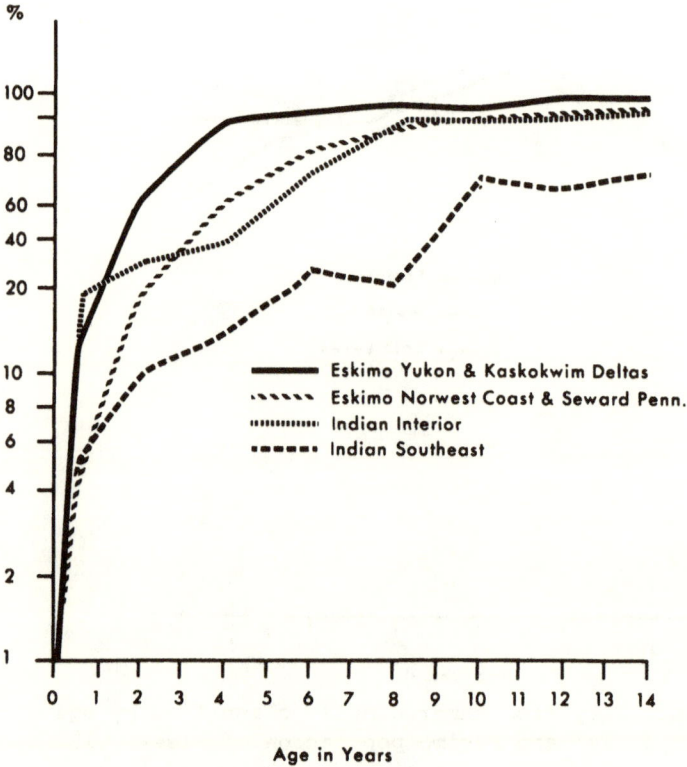

Figure 2   Tuberculin sensitivity in Eskimo and Indian
children of Alaska, 1948-51

In view of this high morbidity it is not surprising that
infection rates among native children were extremely high.
Figure 2 shows age-classified tuberculin sensitivity data
for Alaskan Eskimo and Indian children (2, 6). During the
1949-51 period, well over 80 per cent of Eskimo children
were infected by the age of five years; this implies an
annual infection rate of 25 per cent, the highest ever recorded in the world.

Thus, prior to the institution of comprehensive antituberculous programs, tuberculosis was an extremely serious
problem among Eskimos in all three countries - Greenland,
Alaska, and Canada.

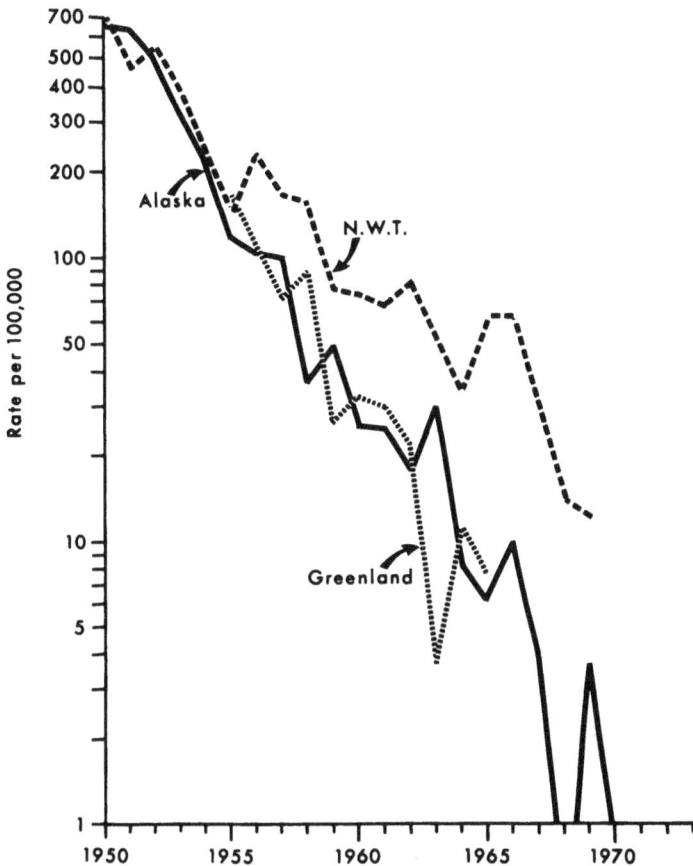

Figure 3 Tuberculosis death rates in arctic natives (Alaska, Greenland, and the Northwest Territories)

ANTITUBERCULOUS PROGRAMS AND THEIR IMPACT

In Greenland, a comprehensive program was started around 1950; the Alaskan program followed about five years later, while the one in Canada only became fully operational in the early 1960s. In all three countries, great emphasis was placed on the early diagnosis of cases of tuberculosis and their removal for treatment. Other aspects of the programs differed from country to country. Greenland emphasized BCG vaccination, while in Alaska BCG vaccination was used less frequently; very extensive chemoprophylaxis was used instead. In the Canadian program both BCG and chemoprophylaxis

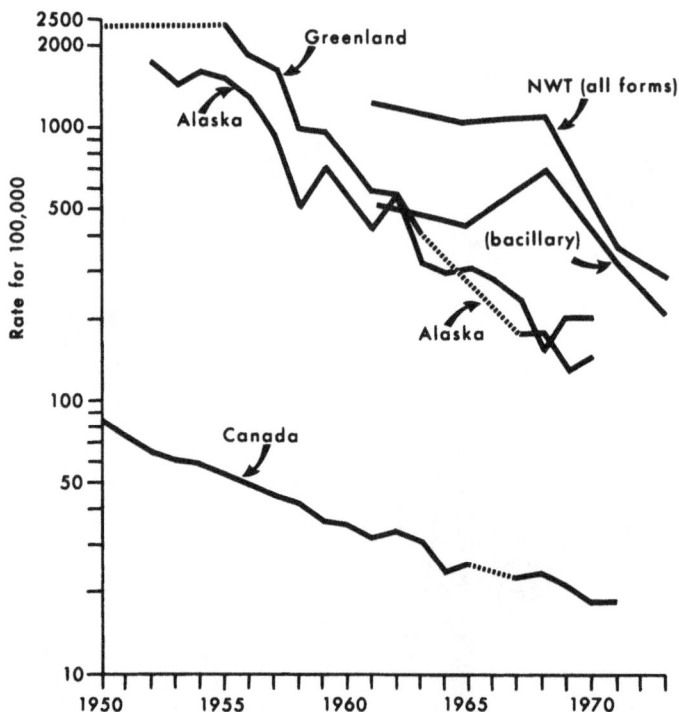

Figure 4   Incidence of tuberculosis in arctic natives
(Greenland, Alaska, Northwest Territories) and in Canada as
a whole

were used. Establishment of these programs was followed
by a decline in tuberculosis as measured by the three
indices of mortality, morbidity, and infection rates.

   Mortality declined very rapidly in all three countries
(Figure 3). In Alaska, the mortality rate, which had been
over 600 per 100,000 in 1950, dropped to about 10 per
100,000 by 1965 and there were no deaths from tuberculosis
in 1968 or 1970. In Greenland, the mortality curve behaved
in exactly the same way. Canada has been lagging somewhat
behind - with rates around 250 in 1956, dropping to about
14 per 100,000 in 1969.

   Incidence rates show a similar decline (Figure 4). In
Greenland and in Alaska the respective incidence rates were
2,500 and 1,700 per 100,000 in 1955. Over the next ten
years, there was a sevenfold decline to somewhere between

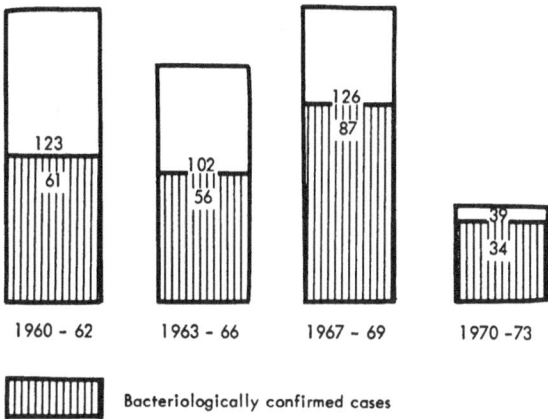

Figure 5 Mean annual incidence of tuberculosis (all forms) in Canadian Eskimos, Northwest Territories, 1960-73 (rates per 10,000)

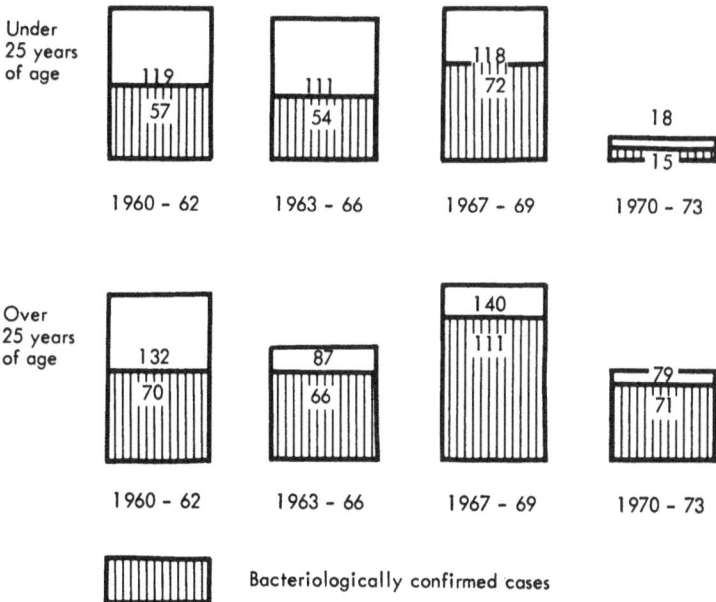

Figure 6 Mean annual incidence of tuberculosis in Canadian Eskimos, classified by age, Northwest Territories, 1960-73 (rates per 10,000)

200 and 300 per 100,000 in 1965. In the Northwest Territories, the morbidity in the late 1960s was still extremely
high, with an annual incidence rate of about 1 per cent;
however, it had dropped to below 300 per 100,000 by 1973.
Nevertheless, tuberculosis rates for Canada as a whole are
still 40 times lower. On the other hand, the over-all Canadian rate is declining more slowly than that for Eskimos.
Data for the years 1960-73 are analysed in more detail in
Figure 5. The over-all mean annual rate was 123 per 10,000
in the early 1960s and a little higher, 126, in the late
1960s. The rates for the late 1960s reflect the intensifica-
tion of case finding. A few years ago the apparent lack of
progress in the fight against tuberculosis was disturbing.
Then in the early 1970s came the sudden drop from 126 to
39 cases per 10,000. The proportion of bacteriologically
confirmed cases increased over this period of study.

The decline in new cases is much more substantial in persons under the age of 25 than in those over 25 (Figure 6).
One of the reasons for this is that primary tuberculosis has
virtually disappeared. The rates during the three periods of
the 1960s were well over 30 per 10,000, but they dropped to
0.1 per 10,000 in the early 1970s (Figure 7). This indicates
a marked reduction in the risk of tuberculous infection,
achieved by early diagnosis with cure by appropriate chemotherapy. There has been a parallel change in Alaska; Comstock and Philip (3) estimated the annual risk of infection

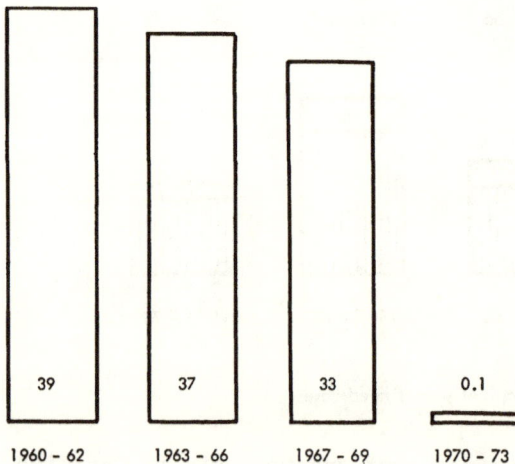

Figure 7   Incidence of primary tuberculosis in Canadian Eskimos, Northwest Territories, 1960-73 (rates per 10,000)

was about 25 per cent in 1950, but had diminished to about 0.3 per cent in 1970.

CONCLUSIONS

One may draw two conclusions of general interest from these studies. First, it is possible to diminish a tuberculosis problem rapidly by an antituberculous program. Secondly, the most important facet of such a program is the diagnosis of cases early enough to prevent them becoming important sources of infection. Such measures as chemoprophylaxis and BCG vaccination, although valuable, probably do not have a great immediate impact on the problem.

REFERENCES

1. Fellows, F.S., "Mortality in the native races of the territory of Alaska with special reference to tuberculosis," Public Health Rept. 49 (9): 289-98 (1934)
2. Fraser, R.I., Comstock, G.W., and Kaplan, G.J., "Tuberculosis in Alaska, 1970," Am. Rev. resp. Dis., 105: 920-26 (1972)
3. Comstock, G.W., and Philip, N.R., "Decline of the tuberculosis epidemic in Alaska," Public Health Rept., 76: 19-24 (1961)
4. Jensen, O., "Tuberkulosesituationen i Julianehab Distrikt, Grondland."
5. Johnson, M.W., "Tuberculosis in Alaska: Experience with twenty year control program, 1950-1970," Second International Symposium on Circumpolar Health, Oulu, Finland, 21-24 June 1971
6. Weiss, E.S., "Tuberculin sensitivity in Alaska," Public Health Rept., 68: 23 (1953)
7. Wherrett, G.J., "A study of tuberculosis in the Eastern Arctic," Canad. J. Public Health, 60: 7 (1969)

Methodology and results of phenotyping isoniazid inactivators

L. EIDUS, O. SCHAEFER, and M.M. HODGKIN

The rates of acetylation of isoniazid (INH), phenelzine (Nardil), hydralazine (Apresolin), sulphadimidine, and diaminodiphenylsulfone (Dapson) are genetically determined. Because of the clinical implications of differences in inactivation rates of these drugs, methods for classifying slow and fast acetylators were introduced.

Early phenotyping procedures estimated either the half-life of isoniazid in the blood or a single blood concentration at a fixed interval after a test dose of isoniazid. In 1970, a reliable urine test was devised (1). This method, later termed the SpM test, calculates an inactivation index, that is the proportion of acetylisoniazid to free INH and acid labile hydrazones in the urine specimen. A spectrophotometer is utilized for the determination of INH in the ultra-violet range and an adaptation of the Eidus-Hamilton colour reaction is employed for the estimation of acetylisoniazid (AcINH) (10). Because the separation between slow and fast acetylators increases with time, urine samples are collected for 6 to 8 hours after administration of the test dose of the drug. Indices of 3 or lower indicate slow inactivators, whereas fast metabolizers exhibit values of 5 or more.

With the advent of intermittent treatment of tuberculosis, the need for a simple screening test of INH therapy has increased. Hence, this institute developed a simple qualitative procedure (EF test) capable of distinguishing slow and fast inactivators (2, 5). It is based on the same principle as the original method, but does not require use of a spectrophotometer, and can be performed with simple equipment. Two 1 $m\ell$ aliquots (a and b) of a urine sample are acidified with 0.5 $m\ell$ of 0.5N hydrochloric acid to liberate free INH from its hydrazone bindings. The excreted acetylisoniazid is determined on aliquot "a". In aliquot "b", the free isoniazid is converted to its acetyl derivative by one drop of acetic anhydride. It therefore contains excreted AcINH plus free INH acetylated in vitro. The same red colour reaction (10) is used for both aliquots, which can be compared visually or with an inexpensive colorimeter. In

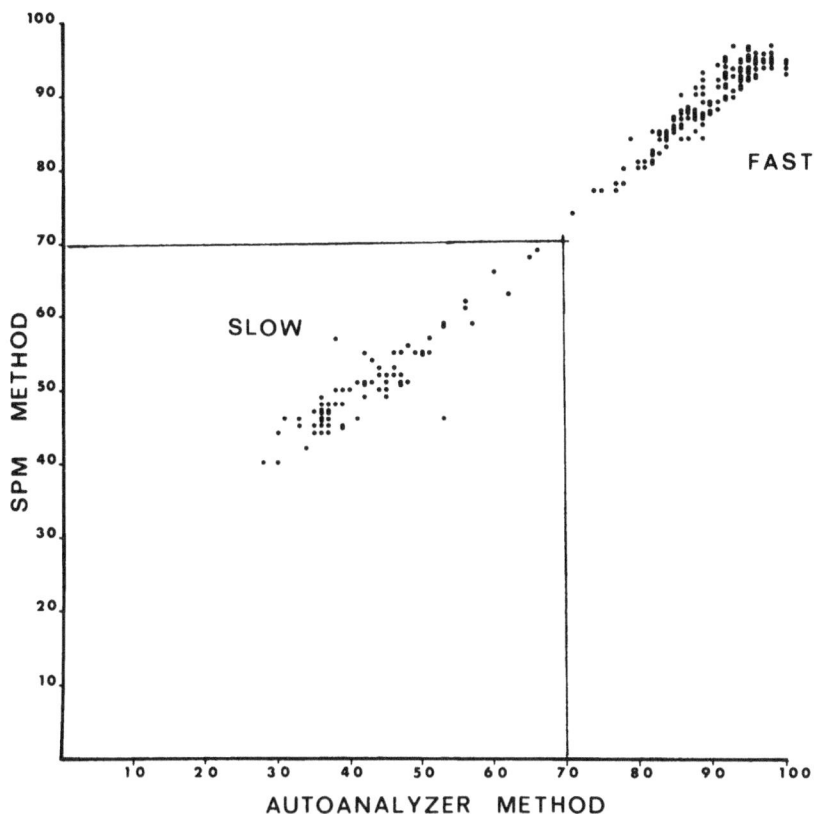

Figure 1   Acetylisoniazid as a percentage of total hydrazides in urines of 198 subjects - comparison of results by
SpM and automated methods

the latter case, an inactivation index can be calculated or
the percentage of acetylisoniazid to total hydrazides estimated (5).

By following another version of the Eidus-Hamilton test
for N acetylisoniazid (9) and, thereby, avoiding the use of
organic solvents, the screening test was adapted to an Auto
Analyzer. This permits the analysis of 60 samples per hour.
Figure 1 compares the results obtained by the automated and
SpM methods. Both procedures identically classified 198
patients into 71 slow and 127 fast acetylators, with a good
correlation between results obtained by the two methods.

The principle employed in the Auto Analyzer can also be
utilized in a simple manual procedure. It uses the same

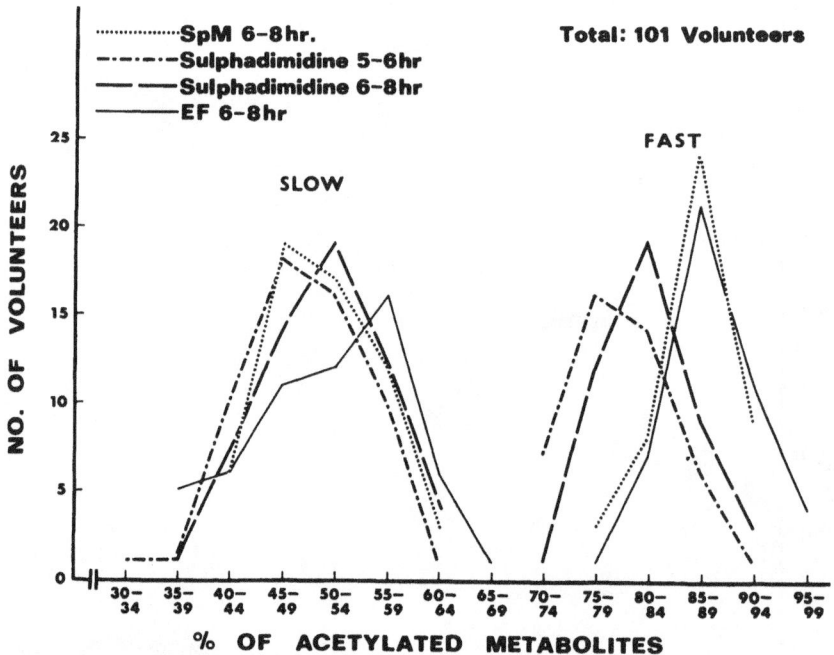

Figure 2   Comparison of various urine tests for phenotyping isoniazid inactivators

dilution scheme, concentrations, and proportions of reagents as the Auto Analyzer method (9). In the manual test, 1 ml of each of the diluted aliquots, "a" (AaINH) and "b" (AcINH plus INH acetylated in vitro), is transferred to matched test tubes. To each aliquot, 1 ml of 4 per cent potassium cyanide and 4.83 ml of 1.6 per cent chloramine-T solution are added. A red colour develops in 5 minutes. Distilled water is then added to tube "b" from a burette until its colour matches that of tube "a". Then,

$$\text{AcINH\%} = \frac{\text{aliquot "a" in ml} \times 100}{\text{aliquot "b" in ml} + \text{amount of water in ml}}$$

These various modifications of the urine test were designed to suit conditions prevailing in different laboratories. While these developments were in progress, other researchers investigated the possibility of using sulphadimidine instead of isoniazid as the test substance (4, 7). A comparison of the SpM, EF, and two versions of the sulphadimidine tests was thus carried out in 101 volunteers (6).

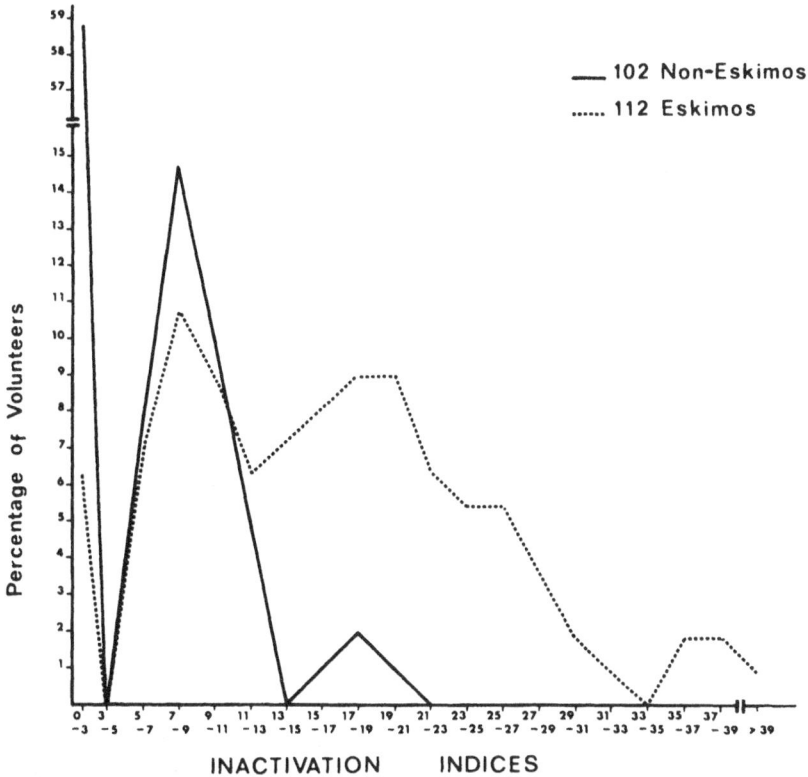

Figure 3   Distribution of inactivation indices (II) in Eskimos and Canadian students

For the INH phenotyping methods, an oral dose of 10 mg/kg
ordinary* isoniazid was administered, and 6-8 hour urine
specimens were divided into aliquots to carry out the SpM
and EF tests. After an interval of two weeks, the same volunteers were given 44 mg/kg of sulphadimidine. Urine speci-
ments were obtained during the periods 5-6 and 6-8 hours
after drug intake. Using 70 per cent as the demarcation
line between the two phenotypes, all methods divided the
101 volunteers into 60 slow and 41 fast acetylators. The
SpM, EF, and two versions of the sulphadimidine methods all
exhibited a good resolving power (Figure 2); however, the
SpM test achieved the greatest separation of the two inactivator groups (6).

  * See succeeding paper on slowly releasing isoniazid.

TABLE 1
Isoniazid inactivation patterns of selected populations

Population	Test method	Distribution of phenotypes (%)			Authors
		"Fast"	Mod. fast	Slow	
Can. Eskimos	Urine	60.7	33.0	6.3	Present
Japanese (in Tohoku)	Blood	58.5	34.0	7.5	Sunahara (8)
Ainus	Blood	51.2	36.0	12.8	Sunahara (8)
Koreans	Blood	44.6	44.6	10.8	Sunahara (8)
Thais	Blood	19.5	52.8	27.8	Sunahara (8)
Americans	Blood	9.0	36.5	54.5	Levy et al.*
Can. students	Urine	3.9	37.3	58.8	Present

* Reclassified by Sunahara et al. (8) according to the criteria of their blood test.

The frequency distribution of inactivation indices (SpM method) was compared in 102 Canadian students (Caucasians) and 112 Eskimos (3). While 58.8 per cent of Canadian students are slow acetylators, only 6.3 per cent of the Eskimos belong to this group (Figure 3). The indices of slow acetylators in both populations are confined to a narrow zone, but those of fast metabolizers exhibit a widespread distribution. A large proportion (38 of 42 Caucasian fast metabolizers) have indices over 5 but below 13 with a peak frequency at 7-9 position; 4 fall in the range 13-21, with a low peak in the region 17-19. The curve of Eskimo fast inactivators also shows two peaks in the same positions, but the second mound forms a high plateau with a gradual and far extending slope. Hence, the distribution of inactivation indices for Eskimo fast metabolizers is different, the majority falling in the region over 13. In another study, the subdivision of fast acetylators was observed at an index of 12.75. It may be that homozygous fast acetylators inactivate isoniazid more rapidly than the heterozygous ones. The demarcation line between moderately fast (intermediate) and "fast" acetylators is not sharply defined. Nevertheless, such a subclassification has practical value in planning treatment and chemoprophylaxis.

The isoniazid inactivation patterns of selected populations are compared in Table 1. The phenotype distributions yielded by the blood test in Japanese in the Northern Province of Tohoku and the Americans reclassified by Sunahara (8) concur with those obtained by the SpM urine test in Eskimos and Canadian students.

ACKNOWLEDGMENT

This study was supported by the WHO and the National Health Grant 606-7-776.

SUMMARY

Some 63.4 per cent of Canadian Indians and almost all Eskimos rapidly inactivate isoniazid by acetylation. In order to facilitate drug prescription, simple urine tests were designed for phenotyping isoniazid inactivators. The classification of slow and fast acetylators can be based on either the proportion of acetylisoniazid (AcINH) to isoniazid or the percentage of AcINH to total hydrazides in urine samples collected for 6 to 8 hours following a test dose of isoniazed. The several methods described employ the same principle, but the procedures are modified to satisfy different objectives. The spectrophotometric method is capable of subdividing fast inactivators into moderately fast and "fast" acetylators. The screening procedure identifies slow and fast inactivators without further subclassification. Two modifications of this test have been devised, one using an Auto Analyzer. The methods are compared, and their individual merits discussed.

REFERENCES

1. Eidus, L., Harnanansingh, A.M.T., and Jessamine, A.G., "Urine test for phenotyping isoniazid inactivators," Am. Rev. resp. Dis., 104: 587-91 (1971)
2. Eidus, L., and Hodgkin, M.M., "Screening of isoniazid inactivators," Antimicrob. Agents & Chemother., 3: 130-3 (1973)
3. Eidus, L., Hodgkin, M.M., Schaefer, O., and Jessamine, A.G., "Distribution of isoniazid inactivators determined in Eskimos and Canadian college students by a urine test," Revue can. Biol., 33: 117-23 (1974)
4. Evans, D.A.P., "An improved and simplified method of detecting the acetylator phenotype," J. med. Genet., 6: 405-7 (1969)
5. Hodgkin, M.M., Hsu, A.H.E., Varughese, P., and Eidus, L., "Evaluation of a new method for phenotyping of slow and rapid acetylators," Int. J. clin. Pharmacol., 7: 355-62 (1973)

6. Jessamine, A.G., Hodgkin, M.M., and Eidus, L., "Urine tests for phenotyping slow and fast acetylators," Canad. J. Public Health, 65: 119-23 (1974)

7. Rao, K.V.N., Mitchison, D.A., Nair, N.G.K., Prema, K., and Tripathy, S.P., "Sulphadimidine acetylation test for classification of patients as slow or rapid inactivators of isoniazid," Br. med. J., (iii): 495-7 (1970)

8. Sunahara, S., Urano, M., and Ogawa, M., "Genetical and geographic studies on isoniazid inactivation," Science, 134: 1530 (1961)

9. Varughese, P., Hamilton, E.J., and Eidus, L., "Mass phenotyping of isoniazid inactivators by automated determination of acetylisoniazid in urine," Clin. Chem. 20: 639-41 (1974)

10. Venkataraman, P., Eidus, L., and Tripathy, S.P., "Method for estimation of acetylisoniazid in urine," Tubercle (Lond), 49: 210-16 (1968)

Intermittent chemotherapy of tuberculosis patients rapidly inactivating isoniazid

M.M. HODGKIN, L. EIDUS, O. SCHAEFER, B. POLLAK, and D. LEUNG

Patients on domiciliary programs tend to be irregular in self-administration of medicaments and often discontinue drugs prematurely. Hence, fully supervised intermittent chemotherapy has been recommended to ensure a complete course of medication.

Among primary antituberculous agents, only isoniazid (INH) in combination with streptomycin was effective in twice-weekly treatment. The same regimen when administered once a week, after an initial phase of one month of daily treatment, achieved bacteriological quiescence in 95 per cent of patients metabolizing isoniazid at a slow rate, but in only 76 per cent of those acetylating the drug rapidly (6, 9). From data obtained in south India, one would predict an even lower bacteriological conversion rate in Eskimos who are predominantly fast acetylators with the highest acetylation capacity (3, 5).

Once-weekly intermittent chemotherapy is an asset when treating patients who live in remote areas, and since an efficient INH-streptomycin regimen is already available for slow acetylators (7), an effort was made to develop a new Matrix therapy that would allow intermittent chemotherapy of fast inactivators. The preparation investigated contained approximately 37 per cent of ordinary INH and 63 per cent of a slowly releasing Matrix component (supplied by ICN Canada Ltd., Montreal).

Thirty-five volunteers were divided by a urine test (2, 3) into 11 slow, 12 moderately fast (intermediate), and 12 fast acetylators. Indices of 3 or lower were considered to indicate slow metabolizers, values between 5 and 12.75 to identify moderately fast inactivators, and those >12.75 to distinguish fast acetylators.

The average age (41.5-48.6) and weight (58.1-64.3) of all the three groups were similar. As for inactivation indices, the slow acetylators had an average of 1.2, ranging from 0.9 to 1.6; the indices of the moderately fast group were scattered between 5.3 and 12.7, yielding an average of 9.1; while the fast acetylators exhibited a widespread distribution from 12.8 to 30.6 with a mean of 17.6.

All volunteers received a single dose of 15 mg/kg ordinary isoniazid, the amount usually employed in intermittent chemotherapy. Thereafter, the two fast metabolizer groups were given a double and triple dose of Matrix preparation, i.e., 30 and 45 mg/kg, separated by adequate intervals. Blood was collected 1, 2, 4, 6, 8, and 12 hours following drug intake, while urine was collected over six hourly intervals for 30 hours. Concentrations of free isoniazid and acid labile hydrazones were estimated in plasma (1) to draw the average plasma concentration-time curves and calculate the area under the curves (AUC). Urinary concentrations of free INH (1), acetylisoniazid (10), and isonicotinic acid (8) were determined to compute the recovery rates of the drug.

In the 0 to 6 hour period, urinary recovery rates are higher in fast metabolizers than in slow inactivators (Table 1). This has been observed previously (4), and is attributable to a greater production of INH metabolites by fast acetylators, with more rapid urinary excretion of these compounds than of free INH.

The recovery of Matrix isoniazid is relatively low in the first six hours. However, the absorption of Matrix isoniazid continues throughout the enteric tract and is

350 Pulmonary function and chest diseases

TABLE 1
Urinary recovery rates (percentage of test dose administered) for
15 mg/kg of ordinary isoniazid (O) and 45 mg/kg of INH matrix (M)

| Inactivator group | INH prep. | Dosage (mg/kg) | Recovery | | | Cumulative rec. rates over 30 hr |
			0-6 hr	6-12 hr	12-24 hr	
Slow	O	15	37.9	28.0	16.6	85.1
Mod. fast	O	15	45.0	23.0	6.7	75.3
	M	45	27.6	24.6	17.9	73.6
"Fast"	O	15	50.5	21.5	6.0	78.6
	M	45	27.8	24.4	18.1	73.7

ultimately as complete as that of the normal preparation.
This is reflected in the similarity of cumulative recovery
rates over 30 hours. The delayed absorption of the Matrix
preparation allows administration of a three times higher
dose in fast inactivators without elevating peak levels beyond the limits of tolerance and safety.

Blood level curves (Figure 1) show that a 15 mg/kg dose
of ordinary INH produces a gradual elimination slope in
slow inactivators, and steep ones in the two fast acetylator groups. The gap between the elimination lines of slow
and fast metabolizers is much wider that between the two
fast inactivator groups.

A double dose of INH-Matrix modifies the elimination pattern of the fast acetylator groups so that the slope becomes similar to that of slow inactivators receiving ordinary INH. A triple dose of Matrix procures adequate peak
levels in moderately fast inactivators with a slope almost
coinciding with that of the slow metabolizers. In fast acetylators, the blood concentrations reached with the 45
mg/kg dose of INH-Matrix are still lower than the corresponding ones attained in the moderately fast group, but the
elimination pattern is similar.

The area under the plasma concentration-time curve (AUC)
is summarized in Table 2. A 15 mg/kg dose of ordinary isoniazid produces an average AUC of 133.4 in slow acetylators,
whereas in the moderately fast and fast groups the corresponding AUCs are only 55.5 and 38.8, respectively, 41.6
and 29.1 per cent of the AUC in slow inactivators.

A double dose of the Matrix preparation (30 mg/kg) does
not improve the area under the curve in moderately fast or
fast acetylators. On the other hand, a further increase of
the Matrix isoniazid dosage to 45 mg/kg expands the AUC values of the two fast metabolizer groups by over 100 per cent.

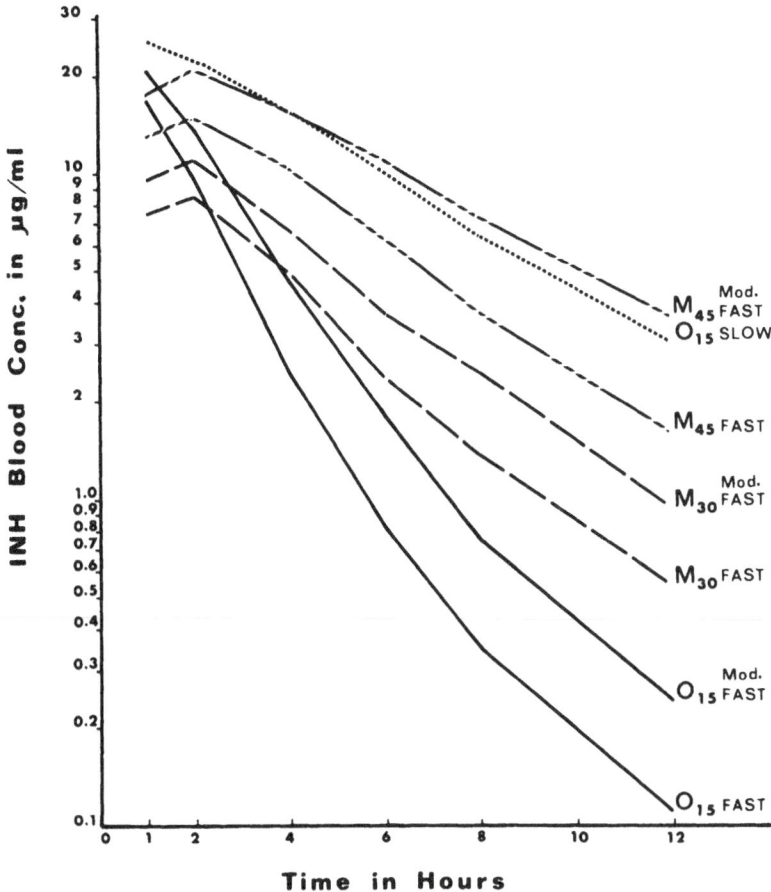

Figure 1   Average blood levels achieved with 15 mg ordinary INH per kg (O) in slow and fast inactivators as well as with 30 and 45 mg Matrix preparation per kg (M) in fast acetylators

With a triple dose of INH-Matrix, the average AUC of moderately fast acetylators becomes 96.5 per cent of that obtained in slow inactivators with ordinary isoniazid, but in fast acetylators it is still only 61.7 per cent of that achieved in slow inactivators with ordinary INH. Whether the latter level would be sufficient to reach the therapeutic goal, or whether a further slight increase of the blood concentrations would be necessary, can only be established by clinical trials.

352 Pulmonary function and chest diseases

TABLE 2
Area under curve (μg/ml.hr) in 12 hours following administration
of selected preparations of INH

Inactivator group	No. of volunteers	15 mg/kg 0*	30 mg/kg M*	45 mg/kg M*
Slow	11	133.4		
Mod. fast	12	55.5	55.8	128.7
		(41.6%)**	(41.9%)	(96.5%)
"Fast"	12	38.8	39.8	82.3
		(29.1%)	(29.8%)	(61.7%)

*   0 = ordinary INH; M = INH matrix.
** AUC values expressed as a percentage of the average AUC
obtained with 15 mg/kg of ordinary INH in slow acetylators (133.4).

A pilot study on a small group of Eskimo fast acetylators (average inactivation index of 22.9) revealed that increase in dosage from 45 mg/kg to 50 mg/kg of Matrix isoniazed expanded the average AUC to 86.3 per cent of the AUC achieved with ordinary isoniazid in slow inactivators. Thus we conclude that Matrix isoniazid can be used for intermittent chemotherapy of the entire range of fast acetylators. Among Caucasian rapid metabolizers, the incidence of fast acetylation is only 3.9 per cent (3), and a triple dose of the new preparations will procure a favourable response in almost all patients; however, the dosage can be increased slightly, if required, for Eskimos, of whom 60.7 per cent are fast inactivators.

ACKNOWLEDGMENT

This study was supported by the WHO and the National Health Grant 606-7-776.

SUMMARY

Domiciliary treatment of tuberculosis is often unsatisfactory, owing to the irregular drug intake of the patients. Fully supervised intermittent chemotherapy may avoid this shortcoming. A once-weekly drug-regimen comprising large doses of isoniazid (INH) plus streptomycin was found efficient only in slow metabolizers of INH. As the majority of the circumpolar population consist of fast acetylators, a slowly releasing INH-Matrix preparation was devised to compensate for rapid inactivation of the drug. Because of protracted absorption of this formulation, large doses can be administered. When a triple dose of Matrix isoniazid (45 mg/kg) is given to moderately fast acetylators, blood levels are identical with those achieved in slow inactivators with 15 mg/kg ordinary INH. The pharmacokinetics of the Matrix preparation and its therapeutic implication are discussed.

REFERENCES

1. Eidus, L., and Harnanansingh, A.M.T., "A more sensitive spectrophotometric method for determination of isoniazid in serum or plasma," Clin. Chem., 17: 492-4 (1971)
2. Eidus, L., Harnanansingh, A.M.T., and Jessamine, A.G., "Urine test for phenotyping isoniazid inactivators," Am. Rev. resp. Dis., 104: 587-91 (1971)
3. Eidus, L., Hodgkin, M.M., Schaefer, O., and Jessamine, A.G., "Distribution of isoniazid inactivators determined in Eskimos and Canadian college students by a urine test," Revue can. Ciol., 33: 117-23 (1974)
4. Eidus, L., Ling, G.M., and Harnanansingh, A.M.T., "Isoniazid excretion in fast and slow inactivators and its practical aspect for phenotyping," Arzneimittel-Forsch.(Drug Res.), 21: 1696-9 (1971)
5. Jeanes, C.W.L., Schaefer, O., and Eidus, L., "Inactivation of isoniazid by Canadian Eskimos and Indians," Can. Med. Assoc. J., 106-331-5 (1972)
6. Menon, N.K., "Madras study of supervised once-weekly chemotherapy in the treatment of pulmonary tuberculosis: Clinical aspects," Tubercle (Lond) Suppl., 49: 76-8 (1968)
7. Mitchison, D.A., "II Clinical applications of antibiotic and chemotherapeutic agents," Proc. R. Soc. Med., 64: 537-40 (1971)
8. Nielsch, W., "Nachweis und Bestimmung von pyridin-4-Derivaten," Chemikerzeitung, 82: 329-41 (1958)
9. Tripathy, S.P., "Madras study of supervised once-weekly chemotherapy in treatment of pulmonary tuberculosis: Laboratory aspects," Tubercle (Lond) Suppl., 49: 78-80 (1968)
10. Venkataraman, P., Eidus, L., and Tripathy, S.P.," "Method for estimation of acetylisoniazid in urine, Tubercle (Lond) 49: 210-16 (1968)

Pathogenesis of urogenital tuberculosis: an experimental study in guinea pigs

B. WINBLAD and M. DUCHEK

In Nordic countries, the control of tuberculosis as a disease and as a cause of death has been so effective in the
last few decades that the number of newly detected cases of
active tuberculosis is now among the lowest in the world.
However, the decline of post-primary tuberculous manifestations, including urogenital tuberculosis (UGT), has been
less favourable. Recently Fritjofsson and Kollberg (5) examined the incidence of UGT in two Swedish counties. The
number of new cases was practically constant during the 10-
year period 1960 to 1969, averaging four new cases of active
UGT per 100,000 inhabitants per year in the northern county
and 2/100,000 per year in the southern county.

The pathogenesis of UGT is incompletely known. The primary manifestation of urinary tract tuberculosis arises
from haematogenous spread to the kidney. Subsequent spread
through the urinary tract and to the genitalia has been
considered as occurring via the urinary (canalicular) route
(6, 7), but the additional possibility of lymphatic spread
has been implied in some publications (1, 6). Tubercle bacilli may spread from the prostate and/or the seminal vesi-
cles to the scrotal organs by way of the ductus deferens
(10). We have now undertaken an experimental study (2,3,4,
9) to test whether there are other paths of infection than
the usually accepted canalicular one.

Eighty male guinea pigs were divided into eight equal
groups and inoculated via the urinary or genital organs
with 0.05 ml of a standardized dilution of a human strain
of tubercle bacilli ($H_{37}Rv$). To prevent leakage and spread,
a strongly bactericidal plastic film was applied over the
site of injection before the needle was withdrawn.

All animals were killed after 3-8 weeks and the extent
of the tuberculous infection was determined macroscopically,
histologically, and bacteriologically. The diagnostic results obtained by the use of haematoxylin-eosin staining,
staining according to Ziehl-Neelsen, and fluorescent staining were compared with each other and with the results of
culture on Löwenstein-Jensen medium. Fluorescent staining
with Auramin-rhodamine was found superior to the classical

TABLE 1
Tuberculous changes in the urogenital tract of male guinea pigs
following inoculation into the left ureter (groups A_1 and A_2) or the
urinary bladder wall (groups B_1 and B_2)

Group	No. of animals	LE	LSV	P	B	RSV	RE	LUD	LUP	LK
A_1 Intact ureter	10	2	2	4	4	3	2	8	9	5
A_2 Ligation of ureter	8	3	2	2	2	0	2	5	8	7
B_1 Intact ductus deferens	9	1	1	8	9	0	3			
B_2 Resection of ductus deferens	9	4	0	5	9	0	7			

Site of inoculation *

* LE, left epididymis; LSV, left seminal vesicle; P, prostate;
Bl, urinary bladder; RSV, right seminal vesicle; RE, right epididymis;
LUD, left ureter distal; LUP, left ureter proximal; LK, left kidney.

Ziehl-Neelsen method and about as effective as culture for
the demonstration of microorganisms. The bacteria were
more clearly visible if epi-illumination was used instead
of transillumination, especially at higher degrees of mag-
nification. The conventional histological method, using
haematoxylin-eosin, in combination with fluorescence microscopy provided an adequate means of mapping the spread of
tuberculous infections (8).

In the first two groups of animals, tubercle bacilli
were injected into the upper part of the intact ureter (Al)
and the ligated ureter (A2). Ligature of the ureter was
carried out under a dissecting microscope, carefully spar-
ing the vessels surrounding the ureter. The results (Table
1) show that in both groups there was spread to the lower
part of the ureter. Macroscopically, longitudinal greyish-
white streaks were observed on the outer wall of the ureter,
both proximal and distal to the ligatures and extending out
to the enlarged para-aortic lymph nodes. Microscopically,
tuberculous changes were seen in and around lymphatics in
the periureteral tissue (Figure 1). There was spread to
both the left and the right epididymis, in three animals in
each group to the left and in two to the right. Urinary
cultures were positive in five animals from group Al and
two animals from group A2. Blood cultures were negative.

In the next two groups (Bl, B2) tubercle bacilli were
injected into the anterior part of the trigonum. In group
B2, both spermatic ducts were carefully dissected free
from their vessels, partially resected and both ends ligated

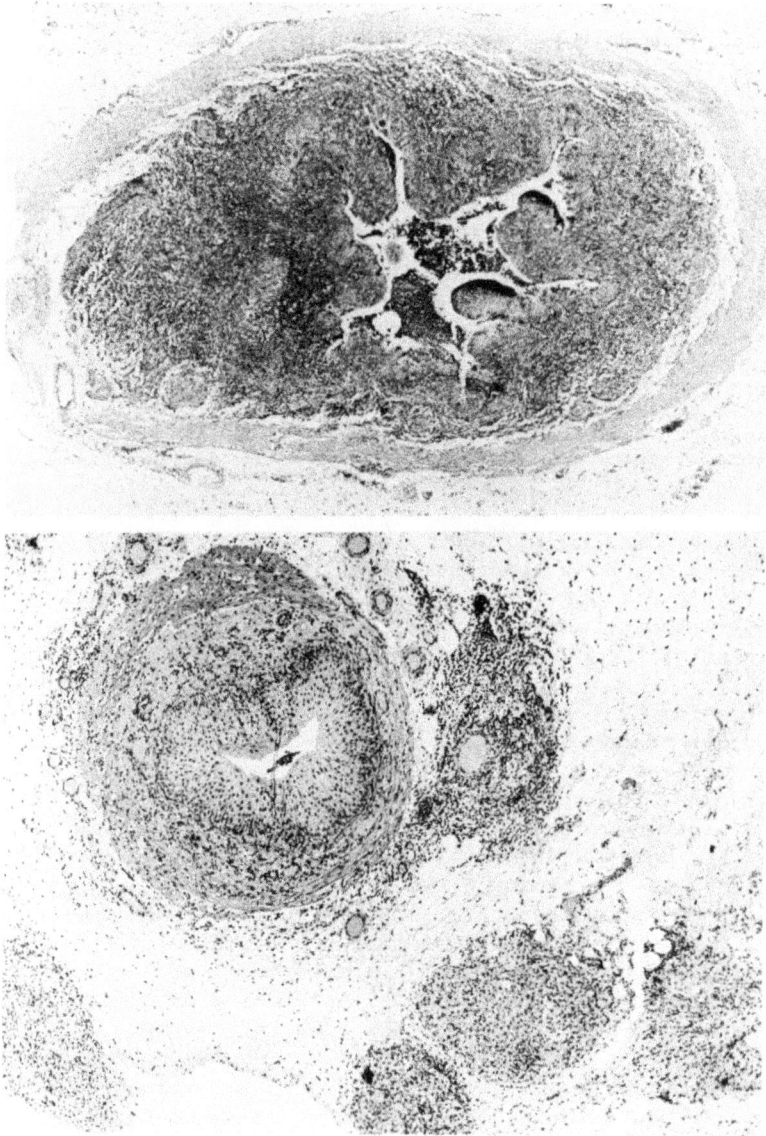

Figure 1 Section of proximal (upper photo) and distal (lower photo) part of ureter 28 days after intraureteral injection of tubercle bacilli in an animal with ligated ureter. Upper photo shows intraureteral inflammatory changes with some epithelioid cell granulomas. Lower photo shows epithelioid cell granulomas and lymphocytes in and around lymphatics in periureteral connective tissue. Haematoxylin/eosin x72.

before inoculation into the bladder wall. All animals showed tuberculous changes at the site of inoculation (Table 1). There was spread to the prostate in nearly all animals. The spread was usually continuous, but in some animals there was evidence of lymphatic spread. Tuberculous changes were observed in the epididymes, unilaterally or bilaterally in three of nine animals in group B1 and in eight of nine animals in group B2. Spread to the epididymis usually occurred by way of the lymphatics. Urinary cultures were positive in four animals in each group. Blood cultures were negative.

In the last four groups (Table 2), inoculation of tubercle bacilli was performed into the left epididymis or seminal vesicle. In half of the animals (groups C2 and D2), the ductus deferens was resected before inoculation. When inoculated into the left epididymis, there was spread to the prostate and/or seminal vesicle in only two of 10 animals. However, when inoculated into the left seminal vesicle, there was spread to the epididymis on the same side in six or ten animals (groups D1 and D2 respectively). Macroscopically, greyish-white streaks were seen along the spermatic duct joining the seminal vesicle with the epididymis. Microscopically, there were epithelioid cell granulomas in and around the lymphatics outside the spermatic duct. No changes were seen in the lumen of ductus deferens (Figure 2).

TABLE 2
Tuberculous changes in the genital tract of male guinea pigs following inoculation into the epididymis or the seminal vesicle

Group	No. of animals	Site of inoculation *				
		LE	LSV	P	B	RSV
C_1 Intact ductus deferens	9	9	0	2	0	1
C_2 Resection of ductus deferens	10	10	1	2	0	1
D_1 Intact ductus deferens	10	6	10	10	0	1
D_2 Resection of ductus deferens	10	10	10	10	1	1

* LE, left epididymis; LSV, left seminal vesicle; P, prostate;
B, urinary bladder; RSV, right seminal vesicle.

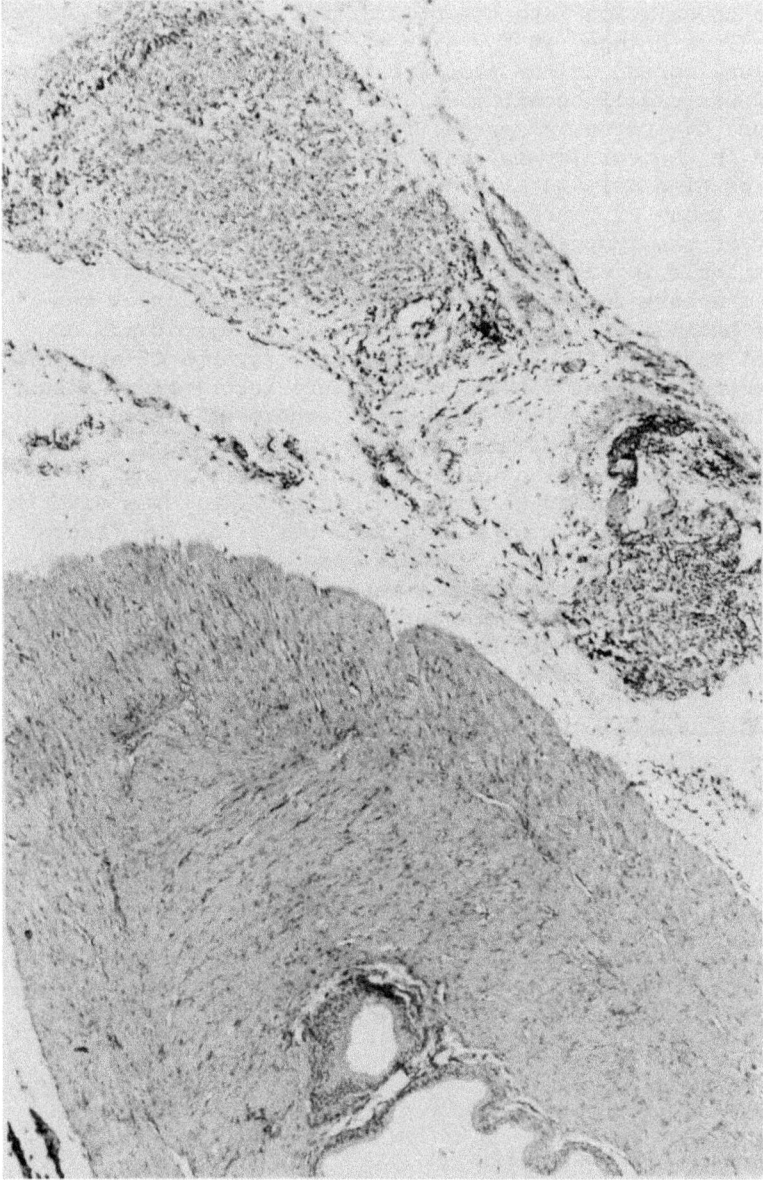

Figure 2 Cross-section of ductus deferens (DD) and surrounding tissue. Inflammatory granulomatous areas in the
loose periductal tissue. Ductus deferens is not engaged.
Haemotoxylin/eosin x 63.

CONCLUSIONS

1. Tuberculosis spreads from the urinary passages to the genitalia, and within the genitalia regardless of whether the ureter or ductus deferens is intact or not.
2. The lymphatics constitute an important route of spread within the urogenital system.
3. Spread is more common from the pelvic to the scrotal genitalia than in the opposite direction.

   It is hazardous to apply these conclusions directly to man. The experiments have concerned primary tuberculous infection by a relatively large number of bacteria in a previously non-immunized guinea pig. In man, genital tuberculosis is a late manifestation of the disease, and almost always occurs in previously immunized territory. Studies are now in progress to see whether a secondary tuberculous infection in an immunized animal takes the same over-all course and spreads by the same routes as in a non-immunized host.

ACKNOWLEDGMENT

These investigations were supported by grants from the Swedish National Association against Heart and Chest Diseases, Carin Tryggers Foundation and the Medical Faculty of the University of Umeå, Sweden.

SUMMARY

An experimental study of the spread of urogenital tuberculosis was undertaken in 80 male guinea pigs. These were divided into eight equal groups and tubercle bacilli ($H_{37}Rv$) were inoculated into the ureter, urinary bladder, vesicula seminalis, and epididymis. In order to investigate whether infection can spread if the canalicular route is excluded, half of the animals in each group were prepared by ligature of the ureter or resection and ligature of the ductus deferens. Spread of infection to the lower urinary tract and the genitalia occurred irrespective of whether the ureter or ductus deferens was intact or not. It is concluded that lymphatic spread is possible and occurs more often than urinary, canalicular spread.

REFERENCES

1. Bauereisen, A., "Beitrag zur Frage der aszendierenden Nierentuberkulose," Zeitschr. f. gynäkol. Urologie, 2: 132-53, 276-84 (1911)
2. Duchek, M., and Winblad, B., "An experimental method for studying the spread of genital tuberculosis," Urol. Res., 1: 32-6 (1973)
3. Duchek, M., and Winblad, B., "Spread of tuberculosis from the urinary bladder to the male genital organs. An experimental study," Urol. Res., 1: 141-4 (1973)
4. Duchek, M., and Winblad, B., "Experimental male genital tuberculosis, the possibility of lymphatic spread," Urol. Res., 1: 170-6 (1973)
5. Fritjofsson, A., and Kollberg, S., "The incidence of urogenital tuberculosis," Intern. Urol. Nephrol., 5: 291-6 (1973)
6. Ljunggren, E., "Urogenital tuberculosis," in Encyclopedia of Urology, IX/2, 1-222 (Berlin: Springer, 1959)
7. Mazurek, L.J., "The importance of the urethro-seminal reflux in the pathogenesis of the genital tbc in the male," Urologia, 30: 220-9 (1963)
8. Winblad, B., and Duchek, M., "Comparison between microscopical methods and cultivation for demonstration of tubercle bacilli in experimental tuberculous infection," Acta path. microbiol. scand., Sect. A, 81: 824-30 (1973)
9. Winblad, B., and Duchek, M., "Spread of tuberculosis from obstructed and non-obstructed upper urinary tract," Acta path. microbiol. scand. Sect. A, In press (1975)
10. Zádor, O., Baranyi, E., Földes, Gy., and Csontai, A., "Über die Pathogenese der Genitaltuberkulose beim Manne," Urologia, 34: 4-14 (1967)

Commentaries

"Pulmonary disease in Alaska," by R.I. Fraser (Alaska Division of Public Health). Chronic pulmonary disease is seen as an increasingly major public health problem in rural Alaska. The conditions grouped in this category include: (1) post-tuberculosis bronchiectasis and loss of lung

volume from lung destruction due to tuberculosis, resec-
tional surgery, or old thoracoplasties; (2) non-tuberculous
bronchiectasis resulting from necrotizing viral and bacterial pneumonia in children; and (3) emphysema and chronic
bronchitis resulting from cigarette smoking. Population
characteristics in Alaska pose challenges for the administration of inhalation therapy in rural communities with the
common problems of equipment, training programs centred on
the village level, and logistics of maintaining equipment
and supplying oxygen. The program in Alaska is evolving in
the direction of increased recognition of the problem, inhalation therapy training for the public health nurses in
the field hospitals, and the development of community-
oriented maintenance programs.

"A review of tuberculosis in Alaska, 1974," by R.I. Fraser
(Alaska Division of Public Health). The Alaskan native
population experienced an epidemic of tuberculosis in the
1950s rare in the annals of recorded medicine. Ambulatory
drug therapy was first utilized in this population, studies
on the effectiveness of isoniazid (INH) prophylaxis or preventive therapy were first carried out in this population
group, and Alaska was among the pioneers of treatment of
tuberculosis in general hospitals. The incidence of tuberculosis has declined considerably over the years. However,
in 1971-73 it has remained fairly stable. The type of cases
recognized in the last three years has been unique in that
60 per cent of the cases have been minimal, with a small
percentage moderately active and far advanced. INH and Ri-
fampin have provided the basic initial therapy program for
the last 2½ years.

"Tuberculosis in Alaska," by J.D. Millar (CDC, Atlanta, Ga.,
USA). The epidemiology of tuberculosis in Alaska illustrates dramatically what can be accomplished under difficult
environmental conditions with limited health resources.
Twenty-five years ago, up to 80 per cent of children in the
Yukon-Kuskokwim delta area were positive tuberculin reactors by the age of five years. In a survey done in 1969-70,
no children under five were found to be reactors. For the
entire state of Alaska in 1973, infection rates were only
0.1 per cent for pre-school children, 0.2 per cent for
school enterers, and 0.3 per cent for 7th and 8th grade
students. The marked reduction in infection rates in

children can be attributed to intensive case finding, hospitalization, and ambulatory treatment programs which during the past two decades have markedly reduced the pool of infectious cases in Alaskan communities. In addition, a large portion of the Alaskan native population, particularly in the Bethel area, participated in the early Public Health Service trails of isoniazid preventive therapy. This community-wide application of preventive therapy has undoubtedly contributed to the decline of the tuberculosis epidemic in Alaska.

Other circumpolar populations share with Alaska a large reservoir of infected persons from years past. Unlike Alaska, however, the persons in these reservoirs are largely untreated. Even where transmission of tuberculous infection has been largely interrupted, cases of tuberculosis will continue to come from this infected pool. The future incidence of disease can be reduced by treatment of these infected persons.

Recently, concern about isoniazid-associated hepatitis has necessitated a reassessment of the use of this valuable drug. Surveillance of approximately 13,000 persons on isoniazid by the US Public Health Service has provided data on the frequency, age distribution, and other epidemiologic characteristics of isoniazid-associated hepatitis. Isoniazid can be used safely and effectively, with appropriate monitoring of patients. As with any drug, the benefits must be weighed against the risks.

"Preventive treatment to reduce the incidence of tuberculosis among Canadian Eskimos," by J.D. Galbraith (Medical Services, National Health and Welfare, Baker Centre, Edmonton, Canada). The incidence of tuberculosis has been very high among Canadian Eskimos, the peak incidence being among young women (Archives of Environmental·Health, Vol. 25, November 1972). Starting in 1967, a prophylaxis program using two antituberculous drugs for a period of 18 months was initiated among the Eskimo population. Up to the end of 1972, 825 Eskimos had completed a course of antituberculous drugs. The indications for prophylaxis included: (1) inactive tuberculosis cases who had either no earlier treatment or whose treatment by present standards was considered inadequate; (2) contact with an infectious case of tuberculosis; and (3) selected tuberculin reactors, mainly children and young persons. Surveillance by follow-up chest X-rays and sputum tests has been thorough and indicates a

reduction in the number of new cases of expected tuberculosis. A review of the 825 persons shows 50 had taken their
drugs for less than six months. This report shows that of
those who had taken more than six months of preventive
drugs three developed active tuberculosis at five, eight,
and fourteen months after the completion of chemoprophylaxis. The average follow-up period at the end of 1973 was
34 months. Of the three cases that developed active tuberculosis after the course of prophylaxis, one case had tu-
bercule bacilli resistant to Isoniazid, Streptomycin, and
Ethambutol. It is realized that in dealing with small numbers of active cases statistical validity is very unreliable
but to date this program appears to have markedly reduced
the incidence of breakdown with tuberculosis in that section
of the population known to be at highest risk.

ARCTIC OPHTHALMOLOGY

Pterygium, climatic keratopathy, and pinguecula of the eyes in arctic and subarctic populations

H. FORSIUS

The eyes are not effectively protected against extremes of cold and wind. Consequently, changes in the external parts of the eye might be expected in Arctic populations. However, we have shown previously (8) that the eyes endure the arctic cold and snow better than any other part of the face. Lesions occur in the corneal epithelium, but heal in a short time. The weather conditions of the spring and summer try the eyes more, and the most probable source of trouble is in radiation from the sun, particularly by ultra-violet (UV) light.

The amount of UV light reaching the ground depends, among other things, on air humidity, cloud cover, and the ozone concentration in the lower layers of the atmosphere. Duke-Elder states that the atmosphere is more permeable to the shorter waves in extreme cold (5). Ultra-violet light seems to result in climatic keratopathy, pterygium, and possibly pinguecula.

The eyelids offer no protection against UV light reflected from snow. The higher the sun rises, the greater is the harm caused to the eyes. In the Alps, where the sun is high and the atmosphere is also rarified, acute snow-blindness may take a violent course, resulting in corneal ulcerations and ultimate blindness. The farther north one goes, the less is the risk, because the sun is lower. Acute snow-blindness is not a major problem in North Greenland, among the northern-most North-American Eskimos, or the Lapps and Finns. Further, arctic and subarctic populations have learned to protect their eyes by using various kinds of shades.

Acute snow-blindness affects mainly the middle portion of the cornea, but milder doses of ultraviolet light may after a time cause changes starting in the periphery of the

cornea. Around the Red Sea, a large proportion of the population suffers from a "climatic" keratopathy (14). Freedman
(9) described a similar disabling lesion of the eye in Labrador ("Labrador keratopathy").

Talbot (17) and Kerkenezov (13) were among the first to
present evidence that pterygium corneae originates from a
lesion caused by ultra-violet light. Cameron's map of pterygium (4) shows this formation is most common in the equator-
ial regions, where it constitutes a major therapeutic problem. The incidence is almost zero among indoor workers in
central and northern Europe, but is also low among outdoor
workers in this part of the world. However, the degeneration again becomes more frequent in arctic and subarctic
regions. Thus, pterygium was detected in 33 per cent of men
over the age of 40 in northern Newfoundland (10).

A pinguecula is seen in almost all subjects over 40
years of age, less frequently among women than men, and more
often in outdoor than indoor workers. It is more pronounced
medially in the young, but flattens out in the higher age
groups when it atrophies (1,2,7,20). Cameron (4) found that
people using spectacles had smaller pinguecula and less
pterygium than those who did not.

MATERIAL

The author has studied Lapps in northern Finland, Eskimos
in Wainwright, Alaska, Igloolik, NWT, and Augpilagtoq,
Greenland, populations in northern and southern Iceland
(Husavik and Reykjavik), and other groups in Finland and
the USSR, giving a total of 2,287 subjects 20 years of age
or older (Table 1). Minor changes observed on a Haag-Streit
biomicroscope have been noted, which may explain differences in frequencies of ophthalmological changes, compared
with reports of other authors. The palpebral aperture was
measured on standard photographs made by the same clinical
photographer (H. Nieminen, Oulu, Finland). The size of the
pinguecula was estimated on a scale of 0 to 3, both medially and laterally, and the mean was noted.

The results have been related to figures from meteorological stations in Finland, Iceland, the USA, and Canada.
The figures from central Finland and Reykjavik, Iceland
were based on examinations carried out at old people's
homes.

TABLE 1

Populations investigated for pterygium, climatic keratopathy, and degree of pinguecula

	Latitude	Age groups										Total		
		20-39 years			40-59 years			60+ years						
		M	F	Total	M	F	Total	M	F	Total		M	F	Total
Skolt Lapps	69°	52	49	101	43	47	90	21	31	52		116	127	243
Mountain Lapps, N. Finland		13	10	23	12	16	28	5	8	13		30	32	64
Finns, Kökar, S. Finland	60°	55	70	125	66	78	144	45	71	116		166	219	385
Finns, Oulu	65°	-	-	-	1	-	1	97	122	219		98	122	220
Icelanders Husavik 1972	66°	65	79	144	84	78	162	65	48	113		214	205	419
Reykjavik 1973	64°	-	-	-	-	-	-	142	156	298		142	156	298
Eskimos Upernavik, Greenland	73°	23	13	36	12	22	34	11	11	22		46	46	92
Wainwright, Alaska	71°	22	21	43	9	12	21	16	5	21		47	38	85
Igloolik, Canada	69°	49	58	107	22	22	44	5	2	7		76	82	158
Cheremis, USSR	57°	189	-	189	131	-	131	3	-	3		323	-	323
Total												1,258	1,029	2,287

TABLE 2
Occurrence of pterygium (Pt), classified by age and population groups

Population		Age groups						Total	
		20-39 years		40-59 years		60+ years			
		Pt	Total	Pt	Total	Pt	Total	Pt	Total
Lapps	♂	2	65	3	55	6	26	11	146
	♀	-	59	2	63	4	39	6	161
Cheremis, USSR	♂	6	189	8	131	1	3	15	323
Eskimos									
Greenland	♂	1	16	1	12	5	11	7	39
	♀	-	13	-	22	-	11	-	46
Alaska	♂	-	22	1	9	4	16	5	47
	♀	-	21	-	12	-	5	-	38
Canada	♂	-	49	2	22	-	5	2	76
	♀	1	58	1	22	-	2	2	82
Icelanders	♂	-	65	3	84	7	207	10	356
	♀	-	79	-	78	-	204	-	361
Finns									
Oulu	♂	-	-	-	1	9	97	9	98
	♀	-	-	-	-	4	122	4	122
Kökar	♂	-	55	3	66	8	45	11	166
	♀	-	70	1	78	7	71	8	219
Total								90	2,280

RESULTS

The frequency of pterygium (Table 2) and climatic keratopathy (Table 3) increases with age. In old people who have
been leading an indoor life for some time, the pterygium
becomes pale and the pinguecula flattens to such a degree
that its existence may be impossible to evaluate. Climatic
keratopathy does not seem to change once established.

The Eskimos and Icelanders live in a tundra area, the
Lapps live in forests near the tree-line, and the Finns and
Cheremis live in forests farther to the south. The frequency of climatic keratopathy is fairly well correlated
with open country, but the occurrence of pterygium and pinguecula seems to be independent of the type of landscape.

Eskimos in South Greenland have pterygium more frequently than those in North Greenland (11), agreeing well with
the theory that UV light is the main cause of this condition. More pterygium was noted in NW Greenland (latitude
73°) than in Alaska (71°) and Canada (69°), but the number

TABLE 3
Occurrence of climatic keratopathy (K) in different age groups

Population		20-39 years K	Total	40-59 years K	Total	60+ years K	Total	Total K	Total
Lapps	♂	2	65	18	55	16	26	36	146
	♀	-	59	8	63	18	39	26	161
Cheremis, USSR	♂	2	189	10	131	-	3	12	323
Eskimos									
Greenland	♂	2	23	4	12	9	11	15	46
	♀	1	13	3	22	7	11	11	46
Alaska	♂	3	10	4	8	7	16	14	34
	♀	-	20	1	12	1	5	2	37
Canada	♂	6	49	13	22	2	5	21	76
	♀	1	58	5	22	2	2	8	82
Icelanders	♂	1	65	16	84	46	207	63	356
	♀	2	79	1	78	14	204	17	361
Finns	♂	-	-	-	1	20	97	20	98
	♀	-	-	-	-	4	122	4	122
Total								249	1,888

of subjects is too small for drawing any conclusions (Table 2). The coldest of the three settlements is Igloolik, NWT, which suggests that none of these degenerations has anything to do with temperature.

Pterygium is rare in Iceland, so that one might expect to find a low frequency of climatic keratopathy. This was not the case, however. There are few whole days with clear skies and the humidity is high in Iceland. Possibly, other components such as dust must co-exist with UV light if a pterygium is to develop, or continuous exposure to sun must be longer than the maritime climate of Iceland affords. The amount of irradiation is in any case sufficient for the formation of band keratopathy. Pterygium occurred medially with few exceptions.

In his study of the Red Sea region, Falcone (6) found that climatic keratopathy, unlike pterygium, was more common laterally. In the Arctic (Table 4), there was no clear difference in the occurrence of keratopathy medially or laterally in the cornea with or without pterygium. There were more pterygium cases without keratopathy than with keratopathy, but keratopathy was much more frequent in the pterygium cases than in the total population. The pterygium cases also had a marked pinguecula more often than the non-pterygium group.

There were no significant differences in the frequencies of climatic keratopathy and pterygium between the Eskimos and the Lapps, and no certain difference between the Eskimos, Lapps, and Icelanders in the frequency of band keratopathy, but for pterygium there were highly significant differences. There is no statistically significant difference in the frequency of pterygium between the Cheremis and the Icelanders, in spite of the striking difference of the keratopathy frequency.

Women suffer less from climate-induced changes in the eyes than men. There were 70 pterygium cases among the men and only 20 among the women; similarly, 181 men had climatic keratopathy compared with 68 women.

DISCUSSION

Climatic band-shaped keratopathy and pterygium, and possibly also pinguecula, may be attributed to excessive exposure to UV light. There ought to be a definite parallelism in their prevalences; however, this is not so. Frequency figures from the Tropics suggest a certain antagonism between the first of these two degenerations. Band-shaped keratopathy is very common in the Red Sea region, where the eyes are probably exposed to the highest concentrations of ultra-violet light in the world. However, among 54 patients with band-shaped keratopathy, in many instances leading to blindness, Bietti et al. (3) found only three definite cases of pterygium. Rodger's material from the same region (15) showed a pterygium frequency of only 2 per cent.

Wyatt (19) reported that 29 out of 320 male residents of the NWT over 40 years of age had climatic keratopathy, against only 3 women out of 332. He also confirmed Freedman's finding that nearly 90 per cent of male Labrador residents over the age of 40 showed climatic keratopathy. Freedman (9) stated that climatic keratopathy was more frequent in Labrador than in the Arctic.

In the populations investigated by our group, both climatic keratopathy and pterygium were found mainly in elderly men living out of doors, although the two conditions were not always encountered in the same individuals.

There is usually a clear zone between the limbus and the band-shaped degeneration; this probably results from a secondary lesion within the area of the climatic keratopathy. It may be that the presence of this zone prevents the formation of a pterygium. Band-shaped keratopathy has various causes, the most notorious of which is chronic

TABLE 4
Climatic keratopathy (K) in different populations (M, medially; L, laterally)

Population	Males				Females			
	K more marked		No difference	Total	K more marked		No difference	Total
	M	L			M	L		
Lapps, N. Finland	18	4	43	65	10	4	19	33
Finns, Oulu	10	3	27	40	1	2	5	8
Iceland	19	5	79	103	4	0	16	20
Cheremis, USSR	11	-	9	20	-	-	-	-
Eskimos	24	7	55	86	7	10	22	39
Total eyes	82	19	213		22	16	62	
%	26.1	6.1	67.8		22	16	62	

TABLE 5
Degree of pinguecula (Ping., arbitrary units) and height of palpebral aperture (Palp.ap, mm)

Age (years)	Lapps, N. Finland			Finns, Kökar			Cheremis, USSR			Eskimos, Greenland			Icelanders, Húsavík		
	No.	Palp.ap	Ping.	No.	Palp.ap	Ping.	No.	Palp.ap	Ping.	No.	Palp.ap	Ping.	No.	Palp.ap	Ping.
20-39	101	8.90	0.93	67	9.19	0.81	159	8.95	1.25	28	9.10	1.76	123	9.43	0.47
40-59	92	8.68	1.61	78	8.66	1.23	111	8.77	1.68	14	8.92	2.08	151	9.07	0.95
60+	48	8.64	1.79	58	8.48	1.30	2	7.04	1.63	4	8.19	1.75	92	8.83	1.23
Total	241	8.76	1.37	203	8.78	1.11	272	8.86	1.43	46	8.97	1.85	366	9.13	0.86

uveitis. In mild cases, climatic band-shaped keratopathy
resembles this condition closely. In both instances there
may be a lucid zone between the limbus band formation.
Round transparent spots are also seen in both conditions.
According to Vogt (18), they originate from vacuolar degeneration.

An astonishing finding was that there was no significant
difference in the height of the palpebral aperture between
the different ethnic groups (Table 5). Mongol eyes look very
narrow because of the elongated shape of the lids, but the
middle of the eye is nevertheless the same size as in Lapps,
Finns, Icelanders, and Cheremis, according to our findings,
and compares with the figures reported for Japanese (14)
and Greenland Eskimos (16). There seems no correlation between the degree of pinguecula and the height of the palpebral aperture (Table 5).

In cases of pterygium and keratopathy, pinguecula was
more developed than in control groups. Subjects developing
climatic keratopathy and pterygium thus seem to possess a
special disposition towards pinguecula formation.

SUMMARY

Ophthalmological investigations on climate-induced changes
in the eyes were performed during population studies on
the Lapps in northern Finland, on the Eskimos at Wainwright
in Alaska, Igloolik in the NWT of Canada, and Augpilagtoq
in Greenland, and also on populations in Iceland, Finland,
and the USSR. The frequency of climatic keratopathy is
fairly well correlated with the openness of the country,
but the occurrence of pterygium and pinguecula are independent of the type of landscape. An excessive amount of ultra-
violet light seems to cause all three conditions, which are
more frequent in males than in females. None of the three
conditions show any correlation with low ambient temperatures. Pterygium is rare in Iceland, but climatic keratopathy is as frequent as for the Lapps and Eskimos. Pinguecula occurs more frequently in both pterygium and climatic
keratopathy subjects than in normal individuals. Pterygium
is more common in keratopathy carriers than in normal subjects. It is suggested that the clear zone between the limbus and the band-shaped degeneration prevents the formation
of pterygium.

REFERENCES

1. Akimoto, M., "Clinical studies on pinguecula. Report I. Shape and incidence of pinguecula regarding the age," Acta Soc. Ophthal. Jap., 67: 143-52 (1968)
2. Akimoto, M., "Clinical studies on pinguecula. Report III. Observation of limbus portion on living body and other studies," Acta Soc. Ophthal. Jap., 70: 433-48 (1966)
3. Bietti, G.B., Guerra, P., and Ferraris de Gaspare, P.E., "La dystrophie cornéene nodulaire en ceinture des pays tropicaux à le sol aride," Bull. Soc. Ophthal. Fr., 68: 101-29 (1955)
4. Cameron, M.E., Pterygium throughout the world (Springfield, Ill.: C.C. Thomas, 1965)
5. Duke-Elder, W.S., "The pathological action of light upon the eye," Lancet 1: 1137 (1926)
6. Falcone, G., "La distrofia corneale dei tropici," Rav. Ital. Tracoma, 6: 3-17 (1954)
7. Forsius, H., and Eriksson, A.W., "Die Frequenz von Pinguecula und Pterygium bei Innen- und Aussenarbeitern," Klin. Mbl. Augenheilk., 142: 1021-30 (1963)
8. Forsius, H., "Climatic changes in the eyes of Eskimos, Lapps and Cheremisses," Acta ophthal., 50: 532-8 (1972)
9. Freedman, A., "Labrador keratopathy," Arch. Ophthal., 74: 198-202 (1965)
10. Gilland, J.G., "The cornea in Canada's northland," Canad. J. Ophthal., 5: 146-51 (1970)
11. Hertz, V., "Meddelelser om Øjensygdomme i Grønland," Ugesk. f. Laeger, 91: 805 (1929)
12. Johnson, G.J., and Ghosh, M., "Labrador keratopathy. Clinical and pathological findings," to be published in Canad. J. Ophthal.
13. Kerkenezov, N., "A pterygium survey of the far north coast of New South Wales," Trans. Ophthal. Soc. Austr., 16: 110-19 (1956)
14. Martin. R., Lehrbuch der Anthropologie (Jena, 1928)
15. Rodger, F.C., "Clinical findings, course and progress of Bietti's corneal degeneration in the Dahlak Islands," Brit. J. Ophthal., 57: 657-64 (1973)
16. Skeller, E., "Anthropological and ophthalmological studies on the Angmagssalik Eskimos," reprinted from Meddelelser om Grønland, 107: (4)
17. Talbot, G., "Pterygium," Trans. Ophthal. Soc. N.Z., 2: 42-5 (1948)

18. Vogt, A., Lehrbuch und Atlas der Spaltlampenmikroskopie
    des lebenden Auges. Teil I (Berlin: Springer, 1930)
19. Wyatt, H., "Corneal disease in the Canadian north,"
    Canad. J. Ophthal., 8: 298-305 (1973)
20. Yamamoto, K., "Observation of the pinguecula," J. clin.
    Ophthal. (Tokyo) 16: 663-73 (1962)

Types of strabismus occurring among Indians and Eskimos of the Northwest Territories

E. ELIZABETH CASS

Among Caucasian races, convergent strabismus is far more prevalent than divergent, whereas, among Asiatic races, it has been reported that divergent strabismus prevails in a proportion of 4 to 1. Among the Algonkian races, I have rarely found strabismus, and convergent concomitant strabismus occurred only in children of mixed blood. The present report concerns the form of strabismus among the peoples of the Northwest Territories.

Difficulties in conducting the examinations included the following factors:

(a) *Distribution of the population.* An enormous area is very lightly populated. The main concentration of people is around Great Slave Lake, surrounding the towns of Fort Smith, Hay River, and Yellowknife. A second concentration of approximately 1,000 people live in Fort Simpson and the satellite settlements. In the Mackenzie Delta, there were between three and four thousand Eskimo, Indian, Métis, and Whites in 1958 when the town of Inuvik, then called East Three, was being built.

(b) *Communications.* Roads are still few, and are only found around Great Slave Lake. Airports are found mainly in the larger settlements, although this situation has improved enormously in the last five years. Jet aircraft can now land at a number of airstrips in the Arctic. The single-engined Cessna, landing on lakes and rivers in the summer, and on land in the winter, has now been replaced by the more comfortable STOL twin Otter (9). At times, the survey

involved use of a dog team and canoe up the Mackenzie, and
travel by bombardier or snowmobile. Because of uncertainties of transport, some patients can only be seen at certain times of the year.

(c) *Climatic conditions*. The NWT is characterized by extremes of climate, -50 to -60°F in winter, and occasionally
above 80°F in summer. Darkness, blizzards, and poor landing
conditions often restrict flying.

(d) *Nomadic nature of the people*. Many of the indigenous
population are still trappers and hunters, only visiting
their settlements at certain seasons to trade, mend traps
and nets, and to replenish supplies and equipment.

(e) *Multiplicity of languages*. There are about six Indian languages, and sixteen dialects in the NWT, which makes
communication extremely difficult for an itinerant observer.
There are also at least three different Eskimo dialects.
School-children can communicate fairly well in English, but
the older people usually speak only their own language and
are shy about speaking English, even if they know a little.
It is the same with many preschool children. It is a great
asset if you can speak, even badly, a little of the person's
language, to give them confidence.

(f) *Varying cultures*. The cultures of the people vary.
The Loucheux Indians, for example, have strict tribal laws
against intermarriage, even by second cousins. Among the
central Eskimos (from Cambridge Bay to Pelly Bay) there is
still the habit of wife-changing on the trail, and in small
settlements, much inbreeding results in the appearance of
congenital disorders. There is also a complicated adoption
system, and it is difficult to ascertain true parentage.

ETHNIC ORIGINS

Both Indians and Eskimos are of Asiatic origin, travelling
to Canada many centuries ago. The Indians of the NWT all
belong to the Athapaskan group, and like the Chinese and
Japanese, their language has tonal qualities, varying in-
flections giving different meanings to apparently similar
words. The Eskimo were kept from migrating farther south by
the Indians and there used to be constant war between the
two groups.

ATTITUDE OF THE NATIVES

Some of the indigenous peoples still have a mistrust and
dislike of the white person. They are tired of people coming

to do surveys, taking blood and urine specimens, and not
telling them why. In some cases, they are now refusing to
co-operate, or (in order to get rid of the white man quickly) they are telling him what they think he wants to know.
Unless the people are known intimately, it is very difficult to arrive at the truth by questioning. Interpreters
also may be quite inadequate.

MODE OF LIFE

In the northerly regions, and in all the smaller settlements, the Indian and Eskimo used to live by trapping and
hunting, as did many of the Métis (those of mixed blood).
Very few have remained permanently in the smaller settlements; a few have found work in the larger settlements as
janitors in the schools and nursing stations, or as assistants in the Hudson Bay store. Those who live around
Great Slave Lake have gravitated increasingly to the
towns, where they work or more commonly live off welfare.

FOOD

The Indian and Eskimo traditionally live on a high protein,
low starch, salt, and carbohydrate diet, but in the settlements, they often live on a completely inadequate starchy,
fatty and low-protein diet. Scurvy and rickets can be found
in some settlements.

VISION

The older people never had myopia, but when the children
attend residential schools, or come to live in the settlements, myopia develops at an appalling rate. This is not
due to increased close work. Men, women, and children in
the past sewed and did fine work in poorly lighted igloos
and tents without developing myopia. The problem seems related to the change from a high protein, low carbohydrate,
salt diet, to a high starch, inadequate protein diet. A
high proportion of children born after 1940 exhibit myopia,
and the tendency is still increasing.

GROUPS STUDIED

The Indians chosen for study are (1) the Loucheux of the
Mackenzie Delta, including (a) the McPherson group at Fort
McPherson, Inuvik and Aklavik, (b) the isolated Arctic Red

River group, and (c) the Old Crow group, who live in the Yukon, but are related to the McPherson and Arctic Red Loucheux.

The Old Crow Indians are the most isolated and the most healthy. They follow strict tribal laws, and inbreeding is forbidden. The people of Arctic Red are dying out; they did not follow their tribal laws and many have congenital ocular conditions. The McPherson Loucheux have intermarried with Whites and there are many Métis.

(2) The Hare Indians live at Good Hope, five miles below the Arctic Circle. They are a completely different tribe, and have had very little contact with white people. They have no strong tribal laws and are developing congenital conditions. Alcoholic drink is also being imported in increasing quantities, with consequent ocular injuries.

(3) A third group of Indians living 100 miles south of the Arctic Circle, although called Hare Indians, are a mixture of two different tribes with substantial white blood. One group lives at Fort Norman, and the other at Fort Franklin, where they have intermarried with a few Eskimo who came down the Coppermine River, and with some Dogrib Indians who travelled up from the south. They have no strong tribal laws, and have had much contact with the whites. Congenital ocular diseases are on the increase, as also is the consumption of alcohol.

ESKIMOS

The Eskimo who live in the Mackenzie district and travel to islands off the coast are very mixed racially, as whalers have wintered in this area for over a hundred years. The people are used to strangers of all nationalities and have intermarried with them freely. They are mostly in transition, and very few live by hunting and trapping.

Along the coast, at Gjoa Haven, Spence Bay, and Pelly Bay are three much smaller and more isolated settlements on a recent small airline route. Gjoa Haven has increased rapidly from its few initial families, as other groups of Eskimo have settled there. Spence Bay has a large nomadic population, and forms the largest concentration of Eskimo in this area. They have had little contact with Whites until recent years. Pelly Bay is a small and isolated settlement with much inbreeding - it shows a high percentage of congenital ocular disease.

The coastal Eskimo at Spence Bay, Pelly Bay, and Gjoa Haven are generally far healthier than the Western Eskimo,

TABLE 1
Strabismus in Eskimos from various regions – number of cases and per cent of sample

	Western arctic Eskimo		Spence Bay		Gjoa Haven		Pelly Bay	
	No.	%	No.	%	No.	%	No.	%
Congenital	7	0.59	2	0.63	3	1.2	4	2.31
Congenital and familial	13	1.09	0	0	0	0	0	0
Acquired								
(a) following systemic infection	4	0.34	2	0.63	1	0.4	0	0
(b) following local infection of the eye	2	0.17	0	0	0	0	0	0
(c) following trauma	0	0	0	0	0	0	0	0
Concomitant	1	0.09	0	0	0	0	0	0
Total population examined	1,193		315		199		173	
Total with strabismus	27	2.26	4	1.26	4	1.6	4	2.32

Total population 2,759; total examined 1,936; total with strabismus 39 (2.03%).

TABLE 2
Strabismus in Indians from various regions – number of cases and per cent of sample

	Ft. McPherson, Aklavik, Inuvik		Arctic Red		Old Crow		Good Hope		Ft. Franklin		Ft. Norman	
	No.	%	No.	%	No.	%	No.	%	No.	%	No.	%
Congenital	1	0.19	5	2.81	0	0	8	2.5	5	2.46	1	1.02
Congenital and familial	2	0.38	3	1.69	2	0.97	0	0	2	0.99	2	2.94
Acquired												
(a) following systemic disease	0	0	0	0	0	0	1	0.33	1	0.49	1	1.02
(b) following local infection of the eye	0	0	0	0	0	0	3	0.99	0	0	0	0
(c) following trauma	0	0	0	0	0	0	2	0.66	0	0	0	0
Concomitant	1	0.19	0	0	0	0	0	0	0	0	0	0
Cause unknown	0	0	0	0	0	0	1	0.33	0	0	0	0
Total population examined	522		178		205		304		208		99	
Total with strabismus	4	0.77	8	4.50	2	0.94	15	4.9	8	3.94	4	4.10

Total population 2,076; total examined 1,516; total with strabismus 41 (2.09%).

but there have been many cases of birth trauma on the
barrens because of local customs. At parturition, the Eskimo squats to deliver her baby, and another woman gets behind her and puts a knee in her back, squeezing her stomach
hard, sometimes to the point of causing involution of the
uterus. Where birth was difficult, the Shaman (Medicine Man)
sometimes danced on the stomach. Birth trauma, therefore,
was frequent in Eskimos, and there were cases of congenital
strabismus, with no evidence of a family history.

Neither the Eskimo nor the Indian ever develop accommoda-
tive strabismus, unless there is white ancestry. Is this an
expression of genetics or environment? Or is it that a
cross-eyed person has been considered unlucky, and thus sur-
pressed?

TYPES OF STRABISMUS

The main forms of strabismus in the Eskimo are summarized
in Table 1.

In the small isolated settlement of Pelly Bay, where
there is homogenicity and wife changing on the trail, the
only cause of strabismus was congenital. The congenital and
familial strabismus is present among the western Arctic Eskimo, where there is a great deal of heterogenicity. The
parents did not suffer from strabismus.

Acquired strabismus was in some instances due to local
conditions seriously impairing vision in one eye (T.B.,
trauma, or infection), and in other instances to systemic
disease (T.B. meningitis, cerebral tuberculoma, or other
cerebral diseases). The one concomitant strabismus among
the western Arctic Eskimos had an unknown white father.
The mother also came from some other community and no one
seemed to know much about them.

Table 2 presents comparable data for the Indians mentioned in this paper. The Loucheux of the Mackenzie Delta
had not mingled with the Whites to the same extent as the
Eskimo. The percentage of strabismus among the McPherson,
Aklavik, and Inuvik Indians was low. The only one with concomitant strabismus had a white father and was quite different from the rest of the family.

At Arctic Red River where there had been more mixing
with the Whites and much more intermarrying, there was both
congenital and also congenital and familial strabismus,
with a generally higher percentage of congenital diseases.

The only cases of strabismus seen in Old Crow were congenital and familial and were found in two small boys who

TABLE 3
Influence of age of subject on prevalance of strabismus in Eskimos

Form of strabismus	Born before 1940 (N = 556)		Born 1940-59 (N = 972)		Born 1960-70 (N = 408)	
	No.	%	No.	%	No.	%
Congenital	4	0.9	6	0.6	6	1.47
Congenital and familial	3	0.5	8	0.8	2	0.49
Acquired						
(a) following systematic disease	2	0.44	4	0.41	1	0.245
(b) following local infection	0		2	0.20	0	
(c) following trauma	0		0			
Concomitant	0		1	0.10	0	
Total cases	9		21		9	

TABLE 4
Influence of age of subject on prevelance of strabismus in Indians

Form of strabismus	Born before 1940 (N = 619)		Born 1940-59 (N = 809)		Born 1960-70 (N = 88)	
	No.	%	No.	%	No.	%
Congenital	6	0.97	12	1.48	2	2.27
Congenital and familial	2	0.32	8	0.988	1	1.14
Acquired						
(a) following systematic disease	1	0.16	2	0.25		
(b) following local infection	1	0.16	2	0.25		
(c) following trauma	1	0.16	1	0.12		
Concomitant	0	0	1	0.12		
Cause unknown	1	0.16	0			
Total cases	12		26		3	

had a white father and had been adopted into other families.

At Good Hope there had been inbreeding, and a lot of alcoholism; here, there was a high percentage of congenital
strabismus, often associated with other defects. There were
no examples of congenital and familial type, but there were
cases of strabismus following disease and trauma.

At Fort Norman, Fort Franklin, and Arctic Red, none of
which follows the strict tribal laws against homogenicity,
the highest percentages of strabismus were found.

REFRACTION

Refractive errors among the older Indian and Eskimo were extremely rare and none of them, unless they had white blood,
suffered from myopia. Fairly severe compound hypermetropia
was found among the Loucheux Indians and also those living
in Fort Franklin. White explorers in the old days were not
short-sighted. It was the Hudson's Bay Company that brought
myopic clerks to the north.

However, Indian and Eskimo children born after 1940 show
a rapidly increasing prevalence of myopia.

SUMMARY

Visual problems have been studied in 1,936 Eskimos and 1,516
Indians from selected settlements in the NWT. When living
in their natural habitat, both Indians and Eskimos only
suffer a limited range of the various forms of strabismus.
Congenital strabismus is associated with homogenicity,
follows birth trauma and prenatal infections, and is often
accompanied by other congenital defects. Convergent strabismus develops in some cases with untreated trauma or infection causing monocular blindness or impaired vision and
with hypermetropia in the unaffected eye. The prevalence of
tuberculous infections and the inaccessibility of the nomad
people has led to a number of cases of paretic strabismus
following tuberculosis, meningitis, or cerebral tuberculo-
mata. Paretic strabismus has also followed other types of
meningitis. Concomitant strabismus has not been found, except in two isolated cases, both 50 per cent White. The
absence of this condition seems a racial characteristic.

REFERENCES

1. Cass, E.E., "Divergent strabismus," Brit. J. Ophthal.,
   21: 538 (1937)

2. Cass, E.E., "The Increasing Incidence of Myopia in Different Ethnic Groups in the Northwest Territories,
Canada," Read at 3rd Congress, International Society of
Geographical Ophthalmology, May 1973, Cadiz, Spain
3. Davies, L.E.C., and Hanson, S., "The Eskimo of the Northwest Passage," Canad. Med. Assoc. J., 92: 205 (1965)
4. Schaefer, O., "The changing health picture in the Canadian North," Canad. J. Ophthal., 8: 196 (1963)

Commentaries

"Acute glaucoma in the arctic; Studies of the difference
between the Eskimo and Indian peoples, and of the effects
of myopia in each group," by H.T. Wyatt, L.A. Balisky, and
O. Singh (University of Alberta, Edmonton, Canada). The
high risk of acute angle closure glaucoma among arctic Eskimos has been well documented. The same high risk does not
occur among arctic Indians. The high risk among Eskimos is
associated with an unusually high prevalence of shallow anterior chambers, which is not present among Indians. In
both races a high prevalence of myopia among the younger
age groups was found, indicating that the ocular characteristics of both groups are changing. It is suggested that
these changes in the Eskimos will lead to a reduction in
the risk of acute glaucoma in the future.

"The incidence of myopia in Finnish Lappland," by H.S.
Luukka (Department of Ophthalmology, University of Oulu,
Finland). Including Finns, Lapps, and Skolts over 900
people in Lappland have been investigated since 1967. The
refractive power of the cornea was measured with the Javal-
Schiotz keratometer and the anterior chamber depth with the
Haag-Streit 900 pachometer before and after cycloplegy.
Three hundred young male adults (soldiers) have been examined by the same methods as a control group. The prevalence of myopia seems to be higher among young than older
people. The analysis is, however, unfinished. Nutritional
circumstances of most of the people examined here have
been investigated by physiologists in Inari expeditions of

the IBP-HA project. The increase of myopia seems to fit in
with an increase in the change to "civilized" carbohydrate-
rich nutrition of recent years.

"A pedigree study of myopia in Eskimos," by R.W. Morgan
(Department of Preventive Medicine, University of Toronto,
Toronto, Canada). A survey team examined all Inuit aged 15
and over in the Canadian settlements of Gjoa Haven and
Spence Bay. For each person, the visual acuity was recorded.
All persons with a VA of 20/40 or less in either eye were
referred for confirmation and diagnosis by the team ophthalmologist. The prevalence of myopia was 4.3 per cent in persons over age 30, and 31.2 per cent in persons under age
30. For confirmed myopes selected as probands, detailed
pedigrees were constructed. The prevalence of myopia in the
relatives of probands was 15.4 per cent (expected 13.0 per
cent), thus showing a very slight excess. Out of 29 probands in 24 families, only 4 myopic parents were found, thus
indicating a non-genetic aetiology for much of the myopia
in the younger Inuit. Since there was no correlation of myopic status with height, weight, or ponderal index, nutritional factors would not appear to be the primary aetiolo-
gic agents. Theories concerning other environmental influences, including schooling, would appear to have more cre-
dibility.

"Benign conjunctival papillomas in native people," by W.G.
Pearce, S. Nigam, and B. Mielke (Department of Ophthalmology and Pathology, Charles Camsell Hospital and University
of Alberta Hospital, Edmonton, Canada). In mid-1971 the
University Department of Ophthalmology in the Charles Camsell Hospital started providing eye service and education
visits to the Inuvik zone of the Northwest Territories.
During the following three years, four unrelated Eskimo patients resident in this area were found with benign conjunctival
papillomas. Two additional cases were found among Indians
resident in northern Alberta. A search of pathology reports
for the past five years from the University of Alberta
Hospital and the Provincial Department of Public Health,
which primarily serve the white population of northern Alberta, revealed three further cases, one of which was from
an Eskimo and two were probably from Caucasians. Although
there is as yet no firm evidence that this condition has a
higher prevalence among Eskimos or native people generally,
the findings of the present report are suggestive.

OTITIS MEDIA

Ear disease among the Eskimo population of the Baffin zone

J.D. BAXTER

Ear disease is a major health problem among the Eskimo population of Canada.

During 1972-73, surveys were conducted in all thirteen hamlets and settlements in the Baffin Zone with the exception of Port Burwell. The objectives were to assess the extent of ear disease in the Eskimo population, to identify individual problems, and to initiate procedures for their appropriate management. A total of 3,770 Eskimos, 74.8 per cent of the estimated Eskimo population of Baffin Zone, were examined; 74.8 per cent were under twenty-two years and 55 per cent were under twelve years of age.

Relatively little ear pathology is present in Eskimos born prior to 1950 (Table 1). However, about 50 per cent of those born after that date have suffered or are currently suffering from middle ear disease. Approximately 20 per cent under the age of twenty years have scarring of the tympanum as a sequelae to either suppurative or serous otitis media. Acute otitis media was observed in about 6 per cent and serous otitis media in about 12 per cent of children under three years of age. Chronic forms of otitis media were observed almost exclusively among these born after 1950. Attic involvement with cholesteatoma was seen in only two ears.

The number of Eskimos with normal ears varies considerably from settlement to settlement (Table 2), most bilaterally normal ears being seen in Igloolik (81.8 per cent), and fewest at Lake Harbour (30.9 per cent). Almost 40 per cent of the Broughton Island population had minimal scarring, compared with less than 4 per cent at Hall Beach. There was little intersettlement difference in the prevalence of acute otitis media. Serous otitis media was most frequent in Pangnirtung. Chronic forms of otitis media

TABLE 1
Results of otoscopic examinations of the Eskimo population of the Baffin Zone in relation to ear pathology and age (data expressed as percentages)

Condition of ear	Year of birth											Total sample* (N=3,677)
	Before 1900 (N=10)	1900-1909 (N=52)	1910-1919 (N=107)	1920-1929 (N=159)	1930-1939 (N=256)	1940-1949 (N=331)	1950-1954 (N=246)	1955-1959 (N=472)	1960-1964 (N=866)	1965-1969 (N=845)	Post-1969 (N=333)	
Bilaterally normal	90.0	76.9	80.4	85.9	81.1	79.0	69.9	48.0	49.1	47.2	45.1	57.5
Unilaterally normal	0	1.0	2.3	2.2	3.7	3.2	5.5	8.5	5.5	6.6	6.9	5.62
Minimal scarring	10.0	19.2	13.6	7.6	11.7	13.0	12.6	26.0	22.9	21.1	11.6	18.5
Maximal scarring	0	1.9	1.4	3.5	1.4	1.7	2.4	3.5	4.0	1.8	0.3	2.5
Acute otitis media	0	0	0	0	0.2	0	0.2	0.2	0.5	1.0	5.6	0.9
Serous otitis media	0	0	0.9	0.6	0.2	0.9	1.0	1.2	2.3	5.9	12.8	3.4
Chronic otitis media	0	1.0	0.5	0.3	1.4	1.5	5.7	8.5	8.8	8.6	4.4	6.2
Chronic suppurative otitis media	0	0	0	0	0	0.6	1.8	3.3	4.3	3.1	4.3	2.7
Attic involvement	0	0	0	0	0	0	0	0.3	0.1	0	0	0.1
Not visualized	0	0	0.9	0	0.4	0.2	0.8	0.6	2.3	4.7	9.5	2.7

* Results for 98 Eskimo adults seen in Frobisher Bay were not considered to be representative of the total population in the area and are, therefore, not included in this analysis.

TABLE 2
Results of otoscopic examination of the Eskimo population of Baffin Zone classified by community

Condition of ear	Community												
	Arctic Bay (N=233)	Broughton Island (N=258)	Cape Dorset (N=442)	Clyde River (N=265)	Frobisher Bay (N=596)	Grise Fiord (N=87)	Hall Beach (N=205)	Igloolik (N=422)	Lake Harbour (N=181)	Pangnirtung (N=502)	Pond Inlet (N=344)	Resolute Bay (N=142)	Total (N=3,677)
Bilaterally normal	59.2	33.9	65.8	65.7	40.4	58.6	76.6	81.8	30.9	56.6	60.8	56.0	57.5
Unilaterally normal	4.1	6.0	7.7	4.5	6.5	2.9	7.1	5.0	4.7	7.2	4.1	0	5.6
Minimal scarring	23.8	39.7	9.2	19.6	22.4	24.7	3.9	5.5	35.1	12.9	22.0	27.8	18.5
Maximal scarring	0.4	2.9	1.8	1.1	4.7	0.6	2.2	0.2	6.4	3.8	0.9	2.8	2.5
Acute otitis media	1.3	0.4	0.6	0.8	0	0.6	2.0	1.2	0.6	1.8	1.6	0	0.9
Serous otitis media	3.0	3.3	1.7	2.1	1.9	6.3	0.2	0.8	1.9	12.0	2.5	3.5	3.4
Chronic otitis media	3.7	5.8	9.6	2.3	13.2	2.9	4.9	4.3	7.5	3.0	3.6	3.9	6.2
Chronic suppurative otitis media	3.0	2.1	2.7	1.5	6.4	1.7	1.7	0.6	5.3	0.7	1.6	4.6	2.7
Attic involvement	•0	0.6	0	0	0.2	0	0	0	0	0	0	0	0.1
Not visualized	1.5	5.2	0.9	2.5	4.4	1.7	1.5	0.7	7.7	2.2	3.1	1.4	2.7

were observed most often among the school-children of Frobisher Bay (19.6 per cent), the total population of Cape
Dorset (13.33 per cent), and the total population of Lake
Harbour (12.7 per cent). The settlement in which the fewest
chronic forms of ear disease were seen was Pangnirtung.
Chronic ear disease was more prevalent in southern than in
high northern settlements.

The prevalence of ear disease seems a relatively recent
phenomenon among the Eskimos, affecting the young to a much
greater extent than the old. The onset of chronic otitis
media seems to arise in early childhood, and no new cases
of ear disease occurred among the elementary school population in Frobisher Bay (2) and Grise Fiord over the fourteen-
month study period.

A great deal of scarring of drums was observed in ears
that were essentially disease-free and gave adequate hearing; this indicates that many ears heal spontaneously,
with little or no medical or surgical treatment. One-third
of the Cape Dorset Eskimos who had discharging ears in
1968 (1) were found in 1972 to have scarred tympani, but
their hearing was within normal limits. Similarly, in the
school population of Frobisher Bay, many more ears improved
than deteriorated over a fourteen-month interval, especially
among older children (2). Deterioration appeared to be related to recurring episodes of suppuration, which were more
common among younger children.

The precursors of chronic otitis media, acute, or serous
otitis media were noted almost exclusively in the preschool
age group. In terms of treatment, one may (1) attempt to
prevent acute or serous otitis media, (2) vigorously treat
acute or serous otitis media, to prevent its advance to
chronicity, or (3) attempt to ameliorate chronic disease
either medically or surgically. The first possibility is
the ideal, but factors underlying the incidence of acute
and serous otitis media in Eskimos remain largely a matter
of conjecture. The current high prevalence of chronic disease suggests that acute and serous otitis media affect a
greater proportion of young Eskimos now than some years ago,
but this may not be so. Acute and serous otitis media may
not have progressed so readily to a chronic form twenty or
thirty years ago.

Further evaluation is needed to decide the most appropriate treatment of chronic otitis media among the Eskimos.
Of the various surgical procedures, tympanoplasty should be
reserved for carefully selected cases in which a dry ear is
a prerequisite and appropriate follow-up is assured. Other

forms of ear surgery are rarely indicated, as the disease is primarily in the middle ear and attic involvement and cholesteatoma are not usually observed.

The initial infection stems from the nose and nasopharynx. However, the survey shed little light on factors affecting nasopharyngeal health and function. We obtained no data on the frequency of upper respiratory infections, or the relationships, if any, between ear disease, immune mechanisms, and the emotional characteristics of the Eskimo. We observed no relationship between the condition of the tonsils, which were generally small or medium-sized, and ear disease. Nor did we find evidence of nasal obstruction. The dryness of ambient air may have been an aggravating condition for the nose; a low absolute humidity led to nasal crusting and stagnation of the nasal secretions, possibly contributing thereby to Eustachian tube infection. It would be of interest to determine whether an increase in the humidity of the environment would change the prevalence of ear infections.

Impetigo was observed frequently, suggesting that standards of hygiene in the home are not yet sufficiently high. The prevalence of ear disease may also be related to standards of hygiene, and in this regard further efforts to educate the Eskimo are recommended.

One major disadvantage of the present study is that only cross-sectional data were obtained. Longitudinal studies are recommended, in which the specific effects of disease and its treatment can be manipulated experimentally in various age groups, particularly infants and preschool children.

SUMMARY

An otolaryngological survey of the Eskimo population of the Baffin Zone was carried out between March 1972 and June 1973. Its purpose was to assess the extent of ear disease, to identify individual problems, and to initiate procedures for their appropriate management. Twelve of the thirteen settlements in the zone were visited and 74.8 per cent of the Eskimo population was examined. Fifty per cent of the younger Eskimos examined had suffered or were currently suffering middle ear disease. Approximately twenty per cent under the age of twenty years had minimal or maximal scarring of the tympanum which was the sequelae of either suppurative or serous otitis media. Chronic otitis media was found mainly among the children. Between thirteen and nineteen per cent of the school population in various settle-

ments suffered from the disease. Chronic otitis media or
evidence of previous suppurative ear disease was infrequent
in adults. Chronic ear disease was more prevalent in the
southerly settlements. Longitudinal studies of the Eskimo
elementary school population in Frobisher Bay and Grise
Fiord indicated no increase in the prevalence of chronic
otitis media over a 14-month interval, suggesting that the
onset of the disease is usually in early childhood.

REFERENCES

1. Ling, D., McCoy, R.H., and Levinson, E.D., "The incidence of middle ear disease and its educational implications among Baffin Island Eskimo children," Canad. J.
   Publ. Health, 60: 385-90 (1969)
2. Ling, D., Katsarkas, A., and Baxter, J., "Ear disease
   and hearing loss among Eskimo elementary school-children,"
   Canad. J. Publ. Health, 65: 37-40 (1974)

Ear disease in western Canadian natives – a changing entity – and the results of tympanoplasty

A.J. LUPIN

The high incidence of chronic suppurative otitis media in
various Indian and Eskimo populations has been well described (1-6 and 7-25). The problem is not confined to Canada but also exists among the natives of Alaska, Greenland,
Lapland, US Indians, and natives from the northern regions
of China (29) (Table 1). There are similarities in the disease as it affects natives of the northern regions, although there is a great variability in incidence from
settlement to settlement. Our experience in the western
Canadian Arctic and in northern Alberta approximates that
of other authors. The disease affects about 40 per cent of
the population and is apparently increasing in prevalence,
hardly affecting those born before 1920. The children are
born with intact tympanic membranes, but in the majority
of those affected (89 per cent of cases), the condition
commences before two years of age. Those free of ear disease

TABLE 1
Incidence of middle ear disease (as a percentage) in
selected populations

Alaska natives	30-60
British Columbia Indians	34-54
Baffin Eskimos	30-40
Swedish Lapps	High
Western Canadian Arctic natives	30-40
England (acute otitis media)*	2.8 over all
Navajo Indians	1-6
Edinburgh, Scotland, at turn of the century	38-50

* Under 6 years of age.

at age two seem unlikely to be affected. Recurrent attacks
of otitis media occur, drainage of purulent material being
associated with perforation of the tympanic membrane. The
attacks persist throughout chilhood but appear to slow down
in teenage and later life. In the majority of cases there
is a conductive loss that may vary with the discharge (9);
if the ears are treated by local cleaning and instillation
of ear drops, loss of hearing and otorrhoea are usually the
only disabilities. A small but significant proportion of
cases, however, progress to erosion of the ossicles, adhesive otitis media, or tympanosclerosis. Attic cholesteatomas are unusual. Cholesteatomas (about 3 per cent in our
survey) appear to result from destruction of the annulus by
the disease process, with migration of canal wall skin into
the middle ear; these cases frequently require radical mastoidectomy. Sometimes sensory loss occurs additionally, perhaps as a result of infection, and sometimes the perforations close spontaneously.

Chronic ear disease can be a serious disability for the
young native patient who suffers a significant loss of verbal ability and falls behind in reading, mathematics, and
language (9, 19).

It is hard to blame anatomical factors for the prevalence of the condition in the Eskimo. The bacteriology is
unremarkable and serum immunoglobulins are normal. Secretory lgA may be deficient but this has not been resolved to
date (8). Eustachian function tests (30) have thus far
shown no dysfunction, but there is a need for further study
of this question. If breast feeding is omitted in the first
month of life, there is an associated fivefold increase in
the incidence of otitis media and a tenfold increase in the
incidence of severe cases (1). The most likely correlation

seems between the disease and poverty - overcrowding, poor
sanitation, and lack of personal cleanliness (12,23,29).

Argument has been made for and against T & A (9,19,26,
27). Our experience is that T & A does not affect the occurrence of otitis media attacks. Relatively small doses of
prophylactic ampicillin have had some success in preventing
attacks (20). Hygienic measures and improvements in sanitation have also been helpful in some areas. Aural cleansing
with dry swabs and hydrogen peroxide ear drops are useful
in clearing up particular episodes of otorrhoea, but are
unlikely to prevent further attacks. Hearing aids have been
recommended for these children (9), but we have found it
difficult to persuade children to wear them and the batteries do not function well at cold temperatures. Furthermore
the ear moulds easily get blocked with secretions.

Surgical programs are underway in various parts of the
world, notably Alaska, British Columbia, and among the Navajo populations. Their aim is to close perforations, thereby
both preventing further deterioration and improving hearing.
Various techniques of tympanoplasty exist; the second part
of this paper presents our method and the results obtained.

METHOD OF TYMPANOPLASTY

Selection was made after referral from nursing stations,
schools, local physicians, and others involved in the care
of children with noticed otorrhoea or hearing loss. The
findings were confirmed and a general history and physical
examination performed. Audiology was obtained, particularly
for pure tones. T & A was not performed unless indicated
for serious recurrent tonsillar infections. The operation
was performed under general anaesthesia, using Xylocaine
2 per cent with one in a hundred-thousand adrenaline to in-
filtrate the external ear canal and an area of the scalp
just above the pinna. A horizontal incision was made in
this latter area and a disc of temporalis fascia was removed (Figures 1-4). The incision was closed with unabsorb-
able suture and the fascia retained as a flap. The remainder of the surgery was performed trans-canal and consisted
of creating a posterior canal-wall flap based superiorly
which was elevated in continuity with the skin of the remains of the drum and the skin immediately surrounding the
annulus. Occasionally, drilling of the anterior canal wall
was needed to obtain exposure anteriorly. The surface of
the drum remnant and the edge of the perforation were
carefully denuded of epithelium. The middle ear was filled

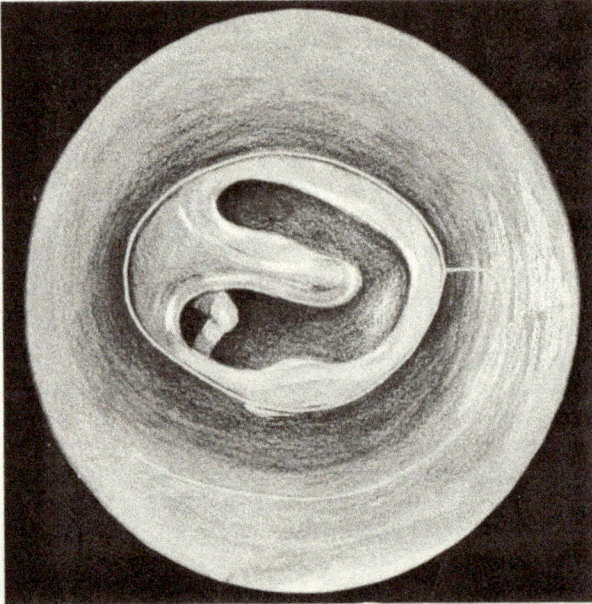

1

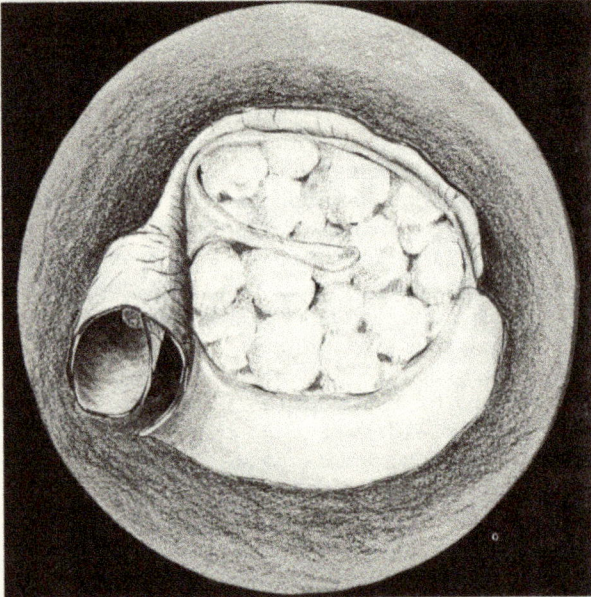

2

Figure 1   Trans-canal view of perforation; incisions outlined

Figure 2   Skin elevated; Gelfoam in place

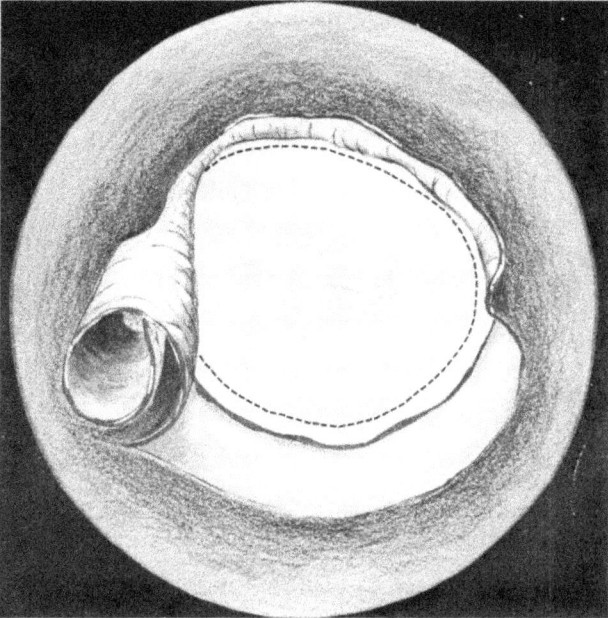

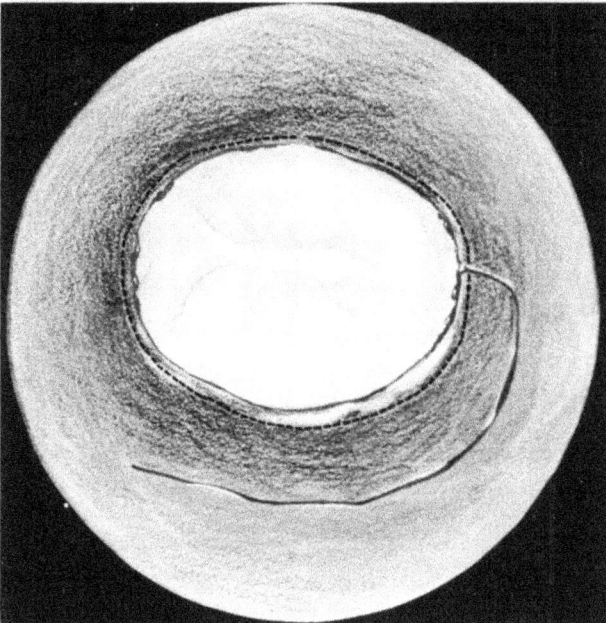

3

4

Figure 3   Fascia inserted
Figure 4   Skin replaced

with gelfoam, soaked in Synalar Bi-Otic drops. The fascia
was placed over the remains of the drum and draped a little
up the canal wall. The skin was returned so far as possible
to its original position, covering the edge of the graft,
and packed in place with more soaked gelfoam.

Postoperative care was minimal. Sutures were removed on
the seventh day. The packing was inspected and if loose it
was removed. Any postoperative breakdown that was recognized was treated by early re-operation.

Follow-up examinations one or more years after surgery
have proved very difficult. Patients change their names and
place of domicile and audiology is complicated by a lack of
quiet facilities and the difficulties of keeping a travelling audiometer calibrated. Criteria of a good hearing result were considered hearing within 10 db of the normal ear,
or better than 35 db if the damage was bilateral.

RESULTS

Of those surveyed in the Arctic, 76.6 per cent had an intact
tympanic membrane one year or more following surgery and of
these 69.5 per cent had improvement in their hearing (Table
2). In northern Alberta 79.2 per cent had intact tympanic
membranes and 75.7 per cent had improved hearing one year
or more following surgery (Table 3). The follow-up rates
are 74.5 and 54.1 per cent respectively. The effectiveness
of the surgery may be better than this, as some cases had
unilateral improvement in hearing and others had failure
followed by success from repeated surgery. The latter were
counted as separate operations and recorded as success and
failure respectively in the analysis. It also proved easier
to follow up cases that had failed, since they remained in
the memory of the nurses at nursing stations and presented
for treatment.

Complications other than failure to heal and postoperative otitis media were few. There were no cases of canal
stenosis, one wound infection of the scalp, and two cases
that developed epithelial pearls on the tympanic membrane
requiring marsupialisation. The surgery is relatively simple and painless for the patient, and revision when needed
is not very different from the original procedure as the
healing process is so effective in the skin of the deep
part of the canal.

TABLE 2
Tympanoplasty survey, 1973

	Number performed	Number surveyed	Intact TM	Hearing improved
Cambridge Bay	19	14	12	10
Fort Smith	9	3	3	2
Gjoa Haven	12	12	7	9
Coppermine and Holman Island	38	26	21	18
Spence Bay	17	17	13	12
Inuvik	9	5	4	4
Aklavik	6	5	3	4
Total	110	82	63	55
As %		74.5	76.6	69.5

TABLE 3
Tympanoplasty survey, 1973, northern Alberta

Settlement	Number performed	Number surveyed	Intact TM	Hearing improved
Athabasca	12	5	4	5
Assumption	6	4	3	3
Atikameg Area	31	21	18	18
High Prairie	13	8	8	7
Foisy Area	19	5	3	2
Calais	13	10	6	5
Duffield	25	5	5	5
Fort Chipewyan	7	6	6	6
Fox Lake	5	5	5	5
Beaverlake Area	17	1	1	0
High Level	1	1	1	1
Hobbema	46	29	22	21
Peace River area	12	11	7	6
Total	207	111	88	84
As %		54.1	79.2	75.7

COMMENT

There is a need for a better assessment of the procedure,
and a prospective study is being initiated which will en-
tail operating on one ear only in cases of bilateral tympanic membrane perforation, allowing the non-operated ear
to serve as a control. However, the physicians' ultimate

aim should be prevention, based on better education and
better living conditions for the native population. "Ear
disease is the inheritance of the poor."

SUMMARY

A review is given of otitis media in northern native populations, including incidence, natural history, the effects on
the individuals affected, and what is known of causative
factors. A brief description is given of the method used in
surgical treatment, and the results obtained. Suggestions
are made for improvement of both follow-up and home conditions for the native population.

REFERENCES

1. Schaefer, O., "Otitis media and bottle feeding," awaiting publication
2. Reed, D., Strive, S., and Maynard, J.E., "Otitis media
   and hearing deficiency among Eskimo children. A cohort
   study," Am. J. publ. Health, 57: 1657 (1967)
3. Palmer, S.J., "Survey of hearing difficulties undertaken among Alberni Indian," Indian Affairs Counselling
   Report, 11 April 1968
4. Cambon, K., Galbraith, J.D., and Kong, G.,"Middle ear
   disease in Indians of the Mount Currie Reservation,
   British Columbia," Canad. Med. Assoc. J., 93: 1301
   (1965)
5. Ling, D., McCoy, R.H., and Levinson, E.D., "The incidence of middle ear disease and its educational implications among Baffin Island Eskimo children," Canad.
   J. publ. Health, 60: 385 (1969)
6. Woodman, B., "Alaskan plan to fight otitis media among
   native people has broad impact," Nat. hear. Aid J.
   (1968)
7. Beal, D., Stewart, K.C., and Fleshman, J.K., "The surgical programme to reduce the morbidity of chronic otitis media in the Alaskan native," Circumpolar Health
   Conference, Oulu, Finland, 1971
8. Berg, D.E., Larse, A.E., and Yarrington, C.T. Jr.,
   "Association between serous and secretory immunoglobulins and chronic otitis media in Indian children,"
   Ann. Otolaryngol., 80: 766-72 (1971)
9. Baxter, J.D., and Ling, D., "Hearing loss among Baffin
   Zone Eskimos - a preliminary report," Canad. J. Otolaryngol., 1: 337-43 (1972)

10. Black, L., "Morbidity, mortality and medical care in the Keewatin area of the central Arctic, 1967," Canad. Med. Assoc. J., 101: 35-7 (1969)

11. Brody, J.A. et al., "Draining ears and deafness among Alaskan Eskimos," Arch. Otolaryngol., 81: 29-33 (1965)

12. Clark, E.T.A., Proc. Roy. Soc. Med., 55: 61 (1962)

13. Clements, D.A., "Otitis media and hearing loss in a small aboriginal community," Med. J. Austr., 1 (16): 665-7 (1968)

14. Hayman, C.R., and Kester, F.E., "Eye, ear, nose and throat infections in natives of Alaska," Northwest Med., 56: 423 (1957)

15. Jaffe, B.T., "The incidence of ear diseases in the Navajo Indian," Laryngol., 79: 2126-34 (1969)

16. Johnson, R.L., "Chronic otitis media in school age Navajo Indians," Laryngol., 77 (11): 1990-5 (1967)

17. Juselius, H., "An audiometric survey of the incidence and causes of hearing defects amongst draftees in the Vasa Military District, Finland 1954-1968," Acta Otolaryngol., 69: 117-22 (1970)

18. Kaplan, G.J., Fleshman, J.K., Bender, T.R., Baum, C., and Clark, P.S., "Long term effects of otitis media: A ten-year cohort study of Alaskan Eskimo children," Pediatrics, 52: 577-85 (1973)

19. Maynard, J.E., "Otitis media in Alaskan Eskimo children: an epidemiological review with observations on control," Alaska Med., 11: 93-8 (1969)

20. Maynard, J.E., Fleshman, J., and Tschopp, C.T., "Otitis media in Alaska Eskimo children. Prospective evaluation of chemophophylaxis," J. Am. Med. Assoc., 219: 597-9 (1972)

21. McDermott, W., Deuschle, K.W., and Barnett, C.R., "Health care experiments at Many Farms. A technological misfit of health care and disease pattern existed in this Navajo community," Science, 1: 23-31 (1972)

22. Rossi, D.F., "Hearing deficiency in Pueblo Indian children," Rocky Mountain Med. J., 69: 65-9 (1972)

23. Wallace, H.M., "The health of American Indian children," US Health Serv. & Mental Health Admin. Repts., 87: 867-76 (1972)

24. Weymuller, E.A., and Reed, D.G., "Otological problems of the Alaskan native population," Laryngoscope, 82: 1793-9 (1972)

25. Zonis, R.D., "Chronic otitis media in the southwestern American Indian," Arch. Otolaryngol., 88 (4): 360-5 (1968)

26. Fritz, M.H., "Tanarra revisited," Northwest. Med., 62:
    589 (1963)
27. Mawson, S.R., Adlington, P., and Evans, M., "A controlled
    study of adeno-tonsillectomy in children," J. Laryngol.,
    82: 963-79
28. Editorial, "Clinic travelling by earmobile to reserva-
    tions in Montana and Wyoming," Northwest Med. (Sept.
    1972)
29. Personal communication, Chinese Medical Delegation to
    Canada 1973
30. Author, unpublished work

Chronic otitis media in the Keewatin district

D. BRODOVSKY, C. WOOLF, L.M. MEDD, and J.A. HILDES

The Keewatin district comprises an area of about 200,000
square miles, situated for the most part on the west coast
of Hudson Bay. Eight small communities include the Belcher
Islands, situated almost 600 miles east of Churchill and
near the coast of Arctic Quebec. The population of approximately 3,000 is largely Eskimo, with a small proportion of
immigrant white workers from southern Canada. The University of Manitoba northern medical unit instituted visits by
consultant otolaryngologists because of the reported high
prevalence of chronic otitis media in other northern populations (1,2,3). These visits were directed primarily towards the assessment of individual cases referred by nurse-
practitioners, but as the magnitude of the problem became
evident an attempt was made to screen as many people as
possible, particularly children.

MATERIALS AND METHODS

Records were maintained on all cases seen in clinic by the
two visiting consultants. In addition, surveys of all
available school-children were undertaken in the classrooms
during each visit, and a number of adults were examined.
Some of the latter were self-selected or referred by the
nurse, but asymptomatic adults were also examined as time

TABLE 1
Prevalence of perforations of the tympanic membrane

Settlement	No. of subjects		
	Examined	With perf.	%
Baker Lake	174	75	43
Rankin Inlet	204	68	33
Eskimo Pt.	311	78	25
Coral Harbor	86	26	30
Chesterfield	72	28	39
Repulse Bay	52	18	35
Belcher Island	49	20	41
Whale Cove	18	5	28
Total	966	318	33

permitted, particularly a group from Eskimo Point. From
July 1970 to January 1974, a total of 966 patients were examined. Tympanic membrane perforation - dry or purulent -
was used as a specific criterion of disease. Audiometry was
not performed routinely.

RESULTS AND DISCUSSION

A total of 318 patients had perforations of one or both
tympanic membranes (Table 1). There was a high prevalence
in all settlements, the variability in numbers reflecting
the relative populations of these communities which range
from about 250 to 800. The largest samples were for the age
groups 6 to 10 years and 11 to 15 years, since they were
derived chiefly from school surveys. The greatest prevalence of otitis media was in the teen-age groups. Chi
square analysis showed significant differences between the
prevalence in young children (age 6 to 10) and that for the
next two older age groups. The prevalence in adults is also
significantly lower than that of the teen-age groups.
    Bilateral perforations were present in slightly over
half the diseased patients aged 6 to 10, in less than half
of the two teen-age populations, and in virtually none of
the adults. Spontaneous healing is often advanced as the
reason for the reduction in prevalence of both bilateral
and unilateral perforations in adults. However, few objective data on spontaneous healing are available in the literature. In a number of the present patients, surgery was
delayed by limitations of transportation and operating
time. Ninety-one such patients with 142 perforations were

400 Otitis media

TABLE 2
Natural change in perforations awaiting surgery
over period of 18 months

Condition	No. of ears	%
No change	135	74
Improved		
Perf. healed	14	7.7
Perf. smaller	14	7.7
Deteriorated		
New perf.	7	3.8
Perf. larger	12	6.6

examined twice or more over a period of approximately 18
months by the same two ENT consultants (Table 2). In that
period, 13 perforations healed, but seven new perforations
appeared. This is equal to a net decrease of about 2 per
cent annually, insufficient to account for the changes in
the prevalence with age (Figure 1). With regard to the preschool age group (Figure 1), the apparent prevalence is exaggerated because of selection by parents and nurses, but
this does not apply to the school surveys. The peak

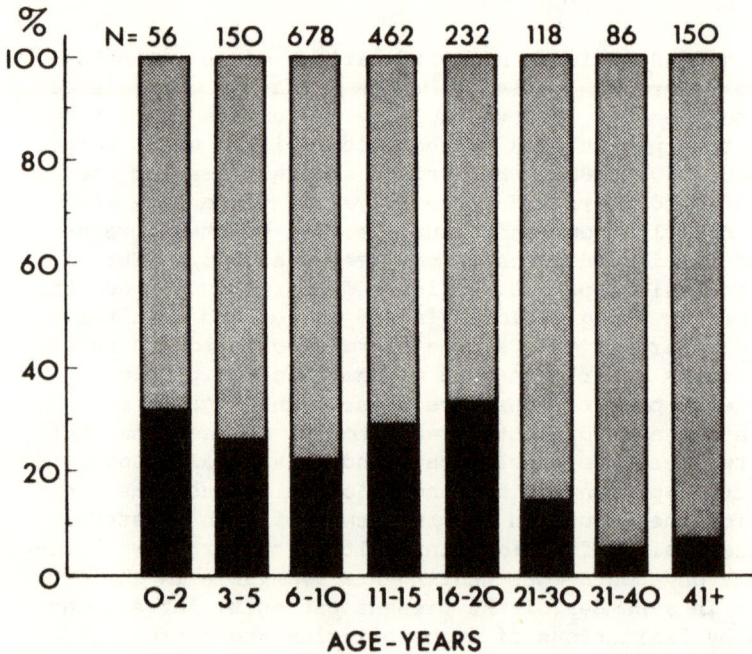

Figure 1 Percentage of ears with tympanic perforation,
classified in relation to age

prevalence in the teens probably relates to environmental factors which affect this particular age group. We think, like others (3, 4), that these children develop chronic otitis media in infancy or early childhood. The current Eskimo teen-agers spent their early years in what was a harsh and disastrous decade for the Keewatin Eskimos. Starvation and a variety of diseases were prevalent, with pulmonary tuberculosis reaching epidemic proportions. By comparison, the Baffin Zone (4) has a much lower frequency of otitis media, including the school-children born between 1955 and 1969 (the ages where the two surveys are most comparable).

The ratio of male to female subjects was 1.2:1, while the ratio of patients with evidence of otitis media was 1.6:1. The significance, if any, of the slightly higher rate of disease in the males is unknown.

A total of 123 patients came to surgery over the past three years. Initially, these patients were evacuated to Winnipeg. However, to simplify and shorten the evacuation period, a unit was established in the Ft. Churchill General Hospital, with surgery undertaken by otolaryngologists from the University of Manitoba. The majority of procedures were Type I tympanoplasties. Follow-up examinations were carried out by visiting consultants on annual or semi-annual visits to the home communities. Data on 112 patients seen at least six months postoperatively are shown in Table 3. The criterion of healing was anatomical closure as determined otoscopically. Improvement denotes a significant reduction, and failure, no change in the size of the perforation.

We wondered if the high failure rate could be attributed to patients in whom the disease process was active or where re-perforation occurred after a successful "take" of the graft. The follow-up period ranged from 6 to over 36 months. The relatively long interval between follow-up examinations does not permit us to estimate the frequency of re-perforation. On the other hand, reconstructive procedures were done to 11 patients after previous failure. Nine of these

TABLE 3
Results of reconstructive surgery

No. of operations	123
No. assessed (6-36 months post-op.)	112
Healed	60%
Improved	13%
Failed	27%

were successful, a higher rate than for the group as a whole. This would suggest that failures are due largely to factors of technique. Until preventive measures can be instituted, surgical intervention seems the best method of managing a disorder which has reached epidemic proportions.

SUMMARY

A survey of 966 Keewatin Eskimos showed a high prevalence of chronic otitis media. Tympanic membrane perforation - dry or purulent - was used as a specific criterion of the disease. The prevalence of perforations was unexpectedly high in the 11 to 15 and 16 to 20 year age groups. Environmental influences may account for this prevalence. Spontaneous healing (2 per cent per annum) does not satisfactorily explain the observed decrease in the incidence of perforations in older age groups. Reconstructive surgery was undertaken in 123 perforated drums, of which 112 have been seen postoperatively; 60 per cent healed completely, 13 per cent were partially successful, and 27 per cent failed. Possible reasons for the apparently high failure rate are explored.

REFERENCES

1. Baxter, J.D., and Ling, D., "Ear disease and hearing loss among the Eskimo population of the Baffin Zone," Canad. J. Otol., 3: 110-22 (1974)
2. Kaplan, G.J., Fleshman, J.K., Bender, T.R., Barem C., and Clark, P.S., "Long term effects of otitis media. A ten-year cohort study of Alaskan Eskimo children," Paediatrics, 52: 577-85 (1973)
3. Lind, D., McCoy, R.H., and Levinson, E.D., "The incidence of middle ear disease and its educational implications among Baffin Island Eskimo children," Canad J. publ. Health, 60: 385-90 (1969)
4. Schaefer, O., "Otitis media and bottle-feeding - an epidemiological study of infant feeding habits and incidence of recurrent and chronic middle ear disease in Canadian Eskimos," Canad. J. publ. Health, 62: 478-89 (1971)

The problem of chronic otitis media in northern Finland

A. PALVA

Northern Finland has about 600,000 inhabitants, with ENT care concentrated in four hospitals. Three each have only one otolaryngologist. The University ENT clinic in Oulu began its work in 1964 with two otolaryngologists; it now has eight specialists and eight residents, and operates on most of the chronic ear cases in Northern Finland.

The incidence of chronic otitis is about 1 to 2 per cent in Finnish draftees for military service (1), though in older age groups the figure must be a little higher. There are thus some 12 to 18,000 patients with chronic ear disease in Northern Finland. The surgical capacity of the four hospitals is currently about 350 to 400 ears per year, so that the surgical treatment of all chronic ear cases would take some 50 years. Thus the indications for surgery must be relatively severe.

The primary aim of chronic ear surgery, especially in a sparsely settled area, is to produce a safe, dry ear. Only in cases of bilateral deafness is the improvement of hearing the main indication for surgery. The order of priority for operative treatment is thus:
1. Emergency ears
2. Cholesteatomas with active infection
3. Infections not controlled by conservative treatment
4. Dry ears, bilateral deafness
5. Dry ears, with cholesteatoma
6. Dry ears, unilateral deafness

However, in practice many social considerations such as place of residence and the patient's age influence this order of indications.

Local doctors send almost every new case of chronic otitis to our Out-Patient Department to receive a treatment plan. If operation is necessary but the case is not urgent, the patient is given instructions for treatment and the local doctor takes care of him until there is opportunity to operate. This period may last from one to two years.

One month before the proposed operation the patient is again called to the Out-Patient Department. The condition of the ear is carefully estimated and possible additional

TABLE 1
Bacteria in the "chronic ear" (percentage
incidence for 956 patients at initial
visit to University ENT clinic)

Pseudomonas aeruginosa	20.7
Staphylococcus aureus	18.0
Proteus strains	12.8
Staphylococcus albus	8.5
Klebsiella-Aerobacter sp.	4.9
Difteroides	4.5
E.coli	3.7
Fungi	1.4
Mycobact. tuberculosis	0.9

TABLE 2
Results of local preoperative treatment in 685 ears (a comparison
of bacteriological findings of the initial test and after preoperative treatment)

Organism	Initial test		Preoperative test	
	No.	%	No.	%
S.aureus	140	20.5	70	10.2
S.albus	64	9.4	33	4.8
E.coli	27	3.9	11	1.6
Klebsiella-Aerobacter sp.	29	4.2	20	2.9
Proteus	85	12.4	46	6.7
P.aeruginosa	130	19.0	69	10.1
A.faecalis	21	3.1	14	2.0
Others	122	17.8	56	8.2
Fungi	10	1.5	10	1.5
Negative culture	94	13.7	99	14.4
Ear dry	111	16.2	323	47.2

TABLE 3
Complications of chronic otitis
media among 2,192 operated cases

Labyrinthine fistula	46
Labyrinthitis	24
Facial paralysis	14
Meningitis	4
Brain abscess	2
Sigmoid sinus thrombosis	1
Total	91

conservative treatment is prescribed to reduce active infection and give better prospects for tympanoplasty.

Table 1 shows the most important microorganisms in a series of 956 ears studied during the initial visit (4, 7). The bacteriology is very heterogeneous. The most problematic is Pseudomonas, the main pathogen in revision and emergency ears. Fungi play only a minor role, but tuberculosis must still be kept in mind because of its special treatment (11). The effectiveness of preoperative local treatment is shown in Table 2. Dry ears increased from 16 to 47 per cent, and most bacterial infections diminished by a half. However, the percentage of fungal infections remained unchanged.

During the years 1964-73, 2,192 chronic ears were operated on and about 600 patients remain on the waiting list. Annual figures for the various types of operation (Figure 1) show that radical mastoidectomy is usual in cases of cholesteatoma or draining ears. All operations are performed by a closed technique, without an open cavity (3,5,6,9,10). The myringoplasties include other types of tympanoplasty without eradication of the mastoid cells. The percentage of myringoplasties is increasing and that of cholesteatomas seems to remain steady. About half of the cholesteatomas are primary ones.

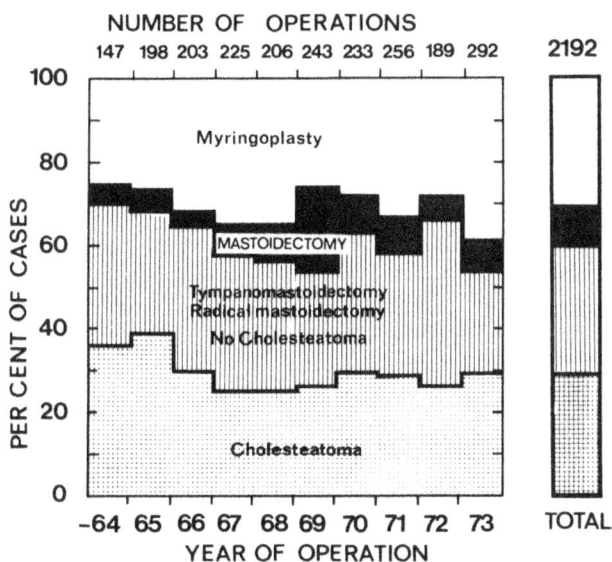

Figure 1 The annual frequency of various types of chronic ear surgery

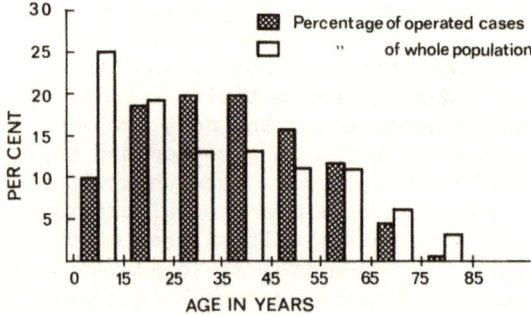

Figure 2   The age distribution of the operative material in relation to the age distribution of the whole population in Finland

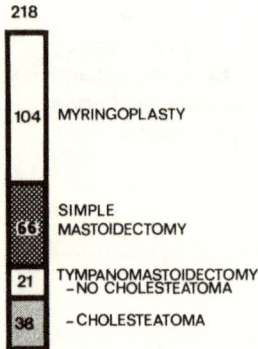

Figure 3   Types of chronic ear surgery applied to children under the age of 15 years

Complications occurred in about four per cent of cases (Table 3). Labyrinthine fistula was observed in 46 patients, and labyrinthitis causing deafness was also common. Serious complications were very rare, and all except labyrinthine fistula cases (8) were operated on as emergency ears.

Figure 2 shows the age distribution of our operative material relative to the age distribution of the entire population in Finland. Children account for only ten per cent of the operations, although we are very active in arranging operations on them (Figure 3). Most mastoidectomies are performed on patients under the age of two years and myringoplasties during school age. The small number of children requiring operation reflects effective treatment

of acute otitis and careful screening both at preschool
children's health clinics and later at school. The children's health clinic system and audiological screening began
in the mid-1940s and during the period 1954-68, the incidence of chronic otitis among draftees dropped from 3 to 1
per cent (2). In the 1930s this figure had been about 10 per
cent! The incidence of adhesive otitis media has remained
unchanged, at 1.5-2 per cent.

In Lapland this year about 1,000 of 20,000 children aged
7 to 15 years had deterioration in hearing. Only 8 of these
were cases of untreated chronic otitis, and only 3 of them
were draining. Secretory otitis media and adhesive otitis
are nowadays the main ear problems among children in northern Finland.

According to these findings, chronic otitis should diminish gratifyingly as the proportion of new cases treated in
childhood increases. However, this does not solve the whole
problem. Primary cholesteatomas, resistant microorganisms,
immunological defects, and acute necrotizing otitis will
still contribute chronic ear problems.

SUMMARY

The incidence of chronic otitis media in Finland is about
2 to 3 per cent. This implies there are 12-18,000 patients
in northern Finland. Careful selection of patients for surgery is therefore necessary. Patients with existing or
threatened complications are the most urgent cases, and comprise about 6 per cent of operations. An analysis of 2,192
chronic ear operations between 1964 and 1973 shows that the
number of myringoplasties and other tympanoplastic procedures (20 to 40 per cent) is increasing. In all other cases,
active disease necessitated eradication of mastoid cells.
The incidence of cholesteatoma was 30 to 40 per cent. The
most important pathogenic microorganisms were Pseudomonas
(20 per cent), Staphylococcus aureus (18 per cent), and
Proteus strains (11 per cent). Fungi were found in only 1.5
per cent and tuberculous otitis media in 0.9 per cent of
cases. The primary aim of surgery, especially in a thinly
settled area, is a safe and dry ear. Only in cases with bilateral deafness is the improvement or restoration of hearing the main indication for surgery.

408   Otitis media

REFERENCES

1. Juselius, H., "An audiometric survey of the incidence and causes of hearing defects among draftees in Finland, 1954-1955," Acta Otolaryngol., 55: 393-404 (1962)
2. Juselius, H., "An audiometric survey of the incidence and causes of hearing defects among draftees in the Vasa military district, Finland, 1954-1968," Acta Otolaryngol., 69: 117-22 (1970)
3. Palva, T., Palva, A., and Salmivalli, A., "Radical mastoidectomy with cavity obliteration," Arch. Otolaryngol., 88: 119-23 (1968)
4. Palva, T., Kärjä, J., Palva, A., and Raunio, V., "Bacteria in the chronic ear. Pre- and postoperative evaluation," Pract. oto-rhinolaryngol., 31: 30-45 (1969)
5. Palva, T., Palva, A., and Kärjä, J., "Myringoplasty," Ann. Otol. Rhinol. Laryngol., 78: 1074-80 (1969)
6. Palva, T., Palva, A., and Kärjä, J., "Cavity obliteration and ear canal size," Arch. Otolaryngol., 92: 366-71 (1970)
7. Palva, T., Kärjä, J., and Palva, A., "Bacterial analyses in chronic otitis media," ORL Digest, 33: 19-26 (1971)
8. Palva, T., Kärjä, J., and Palva, A., "Opening of the labyrinth during chronic ear surgery," Arch. Otolaryngol., 93: 75-78 (1971)
9. Palva, T., Palva, A., and Kärjä, J., "Musculoperiosteal flap in cavity obliteration. Histopathological study seven years postoperatively," Arch. Otolaryngol., 95: 172-7 (1972)
10. Palva, T., Palva, A., and Kärjä, J., "Occicular reconstruction in chronic ear surgery," Arch. Otolaryngol., 98: 340-8 (1973)
11. Palva, T., Palva, A., and Kärjä, J., "Tuberculous otitis media," J. Laryngol. Otol., 87: 253-61 (1973)

Audiological problems of the Eskimo population in the Baffin zone

D. LING

Five teams surveyed all 13 hamlets and settlements of the Baffin zone, with the exception of Port Burwell, during the period March 1972-September 1973 (1). Of the total population of 5,041 Eskimos, 3,574 were rated as to hearing ability, most by means of audiometric screening. This paper summarizes audiological findings and describes procedures initiated to prevent and treat the type of audiological problems discovered. Results obtained during a follow-up visit to each settlement are also reported.

HEARING ASSESSMENT

A high level of ambient noise was present wherever we worked in the nursing station or the school. Our procedure was therefore to screen at 30 dB over the frequencies 500, 1,000, 2,000, and 4,000 Hz, and if subjects failed to respond at any one of these frequencies, to obtain a full audiogram. For children under five yeras of age, speech tests using rhyming words or mothers' reports on hearing status were accepted. Significant hearing loss was considered to be present if subjects over five years had thresholds greater than 35 dB (ISO) at any two frequencies or if children under five years were reported by their mothers to have hearing difficulty.

Sensorineural hearing loss was by far the most common audiological problem. Bilateral impairment of this type was found in 13.9 per cent of adult males and 21 per cent of adult females, but less than 1 per cent of children under 18 years of age, and was associated with extensive exposure to noise from snowmobiles and rifles. The proportion of Eskimos who had serious hearing loss varied considerably from one settlement to another. The number affected in each settlement was roughly proportional to the amount of hunting done and the distance travelled to the hunting grounds. The proportion in Pangnirtung was extremely high; that in Grise Fiord relatively low.

Significant bilateral conductive hearing impairment was found in 5.4 per cent of the population. Very few adults

over 30 had conductive hearing loss. It was much more common
in the 18 to 30 year old age group, of whom about 15 per
cent were affected, than in children 18 and younger, of whom
less than 2 per cent had significant hearing loss. The reason for the lower prevalence in the children is not that
there was less ear disease in this group; on the contrary,
there was more, but when the disease is active, hearing levels are not so severely affected as when perforations are
dry, or adhesions have been established. As with sensorineural hearing loss, the proportion of conductive impairment
varied considerably from one settlement to another. Cape
Dorset and Frobisher Bay (including Apex) were outstanding-
ly worse than Pond Inlet, Clyde River, or Arctic Bay.

Mixed (sensorineural and conductive) hearing loss was relatively uncommon, occurring in less than 1 per cent of
cases in any age group; this suggests that conductive lesions
tend to serve as a protective mechanism against noise damage.

Congenital hearing loss was found in only six Eskimos.
We heard of four more congenitally deaf children who were
away at schools in the South. The prevalence of congenital
sensorineural impairment thus appears to be 0.2 per cent,
similar to the national average.

PREVENTION OF HEARING IMPAIRMENT DUE TO NOISE EXPOSURE

There are two main sources of noise in the Eskimo's life:
the snowmobile and the rifle. The reduction of snowmobile
and rifle noise at source is unrealistic, since hunting is
necessary to the Eskimo way of life. The alternative is to
use earplugs, earmuffs, or noise-reducing helmets. We selected earplugs and, through the Frobisher Bay General Hospital, had them distributed to Eskimos in various settlements.
In two settlements, earplugs were regularly worn by most
hunters, but in other settlements, although earplugs had
been made available, they were not worn. The difference apparently reflected the enthusiasm generated by the nurse
and her Eskimo assistant who distributed the earplugs. Of
some 30 young adult hunters who wore earplugs when hunting,
none had a worse threshold, and most had thresholds which
had improved by some 5-10 dB in comparison to those obtained one year earlier. In contrast, all of the 20 or so
who had not worn earplugs when hunting had lost hearing over
the one- to two-year period since previous audiometric testing. Further educational efforts are needed to ensure that
all Eskimo hunters are made aware of the implications of
noise for their hearing.

HEARING AIDS

We considered all subjects who had either an average bilateral conductive loss>35 dB or an average bilateral sensorineural loss>35 dB at 1,000 Hz and > 40 dB at 2,000 Hz to
be potential candidates for hearing aid usage. Behind-the-
ear type hearing aids with HAIC gains of 40 to 50 dB, frequency range 250-4,200 Hz and maximum output of 120 dB were
used, with standard earmoulds to test each candidate. Speech
tests in Eskimos were then employed to determine whether the
candidate could read better with the hearing aid than without it. Where improvement in hearing for speech was considerable (183 cases), a hearing aid was recommended.

Immediately following our survey, enough hearing aids
were purchased to meet the needs of four settlements and to
fit a number of elementary school-children in Frobisher Bay.
A few months after these aids had been distributed, we visited all settlements again, first to evaluate the use of
hearing aids already supplied and secondly to re-examine
those Eskimos initially considered as candidates for hearing
aid usage (2).

In general, we found that the hearing aids had been accepted and were in use. Few Eskimos wore them all the time,
but most used them on occasions that demanded better hearing, e.g., church, settlement meetings, and family gather-
ings. In most settlements, the nursing staff had taken considerable care in issuing hearing aids, had interpreted instructions for the recipients, had ensured that batteries
were available, and had seen that earmould tubing was adequately adjusted.

ACKNOWLEDGMENTS

The writer would like to thank Drs D. Cameron and J.D.
Baxter and the staff of the Department of Otolaryngology,
Royal Victoria Hospital, for their help and support during
the various surveys. Thanks are also due to numerous people,
particularly nurses and teachers in the settlements. The
work was supported in part by National Health Grant 604-7-
725.

SUMMARY

An audiometric survey has been carried out on 3,574 of
5,041 Eskimos in the Baffin zone. Pure-tone audiometric
screening tests were undertaken at 30 dB (ISO) on children

attending school and on most adults in each community.
Middle ear impedance measures were also made on over 350
children and adults. Significant hearing loss secondary to
otitis media was found mainly in children, several of whom
were educationally handicapped by severe conductive impairment. Among adults, hearing impairment secondary to noise
exposure (principally from snowmobiles and rifles) affected
about 85 per cent of males and 15 per cent of females. Hearing aids were required by about 5 per cent of the total
population.

REFERENCES

1. Baxter, J.D. and Ling, D., "Ear disease and hearing loss
   among the Eskimo population of the Baffin zone," Canad.
   J. Otolaryngol., 3: 110-122 (1974)
2. Ling, D., Baxter, J.D., and Naish, S.J., "Provision of
   hearing aids and ear defenders for Baffin zone Eskimos,"
   Institute of Otolaryngol. Monogr., McGill University,
   1974

Commentaries

"The relationship between suboptimal nutrition and chronic
otitis media in Inuit children in the eastern Arctic," by
P.J. Manning and M.E. Avery (Frobisher Bay General Hospital,
Frobisher Bay, NWT, Canada and Montreal Children's Hospital,
Montreal, Canada). An examination of the prevalence of chronic otitis media among all age groups in eastern Arctic
settlements reveals evidence of significant variation in
the incidence of the disease in these communities. Some evidence is presented that the disease process was not historically always prevalent among Inuit people in this area, but
is of comparatively recent onset and may still be on the increase. These factors lend weight to the hypothesis that the
causative factors are environmental, rather than genetically
determined. Deterioration in nutritional status of affected
groups is proposed as the environmental factor most logically implicated as a causative factor.

"Reconstructive middle ear surgery in Alaskan natives," by
J.D. Williams (The Alaska Clinic, Anchorage, USA). Changes
in surgical technique have produced an increase in tympanoplasty survival rates as well as improved hearing levels and
a significant reduction in post-operative complications.

DENTAL HEALTH

Inuit culture change and oral health: a four-year study*

J.T. MAYHALL

The effects of culture change on the oral health of the
Inuit (Eskimo) have been the subject of several studies.
These have been primarily intercommunity comparisons, in
which degrees of acculturation were inferred from dietary
differences (4,7,9,10). A few longitudinal studies have
charted the oral health within one community during a
period of rapid cultural change partially reflected by altered diet (1,3,6). The present study reports such observations over a four year period (1969-73) in two Northwest
Territories communities (Hall Beach and Igloolik), both located in the Foxe Basin area north of Hudson Bay.

When the two communities were first examined in 1969,
Hall Beach was the centre of population for those individuals and their families employed at the DEW line radar base,
and consequently they appeared to be exposed to a southern
Canadian type of diet. Igloolik, although larger, was more
isolated and a smaller percentage of the family heads were
engaged in wage employment.

By 1973, when the residents were again examined, differences between the communities were being rapidly oblitera-
ted. Igloolik had become the district administrative centre, and the chances for wage employment were greatly expanded, with associated opportunities to purchase an increased amount of processed food. Hall Beach, on the other
hand, displayed a decrease in wage employment because of
the phasing-out of DEW line employment for the Inuit. In
1969, DEW line employees and their families lived at the
radar site, but by 1973 they had been moved to the village,
away from the readily available southern Canadian foods.

* This study forms part of the multidisciplinary Canadian
International Biological Program, Human Adaptability Project.

In 1969, parents questioned about their children's dietary habits indicated that their offspring were consuming
essentially the same food as they. But, by 1973, almost all
parents noted that their children were subsisting primarily
on commercial foods, and, when money was available, enormous quantities of soft drinks and candies were being consumed. In fact, the most dramatic shifts in diet from native to commercial foods were noted in these caries-prone
age groups.

EXAMINATION

All residents of both communities were asked to participate
in the study of 1969 and 1973. At both times, nearly all
of the residents present in the area co-operated. Each examination included a discussion about food consumption for
each member of the family, an oral examination using a
mirror explorer and good artificial light, as well as other
routine diagnostic procedures not reported here. No radiographs were available for this examination.
    In 1969, Dr Otto Schaefer conducted the diet survey with
the aid of a knowledgeable interpreter, and in 1973 the
author was aided by Mr Simon Iyerak, an Inupik speaker.
Briefly, the subject was asked to appraise what proportion
of his diet was made up of processed food and what portion
came from the land.

DENTAL CARIES

Tables 1 and 2 illustrate dental caries rates for the two
communities, as reflected through the number of decayed,
filled, and missing permanent teeth and the number of decayed and filled deciduous teeth (DMFT). At all ages, both
communities show appalling increases in the caries rates
over only four years. Earlier, it was hypothesized that the
most rapid cultural change was to be found in Igloolik,
with Hall Beach also changing, but not as rapidly. The
caries rates fit this trend, increases for males and females being 59.7 per cent and 77.9 per cent at Igloolik and
43.1 and 64.2 per cent at Hall Beach.
    An earlier cross-sectional study (5) also demonstrated
the effects of dietary differences within the Igloolik community in 1969. When those subsisting primarily on purchased food were compared with those obtaining their food
from the land, increases of DMFT for the "acculturated"
Eskimos were of the order of 2.8 times (2.34 teeth affected

TABLE 1
Caries experience among Igloolik Inuit (males and females)

Age	1969		1973		
	N	Mean*	N	Mean*	% change
0-5	132	2.84	69	7.37	+159.5
6-10	58	4.67	101	5.75	+ 23.0
11-15	41	2.75	56	5.14	+ 87.0
16-20	30	3.13	30	6.44	+105.6
21-25	38	2.79	24	8.79	+215.1
26-30	35	4.31	19	5.99	+ 39.2
31-35	30	3.76	25	5.80	+ 54.3
36-40	13	1.84	15	5.00	+171.6
41-45	10	3.60	5	4.60	+ 27.8
46-50	10	7.10	6	7.50	+ 5.6
51-55	14	7.14	8	13.87	+ 94.3
56-60	5	8.40	8	11.00	+ 31.0
61+	7	16.29	5	7.20	- 55.8
All ages	423	3.81	371	6.51	+ 71.0

* Permanent decayed, missing, and filled teeth per individual
plus deciduous decayed and filled teeth per individual.

TABLE 2
Caries experience among Hall Beach Inuit (males and females)

Age	1969		1973		
	N	Mean*	N	Mean*	% change
0-5	54	2.87	29	6.31	+120.0
6-10	18	4.17	38	5.87	+ 40.8
11-15	18	3.94	21	5.76	+ 46.1
16-20	18	4.44	12	5.67	+ 27.6
21-25	15	8.06	16	12.44	+ 54.3
26-30	6	4.83	8	8.37	+ 73.4
31-35	7	13.14	11	13.82	+ 5.1
36-40	7	7.00	6	6.00	- 14.3
41-45	7	6.43	9	12.45	+ 93.6
46-50	3	8.00	6	7.83	- 2.1
51-55	2	18.50	2	25.00	+ 35.1
56-60	1	8.00	0	-	-
61+	4	18.00	3	23.33	+ 29.6
All ages	160	5.36	161	8.25	+ 53.9

* Permanent decayed, missing, and filled teeth per individual
plus deciduous decayed and filled teeth per individual.

versus 6.47 teeth affected). In both cross-sectional and longitudinal studies, the genetic components remained constant, thus eliminating one deficiency of previous inter-community comparisons of dental health. We can see clearly that with an increased consumption of processed foods, the dental caries rates increase.

PERIODONTAL DISEASE

A recent re-evaluation of a group of inland Alaskan Eskimos pointed out that over an eight year interval the prevalence of periodontal disease had increased significantly (3). The Foxe Basin residents were examined in 1969 and again in 1973, using the same criteria (i.e., Russell's Periodontal Index (8)). Kristoffersen and Bang (3) noted that Alaskans experienced little periodontal disease when they were first examined in 1957. Hypermobile teeth were not observed and tooth loss was minimal even in older individuals. Table 3 indicates that the Foxe Basin Inuit are still relatively free of periodontal disease, although there are large increases in the initially low rates for the 11 to 15 years age group. Again, when the cross-sectional data from 1969 (5) were evaluated, there were no statistically significant differences of periodontal disease between the different dietary groupings. It is probably too early to detect significant differences of periodontal disease, but this is an aspect of oral pathology that should be followed closely in the future as cultural changes continue in the Foxe Basin area.

TABLE 3
Foxe Basin Inuit periodontal index score (males and females)

Age	1969			1973		
	N	Mean	s.d.	N	Mean	s.d.
6-10	45	0.03	0.09	117	0.04	0.10
11-15	57	0.07	0.14	76	0.13	0.26
16-20	43	0.09	0.23	42	0.06	0.16
21-25	47	0.03	0.09	40	0.01	0.02
26-30	31	0.10	0.23	26	0.08	0.28
31-35	36	0.07	0.29	36	0.06	0.27
36-40	18	0.16	0.45	21	0.16	0.67
41-45	13	0.06	0.12	14	0.19	0.28
46-50	11	0.60	1.61	12	0.56	1.32
51+	27	2.04	3.17	26	1.41	2.55

418   Dental health

ORAL HYGIENE

Oral hygiene was measured during both the 1969 and 1973 examinations, using the Oral Hygiene Index proposed by Greene
and Vermillion (2). The Debris Index (DI) and the Calculus
Index (CI) measure the number of thirds of the clinical
crowns of teeth present covered with soft debris or supra-
gingival calculus respectively. Both lingual and buccal surfaces of all teeth were examined. The results are presented
in Table 4. It has been almost axiomatic that with a decreased intake of fibrous foods, such as meat, the teeth
should be dirtier, but that commonly held opinion is not
supported in this study. In fact, over the four year interval, the amounts of calculus and debris evident were reduced. This should not be surprising in the light of the
cross-sectional results from 1969 (5). In that study, no
significant differences of calculus and debris deposition
were discernible between the different dietary groups. The
reductions seen in this study may be due partially to better
dental care during the intervening period and much more emphasis by the government dentist, nurses, and myself on the
benefits of good oral hygiene.

ORAL HEALTH AND ORAL HYGIENE

Pearson's product-moment coefficients were determined for
the adult subjects, showing relationships between debris
and calculus levels in 1969 and 1973; highly significant

TABLE 4
Foxe Basin Inuit oral hygiene (males and females): data for debris index
(DI) and calculus index (CI); see text

Age	1969					1973				
	N	DI	s.d.	CI	s.d.	N	DI	s.d.	CI	s.d.
6-10	45	1.11	0.66	0.02	0.07	117	0.50	0.60	0.00	0.00
11-15	57	0.96	0.67	0.02	0.07	76	0.32	0.45	0.01	0.06
16-20	43	0.89	0.50	0.11	0.17	42	0.18	0.35	0.02	0.07
21-25	47	1.14	0.53	0.46	0.35	40	0.11	0.21	0.11	0.20
26-30	31	1.47	0.64	0.63	0.39	26	0.24	0.39	0.27	0.34
31-35	36	1.68	0.57	0.81	0.29	36	0.22	0.30	0.43	0.39
36-40	18	1.87	0.74	0.86	0.30	21	0.45	0.54	0.59	0.42
41-45	13	1.60	0.46	0.92	0.20	14	0.62	0.55	0.62	0.43
46-50	11	1.97	0.65	1.00	0.34	12	0.55	0.53	0.83	0.50
51+	27	2.31	0.75	1.31	0.65	26	0.99	0.89	0.92	0.56

correlations were found in each year (1969: $r = 0.613$, df = 189; 1973: $r = 0.614$, df = 175), emphasizing the relationship between poor oral hygiene and the amount of calculus deposition. There was also a smaller but highly significant relationship between the amount of debris on the teeth and the degree of periodontal disease ($r = 0.337$, df = 258). However, the amount of debris was unrelated to DMFT rates ($r = 0.081$, df = 408).

The periodontal index was significantly correlated with the number of missing teeth in those over twelve years of age (1969: $r = 0.538$, df = 258; 1973: $r = 0.433$, df = 259). This suggests that the higher DMFT rates in older individuals (Table 3) are the result of previous periodontal disease and not caries.

RECOMMENDATIONS

After completing the initial examinations in 1969 (5) I stated that "...the caries rate will continue to increase unless preventive measures are employed," but the increase over the short period of this study is truly shocking. McPhail and his co-workers (4) recommended that the serious state of dental health in the district of the Northwest Territories they studied "...dictates an immediate increase in the amount and regularity of emergency care and basic treatment and ... preventive measures." The same recommendations are applicable to the Foxe Basin. In this area, it is not too late to prevent periodontal disease and dental caries instead of merely repairing the damage caused by these destructive processes.

ACKNOWLEDGMENTS

I wish to thank the following people for their continuing support and encouragement: Dr J.A. Hildes, Professor D.R. Hughes, Dr O. Schaefer, Mrs M.F. Mayhall, and Mr Simon Iyerak. This study was supported by a grant from the National Research Council of Canada through the Canadian International Biological Program, Human Adaptability Section.

SUMMARY

Examination of the Inuit (Eskimo) of the Foxe Basin area of the Northwest Territories in 1969 and again in 1973 revealed results which are comparable to results from Igloolik, NWT in 1969. In both studies, dental caries rates are

extremely high among individuals who, in a rapidly changing
culture, have moved from a native diet to one with a high
proportion of processed foods. No major changes of oral hygiene, calculus deposition, or periodontal disease are seen,
although other studies indicate it may be too early to expect dramatic changes in periodontal disease. It is recommended that preventive measures be instituted now, to fore-
stall pending increases in the oral pathology of these
Inuit.

REFERENCES

1. Bang, G., and Kristoffersen, T., "Dental caries and
   diet in an Alaskan Eskimo population," Scand. J. Dent.
   Res., 80: 440-4 (1972)
2. Greene, J.C., and Vermillion, J.R., "The oral hygiene
   index: a method for classifying oral hygiene status,"
   J. Am. Dent. Assoc., 61: 172-9 (1960)
3. Kristoffersen, T., and Bang, G., "Periodontal disease
   and oral hygiene in an Alaskan Eskimo population," J.
   Dent. Res., 52: 791-6 (1973)
4. McPhail, C.W.B., Curry, T.M., Hazelton, R.D., Paynter,
   K.J., and Williamson, R.G., "The geographic pathology
   of dental disease in Canadian central arctic populations," J. Canad. Dent. Assoc., 38: 288-96 (1972)
5. Mayhall, J.T., "The effect of culture change upon the
   Eskimo dentition," Arctic Anthropol., 7: 117-21 (1970)
6. Möller, I.J., Poulsen, S., and Nielsen, V. Orholm, "The
   prevalence of dental caries in Godhavn and Scoresbysund
   districts, Greenland," Scand. J. Dent. Res., 80: 169-80
   (1972)
7. Price, W.A., "Relation of nutrition to dental caries
   among Eskimos and Indians in Alaska and Northern Canada," J. Dent. Res., 14: 227-9 (1934)
8. Russell, A.L., "A system of classification and scoring
   for prevalence surveys of periodontal disease," J.
   Dent. Res., 35: 350-9 (1956)
9. Russell, A.L., Consolazio, C.F., and White, G.L.,
   "Dental caries and nutrition in Eskimo Scouts of the
   Alaska National Guard," J. Dent. Res., 40: 594-603
   (1961)
10. Russell, A.L., Consolazio, and White, G.L., "Periodon-
    tal disease and nutrition in Eskimo Scouts of the Alas-
    ka National Guard," J. Dent. Res., 40: 604-13 (1961)

The dental disease status of Indians resident in
the Sioux Lookout zone of northern Ontario

K.C. TITLEY and J.T. MAYHALL

The delivery of dental services, the geography of the area,
and the location of communities in the Sioux Lookout zone
of Northern Ontario have been described previously by
Titley (5). Apart from a pilot survey in 1970 (2) of a small
number of children from two communities, no knowledge of the
levels of dental disease in Indians resident in the area existed. In May 1973, however, funds were made available to
carry out a more complete dental survey of Indian communities in the Sioux Lookout zone.

MATERIALS AND METHOD

Over a one-month period, three second-year dental students
from the Faculty of Dentistry, University of Toronto, were
trained to examine patients for clinical caries, occlusion
according to angles classification, oral hygiene according
to the modified debris index of Greene and Vermillion (1),
stain according to presence and colour, and periodontal disease according to a modification of the Russell index (4).
In addition, the students were instructed in the taking of
bitewing and upper and lower anterior occlusal radiographs.
      Examinations were carried out using disposable mouth
mirrors and sickle probes (3) either in natural daylight or
artificial light, and findings were recorded with an elec-
trographic pencil on WHO type A Dental Health Evaluation
cards.
      Three Siemens Heliodent X-Ray machines were purchased,
but only arrived midway through the survey so that only 25
per cent of the people surveyed were radiographed.
      Through the months of June, July, and August 1973, the
students moved freely within the zone, carrying out dental
examinations and dispensing toothbrushes, paste, and oral
hygiene instruction to the Indians. At each community they
met the Chief to explain what they were doing and asked
permission to carry out the survey - on no occasion were
they refused. The two principal investigators (K.C.T. and
J.T.M.) visited the students on location midway through
the summer to check on their progress.

TABLE 1
Percentage survey of nursing stations and satellites

	N	% of total population	% survey of nursing station and satellites
Big Trout Lake (5)	1,721	24.1	30.1
Pikangikum (1)	820	11.5	53.3
Sandy Lake (3)	1,463	20.5	54.4
Round Lake (3)	930	13.0	45.4
Landsdowne House (1)	700	9.8	74.0
New Osnaburgh (2)	833	11.7	43.7
Fort Hope (1)	684	9.6	29.1
Total	7,151	100.0	

Note: 45.5 per cent of the total population was surveyed.
Number of satellite communities in parentheses.

RESULTS

The Sioux Lookout zone is divided into seven areas consisting of a nursing station serving that community and at least one or more satellite communities (Table 1). There is a total of 23 communities, with populations ranging from 17 to 1,002. All communities, except the New Osnaburgh nursing station, are accessible only by air.

The total population of the zone in 1973 was 7,151 treaty Indians. An average of 45.5 per cent took part in the survey (Table 1), but this figure varied from one community to another, being dictated by aircraft scheduling and, in some cases, accessibility of satellite communities.

The Sioux Lookout caries experience is presented in Table 2. All DMF figures are the results of clinical survey alone; radiographic data have not been included. Decayed, missing, and filled teeth (DMFT) figures for permanent teeth are divided into two groups and afford comparison between teenagers under 17 years of age and adults of more than 20 years of age. In view of variations in the time of exfoliation of deciduous teeth, decayed, extracted, and filled teeth (DEFT) figures are recorded only up to 11 years of age. Mean DMFT and DEFT figures reveal no difference with respect to community size or availability of nursing stations. The mean DMFT for permanent teeth more

TABLE 2
Summary of Sioux Lookout caries experience, 1973

	Permanent teeth, ages 0-17 years			Permanent teeth, ages 20+ years			Deciduous teeth, ages 0-11 years		
	Mean DMFT*	Mean decayed	Mean filled	Mean DMFT*	Mean decayed	Mean filled	Mean DEFT*	Mean decayed	Mean filled
Communities with nursing stations	5.70	2.90	2.05	13.37	5.39	1.09	8.05	5.13	0.71
Communities without nursing stations N>200	5.75	2.21	2.80	11.57	4.88	0.74	7.36	4.22	0.84
Communities without nursing stations N<200	5.54	2.29	2.33	12.63	4.95	0.84	7.23	4.20	0.67
Mean totals for Sioux Lookout zone	5.59	2.63	2.27	12.81	5.17	0.95	7.90	4.97	0.78

* DMFT = decayed, missing, or filled teeth; DEFT = decayed, extracted, or filled teeth.

than doubles at 20+ years compared with age 0-17 years. However, the sum total of mean decayed and mean filled teeth is similar in these two age categories, which implies that the increase in DMFT at age 20+ years is due to missing (i.e. extracted) teeth.

For the past three years, treatment priority has been given to the permanent teeth of the teenage population (5). Thus, 2.63 teeth on average are decayed and 2.27 are filled at ages 0-17 years, compared with 5.17 teeth decayed and 0.95 filled for ages 20+ years. Some 46 per cent of decayed permanent teeth have been filled in the teenage sample surveyed, whereas only 16 per cent have been filled in the adult population. It might also be noted that only 14 per cent of decayed deciduous teeth have been filled.

As indicated above, radiographic results have not been included. While examining the radiographs for caries, however, it was decided to record incidental pathology (Table 3). It is rather disturbing to find that among 757 patients there was periapical pathology involving 92 permanent and 87 deciduous teeth. It is conceivable that more pathology of this type exists in these patients since bitewing radiographs do not show the periapical areas. In 107 instances, pre-molars were prevented from erupting; this may indicate that, in the absence of space maintenance, serial extraction may be the treatment of choice for some of these patients.

TABLE 3
Incidental findings of patients radiographed in survey

No. of patients	757
Total radiographs	2,596
Bitewings	1,298
Anterior occlusals (maxilla)	649
Anterior occlusals (mandible)	649
Incidental findings	
1. Periapical rarefying osteitis	
Permanent teeth	92
Deciduous teeth	87
2. Premolars prevented from erupting owing	
to premature loss of primary teeth	107

CONCLUSIONS

A high level of dental disease exists in the Sioux Lookout area. Neither community size nor the presence of a nursing station appears to influence DMF figures. According to the sample surveyed, only a small proportion of dental disease has been treated. Examination of radiographs taken for diagnosis of caries revealed significant amounts of pathology.

ACKNOWLEDGMENT

Research for this study was supported in part by a research grant from Colgate-Palmolive Company.

REFERENCES

1. Greene, J.C., and Vermillion, J.R., "The simplified oral hygiene index," J. Am. Dent. Assoc., 68: 7 (1964)
2. Hargreaves, J.A., and Titley, K.C., "The dental health of Indian children in the Sioux Lookout Zone of Northestern Ontario," J. Canad. Dent. Assoc., 39: 709 (1973)
3. Miller, J., and Atkinson, H.A., "A replaceable probe point," Brit. Dent. J., 90: 157 (1951)
4. Russell, A.L., "A system for classification and scoring for prevalence surveys of periodontal disease," J. Dent. Res., 35: 350 (1956)
5. Titley, K.C., "The Sioux Lookout dental care project: a progress report," J. Canad. Dent. Assoc., 39: 793 (1973)

Epidemiology of oral conditions in Skolt Lapps

HASSE HANSSON

Odontological investigations were carried out among the Lapps in northern Finland between 1967 and 1970. The largest group examined were the Skolts. Since the sixteenth century, these Lapps have formed an isolated group divided into four family districts in Petsamo. The present population of about 600 persons is descended from less than one hundred individuals in the seventeenth century. One can

follow family relationships back to the seventh decade of
the nineteenth century from the registar of the Orthodox
church and further back to the middle of the eighteenth
century using the pedigrees of Nickul compiled in 1934. The
marriage pattern is characterized by kinship between the
spouses, usually in the third to fourth generation. First
cousin marriages are very rare. The three districts where
examinations took place were Nellim (1967), Sevettijärvi
(1968), and Inari (1969-70).

EXAMINATION OF DENTITION

The dental examination recorded the numbers of undecayed
teeth, teeth decayed by caries, teeth filled, and teeth
filled and decayed. In children, the status of deciduous and
permanent teeth was recorded separately. Special attention
was paid to the age at eruption of permanent teeth. Where
teeth were missing, it was determined if extraction, hypodontia, or pathological change was the cause.

THE PRIMARY DENTITION

The literature contains numerous detailed studies of the
time and order of eruption of the permanent teeth, but similar data on the primary teeth are more scarce. The present
cross-sectional study was based on 127 boys and 137 girls
aged 0 to 13.5 years. A tooth was considered erupted when
any part of it had broken through the gum.
  We found the boys got their primary teeth earlier than
the girls. This is in line with reports by Robinov (3) and
Ferguson et al. (1). According to their reports, boys are
earlier not only with respect to the time of eruption of
the first tooth but also in the number of teeth at one year
of age. In comparison with a Swedish population, the eruption in the Skolts is 1 to 2 months earlier for all teeth.
  Figure 1 shows that among the boys the deciduous teeth
are lost earlier from the lower than from the upper jaw.
The same holds true for the girls.

THE PERMANENT DENTITION

We studied the relation between age and number of erupted
permanent teeth and calculated the degree of variation at
any age. Such values are useful when studying child development and evaluating the prevalence of caries in the
permanent teeth.

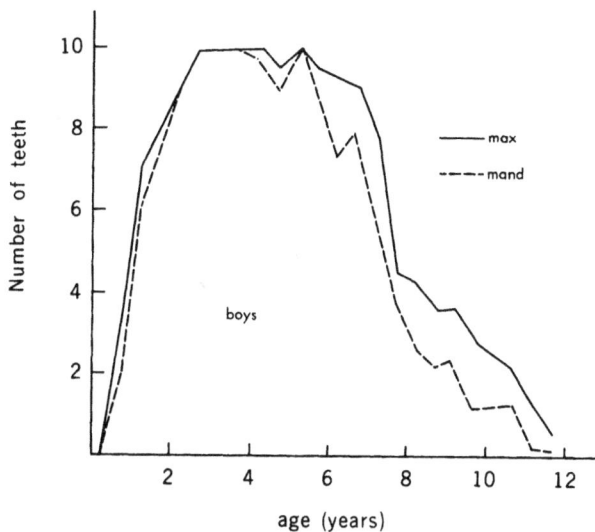

Figure 1   Number of deciduous teeth in Skolt boys - data
for maxilla and mandible

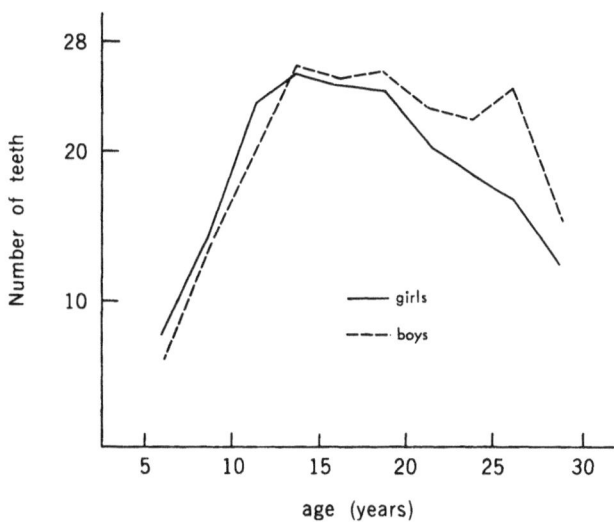

Figure 2   Number of permanent teeth in Skolt boys and girls

Eruption occurs earlier in girls (Figure 2). The "plateau" expected (2) after the eruption of the six first
pairs of teeth (first upper and lower molars, first and
second upper and lower incisors) is more or less smoothed
out because of the large age intervals (2.5 years) used in
this figure. However, it is seen in Figure 3, referring to
Skolt girls with age intervals of 0.5 years. The same holds
true for boys. The difference between upper and lower jaw
development (Figure 3) depends on the fact that the first
lower molar and the first and second lower incisors erupt
1 to 3 months earlier than the corresponding teeth in the
upper jaw. The same pattern is also seen in boys. After the
age of twenty, a striking reduction in the number of permanent teeth occurs. This is especially true for the girls,
but we found it also among the boys.

Figure 4 shows the number of edentulous individuals at
different ages. Already, in the age group 30 to 44, almost
35 per cent of the females and 16 per cent of the males
have lost their teeth. This trend continues in subsequent
groups. The final bars to the right of the figure show data
for the whole population. Total loss of teeth is most common among females at all ages. The age group 65 and over
has grown up under more favourable nutritional conditions
than the younger Skolts and this may partly explain why
fewer of the oldest age group are edentulous.

Among edentulous Nellim Skolts more than 20 years old,
there are 8 persons (8 per cent) who are completely edentulous, while 22 persons (24 per cent) have complete but ill-
fitting dentures (Table 1). The patients without dentures
always show a healthy oral mucosa, but 50 per cent of those
having dentures suffer mild to severe stomatitis (denture
sore mouth). Dentures have been judged as ill-fitting where
the occlusion was wrong or the dentures were in need of re-
basing because of poor stability or retention.

In the edentulous group at Sevettijärvi, 7 persons
(about 4 per cent of the total population more than 20
years old) have no dentures and 12 (9 per cent) have full
dentures; however, 7 of the 12 suffer from stomatitis and
most of the dentures again are of a rather poor quality.

HYPODONTIA

Hypodontia is frequent in small, isolated, and inbred populations. The phenomenon was studied on 500 ortopantomograms
taken in 1970. Individuals between 5 and 20 years of age
were studied and third molars were excluded from the survey.

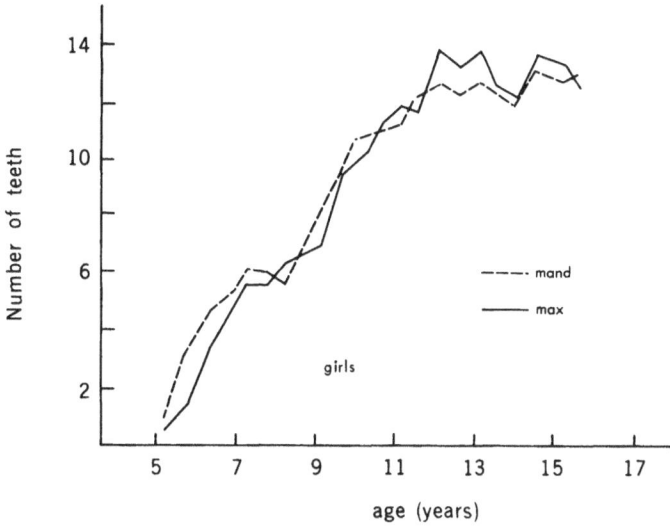

Figure 3 Number of erupted permanent teeth in Skolt
girls - data for mandible and maxilla

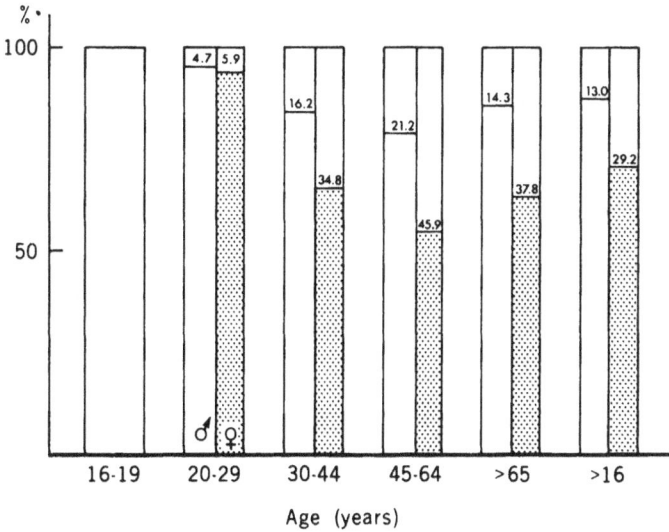

Figure 4 Percentage of edentulous Skolts at ages specified

TABLE 1
Details of edentulous Skolts at Nellim and Sevettijärvi

	Nellim			Sevettijärvi		
	M	F	Total	M	F	Total
Edentulous with no dentures	2	6	8	1	6	7
DSM (denture sore mouth)	0	0	0	0	0	0
Edentulous with complete dentures	8	14	22	3	9	12
DSM	1	10	11	3	4	7
Incorrect dentures	8	14	22	2	7	9

Intra-oral radiographs taken in 1967 and 1968 helped to confirm many cases of hypodontia. Permanent first molars were excluded in this connection owing to a very high frequency of extractions. Three categories of hypodontia were recognized:

Group I: certain hypodontia;

Group II: probable hypodontia. Both radiographs and anamnesis indicate hypodontia, but accidental loss of the tooth during extractions of deciduous teeth cannot be ruled out.

Group III: possible hypodontia. Both radiographs and anamnesis indicate hypodontia, but because of the individual's age or a high incidence of caries an extraction could have been forgotten by the individual.

Results are shown in Table 2. In Grahnen's study of Swedes the corresponding figure was only 5.5 per cent. As anticipated, the number of missing teeth was usually one or two (Table 3).

ORAL HYGIENE INDEX

In earlier epidemiological surveys, the standard of oral hygiene was estimated in some arbitrary way (good, medium, poor) if it was recorded at all. Such assessments can give valid results if the criteria are well defined. Ramfjord developed more precise numerical systems (0 through 3) for assessing the amount of plaque formation. In the present study, the following surfaces were examined: the facial surface of the upper first molars, upper right, and lower left incisors, and the lingual surface of the lower first molars. Oral debris is the soft substance loosely attached to the

TABLE 2
Frequency of hypodontia in the Skolts
(permanent dentition, third molars
excluded)

Group I	12.8%
Group II	4.1%
Group III	2.3%

TABLE 3
Number of missing teeth in individuals with
certain hypodontia (Group 1)

No. of missing teeth	No. of patients
1	8
2	13
3	4
4	3
Total	28

teeth; this was scored: 0 - no debris, 1 - soft debris
covering no more than a third of the tooth surface, 2 -
soft debris covering 1/3 to 2/3rds of the tooth surface,
and 3 - soft debris covering more than 2/3rds of the tooth
surface.

The material was divided into two groups, those with
fairly good oral hygiene (index 0 and 1) and those with
poor oral hygiene (index 2 and 3). About 90 per cent of
males over the age of 16 have poor oral hygiene, and in the
younger age groups, 70 to 80 per cent have poor oral hygiene. The females show a somewhat better situation; only
one-third of the youngest age groups have poor oral hygiene
and in the age groups 16 to 19 and 20 to 29, about 50 per
cent have fairly good oral hygiene. However, among the older females, the majority have index figures of 2 or 3.

SUMMARY

The epidemiology of oral conditions among the Skolt population in northern Finland was studied between 1967 and 1970.
Eruption of the primary and permanent dentition is described and compared with that of other populations. The
study covers both remaining and missing teeth, and the number of edentulous individuals, and relates these to age and
sex. The presence or absence of dentures is also reported

with the clinical condition of the oral mucosa and the quality of the dentures. Hypodontia is studied on 500 ortopantomograms. The incidence (12.8 per cent) is high enough to
merit a genetic analysis.

REFERENCES

1. Ferguson, A.F., Scott, R.B., and Bakwin, H., "Growth
   and development of negro infants. VIII. Comparison of
   the deciduous dentition in negro and white infants," J.
   Paediat., 50: 327 (1957)
2. Fulton, J.T., and Price, B., "Longitudinal data on eruption and attack of the permanent teeth," J. Dent. Res.,
   33: 65-79 (1954)
3. Robinov, M., Richards, T.W., and Anderson, M., "The
   eruption of deciduous teeth," Growth, 6: 127-33 (1942)

Commentaries

"Epidemiologic studies of facial pain and mandibular dysfunction in Lapps in northern Finland," by Martti Helkimo
(Department of Stomatognathic Physiology, Faculty of Odontology, University of Goteborg, Sweden). Results are given
of an epidemiologic clinical study of functional disorders
of the masticatory system in two populations of Lapps (245
genuine Skolt-Lapps and 76 genuine Inari-Lapps aged 15-65
years) in the district of Inari in northern Finland. A
thorough case history in accordance with a standardized
questionnaire was taken and clinical examination was performed. The frequency of various symptoms of dysfunction
was high in both populations; 57 per cent made complaints
of symptoms of dysfunction in the case history, and 47 per
cent had one or more clinically demonstrable severe symptoms. The most common sites of the symptoms were the tem-
pero-mandibular joint and the cheeks. Oral parafunctions
were reported by 42 per cent, frequent headache by 21 per
cent, and general muscle and joint symptoms by 31 per cent.
With but few exceptions the same prevalence of symptoms was
found in both Lapp populations examined. Contrary to results from clinical materials of patients with TMJ disorders

a remarkably even sex and age distribution of dysfunction
was found in this population study.

Considering the fairly widespread opinion that mandibular dysfunctions are ascribable, above all, to the mental
and physical stress and strain of modern civilization the
high frequencies of symptoms found in this study are remarkable. As to psychiatric and socio-medical studies of
people living in the subarctic environments, however,
stress factors are not uncommon although they perhaps are
of different character than in "modern" man. Considering
this fact and the poor dental state of the population, the
results presented in this study are less surprising.

"A method of delivery of dental care in remote areas of the
Canadian north," by K.W. Davey (School of Dental Therapy,
Medical Services, Northern Region, Health and Welfare
Canada, Fort Smith, NWT, Canada). The first Canadian venture into the utilization of dental auxiliaries as an effective force in delivering dental care to people in remote areas began in Fort Smith. Using the New Zealand dental nurse program as a model, the Canadian plan utilized
dramatic modifications to help meet the dental needs as
presented in the Canadian arctic and subarctic. Canadian
graduates are called dental therapists and the program at
the School of Dental Therapy is organized around the stan-
dardization of procedures, the control of treatment, and
the mobility of clinics.

"Racial odontology and the origin of Skolt Lapps," by P.
Kirveskari (Institute of Dentistry, University of Turku,
Turku, Finland). The discovery of so-called racial traits
in human dentition raised high hopes among anthropologists
for the value of teeth in hominid taxonomy. Without exact
knowledge about the mode of inheritance of dental traits,
their true value has been difficult to assess. However, the
availability of standards for classification and progress
made in genetic studies give reason for optimism about the
future role of dental traits in taxonomy.

If Lapp origins can be derived from the major racial
stocks, the Caucasoid and the Mongoloid race obviously must
be considered. The "Mongoloid dental complex" is a well-
established entity consisting of a number of typical trait
frequencies. In spite of general agreement on typically
"Caucasoid" frequencies of racial traits, the actual know-

ledge about trait distributions in Caucasoid populations is
far less complete than that in Mongoloid populations.

The dentition of Skolt Lapps shows a combination of
trait frequencies that is typical neither of the Mongoloid
nor of the Caucasoid race. However, the most reliable racial traits, the shovel-shape of the anterior teeth, and
lower cusp number of lower molars, both indicate Caucasoid
affinities in Skolt Lapps. The absence of Carabelli's cusp
and the presence of the deflecting wrinkle are commonly interpreted as Mongoloid traits. Other traits, such as the
sixth cusp and the distal trigonid crest, conform to the
Caucasoid pattern. In general, Skolt Lapp teeth are morphologically much closer to the Caucasoid than to the Mongoloid
dental complex.

"Interregional comparisons of dental health in northern
Canadian populations," by C.W.B. McPhail (Department of
Social and Preventive Dentistry, University of Saskatche-
wan, Saskatoon, Canada). Paper not submitted.

"Oral pathology in 3,000-year-old skeletal Eskimo material,"
by Björn Hedegård. Paper not submitted.

CHILD HEALTH

The Northwest Territories perinatal and infant
mortality study: infant mortality in the
Northwest Territories, 1973

B. BRETT, W.C. TAYLOR, and D.W. SPADY

Over the past fifteen years, there has been a significant
decrease in the infant mortality rate in the Northwest
Territories, but it is still appreciably higher than for
the rest of Canada. The White child in the NWT has an infant mortality rate similar to that of the rest of Canada,
but Indian and Eskimo children sustain a greater if decreasing risk (Figure 1).

If deaths are subdivided into stillbirths (deaths of
foetuses > 500 grams with gestation > 20 weeks), perinatal
deaths (deaths in the first 7 days of life, including stillbirths), and neonatal deaths (deaths of live infants in the
first 28 days of life), it is seen (Figure 2) that, while
there have been reductions in the neonatal death rate, the
greatest change is in the post-neonatal death rate (from 28
to 365 days of life).

In 1973, there were 1,188 births in the NWT (Table 1),
with 34 infant deaths (deaths of live-born infants in the
first year of life) and 12 stillbirths. There is a preponderance of deaths in the Indian and Eskimo groups, with the
white population in the minority. The neonatal death rate
was 15.2/1,000 live births, with Indians and Eskimos at
greater risk of death during this period. Fifteen of the
18 neonatal deaths occurred in the first 7 days of life;
together with 12 stillbirths, there were thus 27 perinatal
deaths; 17 of these were children under 2,500 grams in
weight, an important factor to consider in analysing causes
of death. Other important factors were:

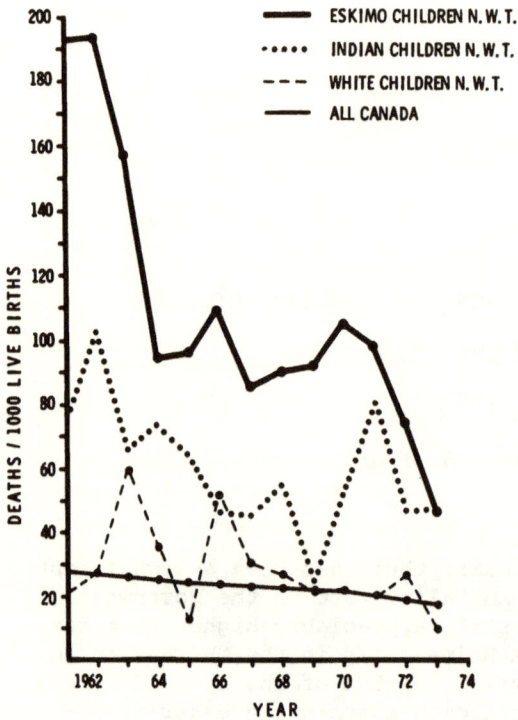

Figure 1   Infant mortality rates in the Northwest Territories, 1962-73. Data obtained from Annual Reports on Health Conditions in the Northwest Territories, Chief Medical Health Officer, Government of the Northwest Territories

TABLE 1
Birth and death statistics in the Northwest Territories, 1973; figures in parentheses refer to the rate per thousand live births (data obtained from the data collected by the NWT Perinatal and Infant Mortality and Morbidity Study)

	Total	Indian	Eskimo	White
Births	1,188	193	447	548
Infant deaths	34 (28.6)	9 (46.4)	20 (44.7)	5 (9.1)
Neonatal deaths	18 (15.2)	5 (25.9)	9 (20.1)	4 (7.3)
Perinatal deaths	27 (22.5)	6 (31.0)	14 (30.8)	7 (12.7)
Stillbirths	12 (10)	1 (5.1)	7 (15.4)	4 (7.2)

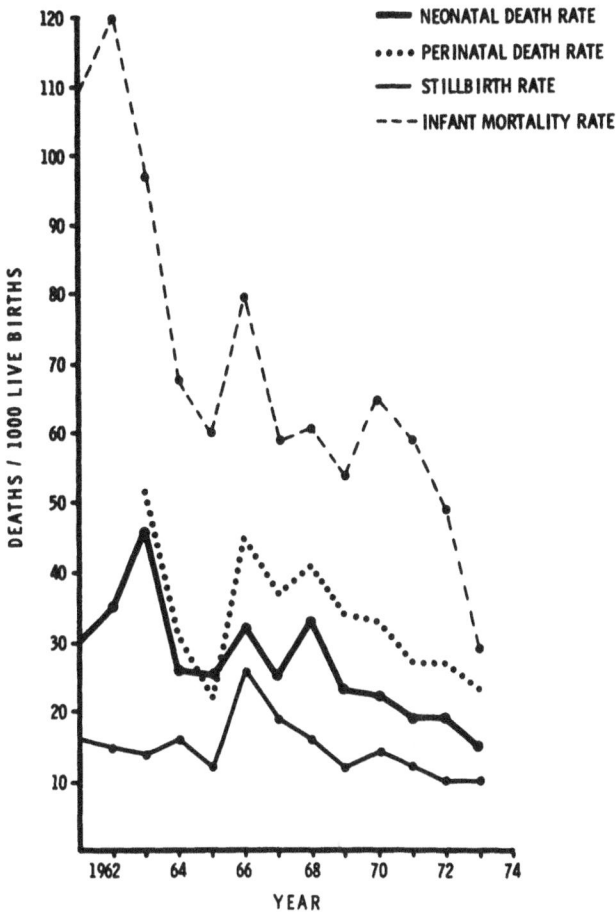

Figure 2   Mortality rates at different times in the first
year of life, Northwest Territories, 1962-73. Data obtained
from Annual Reports on Health Conditions in the Northwest
Territories, Chief Medical Health Officer, Government of
the Northwest Territories

(a)   *Inadequately utilized antenatal care services.*
Of 30 neonatal and stillbirth deaths, only 7 received adequate antenatal care (arbitrarily defined as a first visit
to a health worker by 12 weeks of gestation with at least
5 visits prior to birth). The average number of antenatal
care visits was about four. This should not be taken to mean
that adequate antenatal care services were unavailable but
rather that they were not utilized. A number of problems

arise from lack of good antenatal care: (i) determining
gestational age. If the health worker sees the patient only
infrequently, she may miss quickening at 18 to 20 weeks, an
important sign if the mother does not remember the date of
her last menstrual period. This can make it difficult to
determine when the pregnancy is at term. (ii) the detection
and follow-up of the "high risk" mother with previous ob-
stetrical accidents or chronic ill health is made more difficult when antenatal care is lacking. Conditions which
have occurred in mothers of infants dying in the perinatal
period include epilepsy, rubella in the first trimester,
toxaemia, achondroplasia and mental retardation, pyelonephritis, previous abortions and stillbirths, previous congenital anomalies, and gonorrhoea.

The purpose of antenatal care is to follow the pregnancy
and ensure that all is well. If the uterus is not growing
at the right rate, it may suggest intrauterine death or
twins, both situations that require specialized care.

Another form of prenatal care is that rendered to a high
risk mother who has been transferred to a referral centre
for care and delivery. In a number of cases, these mothers
have not been closely assessed and followed after transfer
to the major centre. Therefore, the risks have not been
lessened and the purpose of the transfer has been lost.
Mothers who are transferred should be referred to a specific doctor, admitted for evaluation on arrival at the hospital, and then discharged to a responsible community agency where they can remain under close continuing prenatal
care until delivery. If this is impracticable, they should
stay in hospital till birth.

(b) *Accidents.*   Skidoo accidents appeared to precipi-
tate two infant deaths. Uterine and placental trauma leads
to early labour and then foetal or premature death. Slip-
ping on the ice or mud may have similar consequences.

(c) *Substandard paediatric care.*   The care rendered to
sick newborn and young infants was at times less than optimum, if compared with the standards of major southern Canadian hospitals. Such a comparison is perhaps unfair because
of the ready availability of expert and continuing attention in southern centres. There was sometimes lack of
aggressiveness in treating a sick baby, failure to recognize sickness, and utilization of inappropriate therapy. In
a number of cases, these were very small infants who should
have had expert care from birth. Unfortunately, such expert
care is not readily available in the north.

(d) *Failure to diagnose a potentially treatable condition.* In two neonatal deaths, congenital heart disease was a major factor. In one case, this was potentially treatable, but in a small community hospital or nursing station it requires experienced clinical judgment to detect such problems.

Between the ages of 28 and 365 days, 16 children died. The population most at risk was the Eskimo, with the Indians next and the White child at very low risk. Some of the factors leading to deaths in this age group were:

(a) *Infections.* Fourteen of the 16 children who died had infection as a major or contributing cause of death. Respiratory tract infection accounted for 9 deaths. Meningitis contributed to 3 deaths, with myocarditis and gastroenteritis completing the picture. On occasion, these infections were superimposed on other conditions such as congenital heart disease or malnutrition.

(b) *Malnutrition.* Malnutrition played a decisive role in at least one death and a contributing role in two others. It is possible that malnutrition was involved in yet more deaths, but it is difficult to assess nutritional status after the fact and from a distance, especially when height and weight are not recorded consistently on the child's chart.

(c) *Poor health care.* A disturbing feature of a number of cases was that they had been seen by a health care worker, and occasionally were in hospital, and yet for various reasons had not received definitive investigation and therapy. This was a contributory cause of death in one case of meningitis and one case of gastroenteritis. Many children seemed to be followed by a health worker for one to two weeks prior to death for "colds" or "upper respiratory infections." They got worse and died. Possibly, such infants who ordinarily could be cared for at home should be more readily admitted to hospitals and nursing stations until they are nearly well.

(d) *Parental neglect.* Neglect contributed to the deaths of at least four children, in two of which death was due to suffocation by the parent sleeping with the child. Alcoholism also played a role in these deaths. There were two cases of sudden infant death, one of which is likely to have been a "battered child."

Throughout this study, a recurring theme was transportation. In many instances patients were transferred from outlying stations to local hospitals, and from local hospitals to major referral centres in the south. However, criticism is necessary in that transferral of patients was not used often enough. A number of infants could be alive today, or would have had a better chance of survival, had they been transferred to a major centre as soon as it became obvious that optimum medical management could not be carried to completion at the home base. This is especially true of sick and of healthy but small newborn infants. One factor which presently inhibits the transfer of infants is the lack of a satisfactory transport incubator.

ACKNOWLEDGMENT

Data for this report have been obtained from the annual reports on Health Conditions in the Northwest Territories 1962-1972, Chief Medical and Health Officer, Government of the NWT and from the data collected by the NWT Perinatal and Infant Mortality and Morbidity Study.

SUMMARY

The infant mortality rate in the Northwest Territories, while still appreciably higher than for the rest of Canada, has shown a dramatic decline over the past 10 to 15 years. The greatest change has been in the post-neonatal death rate. In 1973 there were 1,188 births, 12 stillbirths, and 34 infant deaths, 27 being in the perinatal period. Contributing causes of death were low birth weight, inadequately utilized antenatal care services, accidents during pregnancy, non-availability of expert emergency medical care of the newborn, and failure to diagnose potentially treatable conditions.

Sixteen children died in the post-neonatal period. Factors leading to deaths in this age group were infection, malnutrition, lack of expert medical care, and parental neglect. While air transportation is already utilized extensively in the north, it could have been used even more frequently with advantage to these patients.

Design of the Northwest Territories perinatal and
infant mortality and morbidity study

M. HOLUBOWSKY

Like every other country in the circumpolar group, we are
concerned with infant mortality rates as an indication of
our success, or lack of success, in bettering health care
delivery to our residents. We are highly concerned with
perinatal problems and infant morbidity. Accordingly, a
Northwest Territories Perinatal and Infant Mortality and
Morbidity Study Committee was organized in December 1971
with Dr H.B. Brett, Regional Director for the Northwest
Territories Medical Services, as principal investigator.
The project involves, among others, a neonatologist, a
sociologist, a pathologist, an obstetrician, a nutritionist,
and a representative of the Northwest Territories Medical
Association.

The study, financed by a $110,000 federal health grant,
began officially on 1 April 1973 and will finish in April
1975. It is examining the prenatal care, the birth process, and morbidity patterns of all infants, Indian, Eskimo, and other, born over a 12 month period; each infant
is being followed for a 12 month period after birth. Hence,
consideration is given not only to the possible causes of
death in infancy but to the health status of surviving infants. The objectives are:

(1) To identify the exact causes of death in stillbirths,
neonatal deaths, and infant deaths.

(2) To identify the frequency and nature of morbidity
occurring in the first year of life.

(3) To identify factors associated with infant deaths
and morbidity, such as nutrition, socio-economic status,
and heredity.

(4) To assess the adequacy of care and management of the
infant in the home, the nursing station, and hospital.

(5) To make recommendations to reduce infant mortality
and morbidity.

Detailed data collection forms record (1) Prenatal Re-
Cord, (2) Summary of Labour and Delivery, (3) Apgar Score
Charts, (4) Newborn Record, (5) Nutritional Background Record, (6) Sociological History of the Child. Other exis-
tent records are also photocopied. These include: Growth

Charts, Progress Notes, Immunization Records, Treatment Record, Admission and Discharge Summaries, and Denver Developmental Screening Records. The record sheets are relatively easy to complete, and could continue to be used as standard forms after the study period is completed.

To facilitate data collection in the rural areas, an instruction was developed, with audio-visual transparencies of pertinent materials; visits were also made to all doctors, nurses, and hospitals in the Northwest Territories. Follow-up visits were often needed, because the turnover of doctors and nurses is great. Repeat visits are also being made to units where data collection seems incomplete or incorrect.

Files on each child born within the study period are opened under name, date of birth, location, and medicare number. The medicare number is important since it allows us to trace patient-doctor contacts through the computer data banks of the Hospital Insurance Service.

Many problems have arisen during this study, for example:

(a) Babies have been born to Northwest Territories residents with birth taking place in the South, and the baby being adopted back into another family in the North.

(b) Problems have arisen in obtaining parental consent and subsequent transport of babies to southern pathology departments for proper autopsy examination.

(c) Variations in spellings of native names, due in part to attempts at standardizing the Inuit alphabet.

(d) A major mail strike with loss of some records.

(e) Mobility of the population.

Our population of some 1,200 babies is small in comparison to the sample size of some other studies, but it is total and our analysis should thus be valid and informative. A particularly vital function of our study is a Sub-committee on Deaths. This Committee reviews every stillbirth, neonatal and infant death in detail, and recommendations on each case reviewed are disseminated to all participants in the study.

SUMMARY

Details of organization and implementation of the NWT perinatal and infant mortality and morbidity study are given, together with a discussion of problems encountered in the first year of data collection.

The effects of social and economic background on the hospitalization of children during the first five years of life

P. RANTAKALLIO and M. VÄÄNÄNEN

This paper studies hospital use by the children of Northern Finland from birth to the age of five, between 1966 and 1971. The aim was to find possible social and climatic factors influencing the incidence of disease in this age group. The study was started during the pregnancy of 12,068 mothers, covering 96 per cent of all births in the district (2).

The study area is shown in Figure 1. It is situated between 63° 30' and 70° 0' North. Hospital admissions were investigated in the children's departments of the four central hospitals. Outside these hospitals there is only one practising paediatrician. However, many smaller local hospitals are attended by general practitioners and care for children with minor illnesses. The study does not include either admissions to the smaller hospitals or those received by departments outside the children's departments of the central hospitals.

Children numbering 2,230 had been in one or other of the four children's departments during the first five years of their lives, and hospital visits totalled 3,513. Hospital admissions were most frequent during the first year of life (47 per cent of all cases, 22 per cent occurring during the first 28 days of life).

The most common complaint was respiratory disease (23.8 per cent of all hospital visits). The second commonest group was diseases of the neonatal period (14.9 per cent of all hospital visits), and the third commonest group included infectious and parasitic diseases (11.8 per cent of all visits).

The distribution of hospital visits was next analysed separately for children living in the northern and southern provinces of the study area. Details of climate and its effect on the perinatal period have been given earlier (3). Diseases of the digestive organs and haematopoetic diseases were more common causes of hospital admission in the North than in the South, while the opposite was true for diseases of the newborn period and congenital malformations. However, these differences were most probably caused not by varia-

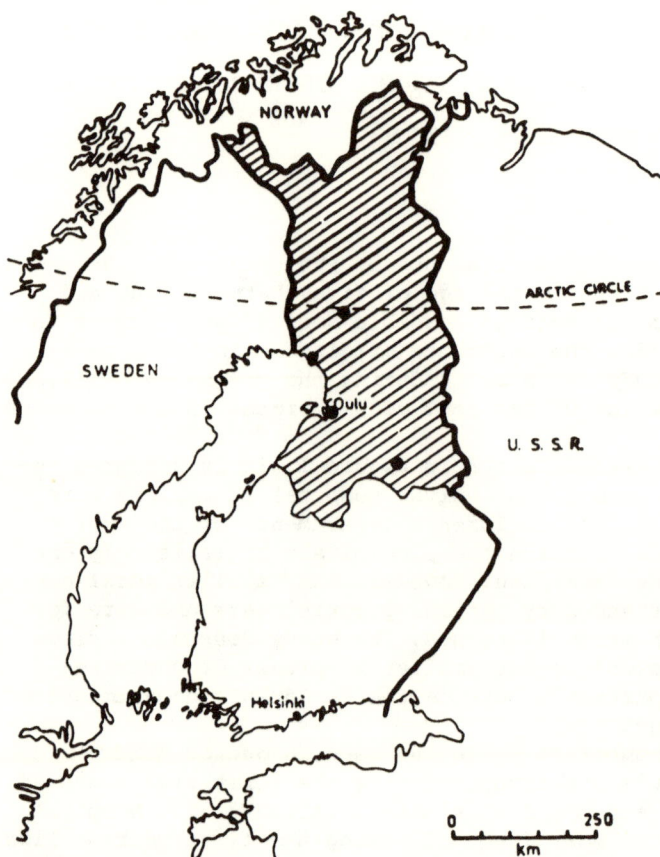

Figure 1   The study area, showing the location of the four
central hospitals

tions in climate but by such factors as differences in the
utilization of hospital beds secondary to the longer mean
distances of Northern province patients from the hospital.

About 50 per cent of all hospital cases lived in the
Northern province, whereas only a third of the population
lived there. Ninety-four per cent of hospital visits of
children from the Northern province were to their provincial hospitals, so that here again it is mainly a question
of the larger number of hospital beds in the Northern province.

Liveborn infants numbering 217 died before the age of
5. The most common causes of death were diseases of the

newborn period (49.8 per cent), the second commonest group
was congenital malformations (19.9 per cent), and the third
commonest diseases were those of the respiratory organs
(6.6 per cent).

There was no significant difference of mortality rate
between the two provinces, the rate being 19.9 per thousand
in the northern and 18.5 per thousand in the southern area
during the first five years of life.

The children living in towns were more frequent users of
the central hospitals than those living in the country; 41
per cent of hospital cases were town dwellers, whereas the
figure for the total population was 33 per cent. Therefore,
when hospital cases were compared with the remainder of the
population, such characteristics of town dwellers as
smaller families and better social standing were accentua-
ted in the hospitalized children. Of those who died, 63.5
per cent had been patients in some children's department.
From the others, one-third had died in some other kind of
hospital. The places of residence of the children were divided into four classes according to their economic, cultural and social level (1). Ratings were significantly
lower among the children who died than among the others and
it was lower among the dead children who had not been patients in a children's department than among those who had
been. Thus the fate of children originating from the less
developed areas was poorer than that of children living in
more developed areas.

In order to obtain more valid information on the social
background of the children who had been patients in the
children's hospitals, a mate for each child was chosen from
those who had not been in a children's hospital but were
living in a similar district. About 40 variables concerning
the biological characteristics of the mothers, the use of
health care systems during pregnancy and labour, characteristics of the child as a newborn infant, and the social
and economic standing of the family were studied. There
were highly significant differences between the hospital
group and their mates (Table 1) with respect to the characteristics of the child and the health care of the mother
during pregnancy; however, factors concerned directly with
the social and economic situation of the family were similar for the two groups. The same is true at the significant
difference level (Table 2) and only among "almost significant" differences is there a factor which measures directly
the social standing of the family (Table 3). Table 4 lists
a further 32 factors, grouped under general headings, in

TABLE 1
Highly significant differences between children admitted to
hospital and their mates (the characteristics of the hospitalized children are indicated in parentheses)

1. Birth weight of the child (low)
2. Length at birth (short)
3. Preterm birth (more)
4. Mother has history of previous low-birth-weight infant(s)
   (more)
5. Physician participated in the delivery (more often)
6. Mother needed hospital admission during pregnancy (more)

TABLE 2
Significant differences between children admitted to hospital and
their mates (the characteristics of the hospitalized children are
indicated in parentheses)

1. Number of antenatal visits (less)
2. Perinatal mortality of the mother's previous children (higher)
3. Percentage of mothers who smoked (more)

TABLE 3
Almost significant differences between children admitted to hospital
and their mates (the characteristics of the hospitalized children
are indicated in parentheses)

1. Percentage of deliveries occurring in central hospitals (higher)
2. Need for bed rest at home during pregnancy (more often)
3. Percentage of mothers belonging to social class IV (higher)

TABLE 4
Variables where children admitted to hospital did not differ
from their mates

Variables	Number of questions
Biological characteristics of the mother	7
Social standing	3
Working	4
School attendance	2
Attitudes	2
Participation in preventive health care	1
Nature of place of residence	4
Internal migration	2
Standard of living	2
Housing standard	5
Total	32

which no significant difference was found between the hospital group and their mates.

Discriminant function analyses showed that children who had been admitted to hospital at some time during their first 5 years could not be discriminated very well from other children living in the similar district if the variables used concerned the family background of children (Rantakallio, to be published). The explanation seems to be that children living in poorer socio-economic conditions are more likely to get sick, but are less capable of getting high quality health care.

SUMMARY

Data for 1966-71 show that every fifth child in Northern Finland has been admitted to a children's hospital during its first five years of life. The children living in towns use children's hospitals more often than those from rural areas, but the mortality rate is higher among children from less developed areas. The three most common disease groups causing hospital admissions are those of the respiratory organs, the newborn period, and infectious diseases. The three most common causes of death are diseases of the newborn period, congenital malformations, and diseases of the respiratory organs. The mortality rate in the northern and southern parts of the study area is the same. However, the children in the Northern province are taken to hospital more often and there are some differences in the incidence of the various diseases, most likely caused by factors other than climate. When children who had been admitted to a children's department were compared with children from a similar district who had not entered hospital, many significant differences were found with respect to the biological characteristics of the child and the health condition and care of the mother during pregnancy, but factors concerning the social background of the family seemed unimportant.

REFERENCES

1. Palmgren, K., "Regional differences in the degree of development in Finland," Publications of the National Planning Bureau, Series A: 15, 1-160 (1964)
2. Rantakallio, P., "Groups at risk in low birth weight infants and perinatal mortality," Acta paediatr. scand. suppl., 193: 1-71 (1969)

3. Rantakallio, P., "The effect of a Northern climate on
   seasonality of births and the outcome of pregnancies,"
   Acta paediatr. scand., suppl., 218: 1-67 (1971)

Changing health hazards in infancy and childhood in northern Canada

MARCIA C. SMITH

Canada's Northwest Territories has an area of 1.3 million
square miles. The 1971 Census listed the population at
34,810, with 33 per cent of Inuit origin, 21 per cent Indian, and 46 per cent non-native. Continuing development of
the north has brought vast changes in the life-style of the
original inhabitants, and continues to influence traditional ways. This paper is a brief review of the impact of such
influences on the health of children.

BIRTH

Average birth weights show distinctive ethnic differences
(Table 1). The Inuit have the smaller infants and the non-
native people the larger ones, with Indian infants just
slightly heavier than Inuit. The incidence of infants with
low birth weights shows a similar pattern (Table 2). The
non-native group has a rate that is less than the Canadian
average, suggesting that environment has less influence
than life-style. The apparent advantage of the northern
white people may be related to their pre-selection from
professional and management groups.

Infant death rates parallel the ethnic pattern of birth
weights (Table 3). Keeping in mind the small numbers involved (a total of 57 infant deaths in 1972), one must interpret the data with caution. The apparently small perinatal death rate for the Indian group could reflect incomplete reporting of stillbirths. However, the largest source
of infant mortality among Indians and Inuit is the group
aged one to twelve months. The complex relationship between
susceptibility to illness and death and low birth weight
should be explored further in northern populations.

TABLE 1
Average birth weight (lb) for infants born
in the Northwest Territories

	Inuit	Indian	Others
1970	7.00	7.05	7.40
1971	6.95	7.00	7.35
1972	7.00	7.15	7.40

TABLE 2
Incidence of low-birth-weight infants ($< 2,500$ g)
in the Northwest Territories (rate per 100 live
births)

	Inuit	Indian	Others	Canada
1970	12.9	11.1	8.5	8.7
1971	11.8	10.9	6.1	
1972	12.0	9.5	7.7	

TABLE 3
Infant death rates in the Northwest Territories (1972)

	Inuit	Indian	Others
A. Perinatal*	41	9	20
B. Neonatal**	24	19	14
C. Postneonatal***	49	28	12
Infant (B + C)	73	47	26

* Deaths within the first seven days of life, including stillbirths.
** Deaths per 1,000 live births in the first month of
  life.
*** Deaths per 1,000 live births in first 1-12 months
  of life.

TABLE 4
Causes of death during childhood (0-14 years), data for
Northwest Territories, 1969 and 1971

	1969 (N = 88)	1971 (N = 79)
Injuries and accidents	15%	28%
Diseases of infancy	33%	38%
Pneumonia	27%	14%
Gastrointestinal diseases	5%	9%
Other	20%	11%

DEATH

Causes of death during childhood show some interesting
changes from 1969 to 1971 (Table 4). Deaths from pneumonia
decreased by 13 per cent, while deaths from accidents increased by a similar amount. The majority of deaths were
related to four causes: diseases of infancy and malformations, injuries and accidents, pneumonia, and gastrointestinal conditions.

ACCIDENTS

To examine household and community hazards, reported accidental deaths were reviewed. As the number in a given year
was rather small, deaths for three years were grouped together (Table 5). More than half (55 per cent) of fatal accidents were in the preschool age group.
    A house fire in the north is usually catastrophic, and
every year several families perish in this way. Motor vehicle accidents, involving cars and not snowmobiles, claim
the lives of both preschool and older children. Drownings
account for one-fifth of accidental deaths, all in the
school age group. They occur in creeks, rivers, public
swimming pools, and cracks in sea ice, and may involve gross
errors of judgment, such as driving a car on thawing ice.
More boys are drowned than girls, perhaps because of their
predilection for playing in boats.

TABLE 5
Deaths from accidents among children living in
the Northwest Territories, 1971-72-73 (N = 56)

Age	Cause	Number
<1 year	"Crib death"	5/11
	Suffocation	3/11
	Burns/fire	3/11
Preschool	Burns/fire	6/20
	Motor vehicle accidents	5/20
	Other	5/20
School age	Drowning	12/25
	Motor vehicle accidents	3/25
	Shooting	2/25
	Burns/fire	2/25
	Other	6/25

TABLE 6
Pediatric hospital admissions from the Northwest Territories
(excluding newborns)

Diagnosis	1970 (N = 1,956)	1972 (N = 2,064)
Respiratory and related	41%	41%
Gastrointestinal conditions	10%	8%
Accidents	9%	7%
Skin conditions	6%	6%
Central nervous system	5%	7%
Other	29%	31%

Crib deaths are a significant statistic in the first
year of life. In addition, death may occur from strangling
by tight clothing, discharge of firearms, and attacks by
dogs, special hazards for children living in the northern
environment.

HOSPITAL ADMISSIONS

A serious illness or a condition requiring specialized care
is a new kind of hazard. Often, a child must be separated
from his family and sent a long distance to the hospital.
Over two thousand separations occurred in 1972. Two-thirds
of these children (excluding newborns) were less than five
years of age; one-third had not reached their first birth-
day.
   Respiratory and related conditions accounted for two-
fifths of the hospital admissions (Table 6). Gastrointestinal conditions, accidental injuries, and skin conditions
together accounted for another fifth. Minor surgery, dental
caries, and tonsillectomy contributed to the elective admissions.
   The average hospital stay was longest for the infant
(14 days in 1972); older children stayed from nine to
twelve days on average. This is perhaps related not so much
to the nature of the illness as to the highly protective
attitude of attending physicians, who feel that a hospital
environment is better than home for the child.

SUMMARY

The risks of birth, illness, and death continue to change
for the paediatric populations of the Canadian North.
While infant mortality has been declining, it is still high

compared with the rate for Canada as a whole, with distinctive differences between native and non-native groups. Injuries and accidents are important preventable causes of
death. Hospital admissions are most often for respiratory-
related infections and involve a large proportion of the
preschool age group.

Socio-economic correlates of mortality and morbidity among Inuit infants

C.W. HOBART

The Inuit infant death rate in the Canadian Arctic has always been high (Table 1). Ten and more years ago, ready explanations included inadequate housing, frequent travel,
imminent shortage of food (Inuit starved to death in the
Keewatin region of the Canadian Arctic as recently as 1958
(3)) and inadequate, often inaccessible health care. However, in the last 5 to 8 years both the conditions of life
and the availability of health care have improved dramatically. As a result of the Inuit low-cost housing program,
it is no longer necessary for the Inuit to live in snow
huts, snow-banked tents, or make-shift shacks. Almost all
have a three-bedroom, suburban style bungalow, with forced
air heat. The threat of starvation is permanently abolished,
infants are rarely subjected to the stresses of winter sled
travel, and most Eskimos have easy access to well-equipped
settlement nursing stations. The nursing stations not only
provide prompt diagnosis and treatment of illnesses, but
also offer pre- and post-natal orientation programs, immunization programs, and well-baby clinics. Patients who
cannot be treated locally are flown to hospital, often in
specially chartered aircraft.

The continuing high mortality rates may thus reflect
patterns of life which Inuit brought with them "off the
land," or patterns that have evolved since moving into the
settlements. The present pilot research study was designed
to test this hypothesis.

TABLE 1
Infant deaths and death rates* classified by ethnic group, Northwest
Territories[1]

Year	Native Indian		Inuit		White/Other		NWT Total		Rate for Canada
	No.	Rate	No.	Rate	No.	Rate	No.	Rate	
1970	14	53.1	60	105.0	10	21.7	84	64.7	
1969	6	24.2	50	90.5	8	20.5	64	53.7	19.3 [2]
1968	14	54.9	51	89.1	12	27.4	77	60.9	20.8
1967	11	45.1	46	83.8	10	29.6	67	59.3	22.0
1966	11	46.2	58	108.8	16	52.4	86	79.9	23.1
1965	13	64.0	50	95.4	5	12.0	68	59.5	
1964	16	73.9	52	92.1	16	35.1	84	68.1	24.7
1963	14	65.5	80	157.0	24	60.0	118	104.0	26.3
1962	23	103.0	98	194.0	10	27.0	131	120.0	23.0
1961	17	77.0	94	185.0	8	21.0	119	108.0	27.0
1959-60				208.5					
1955-58				231.5					
1951-54				164.5					

*Infants dying under 1 year per 1,000 live births.

RESEARCH DESIGN AND DATA COLLECTION

Since there are only about 60 Inuit infant mortalities a
year, it was necessary to introduce a more sensitive index
of health than survival, and to increase the number of cases by sampling over several years (1 January 1969 to
1 January 1972). A morbidity-mortality index was devised,
and relevant data were collected on all infant mortalities,
and on a matched comparison group which survived.

Prior to selecting the sample, community-specific Inuit
infant mortality rates were calculated. Data were then collected from two communities having high infant mortality
rates (over 100.0), three communities having medium rates
(70.0-99.9), and three communities having low rates (below
70.0).

High mortality rates		Medium mortality rates		Low mortality rates	
Frobisher Bay	124.4	Cambridge Bay	95.2	Pond Inlet Igululk	
				Hall Beach	68.9
Inuvik	116.4	Spence Bay		Tuktoyaktuk	47.6
		Gjoa Haven		Coppermine	
		Pelly Bay	88.3	Holman Island	44.1

A total of 134 infants and their families, 67 mortalities and 67 survivors, were studied. Survivors were matched
with mortalities for age, sex, and community of residence.
Data were collected from four sources: death certificates,
the families of the infants concerned and/or native informants, Nursing Station personnel and Nursing Station records, and other informed observers such as priests and
missionaries.

Background information related to education of the parents, adequacy and crowding of housing, temporal proximity
to the nursing station and to a hospital, income level of
the family, nature of the baby care provided by the mother,
continuity of contact between baby and mother, adjustment
of parents to settlement living, and alcohol consumption by
the parents.

In most cases, the expected relationship is obvious; low
mortality and morbidity are hypothesized as associated with
adequate housing, proximity to health care facilities,
higher income, uninterrupted contact between mother and baby, and non-consumption of alcohol. However, the influence
of other factors is less obvious: are higher educational
attainment and adjustment to settlement living directly, or
inversely, associated with a low morbidity-mortality? If
sophistication and acculturation have had disorganizing
consequences, eroding the traditional devotion of the Inuit
mother to her baby, we would expect an inverse association.
If they are associated with a more sophisticated and medically informed understanding of the needs of the baby, the
symptoms of illness, and the services available at the
nursing station, one would expect the reverse.

Dependent variables were mortality, a life-long weighted
monthly morbidity index and a life-long weighted monthly
morbidity death index. The morbidity index considered only
medicated illnesses and weighting these by a factor of one
if the baby remained at home, by a factor of two if there
was admission to a nursing station, and by a factor of
three if there was evacuation to hospital. The total figure
so derived was divided by the number of months of life as a
measure of the time the infant had been at risk. The third
index was identical with the second except that 1.0 was
added if the infant died.

RESULTS

Relationships between independent and dependent variables
have been analysed by cross tabulation (Table 2). Babies

TABLE 2
Relationships between socio-economic variables and mortality, morbidity/month, and morbidity-mortality indices

Independent (socio-economic) variables	Indices of ill-health			Relationship to ill-health
	Mort.	Morb./ month	Morb.- mort.	
Deceased siblings	–	+10*	–	Direct
Natural mother cared for baby	–	–5	–	Inverse
Baby adopted out	+5*	+10	+10	Direct
Age of mother	10	–	–	Middle-age, least illness
No. of children in mother's care	∩5	∩5	∩5	Small and large families show least illness
Mother does skin sewing	U10	U5	U5	Most illness if mother does no or much skin sewing
Mother's education	–	–	10	If no education or much education least illness but most severe illness
Mother's smoking habits	–	U10	U10	None and much, most illness
Mother drinks alcohol	+10	–	+10	Direct
Father's employment	–	–5	–10	No employment - most illness
Father's occupation	ir 5**	ir 10	ir 10	Hunters most, labourers least illness
Father hunts	–	+10	+10	Direct
Father's education	–	+10	+10	Direct
Clothing quality	–10	–10	–10	Inverse
No. of bedrooms	–5	–	–10	Inverse
No. of children in home	U10	U10	–	Many and few, most illness
No. of people in home	–	U5	U10	Many and few, most illness
Persons per bedroom	5	10	5	Inverse
Modernity of heating	–1	–5	–1	Stove only, most illness
Modernity of toilet	–5	–	–5	Inverse
Use of dipper to obtain water	–	+10	+10	Direct
Crowding in housing	U10	U10	U5	Average crowding, least illness
Housing quality	–5	–10	–5	Inverse
Cleanliness of house	–	–2	–10	Inverse
Baby breast-fed	–1	–1	–1	Longest fed, least illness
Baby bottle-fed	+1	+1	+1	Bottle only, most illness
Source of food (store or native)	ir 5**	ir 10	ir 10	Both sources, least illness
Eating of cariboo meat	–	U10	U1	Much and most, much and no illness
Travel time to hospital	–	–	–10	Inverse

* Signifies p level, expressed as a percentage.
** ir signifies an irregular pattern. ∩ signifies an upward curvilinear pattern. U signifies a downward curvilinear pattern.

fare best when cared for continuously by their natural
mothers, when their mothers are neither too old, ill-educa-
ted, traditional, and worn out with much child-bearing, or
too young, acculturated, well-educated, and immature and
when their mothers do not drink alocohol. The characteristics of the fathers present the same pattern, optimum infant health being associated with neither too much tradi-
tionalism nor an excessive acculturation. In terms of
housing, good health in the baby is directly associated with
all measures of housing quality and cleanliness. However,
the traditionalism- acculturation-influence is again apparent in that both under- and over-crowded homes experience more illness in the baby than homes with average
crowding. In terms of nutrition, the duration of breast
feeding is directly related, and early commencement of
bottle feeding is inversely related to the baby's health.
Dependence on a mixture of native and store foods is associated with better infant health than is dependence on
either one alone.

When data for small communities like Gjoa Haven and
Pelly Bay and larger ones like Inuvik and Frobisher Bay are
tabulated separately (Table 3), many of the same relationships are seen. In both large and small communities, there
is a direct relationship between our criteria of infant
morbidity and mortality and such factors as previous childhood deaths in the family, a history of the mother having
lived in a hunting camp, the hand-dipping of water in the
home, the raising of many children, and crowding relative
to other homes in the settlement. Both categories of community also show an inverse relationship between the mortality and morbidity criteria and the birth weight of the
baby, steady employment and skilled occupation of the father, age at commencement of bottle feeding, and the quality and cleanliness of the house.

For *large settlements*, morbidity-mortality was associated directly with the mother working, the babies being
cared for away from home, many children in the home and
drinking by both the mother and the father.

For *small settlements*, morbidity-mortality was associated directly with adoption of the baby, hunting activity
by the father, and crowding of the house (number of bed-
rooms and people per room). The criteria were inversely
associated with families being headed by the natural father, modern sanitation (indoor, vented toilet facilities),
and duration of breast feeding of the infant, and were
associated in a curvilinear fashion with maternal age,

TABLE 3
Number of relationships between independent (socio-economic) variables
and dependent variables significant at 10 per cent level or beyond

| Independent (socio-economic) variables | Settlement size | | Relationship to ill-health |
	Inuvik and Frobisher Bay (N = 52)	Small settlement (N = 56)	
Child and family			
Birth weight	2* inverse	3* inverse	Inverse in large and small settlements
Dead siblings	1 direct	1 direct	Direct in large and small settlements
Care provided by natural mother	1 inverse	Few non-natural mothers	Inverse in large settlements
Child adopted out	-	3 direct	Direct in small settlements
Child cared for away from home	1 direct	-	Direct in large settlements
Mothers			
Age of mother	-	1 middle-aged least illness	In small settlements, middle-aged, least illness
No. of children in the home	2 direct	-	Direct in large settlements only
Sewing of skins by mother	Curvilinear 1 some handicraft least illness	1 direct	Much sewing most illness, some sewing least illness in both large and small settlements
Mother works	1 direct	-	Direct in large settlements
Mother lived in hunting camp	1 direct	1 direct	Direct in large and small settlements
Mother's education	2 some schooling least illness	2 inverse	Much schooling associated with more illness in large settlements
Mother sews children's clothes	1 inverse	1 direct	Inverse in large, direct in small
Mother carries child in amauti	1 inverse	1 direct	Direct in small, inverse in large
Mother wears zippered parka	1 direct	1 direct some illness	Direct in large, curvilinear in small settlements

TABLE 3 (continued)

| Independent (socio-economic) variables | Settlement size | | Relationship to ill-health |
	Inuvik and Frobisher Bay (N = 52)	Small settlement (N = 56)	
Mother smoked while pregnant	1 direct	± smoke illness	Direct in large, curvilinear in small settlements
No. of children previously raised by mother	3 direct	3 direct	Direct in both large and small settlements
Mother drinks alcohol	2 direct	-	Direct in large settlements
Fathers			
Head of family is natural father	-	2 inverse	Inverse in small settlements
Father has steady work	1 inverse	3 inverse	Inverse in both large and small settlements
Father's occupation skilled work	2 inverse	2 inverse	Inverse in both large and small settlements
Father's commitment to hunting	(inverse) $p = 0.20$	2 direct	Direct in small settlements
Father's schooling	1 direct	1 inverse	Direct in large, inverse in small
Father drinks alcohol	1 direct	-	Direct in large settlements
Housing			
No. of bedrooms	-	2 inverse	Inverse in small settlements
No. of children in house	2 direct	∩ least & most most illness	Direct in large, curvilinear in small settlements
No. of people in house	2 direct	1 inverse	Direct in large, inverse in small
People per bedroom	-	2 direct	Direct in small settlements
Modernity of toilet	-	1 inverse	Inverse in small settlements
Use of hand-dipped water	1 direct	1 direct	Direct in both large and small settlements
Crowding in housing	2 direct	3 direct	Direct in both large and small settlements

TABLE 3 (continued)

| Independent (socio-economic) variables | Settlement size | | Relationship to ill-health |
	Inuvik and Frobisher Bay (N = 52)	Small settlement (N = 56)	
Modernity of heating	1 bad heat ± illness	2 inverse	Curvilinear in large, inverse in small settlements
Housing quality	1 inverse	3 inverse	Inverse in both large and small settlements
Cleanliness of housing	1 inverse	1 inverse	Inverse in both large and small settlements
Nutrition			
Baby breast-fed	–	3 inverse	Inverse in small settlements
Age began bottle-feeding baby	3 inverse	3 inverse	Inverse in both large and small settlements
Food source natural	1 ± illness	2 direct	Curvilinear in large, direct in small
Eat meals often	1 direct	–	Direct in large settlements
Eat sweets	1 direct	No sweets or many sweets most illness	Direct in large, curvilinear in small settlements

* Indicates number of significant relationships, 3 being the maximum.

so that both younger and older mothers had more morbidity-mortality.

As anticipated, the data show that some variables have different effects in different-sized communities. The amount of the father's schooling and the family size are directly associated with morbidity and mortality in large settlements, but inversely associated in smaller communities. The mother's carrying of the child in an *amauti* and sewing for her children, and (more weakly) the father's interest in hunting are inversely associated with the criteria in large communities, but *directly* associated in the small settlements. These relationships suggest that acculturation of the father is inversely associated with the criterion in larger settlements but not in small, while the reverse is true of the mother.

DISCUSSION

Certain influences are clearly detrimental to infant health:
for the mother to have a hunting camp background and to
have raised many children already, both indicative of tradi-
tionalism; employment of the mother (in large settlements
only, because there is virtually no such employment in small
settlements); drinking by mothers and fathers (also restricted to the large settlements, where liquor is readily available); dirty homes; early introduction of bottle feeding;
and hand dipping of water for household use.

Other influences are beneficial: steady and skilled employment of the father, and modern uncrowded homes with more
modern toilet facilities. The remaining relationships are
somewhat paradoxical, perhaps because of correlations between the background variables. A traditional, more impoverished life-style is antithetical to infant health, explaining the inverse relationship between infant health and
the father's involvement in hunting, the mother's lengthy
carrying of the baby in the *amauti*, and the mother's sewing
of skins and children's clothes in the small settlements.
However, in the larger settlements, these same traditional
features contribute to health, either through a direct consequence (more meat to eat in a hunting household, more
protection from the cold in the *amauti*), or because the activity indicates a traditional patient and nurturant concern for children.

Some deleterious practices show a curvilinear relationship to infant health, since they are associated with prosperity and the protection prosperity brings, as well as
having more direct negative consequences for health. This
is true of smoking by the mother and family consumption of
sweets. In larger settlements, both of these indices are
inversely associated with infant health because they lose
their significance as indices of affluence.

In larger settlements, education of the father is inversely associated with infant health, at least in part, because of its association with drinking and unsteady employment. However, in small settlements, the mature population
has relatively little education, and the relationship between educational attainments and infant health is reversed.
Education of mothers shows a similar pattern, except that
in large settlements, the least as well as the best educated mothers have more unhealthy babies.

SUMMARY

The study examines socio-economic correlates of infant morbidity and mortality. High employment of males, good uncrowded housing with facilities such as tanked water, vented toilets, and modern heating are associated with infant health. An impoverished and thus usually traditional
life-style is associated with ill health, as is employment
of the mother, early bottle-feeding, overcrowded housing,
and the drinking of intoxicants by both parents. Moderate
acculturation (education) is beneficial in smaller and more
traditional settlements, as are the continued adoption of
traditional practices such as the sewing of children's clothing, carrying of the baby in the amauti, and hunting for
wild meat in the larger more acculturated settlements. The
disadvantageous consequences of heavy smoking and consumption of sweets may be masked by their association with
prosperity.

REFERENCES

1. Department of National Health and Welfare, Annual Reports on Health Conditions in the Northwest Territories.
   Northern Health Service (1961-70)
2. Dominion Bureau of Statistics, Preliminary Annual Report. Vital Statistics (1969)
3. Mowat, F., The Desperate People (Little, Brown & Co.,
   1959)

Child abuse in Alaska

G.W. BROWN

In the book *Woman's Life in Colonial Boston,* Carl Holliday
recalls the following experience: "After they had supped the
mother put two children to bed in the room where they, themselves, did lie and they went out to visit a neighbour. When
they returned the mother went to the bed and not finding
her youngest child, a daughter of about 5 years of age, and
after much search, she found it drownded in a well in her

cellar (1)." Child abuse remains a major problem in urbanized societies today, with multiple historical, sociological, genetic, legal, educational, and health aspects (2,3,
4,5). Whenever a child appears in an emergency ward with a
broken femur, a fractured skull, or cigarette burns, a host
of recent and past biological and sociological factors have
led up to this end result. If a father arriving in Alaska
with his family gets such employment that income for rent,
food and clothing is assured, certain forms of child abuse
will not occur. Lack of employment or sudden loss of employment often tips the scales for abuse in an already unstable
family situation (6).

DEFINITIONS

The Alaskan Child Protection Statute defines neglect as "the
failure to provide necessary food, care, clothing, shelter,
or medical attention for a child." Abuse in the Alaskan
statute means "the affliction by other than accidental means
of physical harm upon the body of a child." A child is here
defined as a person under 16 years of age. Several states
are changing their child protection statutes to include emotional abuse, but this has not yet been done in Alaska.
Kempe (2) and Silver (7) have stressed that emotional deprivation of children, whether from ineffective parenthood
or outright rejection, can cause a "failure to thrive syndrome" which is as abusive as physical injury by other than
accidental means.

CLINICAL FEATURES

The profile of an abusing parent is characteristic. Usually,
the parent suffered abuse as a child. The child is seen as
hard to raise, a "bad seed," or adopted, and it may have a
special disability such as a birth defect or a chronic illness. Recent stress has often upset a precarious family
balance, and the family lacks a "lifeline," a community contact to which they can turn for help in time of crisis. In
a survey from Denver, over 90 per cent of child-abusing parents had no significant psychopathology (2). They were ordinary people who for various reasons lost emotional control, struck out and harmed their children. What forms does
abuse take? Cigarette burns are common. Multiple bruising
may be seen, with or without poorly explained fractures in
different stages of healing; the areas involved include the
legs, face, neck, and other body regions not normally accep-

ted for disciplining purposes. Watch must be kept for damage
to internal organs (liver, spleen, and stomach). During infancy, subdural bleeding is a common manifestation of abuse.
Caffey has stressed the danger of the practice of simply
shaking infants (8). A child whose height and weight remain
consistently below that expected from their birth weight
and gestational age should be suspected as suffering from
emotional abuse.

PSYCHOLOGICAL FACTORS

De Mause (9) has reviewed sociological and psychological
factors which cause abuse, neglect, and rejection of the
child. He writes: "In studying childhood over many generations, it is most important to concentrate on those moments
which most affect the society of the next generation; primarily, this means what happens when an adult is face to
face with a child who needs something. The adult has, I believe, three major reactions available: 1. He can use the
child as a vehicle for projection of the contents of his
own unconscious (Projective reaction), 2. He can use the
child as a substitute for an adult figure important in his
own childhood (Reversal reaction), or 3. He can empathise
with the child's needs and act to satisfy them (Empathetic
reaction)."

COMMUNITY RESPONSES TO CHILD ABUSE

What are some possible solutions? It is easy to state that
parents need help in bringing up their children. It is more
complicated to utilize existing resources and develop new
approaches to providing help in face of the breakdown of
Western family units, with great separation of parents,
grandparents, and other traditional extended families.
    The "Child Protection Task Force" is a multi-professional
and lay voluntary organization, authorized by the Board of
Health of the Greater Anchorage Area Health Department to
explore various means of dealing with this problem. Approaches used include: parent aides, volunteers who work
with neglectful parents; foster homes and nurseries for
crisis placement; parent anonymous groups; parent discussion
groups guided by public health nurses, paediatricians, and
psychiatrists; and development of education materials to
supplant the traditional school health education and family
life courses.

Parent aides, or "lay therapists," reach out actively to help families in crisis, particularly families who feel unable to establish friendships (4). In contrast to professional social workers and public health nurses, parent aides are not concerned with how the baby is faring or how the parent is meeting the baby's needs. Rather, parent aides utilize reflective listening. The goal is to convey, over a period of six to eighteen months, that the parent is accepted and liked for himself or herself, without reference to his/her role as a parent. This establishes friendship and subconsciously helps the parent begin to listen to and understand the needs of his own child. In two years' experience with parent aides in Anchorage, nearly 80 per cent of children are safely returned to their homes in less than eight months, without recurrence of abuse.

The Child Protection Task Force has also established a permanent multiprofessional team called the Anchorage Child Abuse Board, Incorporated. Included on this team are a public health nurse, a psychologist, a minister, a child psychiatrist, a paediatrician, an attorney, and a social worker. The team meets once a week and accepts referrals from other community professional agencies or individuals. However, most of the referrals come from the State's Child Protection Unit. When necessary, the team requests further social or psychological evaluation of either parents or children before making recommendations. The board recruits, selects, trains, and provides on-going supervision of parent aides, and has plans for developing crisis nurseries. It also assists the Borough Health Department in the provision of regular parent discussion groups.

STATISTICAL COMPARISON

Alaska's central reporting of child abuse became effective in June 1971. Over the first year (1971-72), the rate was 48 per 100,000 children, compared with a maximum of 40 per 100,000 children in other parts of the US. From January through June 1973, reported physical abuse was 60 per 100,000, while combined statistics for abuse and neglect were rated at 440 per 100,000. New York City reported 480 cases of abuse and neglect per 100,000 children per year from 1970 to 1972.

No one knows the total number of children that die from abuse. The only two causes of childhood death that increased in the US from 1955 to 1965 were motor vehicle accidents and homicide. There are more than three deaths from child abuse every day in New York and Chicago alone.

CULTURAL COMPARISON

Reported rates of abuse in Alaska may be compared with
those for Iceland. There are some geographic similarities.
Alaska has a rapidly growing population of 300,000. Iceland
has a population of 200,000 which has doubled over the last
70 years. Reykjavik had a population of just over 81,000 in
January 1970, but the records of the child welfare board
showed only four cases of abuse over the decade 1960-69.
Two of the mothers concerned had a history of excessive use
of alcohol and one was reportedly brought up by a domineer-
ing mother who punished her physically, a rare occurrence
in Iceland (10).

Four major features of Icelandic society may be emphasized (10): (1) compulsory health insurance has been in effect since 1936; (2) the population has not been exposed to
war for centuries, except for a peaceful occupation during
World War II (there has never been an Icelandic Army);
(3) violent crimes like murder and rape are rare, with only
14 recorded murders over the period from 1945 to 1970;
(4) Icelanders are individualistic, but still possess the
characteristic of a small society in maintaining lasting
ties between relatives and friends. Interest in genealogy
and personal history is common, and people concern themselves with the welfare of their neighbours.

In contrast, Alaska's health system has a private sector,
a special federal medical service for Alaskan natives,
multiple state and federal maternal, child health, and
crippled children's programs, recent federal Medicaid programs, and emphasis on early screening. Families who are in
stress, who have lost extended family contact, who have inadequate income and who lack community resources and friends
often fall between the gaps in this pluralistic health care
delivery system. The Anchorage Child Protection Task Force,
and the related Child Abuse Board, provide one possible
means of overcoming Alaska's problem of delivering care to
the abused child.

ACKNOWLEDGMENT

The author's appreciation is expressed to members of the
Anchorage Child Protection Task Force and Child Abuse
Board, Inc.

SUMMARY

The hallmark of success in child protection work is co-
operation. Child abuse and neglect encompass all health,
educational, and social endeavours. A multiprofessional
team in co-operation with volunteer groups such as parents
anonymous has been successful in several US metropolitan
centres. However, achievements have been sporadic, with
problems arising from a pluralism of health care services
and stubborn individualism. Alaska presents many challenges
to developing health and social services. Rugged individualism prevails, but does not guarantee economic and social
success. Broken homes with killed, maimed, and chronically
mistreated children abound. Chaotic and unplanned development from gold rush days through earthquakes and floods to
the oil pipeline dream has dumped many federal, state, and
private enterprises into a rapidly growing and heterogeneous population. Families of all racial and cultural groups
lack stability. Suicides, murders, and accidents related to
alcohol and drug abuse are relatively more frequent than in
many other parts of the United States.
    Professionals and volunteers in Anchorage, Alaska have
now developed a community-based child protection service.
This has helped both public and professional education and
professional team involvement with specific cases. In contrast, reported incidence of child abuse in Iceland is very
low. This may relate to differences of social, cultural,
governmental, and family structures compared with Alaska.

REFERENCES

1. Holliday, Carl, Woman's Life in Colonial Boston (Boston, 1922), p. 25
2. Kempe, C.H., "Paediatric implications of the battered
   baby syndrome," Arch. dis. child, 46: 28 (1971)
3. Gill, David G., "Physical abuse of children," Peds.,
   44 (4): 857 (1969)
4. Kempe, C.H. and Helfer, R.E., Helping the Battered
   Child and his Family (Philadelphia: J.B. Lippincott,
   Co., 1972), p. 73
5. Grantmyre, Edward, "Trauma X-Wednesday's Child," Nova
   Scotia Med. Bull., February 29-31 (1973)
6. Davoren, Elizabeth, "The role of the social worker,"
   In Helfer, R.E., and Kempe, C.H. (eds.), The Battered
   Child (Chicago: University of Chicago Press, 1968)

7. Silver, Henry K., and Finkelstein, Marcia, "Deprivation dwarfism," J. Paediatr., 70: 317 (1967)
8. Caffey, John, "The parent-infant traumatic stress syndrome," Am. Roentgenol., 114 (2): 217 (1972)
9. DeMause, Lloyd (ed.), The History of Childhood (New York: Physohistory Press, 1974)
10. Karlsson, Asgeir, "The battered child syndrome in Iceland," Nord. Psyk. Tidssk., 25 (2): 112 (1971)

Commentaries

"Hospital outbreak of adenovirus type 3 pneumonia," by D. Wilkinson, O. Morgante, E.R. Burchak, and F.A. Herbert (Edmonton, Canada). Between July 1963 and October 1964, 206 lower respiratory tract infections were studied during hospital admissions of Indian and Eskimo children. From only four was adenovirus type 3 (AV_3) isolated. There appeared to be no increase in AV_3 in the community during the study period. From July 1964 to December 1964 inclusive sto l and nasopharyngeal suction were negative for AV_3 on 37 children on admission. Of four readmissions in November and December, three were positive for AV_3. During November and December 1964 AV_3 was isolated from 12 patients who became ill after admission. Ten of these showed a rise in neutralizing titre to AV_3 in paired bloods. The clinical course of children showed a temperature of 39.4°C lasting 6 days or longer in 8 out of these 10; conjunctivitis in 3, lasting 2 days or less; cyanosis in 6; and wheezing in 7. There were no deaths. Eight other children had similar illness but virus studies were not done. Institutional outbreaks of adenovirus are uncommon and none has been described in Canada previously.

"Bronchiectasis and bronchitis in Indian children following adeno III virus pneumonia in infancy: a long-term follow-up," by F.A. Herbert, E.R. Burchak, and D. Wilkinson (Charles Camsell Hospital and University of Alberta, Edmonton, Canada). Eleven Indian children under 20 months of age who suffered adeno III type pneumonia during an epidemic in

1964 were re-examined eight to ten years later. Plain films of the chest and/or bronchograms were abnormal in nine. Cylindrical bronchiectatic or bronchitic changes were noted in the seven individuals on whom bronchography was performed. These changes were multilobar and multisegmental in all and bilateral in three. In three patients areas of current lung damage could be related to the "original" pneumonia. Blood gases were relatively normal but significant abnormalities of a restrictive and obstructive type were found. Tuberculin tests were negative, and no immunological abnormalities were detected. Despite the foregoing findings, the children seemed clinically well and were leading normal lives.

"Intractable diarrhoea in Baffin Island Eskimos," by D.M. Coulter and J.S. Popkin (Department of Paediatrics, Montreal Children's Hospital, McGill University, Montreal, Canada). During the three-year period from January 1971 to December 1973 intractable diarrhoea was the single most common cause of referral of infants from Frobisher Bay to the Montreal Children's Hospital. Of the 96 Eskimos referred because of medical problems, there were 16 (17 per cent) with this diagnosis. This disorder was also the most lethal in that 3 (19 per cent) of the infants died. The infants ages ranged from 3 weeks to 9 months, and they came from ten different settlements. All had prolonged diarrhoea with volumes up to 1 litre per day, resistant to oral management and intravenous fluid maintenance with dextrose and electrolytes. Despite thorough bacterial and viral investigations pathogenic organisms were isolated in only one case. Of three infants seen in 1971, two died. The survivor was the sole infant with pathogenic bacteria isolated from her stools. Since November 1972, 13 infants have been treated with early, total intravenous alimentation (dextrose, amino acids, vitamins, Intralipid). Twelve of these infants survived, one dying of a central venous catheter mishap. More aggressive, earlier introduction of total intravenous alimentation has markedly improved the success rate with these children. Further investigation of the pathophysiology of intractable diarrhoea in Eskimo infants is urgently needed.

MENTAL HEALTH AND
CULTURAL CHANGE

Eskimo personality and society – yesterday and today

O. SCHAEFER and M. METAYER

Father Metayer is still a patient in Charles Camsell Hospital, recovering from major surgery. This has given me the opportunity to continue our discussions of the changing personal and social world of the Inuit which began some ten years ago on Holman Island, where I did a health and nutrition survey and Father Metayer collected Inuit legends and studied their genealogy and kinship relations (Figure 1).

Father Metayer is the author of a number of well-known books: *Arlok L'esquimau* published in French, and *I, Nuligak* and *Tales from the Igloo* available in both English and French. His many years of painstaking research into the traditions and mythology of the Central Arctic Inuit have led to the recent publication of *La tradition esquimaude* by the Centre D'Etudes Nordiques of Laval University, a major three-volume work. His genealogical and kinship studies - likely the most extensive ever undertaken for the Copper Eskimos - still await final work-up and publication. I thus wish to acknowledge here my indebtedness to Father Metayer for much of what I have to say.

In our opening session, Dr Brett and Professor Milan will speak about the changing health picture in the Arctic and the frightening prevalence of violence; violence, poisoning, infanticide, and suicide are now the leading causes of death for most native groups in the NWT, the Yukon, and Alaska. Jean Briggs, who lived with the Inuit at Chantrey Inlet for almost two years, emphasized the pre-eminent place of education against anger and violent behaviour in traditional Eskimo society. Her research on the conscious and subconscious education of infants and children against expressions of anger and violence is well known from her book *Never in Anger*. Dr Brody describes the breakdown of traditional family structure and traditional education in modern Eskimo communities; such a breakdown no doubt helps

to explain the frightening increase of violent behaviour
over the last few years. Drs Lynge and Sølling from Greenland draw attention to the role of alcohol in this connection and Dr Kraus reports on the related suicide problems
of native Alaskans.

It has been said that no people in the world developed
such a fierce individualism as the Eskimo. This is only
partly true. For obvious reasons, a hostile environment
with limited food resources, the Eskimos did not develop a
strong tribal culture or a stratified social structure. The
individual family was very much on its own, but within that
family group the individual person was totally responsive
to the needs of the family group in all his or her actions,
even to decisions involving life and death (such as the
priority of eating in times of famine).

Western man has moved far away from such identification
of the individual with the interest and welfare of the family. In modern society individual or state interests in-
fringe upon and displace family priorities in an extreme
manner. When this life-style is suddenly transferred and imposed upon a people still accustomed to the protective pluralism of the extended family, the individual is left in-
secure, lonely, directionless, and meaningless.

An attempt is made in Tables 1-3 to contrast the social
structure, prevailing values, attitudes and practices, and
personal roles and functions of family members in traditional and modern Eskimo society. This form of tabulation
is naturally far too generalized, and freezes a living con-
tinuum of great dynamic complexity with many local variations into an exaggerated and polarized still-picture. However, it may allow us to see some of the cultural and sociological trends that are having a major impact on the physical, mental, and social health of Eskimo society today.

The trends depicted are not unique to the Eskimo. Similar
observations have been made on various American Indian societies and other cultural minorities subjected to

TABLE 1
Eskimo personality and society, yesterday and today

Eskimos retained in the hostile central arctic a primordial social organization based on the extended family comprising perhaps two brothers
with their wives and children and one or two of their parents. There
were no tribal chiefs. The wisest men were listened to and followed
but without compulsion.

---

acculturation. Nevertheless, the picture is more impressive in the case of the Eskimo, as the impact of acculturation has been more recent and more sudden and has involved greater cultural and sociological differences between the traditional and the assumed cultures.

Figures 1-4 further illustrate the role of the mother in Eskimo society. Figure 1 is an Eskimo carving of Mother and Child by Celina (Repulse Bay, NWT): Celina, an elderly Eskimo lady from Repulse Bay, recreated in this carving her image of the natural and ideal mother-child relationship, emphasizing the infant's central role in the mother's life. Anyone who has seen Eskimo children carried on a mother's back knows that children may peek over the right or left

TABLE 2
Members of the nuclear Eskimo family

In the past	Now
Father	*Father*
Highly respected	Feels useless and worthless
The provider of food, on whose hunting skill the life of every member of the family depended. To be known as a good food provider for his own family, the elderly, and neighbours in need was a source of pride and satisfaction.	Eskimo men have lost the independence of the traditional hunter. Work is often for and under a non-Eskimo agent, doing menial, despised and degrading jobs or, even worse, the Eskimo may be shamed into the status of a welfare recipient. He finds transient emotional redress from feelings of frustration, idleness, dependence, and hurt pride in drinking. Alcohol unmasks pent-up hostility feelings leading to violence. The hangover is accompanied by remorse and suicidal behaviour.
Mother	*Mother*
Loved and needed	Has lost central family role, feeling dispensible and idle.
Preparer of shelter, food and clothing. Indispensible centre of family, always busy making and repairing fur clothing, tents, and utensils, tending seal oil lamps day and night, nursing, training, and playing with children. Giving and receiving stimulation and satisfaction in intense interaction with child carried skin to skin for three years on her back or breast.	Clothing and food bought in store. Infants bottle-fed and deposited with siblings, grandparents or left unattended in corner of bed. Idleness whiled away in movies, dances, bars, and "friends." Becoming impatient and punitive, with less well understood and less well trained children.

TABLE 2 (continued)

In the past	Now
Children	*Children*
Loved and cared for, feeling secure and satisfied, with ideal parent figures to imitate. Grew up on mother's back, first three years in intimate contact, receiving response and satisfaction to every urge, motion, and demand in sheltered and secure position, allowing participation in mother's and family's activities and progressing from playful imitation to useful participation in parent's chores.	Intimate infant-mother interaction and understanding lost. Less secure shelter, inferior nourishment. Emotional and sensory deprivation when left to stare listless at empty ceiling or screaming frustrated in soggy diapers.
	Later
	Loss of parents' ideal image and respect. Feeling useless and frustrated, having lost functional role in Eskimo world while unable to realize desires awakened by school and movies. Becomes confused and rebellious.
Interaction in family	*Interaction in family*
Very close. Complete and un-questioned interdependence but with extreme personal tolerance.	Drifting apart. Not needing each other so much. Expressions of anger and intolerance: wife and child beatings. Children rebelling against elders.

shoulder of the mother, but here the infant's head sits right in the centre of the mother's shoulders and there is no doubt the mother figuratively adjusts her head and whole personality to the centre of her attention: Her Child!

Figure 2 shows a carver's view of how the mother-child relationship has developed: it is a carving from Inujuak (Pt. Harrison, Arctic Quebec). His woman is loaded down by two small children, where there is room for only one. She is burdened by the population explosion of the 1960s, as bottle-feeding replaced traditional prolonged breast-feeding.

In the transitional society of some 6 to 8 years ago, when this carving was made, the woman is literally bent down to the ground by too many children; she feels over-burdened and has lost that close and accommodating relationship to her children, which Celina depicted so well.

Figure 3 shows a young mother, nursing her baby inside her amauti (woman's parka, with room to carry baby on back

TABLE 3
Social values, attitudes, and practices

In the past	Now
Personal qualities, not possessions, counted	*Imitation of materialistic expressions of success in the modern world*
Skill, endurance, and deftness marked the man as a likely good food provider and desirable family father. Cloth-making ability rated highest in social attributes of Eskimo women. (Eskimo proverbs speak of the role of wife in hunter's prowess and endurance, and in guarding against burning down of tent)	Big salary, big house, big motorboat, big motorsled are aspirations and regarded as a measure of social success by the young Eskimo men. Getting a well-paid position and buying fancy clothes, rather than making them, characteristic of Eskimo girls.
Sharing of the hunter's kill or catch	
Observed in all Eskimo groups, but most generously in the central arctic where sharing rather than storing ensured survival of a maximum number of people in the face of unpredictable and often shifting migration routes of game. The unlucky hunter did not starve as long as a luckier neighbour could be reached.	Native meat and fish are still shared, but money derived from trapping and wage employment plus the social benefits and amenities bought with this money are, as "white man's" money or tools, not subject to this sharing concept.
	The desire to acquire more of the imagined white man's materialistic success tends to destroy or pervert the vestiges of the sharing concept. Native meat and fish are often surreptitiously sold to whites to circumvent the compulsion to share. Everybody for himself.
Education	*Education*
Continuous from infancy, by imitating and working with parents. Persuasion to help willingly. No overt coercion. Emphasis on restraining anger and violent behaviour.	School has taken the place of parents, with less respect for personality and more impersonal conformity. Parents have lost respect and authority. Expressions of anger and violence are prominent in movies. Emphasis on: "Do not hide your anger, speak up."

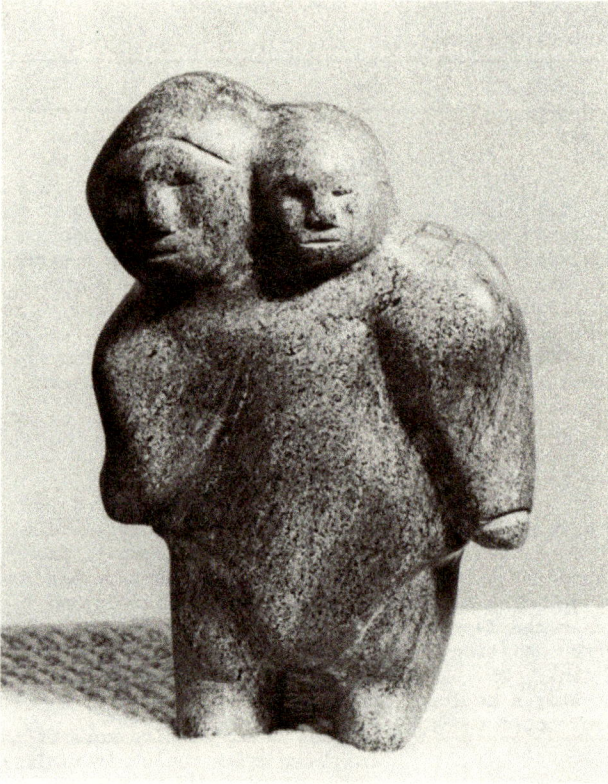

Figure 1

or breast): I saw this beautiful young mother a few days
after she had been delivered in this igloo at Pelly Bay. It
is her first baby. Note how she is completely absorbed in
her main task, satisfying her baby physically and emotionally and oblivious to distractions from the intruder with
his camera and flashlights.

Figure 4 shows another Eskimo mother taking a naked infant out of the amauti to void after nursing. Notice that
only a small piece of cariboo fur is placed at the anus to
give some protection against soiling of the mother's parka
by faeces; this gives little or no protection against
wetting of the amauti by urine. When I questioned the
mother about this, she shook her head in disbelief at such
silly questions: "I am not so dumb. A mother feels and
knows when her baby wants to void." She indicated by imita-

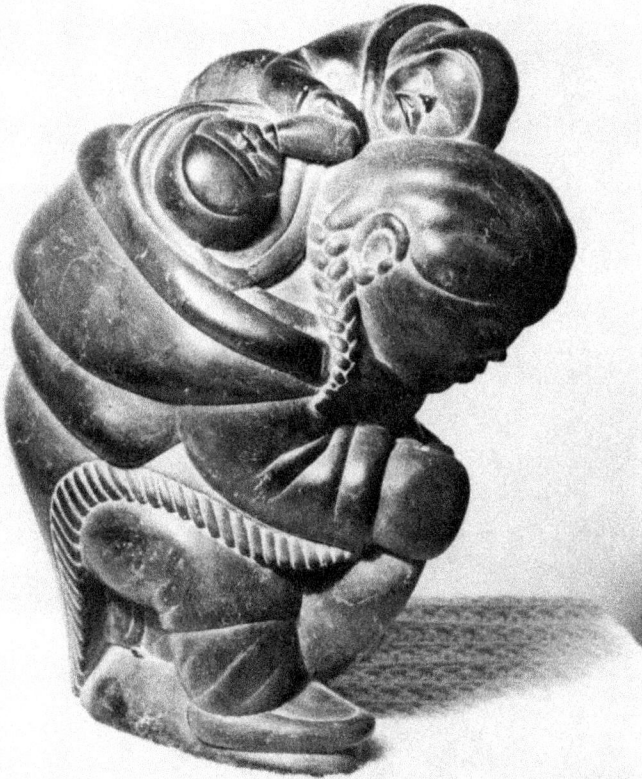

Figure 2

ted movements that an infant normally rests in the amauti with his legs abducted on the mother's back, but makes spasmodic adduction movements with the thighs when the bladder is full and before the sphincter is opened. The interaction and understanding between the baby and mother is so intense and complete that every urge of the infant is attended to immediately, ensuring optimal physical and emotional satisfaction and preventing a build-up of feelings of frustration.

Enuresis or bed-wetting in later childhood is a common paediatric problem in western society. Dr Seitamo has noted a significant increase in the Skolt Lapps troubled by

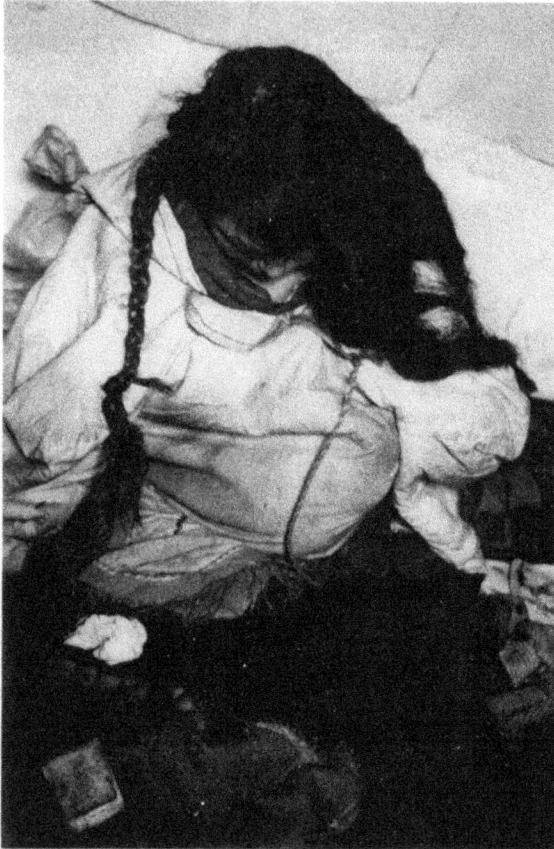

Figure 3

acculturation problems, but it was practically unknown in
a society whose infants were toilet trained almost from
birth. There seem no signs of the alleged psychological
trauma paediatric psychologists of our neurotic western
society have warned us should accompany too early attempted toilet training!

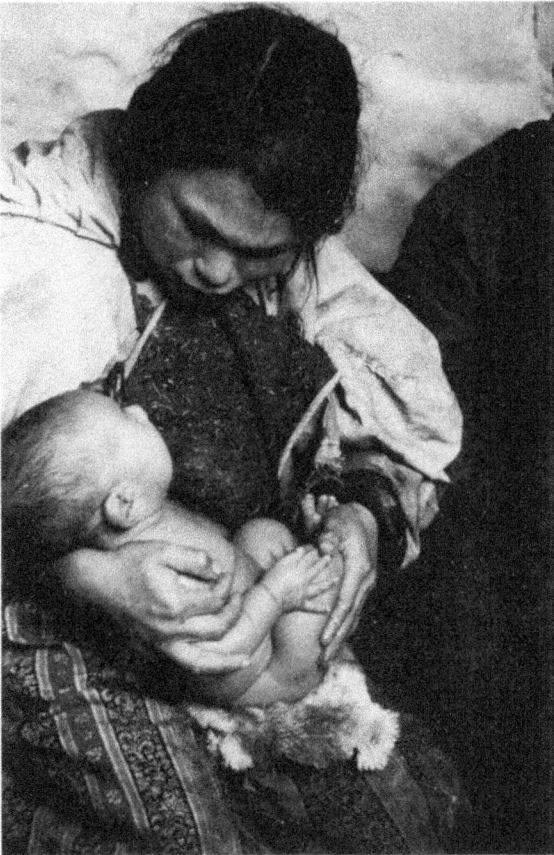

Figure 4

CONCLUSION

The basic elements of traditional Eskimo society, a tightly
knit family structure and personal values, attitudes, and
practices shaped for successful life in a harsh environment,
are falling apart. The older generation feels numbed, be-
wildered, and saddened, while the younger generation is
idle, frustrated, and rebellious.

Men are deprived of their traditional role as meat providers, emasculated and powerless; relief from feelings of
worthlessness and frustration with a temporary illusion of
power are sought through alcohol. This in turn unleashes
pent-up feelings of hostility, aggression, and violence.

Hangovers lead to remorse and even to suicidal behaviour.

Women have lost their indispensable central role in the family, and no longer have an intimate and intense interaction with their children. They suffer from idleness even more than the men.

Children are deprived nutritionally and emotionally from early infancy. They have lost the ideal image of their parents, and no longer learn to become useful by imitating their actions. They often feel misunderstood, useless, and rebellious.

The only social institution of major importance in Eskimo life, the family, is disintegrating. Nothing has yet taken its place. The individual is left lonely, frightened, without direction, and full of anxiety.

An anecdote from my own life with fairly traditional Eskimos further illustrates the consciously patient and personal way of traditional Eskimo education.

When getting ready to leave for a four-week dogsled trip to camps on the Davis Strait, I helped Ituangat, my Eskimo guide, to tie down the load on our long sled. It was much later than I had wanted to leave, and I was in a rush. Joapie, the five-year-old adopted son of Ituangat, groaning and moaning like an old Eskimo, was trying to tighten the ropes. Naturally, he could not make it firm enough, so I pushed him out of my way. All day, Ituangat, with whom I normally exchanged little jokes in my clumsy Eskimo, remained sullen and silent.

On the second day out, my never very profound patience snapped and I exploded, but still no answer. Finally, on the third day after a particularly hard stretch of our route, we were recovering our spirits over a cup of tea and he started on his own: "Doc, I always thought you understood more of us Inuit than the other Kadloonait, but when we left you pushed Joapie out of your way, acting no better than any of them. Did you not notice that I did not push Joapie away? I waited until he was a bit away from me or on your side before re-tightening the ropes. Our boys learn by doing the same as we do and we don't push them away; we don't even let them see or feel if their work has to be redone; they help better when you make them feel they are needed and useful. Joapie will not try to help us for a long time to come now you have pushed him away as useless!"

It is not always so easy to let children help us in modern civilization; certainly not when you are involved with different machinery or a complex operation where a mistake can cost lives, but Ituangat convinced me that there

are many occasions when we should tolerate or better encourage our children's natural desire to imitate the actions
of their elders and to do useful work. Otherwise, we contribute unnecessarily to the growing frustration and deviation
of the younger generation.

Modernity, social structure, and mental health of Eskimos in the Canadian eastern arctic

H.M. SAMPATH

The concept of modernity is a comparatively recent one in
the history of the social sciences. It is usually applied
to traditional societies which are experiencing changes as
a result of contact with Euro-American societies. This contact, which began as early as 500 years ago, gained momen-
tum on a worldwide scale less than 100 years ago, and, in
the Canadian Eastern Arctic, exploded after the end of
World War II. Although seen originally as a purely cultural phenomenon and described as "acculturation," "cultural
change," and the "clash of cultures," there has always been
an awareness of a distinction between social and cultural
factors, so that the combined term "socio-cultural changes"
has found popular usage.

The concept of "social structure" has also been developed
by anthropologists. It is more comprehensive than the concept of "social stratification" which sociologists have utilized quite successfully in studies of modern urban societies. Caudill (4) postulated at least four dimensions of
human behaviour: social, structural, cultural, psychological and biological. He believed that the variance of effects on human behaviour was greatest for the social structural dimension. He suggested that modern social structure
and historical culture should be treated as separate variables, both having fairly independent effects on behaviour
and psychological adjustment.

Modernity affects all four of Caudill's dimensions, but
with regard to the Eskimos in the Canadian Eastern Arctic,
changes of social structure are most dramatic. It has al-

ways been assumed - quite incorrectly - that cultural
change is axiomatically stressful, but as Chance has shown
in Alaska, it can proceed with the minimum of psychological
trauma.

SIKOSULIARMIUT SOCIAL STRUCTURE

Traditionally, Eskimos have been given a territorial identity. The suffix "miut" or "meit" ("inhabitant of"), together
with a place name, was the designation applied to a particular group. But as Graburn (8) pointed out, "these groupings have indefinite boundaries and are of little significance in differentiating the major cultural features of the
area." Boas (3) referred to the Eskimo groups as "tribes,"
and he gave a valuable list showing the geographical distribution of the Central Eskimo tribes. Following Boas, the
Eskimos of Oxford Bay (pseudonym of a Southern Baffin Island
settlement) belong to the tribe called the "Sikosuliarmiut."
    At one time or another, the Sikosuliarmiut occupied at
least 16 coastal sites along this particular part of Baffin
Island. Such sites will be referred to as "camps," the word
"settlement" being reserved for the new, post-contact sites
containing the Hudson Bay Company posts and certain government institutions. An Eskimo camp community was composed of
a more or less transient body of individuals. Membership was
determined or recruited by consent of its former members, as
well as by birth, marriage, and adoption. It was more open
(with or without restrictions) than closed to outsiders, but
it was a comparatively weak social unit. It consisted of a
small number of loosely organized households. The descent
system of its inhabitants was often bilateral, and the post-
marital residence was bilocal, neolocal, or unilocal. There
were no strict kinship bonds among the members of the community; a household could leave a community at any time and
join another by obtaining its members' consent. The new
arrival at once acknowledged his dependence and was then under the influence if not control of the leader of the community which he joined.
    In 1914, Fleming (7), the original Bishop of the Arctic,
made his first trip along the Southern coast of Baffin Island. He visited an unnamed Eskimo camp on "the extreme west
end of Baffin Island," which had a population of 37 people.
This would indicate about eight nuclear families with a
smaller number of households, and agrees with information
obtained from informants in Oxford Bay as well as that from
the earliest available census made by the RCMP in 1965.

There were then five camps around Oxford Bay; two of these
had eight nuclear families, one had seven, one had three,
and one had two. Some of these heads of families were kin
members, e.g. brothers or brothers-in-law, but others were
not. Informants also testified to a great deal of movement
from camp to camp. The camp leader usually remained in the
same camp, but the composition of the camp membership kept
changing. Any member who felt dissatisfied was free to
leave. He could either join another pre-existing camp or
alternatively he could leave with some of his kin and/or
friends and establish his own camp. Thus, one informant -
now a respected elder resident of Oxford Bay - explained
how he lived for two years at a certain camp where a very
well-known figure was the leader; he then decided he wanted
to be "free" and left the camp, taking with him his own
family, his wife's sister's family, and two other men who
were brothers. Together, they established a new camp, with
himself as leader. He developed a good reputation as a
leader and attracted many other families.

Nomadism had an important role in the establishment and
maintenance of interpersonal relations among the Eskimos.
Intercamp migration functioned as an escape mechanism and
tended to avoid serious confrontation between parties. The
individual was free to leave the camp and establish himself
elsewhere. This physical withdrawal was easily possible
when there were other camps in the area, especially before
the Eskimos started to accumulate many material goods. The
older adult Eskimos complain that there are too many people
in the settlement, and that they have lost their freedom of
movement. There is possibly a connection between the physical withdrawal of migration which existed in the camp situation, and the emotional withdrawal which has been noticed
in large settlements like Frobisher Bay.

The highly segmented structure of Eskimo society preclu-
ded the emergence of a truly political leader. However, in
the Oxford Bay area there developed a leader whose status
extended beyond his own camp. He had the reputation of
being an able and skilful hunter, and was able to amass a
great deal of wealth. He could afford to be generous to kin
and to non-kin, and this created a network of obligations
and a certain sense of community throughout the area. He
was also able to keep in a subservient position a number of
other Eskimos who, because of their poverty and low social
status, were referred to as "slaves."

The accumulation of noticeable wealth assumed an added
dimension following contact with white traders. After a

trading session with the Hudson Bay Company, the above-mentioned camp leader would load his komatik with foodstuffs and other desirable goods which he would then distribute to other Eskimos in various camps, ensuring his reputation as a benevolent boss. In this particular camp, therefore, there was a definite social rank order with the wealthy camp leader at one extreme and the poor "slave" at the other.

The flexibility of Eskimo social organization (17) is well illustrated by the changing patterns of social organization observed in Eskimo societies since contact with Europeans was first established. Thus, Balicki (1) described an early phase in the development of Povungnituk, in which the camp leaders played an important role in settlement affairs. Some time later, in the same settlement, Vallee (16) found that the role of the camp leaders had gradually diminished.

Wilmott (18) first conceptualized social differences among Eskimos, distinguishing "camp" and "settlement" Eskimos. Vallee (15) found that the Eskimos of Baker Lake differentiated between "Nunamiut" (people of the land) and "Kabloonamiut" (people of the white man). In this particular settlement, the two groups were developing into social classes, for as Vallee pointed out, "the status of the Nunamiut is being compared unfavourably in terms of prestige to the status of Kabloonamiut."

In Frobisher Bay, the settlement with the largest number of Eskimos in the Arctic, the Honigmanns (9) found that "inequalities in income, jobs, housing, and aspirations have failed to promote stratified social classes," but they distinguished three "personality types" which correspond roughly to degrees of acculturation, which "don't form social classes, though it is tempting to guess that, given time and a rigidification of economic opportunities ... will evolve into social classes." In Inuvik, a large settlement in the Western Arctic, Mailhot (12) found that "social stratification" is emerging - as possibilities of upward mobility for the individual develop. Modernization inevitably produces inequalities, for a variety of new roles are established in the society. As these roles become institutionalized, corresponding status positions emerge and these tend to be fitted into a rank order. The Honigmanns (9) felt that there were cultural barriers which served "to maintain egalitarianism ... most important being the Eskimo's inclination to discriminate qualities of individuals rather than of stereotyped social categories."

Egalitarianism among the Sikosuliarmiut began to disappear long before the settlement was established. It has been mentioned above how one camp boss grew so wealthy and powerful that he actually had "slaves." Social inequality therefore was no new phenomenon to the inhabitants of the settlement.

THE CONTEMPORARY SOCIAL STRUCTURE

The Oxford Bay identification list of 15 January 1970 showed a total population of 592 Eskimos resident in the area. This population was made up of 98 nuclear families who occupied 84 houses, and two families who still lived in a camp. Prior to my arrival, six families had emigrated to settlements from whence they had come the previous year, and one family had moved to Frobisher Bay. These six families consisted of 45 individuals. In addition to births and deaths, the Eskimo population changes when individuals leave the settlement for medical treatment in Frobisher Bay or Southern Canada, to attend school at Churchill or other parts of Canada, for job training or employment elsewhere in Canada, and when Eskimos emigrate from other settlements to Oxford Bay.

The aboriginal Eskimo camp was characterized by the absence of any formal organization. The only recognized status positions outside of the kinship system where those of leader or camp boss, and shaman. Sometimes the same individual held both status positions. However, as we have pointed out above, it would appear that in this region of Baffin Island an embryonic social class system was in the process of being developed following contact with the Hudson Bay Company. The new settlement eventually contained the populations of all the camps in the region. This meant that there were a number of ex-camp leaders residing together in the settlement. At this stage, the settlement was a heterogenous collection of various camp members. Housing was of the traditional type, although one of the wealthy camp leaders moved his frame house from his camp to the settlement. At first, camp neighbours were also settlement neighbours, but even though the settlement population was increasing rapidly, there was nothing that could be called a community organization.

In the early 1950s the government began experimenting with various designs of houses, but it was not until 1966 that 25 units were erected and a rental program introduced. This necessitated the formation of a housing association, with authority to decide on allocation of the available houses. The Association consisted of nine members with a

chairman, secretary, and treasurer, all of whom were Eskimos. There are five settlement organizations in which Eskimos are involved. These are: the Anglican Church (to which
all the Eskimos without exception belong), the Community
Council, the Housing Association, the Community Society,
and the Co-operative. These organizations all originated at
the instigations of non-Eskimos, and with the exception of
the Anglican Church, by government agents. They reflect the
increasing efforts of government to develop a community
identity with greater Eskimo participation in the affairs
of the settlement.

Oxford Bay is now in an interesting phase of development.
It achieved territorial autonomy in September 1970, when the
last surviving satellite camp was abondoned and its inhabitants moved into the settlement. It provides full time employment for a number of individuals and many others earn an
income from their artistic work. All the inhabitants live
in government houses supplied with heat and electricity, and
income from government sources, such as old age pensions,
family allowances, and welfare payments, is available to
those who qualify.

What are some of the factors which lead towards social
inequality? These include: occupation, associations, wealth,
descent, religion, and marriage. The older adult Eskimos
were born in camps, and the act of taking up residence in
the settlement dramatized a repudiation of camp life and a
turning away from native culture. There is no doubt this
has produced guilt feelings, accounting for the great ambivalence which has characterized most aspects of their life
in the settlement.

No account of the social structure of a contemporary Eskimo settlement would be complete without mention of the
non-Eskimo or predominantly white group. The psychiatric
implications resulting from the relationships between these
two groups only compound the mental health picture of the
Eskimos (11).

MENTAL HEALTH SURVEY

A mental health survey was carried out by the author. A total number of 214 adults (age 15 and over), 97 males and
117 females, were interviewed. This represented over 93 per
cent of the adult population. As part of the interview, the
HOS (Health Opinion Survey) questionnaire was administered,
a mental status examination was done, and a diagnosis
(using the APA DSM II) was made.

Mental Status Examination

Of the 214 individuals interviewed, 80 were suffering from a diagnosable mental disorder. This gives a total prevalence rate of 373/1,000, which may appear quite high by North American standards. However, high morbidity rates are not uncommon in similar cultural groups. For example, Leon and Climent (10) found an Indian group in Colombia where 72 per cent of the population were suffering from diagnosable mental disorders.

The prevalence rate for schizophrenia was 28/1,000 and for the affective psychoses the rate was 46/1,000. Such high rates are probably due to genetic factors operating in a small group where in-breeding is high, but social factors such as poverty and overcrowding may be implicated in the high prevalence rate for schizophrenia (as in the lower socio-economic classes in southern Canada).

With regard to the non-psychotic mental disorders, the prevalence rate of 116/1,000 for the neuroses is also very high when compared with North American standards (Baltimore: 52/1,000). However, Leon and Climent (10) found a rate of 364/1,000 with their Colombian Indian group. In Oxford Bay, there were three times as many female as male neurotics. For the personality disorders, the rate was 177/1,000 and there were twice as many males as females in this diagnostic category.

HOS Scores

I have followed Jane Murphy (13) and hypothesized a gradient from "sickness" to "wellness" with four groupings of the total population: severe (10 per cent), moderate (27 per cent), mild (58 per cent), and minimal (7.2 per cent). Classifying by sex, the males showed: severe (7.3 per cent), moderate (25 per cent), mild (60.4 per cent), and minimal (7.2 per cent), while the corresponding values for the female were 11, 27.5, 54.3, and 6.7 per cent. It would appear that the women present more symptoms than the men, confirming other studies in Alaska (2,6,13) and Frobisher Bay (14).

Among the males, severe symptomatology decreases with age, while with the females the reverse is true. It thus appears that adolescence is more stressful for the male Eskimo than for the female, but that in adulthood the female becomes more susceptible than the male. In the 45-54 year age group, the females show over four times as many "severe" symptoms as the males, and the high rate of severe symptoms in the females continues into the 55-64 age group.

DISCUSSION

What is the relationship between the contemporary social
structure of Oxford Bay and the distinctive prevalence pattern of psychiatric morbidity which we have described? We
started with the premise that modernity brought about
changes in social structure. We described how the older
adults of Oxford Bay had to adjust to a whole new set of
formal organizational structures imposed from without, together with many informal organizational structures which
developed quite inevitably when a comparatively large number of individuals with differing loyalties and allegiances
found themselves living together in a confined geographical
area.

Once a settlement is established, there is usually no
regression back to the land, although on at least one occasion such a nativistic type movement was unsuccessfully
attempted in Frobisher Bay (9). The movement is rather from
smaller settlements to the arctic urban centres.

The stress of adjustment is apparently felt most keenly
by the older women, and this is reflected by a good correlation between the gradual increase of symptomatology and
the increase in age (up to age 54). The most stressful area
in the social structural field appears to be that concerned
with the male-female relationship. The HOS scores as well
as the prevalence rates of diagnosable mental disorders
both indicate significant differences between males and females both in the population at large and for individual
age groups. What is happening to the Eskimo male-female
relationship? Eskimo family organization was strongly pat-
riarchical and women occupied a very subservient position.
Lubart (11) postulated a bitter resentment by the women of
the men, because of male superiority in the camp. In the
settlement, where the women have been exposed to a more
"democratic" male-female relationship, there was a great
deal of feminine discontent. The women seem to bear the
brunt of the conflict situation. On the other hand, adolescence was more stressful for the male than for the female,
perhaps because he faces a greater identity problem. The adolescent female has problems as soon as she starts going out
with men, and Lubart believes that since the Eskimo females
use the wealthier and economically more secure white males
as models, the Eskimo males run a distant second place. It
can be postulated that the male Eskimos' resentment of the
white males is displaced to the Eskimo females. This may
help explain the large number of battered Eskimo wives.

When these hostile feelings are introjected, the Eskimo males become markedly depressed.

Settlement life can be seen as a "castrating" factor for the adult Eskimo male. His ability to display his masculinity in the old culturally defined ways is lost. At the same time, the status of the female Eskimo has improved, because the new social structure provides opportunities to develop a great deal of independence; her services are in great demand in many fields of endeavour by the non-Eskimos, both males and females.

The 45-54 year age group shows a significant sex difference of symptomatology. It would appear that the menopause takes a heavier toll in the females. One of the advantages of living in a settlement with a comparatively large population is that the number of available sex partners is increased. The author formed the impression that many of the 45-54 year old men were quite promiscuous. This can be seen as an "acting out" of their feelings towards their menopausal wives. The women themselves - at this age - if they were not already widows, led a rather unhappy life, some dependent on their kinfolk, others living a lonely existence by themselves in small one-room houses.

ACKNOWLEDGMENT

This paper is based on research carried out as part of the project: "Identity and Modernity in the East Arctic" of the Department of Sociology and Anthropology, Memorial University of Newfoundland. It was financed by a grant from the Canada Council, Isaac Walton Killam Memorial Fund.

SUMMARY

The most striking effect of modernization in the Canadian East Arctic is the development of comparatively large communities, composed of a majority of Eskimos and a large minority of non-Eskimos. The traditional small, isolated and kinship-based residential group, with its hunting and trapping economy, has given way to the large, socially heterogeneous permanent community with a wage and welfare economy. The contemporary social structure of these communities is almost caste-like, the larger Eskimo group developing a social stratification based primarily on economic factors, but with traditional social factors playing an important role. How is adaptation to this new social structure affecting the mental health of the Eskimos?

Oxford Bay (pseudonym) is a southern Baffin Island settlement founded by the Hudson Bay Company in 1913. An anthropological study and a mental health survey was carried out in this settlement in 1970. The Eskimo population was then around 500, and 93 per cent of adults (age 15 and over) were formally interviewed. Psychiatric symptomatology was severe in 10 per cent of the population, moderate in 27 per cent, mild in 58 per cent, and minimal in 5 per cent. Females had a greater degree of symptomatology than the males. Thirty-seven per cent of respondents were suffering from severe mental disorder. The prevalence rate for schizophrenia was 28/1,000; for the affective disorders, 46/1,000; for neuroses, 116/1,000; and for personality disorders, 177/1,000.

The most stressful area seems the male-female relationship, with the women bearing the brunt of the conflict. Settlement life can be seen as a "castrating" factor for the adult Eskimo male. The prevalence of psychoses is probably due to genetic factors in a group where in-breeding is high, but social factors such as poverty and overcrowding may also be implicated.

REFERENCES

1. Balicki, A., "Two attempts at community organization among the Eastern Hudson Bay Eskimo," Anthropologica, N.S., 1: 122-39 (1959)
2. Bloom, J., "Psychiatric problems and cultural transitions in Alaska," Paper presented at the American Psychiatric Association Annual Meeting, San Francisco, May 1970
3. Boas, F., The Central Eskimo (Lincoln, Nebraska: University of Nebraska Press, 1964)
4. Caudill, W.A., "The influence of social structure and culture on human behaviour in modern Japan," J. Nerv. Ment. Dis., 157: 240-57 (1973)
5. Chance, N.A., The Eskimo of North Alaska (New York: Holt, Rinehart and Winston, 1966)
6. Chance, N.A., and Foster, D.A., "Symptom formation and patterns of psychopathology in a rapidly changing Alaska Eskimo society," Anthropological Papers of the University of Alaska, Vol. 11, No. 1, December 1962
7. Fleming, A.L., Archibald the Arctic (Toronto: Saunders, 1970)
8. Graburn, N.H., Eskimo Without Igloos (Boston: Little, Brown and Company, 1969)

9. Honigmann, J., and Honigmann, I., Eskimo Townsmen
    (Ottawa: The Canadian Research Centre for Anthropology,
    St. Paul's University, 1966)
10. Leon, C.A., and Climent, C.E., "Assessment of instru-
    ments for studying the prevalence of mental disorder,"
    Soc. Psychiat., 5: 212-15 (1970)
11. Lubart, J., Psychodynamic Problems of Adaptation - Mac-
    Kenzie Delta Eskimos (Ottawa: Northern Science Research
    Group, Department of Indian Affairs and Northern Develop-
    ment, 1971)
12. Mailhot, J., Inuvik Community Structure - Summer 1965
    (Ottawa: Northern Science Research Group, Department of
    Indian Affairs and Northern Development, 1968)
13. Murphy, Jane, An Epidemiological Study of Psychopatho-
    logy in an Eskimo Village (Ann Arbor, Michigan: Univer-
    sity Microfilms, 1960)
14. Sampath, H.M., "Modernity and mental health of Eskimos
    in the East Arctic. A study of treated psychiatric ca-
    ses in an Arctic town," Paper presented at the Canadian
    Psychiatric Association Annual Meeting, Montreal, June
    1972
15. Vallee, F., Kabloona and Eskimo in the Central Keewatin
    (Ottawa: Northern Co-ordination and Research Centre,
    Department of Northern Affairs and National Resources,
    1962)
16. Vallee, F., Povungnetuk and its Cooperative. A Case
    Study in Community Change (Ottawa: Northern Co-ordina-
    tion and Research Centre, Department of Indian Affairs
    and Northern Development, 1967)
17. Wilmott, W.E., "The flexibility of Eskimo social organi-
    zation," Anthropologica, 2: 48-57 (1960)
18. Wilmott, W.E., The Eskimo Community at Port Harrison
    (Ottawa: Northern Co-ordination and Research Centre,
    Department of Northern Affairs and National Resources,
    1961)

Acculturative stress in northern Canada:
ecological, cultural, and psychological factors *

J.W. BERRY

A basic proposition of recent work on the relationship between mental health and culture is that persons and groups
undergoing social and cultural changes will experience
psychological discomfort. This proposition has been subjected to detailed scrutiny in recent years, with the general
consensus that there exists an association between socio-
cultural change and mental health (14, 15).

In northern Canada, many workers have pursued various
aspects of this relationship. Frank Vallée has noted that
discontinuity and incongruence in culture and behaviour between the two systems relate to the observed stress, and he
has distinguished between communal (or societal) problems
and personal (or psychological) problems. Chance (12) has
also emphasized these variables, rather than the mere rapidity of social change. Lubart, Sampath, and Wintrob have
examined clinical features of these personal changes, and
Mackinnon and Neufeldt have also attempted to relate mental
health in the North to various features of existing life-
style and cultural change.

Throughout the history of research on cultural change
and mental health, there has been confusion of terminology.
Antecedent variables have been described as "acculturation,"
"modernization," "education," "wage employment," and "exposure to mass media." Similarly, the dependent variable
has been termed "mental health," "personal adjustment,"
"personal discomfort," and "psychosomatic stress." We prefer the term "acculturative stress" (4) for the dependent
variable; psychological stress may derive from many antecedent factors, but this term applies only to those stresses
that are theoretically or empirically linked to acculturation. Similarily, there are numerous behaviours which may
result from acculturation (such as shifts in previous levels of linguistic, perceptual, or cognitive behaviours),

* An extended version of this paper will be published in
the *Journal of Cross Cultural Psychology*, 1974.

but we will limit the term to those affective states or behaviours usually subsumed under the term "mental health."
Thus limited, the term becomes manageable, and useful in
considering our basic proposition that psychological stresses exist as a function of acculturative influences.

The research to be reported here examines ecological,
cultural, and psychological variables associated with variations in the psychological response to acculturation.

THE MODEL AND SOME HYPOTHESES

Research over the past few years has been guided by a three-
stage model in which behaviour is considered as a function
of culture which is an adaptation to ecology (2,4,9). The
model also takes account of acculturative influences, a
modified contact culture, and a set of acculturated behaviours.

The ecology component of the model considers human organisms in interaction with their habitat. In pursuing primary needs in specific physical environments, certain "economic possibilities" are open, ranging from hunting and
gathering to agriculture and animal husbandry (18). Hunters
and gatherers typically store little food, have low population densities and small settlement units, and are migratory; on the other hand, agriculturalists typically accumulate food, allowing a higher population density, larger
settlement units, and a sedentary life-style.

In the traditional culture component, hunting societies
show a low level of socio-cultural stratification, while
among the agriculturalists stratification is more marked.
Emphases among the hunters are usually upon achievement,
self-reliance, and independence ("assertion"), while among
the agriculturalists they are upon responsibility and obedience ("compliance") (1).

The traditional behaviour component is limited to behaviours theoretically linked to "psychological differentiation" (20), and involve behaviour in the perceptual, cognitive, social, and affective domains. The behavioural and
the eco-cultural dimension are linked, since socialization
emphases upon achievement and independence foster psychological differentiation, while those upon obedience and compliance inhibit differentiation (13 20).

At the acculturation level of the model, we are concerned with the extent of urbanization, western-style education, and wage employment, as well as the "pressures to
change" these activities. In the contact culture component,

we are interested in settlement patterns and population
densities which develop, the new socio-cultural strata which
become differentiated, the social controls which are imposed, and the changes in socialization practices which
emerge. And finally in the acculturated behaviour component,
we are interested in "shifts" in levels of behaviour which
were apparent prior to, or during early stages of, culture
contact, and in the "acculturative stress" behaviours which
emerge in response to the acculturative influences and new
elements in the contact culture.

The basic hypothesis is that acculturative stress varies
as a function of both the traditional culture and behaviours
which characterize a community and the acculturative influences which impinge upon that community. At the community
level, acculturative stress will be greater in communities
where there is a greater cultural and behavioural disparity
between the two groups and where there is stronger pressure
placed upon the traditional community to become acculturated. At the individual level, acculturative stress will be
greater for persons who are less psychologically differentiated; that is, individuals who are less independent on
events in their milieu will be more susceptible to changes
due to acculturative influences, and hence will exhibit
greater acculturative stress.

Typical acculturative influences involve a high population density and settlement size, a set of social controls,
introduced during education, wage employment, and through
the strengthening of government, with some emphasis upon
compliance and obedience during socialization. Communities
that are traditionally low in population density, settlement size, and socio-cultural stratification deviate
most from this pattern. We may thus predict that greater
acculturative stress will be characteristic of migratory,
low population density, and low stratification societies,
while lesser acculturative stress will be characteristic of
more sedentary and stratified societies. The other dimension, pressure to become acculturated, will be low in plu-
ralist societies where ethnic diversity is prized, and acculturative stress will be correspondingly small. At the
other extreme, acculturative stress should be high in assi-
milationist societies (7,8,9). Within all communities,
those individuals who exhibit high psychological differentiation ("field-independent") will show less acculturative
stress than those who are less differentiated.

METHODS

The study involved sampling from two types of communities
in each of three eco-cultural settings; in each setting,
one community was "relatively traditional," and one "relatively acculturated." A non-native comparison sample was
also selected. The "migratory" end of the eco-cultural dimension was represented by the Eastern Cree of James Bay,
the "sedentary" end by the Tsimshian of northern coastal
British Columbia, and an intermediate position by the Carriere of the northern British Columbia interior. The non-
native sample was from an Ontario farming village. There
were, thus, six native and one non-native samples, each of
approximately n = 60.

Our primary interest lay in acculturative stress variables. These include a 20-item psychosomatic check list
(stress) prepared for cross-cultural use (11) from the longer Cornell Medical Index (10), the 14-item marginality
scale (17, 3), and a 24-item scale assessing attitudes towards the larger society (19). Details of ethnic identification were also sought.

Psychological differentiation was assessed using Kohs
Blocks (for perceptual differentiation), Ravens matrices,
and by Reserve for social differentiation (a modification
of Jourard's self-disclosure questionnaire (16)).

RESULTS AND DISCUSSION

Our hypothesis that acculturative stress would be highest
for the low food accumulating group (Cree) was confirmed
for both Stress and Marginality ($p < 0.01$ and < 0.001 respectively), using analysis of variance across the six native samples.

Data from the attitude scales and the identification
questions fall into a similar pattern. The Cree samples
were negative with respect to Assimilation, the Tsimshian
were more positive, with the Carriere falling in between
($p < 0.001$). With respect to Integration, all groups were
in favour of this strategy, but the Cree were most in favour, the Tsimshian least, and the Carriere intermediate
($p < 0.001$). None of the comparisons of attitudes by level
of acculturation were significantly spread. For Identification all groups were predominantly "Indian," but the Cree
were most predominantly "Indian," the Carriere less, and
the Tsimshian least (x^2 = 17.9, $P < 0.01$); similar reciprocal patterns characterize the alternatives of "Canadian"
and "Both."

Taken together, patterns in these variables support our first hypothesis. Those (the Cree) whose traditional migratory life-style differs most from the cultural style of the Euro-Canadian larger society suffer the most acculturative stress, have the least interest in Assimilating (the most in Rejecting major ties with the larger society), and identify most as "Indian" people.

However, acculturative stress is extant in all three groups, when compared with the non-native sample: Stress and Marginality are clearly less in the non-native than in the Amerindian groups.

Within samples, the data strongly indicates a negative relationship between psychological differentiation and acculturative stress. The three measures of differentiation employed are those which varied across the three eco-cultural settings (9). Of 54 correlations, 46 were negative (24 of them significant at the 0.05 level). Within any sociocultural group, individuals who have attained separateness from their fellows, and an independent cognitive style in interaction with their environment, seem less susceptible to the stresses of socio-cultural change.

However, there is a paradox in our data: across samples, those (the Cree) who are (9) more highly differentiated on two of the tasks (Kohs and Reserve) exhibit the highest levels of acculturative stress; conversely those (the Tsimshian) with lowest levels on these two tasks exhibit the least acculturative stress. Nevertheless, within samples, those who are most differentiated are least subject to acculturative stress. On the basis of the Cree data (6), it was tempting to interpret the results in terms of "typicality": those who exhibited high differentiation in a society where it was typical to do so might be less susceptible to acculturative stress. However, this inverse relationship carries through to the other two Amerindian eco-cultural settings, where lower levels of differentiation exist (9). A possible resolution of this paradox lies in the fact that all three Amerindian groups (in keeping with requirements of northern life (5)), although differing among themselves, do exhibit high levels of differentiation when viewed in a worldwide perspective (4). Thus, the "typicality" interpretation may have some validity: those who manifest, within communities, those characteristics that are prototypical in the culture area will be placed in positions minimally susceptible to acculturative stress.

The task of penetrating the global assertions about relationships between acculturation and mental health has begun. The course of acculturative stress has been shown to vary according to our hypotheses. At the community level, acculturative stress is related to cultural and behavioural discontinuities encountered during acculturation, while at the individual level, acculturative stress is related to the psychological differentiation. A third hypothesis was not testable in the present design - that acculturative stress varies with acculturative pressures. This should now be explored in a society with policies of assimilation towards native or ethnic peoples. At the same time, changes in acculturative stress should be monitored as Canada implements its announced policies of cultural pluralism.

ACKNOWLEDGMENT

The assistance is gratefully acknowledged of Bob Annis, Reg Mark, Margery Mark, Rose Pierre, Alec Pierre, Brenda Prince, Fred Sam, Ted Wilson, Shirley Reece, Laurie Price, John Kane, and the Canada Council (grants S70-0103, S71-0330, S72-0184).

SUMMARY

A basic proposition of recent work on the relationship between cultural change and mental health is that persons and groups undergoing acculturation will manifest a certain amount of psychological discomfort and social disintegration. The term acculturative stress is proposed to denote the personal and social conditions of psychosomatic distress, marginality, and deviance, which are observable in situations of acculturation. Levels of acculturative stress are predicted for six Amerindian samples by examining potential psychological discontinuities between those behaviours nurtured in traditional life and those expected in Euro-Canadian settlement life. Specifically, higher levels of acculturative stress are predicted for traditionally migratory populations, and lower levels for traditionally sedentary ones. Three Amerindian cultural groups (the migratory Cree, the sedentary Tsimshian, and the intermediate Carriere), each represented by two community samples (one relatively traditional, and one relatively acculturated), were studied. Samples, stratified by age and sex, were tested and interviewed by members of their own group who had been trained in the role of psychological field worker. Perceptual-cognitive, and socio-emotional behaviours were examined, and tests of acculturative stress were employed.

Results show that across this eco-cultural range, the migratory Cree people are the most susceptible to such stress, the Tsimshian least susceptible, and the Carriere intermediate. Within samples, perceptual-cognitive and socioemotional behaviour are predictive of levels of individual stress. Implications for most Inuit, Algonkian, and Athabaskan peoples in Canada, and for most migratory hunters and gatherers in the circumpolar regions, are that high levels of acculturative stress may be expected. However, intelligent monitoring of the socio-cultural and psychological factors associated with such stress should permit major relief from it.

REFERENCES

1. Barry, H., Child, I., and Bacon, M., "Relation of child training to subsistence economy," Am. Anthropol., 61: 51-63 (1959)
2. Berry, J.W., "Temne and Eskimo perceptual skills," Int. J. Psychol., 1: 207-29 (1966)
3. Berry, J.W., "Marginality, stress and ethnic identification in an acculturated aboriginal community," J. Cross Cult. Psychol., 3: 239-52 (1970)
4. Berry, J.W., "Ecological and cultural factors in spatial perceptual development," Canad. J. Behav. Sci., 3: 324-336 (1971)
5. Berry, J.W., "Psychological research in the north," Anthropologica, 13: 143-57 (1971)
6. Berry, J.W., "Possession of typical cognitive and personality traits, and resistance to acculturative stress," Abstr. Guide 20th Inter-Cogn. Psych., Tokyo (1972)
7. Berry, J.W., "Psychological aspects of cultural pluralism: unity and identity reconsidered," Paper presented at IACCP Regional Conference, Ibadan, April 1973
8. Berry, J.W., "Ecology, cultural adaptation and psychological differentiation: Traditional patterning and acculturative stress," In Brislin, R, Bochner, S, and Lonner, W. (eds.), Cross-Cultural Perseptives on Learning (Sage, 1974)
9. Berry, J.W., and Annis, R.C., "Ecology, culture and psychological differentiation," Int. J. Psychol. (1974)
10. Brodman, K., Erdmann, A.J., Lorge, I., Gershenson, C.P., and Wolfe, H.G., "The Cornell Medical Index health questionnaire III. The evaluation of emotional disturbances," J. clin. Psychol., 8: 119 (1952)

11. Cawte, J., Binanchi, G.N., and Kiloh, L.G., "Personal discomfort in Australian aborigines," Austral. New Z. J. Psych., 2: 69-79 (1968)
12. Chance, N.A., "Acculturation, self-identification and personal adjustment," Am. Anthropol., 67: 372-93 (1965)
13. Dky, Ruth and Witkin, H.A., "Family experiences related to the development of differentiation in children," Child Development, 36: 21-55 (1965)
14. Fried, M., "Effects of social change on mental health," Am. J. Orthopsychiat., 34: 3-28 (1964)
15. Inkeles, A., and Smith, D.H., "The fate of personal adjustment in the process of modernization," Int. J. Comp. Soc., 11: 81-114 (1970)
16. Jourard, S.M., The Transparent Self (New York: Van Nostrand, 1971)
17. Mann, J.W., "Group relations and the marginal man," Human Relations, 11: 77-92 (1958)
18. Murdock, G.P., "World ethnographis sample," Am. Anthropol., 59: 664-87 (1957)
19. Sommerlad, E., and Berry, J.W., "The role of ethnic identification in distinguishing between attitudes towards assimilation and integration of a minority racial group," Human Relations, 23: 23-9 (1970)
20. Witkin, H.A., Dyk, R.B., Faterson, H.F., Goodenough, D.R., and Karp, S.A., Psychological Differentiation (New York: Wiley, 1962)

Psychological adaptation of Skolt Lapp children to cultural change

L. SEITAMO

The aim of this work was to compare the psychological adaptation of Skolt Lapp girls and boys in a situation of cultural change arising from the collision between the Lappish and Finnish culture, with special reference to differences in adult male-female roles. A control group of children from northern Finland was also tested. The data form part of the International Biological Program/Human

Adaptability study (1968-73). Comparisons were made of adaptation to school: (1) intellectual readiness for school work, (2) school motivation, work habits and adaptability, and (3) school achievement.

The theoretical frame of reference is based on learning theories (1,2,4,5,7,8,9). During cultural change, the crucial factors affecting adaptation are the areas of change, the degree and rapidity of change and whether both sexes are affected equally (8). If there are sex differences, then the anxiety and insufficiency evoked by the changes prevent the parent of the sex in question from being able to guide the children in new situations, and from acting as a powerful model for identification and observational learning. The difficulties experienced in adult roles are reflected most clearly in the adaptation of the children of the same sex (5). The adequacy of the school system is also an important factor in adaptation.

METHODS

The subjects were the whole school age group of Skolt children in Sevettijärvi (N = 81; 6-15 years) and a control group from Northern Finland (N = 68). The measures used were:
1. Wechsler Intelligence Scale for Children; Block Design as a measure of culture-free performance. This provides a practical evaluation of potential learning ability rather than a fair culture-free estimate. The tests were performed in Finnish in order to estimate readiness for the existing school system.
2. Teachers' ratings of personality traits (5-point numerical scale, Catell-Pitkänen); children's ratings.
3. School grades.

The cultural description is based on observations, interviews, and the inventory "Children's reports of parental behaviour" (E.S. Schaefer's scale).

CULTURAL DIFFERENCES

The relevant ecological and cultural situation is described thoroughly by Forsius (3) and Seitamo (6, 7).

Adult Male-Female Roles

The role of the Skolt men is undergoing change. The traditional means of livelihood in the wilds have been exchanged

for temporary employment, often far from home. The women's
handicrafts are an important means of livelihood. Both
sexes are dissatisfied with being Skolts; they are the
least prestigious minority group in Northern Finland, characterized by old traditions and a different language. The
Skolt women do not value their menfolk, and the men suffer
from feelings of inferiority and insufficiency in the changing situation. The women dominate the home, are chiefly
responsible for child guidance and help the girls, in particular, to become more Finnicized, because of the higher
social status this entails.

The society of Northern Finland is a hunting-agrarian
society with patriarchal-authoritarian dominance by the
menfolk. This society is also changing, but not so rapidly.
The economic situation has improved, and power and strength
are valued. Both of the parents are responsible for the
education of the children.

Boys-Girls

The Skolt girls are more closely directed and controlled,
and they participate in work; the boys grow up more freely.
No such differences appear with the Finnish children. The
Skolt boys perceive their mother and the Finnish girls
their father - the parent of the opposite sex and the one
who has more power and influence - as less acceptive and
less satisfied with them than does the opposite sex within
these cultures (Schaefer's scale). Thus the factors affecting the socialization process are less favourable for the
Skolt boys and Finnish girls than they are for the opposite
sex within these cultures.

HYPOTHESES

Opposite sex-role trends appear within the Skolt and Finnish cultures: the Skolt boys have more difficulties in
adapting to cultural change than the Skolt girls, their intellectual readiness for the school environment is poorer,
and they have poorer school motivation and achievements.
Within the Finnish group, there are slight tendencies in
the opposite direction. The Skolt groups score lower than
the corresponding Finnish groups, but differences between
the girls are less than those between the boys.

TABLE 1
Means, standard deviations, and significance of differences in means
for intelligence tests and school marks

| | Sevetti | | N. Finland | | Difference between* | | | |
| | | | | | 1:2 | | I:II | |
Variable	1(39)	2(42)	1(33)	2(35)	I	II	1:1	2:2
Block	12.0	11.0	11.5	12.0	0.1	NS	NS	0.1
design	(2.1)	(2.3)	(2.2)	(2.1)				
Picture	11.8	11.6	10.0	10.9	NS	NS	0.01	NS
completion	(2.4)	(2.2)	(2.2)	(2.4)				
Picture	7.4	6.5	8.0	8.6	0.1	NS	NS	0.01
arrangement	(2.3)	(2.2)	(2.2)	(3.2)				
Object	10.8	10.2	10.7	10.8	NS	NS	NS	NS
assembly	(2.8)	(2.8)	(2.7)	(2.9)				
Coding	7.9	5.2	8.0	6.9	0.001	0.1	NS	0.01
	(3.1)	(2.4)	(2.3)	(2.2)				
Vocabulary	7.9	8.0	9.1	10.5	NS	0.01	0.1	0.001
	(2.5)	(3.3)	(2.8)	(2.8)				
Information	9.3	8.9	9.8	10.9	NS	NS	NS	0.01
	(3.1)	(3.0)	(3.6)	(2.8)				
Comprehension	10.5	10.2	11.2	11.7	NS	NS	NS	0.1
	(2.7)	(3.4)	(3.5)	(3.2)				
Similarities	10.7	10.4	11.4	11.1	NS	NS	NS	NS
	(2.3)	(3.1)	(3.3)	(2.6)				
Arithmetic	8.9	8.1	8.1	8.8	0.1	NS	NS	NS
	(2.4)	(1.8)	(1.9)	(1.8)				
Non-verbal	99.9	92.0	96.4	98.2	0.01	NS	NS	0.05
IQ	(14.2)	(11.6)	(11.2)	(14.2)				
Verbal	96.7	94.0	98.9	103.8	NS	NS	NS	0.01
IQ	(13.2)	(14.8)	(15.1)	(12.1)				
Full-scale	98.1	92.5	97.4	101.3	0.1	NS	NS	0.01
IQ	(13.5)	(13.8)	(13.1)	(12.3)				
Reading	7.2	6.7	7.6	7.2	0.1	0.1	NS	0.1
	(1.4)	(1.1)	(0.9)	(0.8)				
Writing	7.1	6.2	7.2	6.7	0.01	0.05	NS	0.05
	(1.1)	(1.2)	(0.9)	(0.8)				
Mathematics	6.5	6.2	6.7	6.9	NS	NS	NS	0.05
	(1.4)	(1.2	(1.2)	(1.4)				
Average	7.3	6.7	7.3	7.0	0.05	NS	NS	NS
	(0.9)	(0.8)	(0.8)	(0.8)				

* p<; I = Sevettijärvi, II = N. Finland, 1 = girls, 2 = boys.

RESULTS

Intellectual Readiness (Table 1)

The readiness of each of the groups for education is about

the same, when the effect of cultural differences are eliminated as far as possible (Block Design). There is a
slight tendency for the Skolt boys to attain a lower level
than the other groups.

In non-verbal functions typical of the school environment (Picture Arrangement, Object Assembly, Coding) the levels of the Skolt boys tend to be lower than those of the
Skolt girls and Finnish boys, while in non-verbal functions
typical of the Skolt culture: exact minute visual perception (Picture Completion), their level is about the same as
that of the Skolt girls, and somewhat, though not significantly, higher than that of the Finnish boys. Their readiness for visuomotor pencil-paper work (Coding) is exceptionally poor.

Verbal functions do not differ significantly within the
Skolt group, though a tendency appears for the girls to
attain a better level. Within the Finnish group the general
tendency is the opposite. Differences between the girls are
small. In exact minute visual perception the Skolt girls
perform significantly better than the Finnish girls, but in
verbal functions they tend to score lower.

The over-all intellectual readiness for school work (IQs)
is poorer for the Skolt boys than for the Skolt girls and
Finnish boys. These general differences are widest in non-
verbal functions, though the difference of verbal functions
between the Skolt and Finnish boys is still more marked.
Within the Finnish group, the trend is the opposite, though
slight. The girls do not differ significantly.

The non-verbal functions do not improve more than the
expected norm-values as a function of school career in any
group, but in the Skolt group most verbal functions improve
significantly. The improvement is more marked among the
boys, indicating that their verbal readiness is especially
poor in the lower classes but improves under the influence
of school.

School Motivation and Work Habits (Tables 2-4)

The Skolt boys' motivation to go to school, as rated by
themselves ("like to go to school" - Skolts: boys 24 per
cent, girls 58 per cent; Finns: boys 65 per cent, girls 87
per cent) and by their teachers, is significantly weaker
than that of the Skolt girls and Finnish boys. The differences within the Finnish group are in the same direction,
but smaller.

TABLE 2
Significance of differences of means on teachers' ratings and discrimination analysis, Sevettijärvi girls (I) versus boys (II)

Rating	p on group rated higher		Correlations between discriminating functions and variables
	I	II	
Likes to go to school	0.001		-0.6
Impolite		0.001	0.59
Insolent		0.001	0.57
Hostile		0.001	0.57
Untrustworthy		0.01	0.49
Hard-working	0.01		-0.46
Unpersevering		0.05	0.42
Vicious		0.01	0.39
Friendly	0.05		-0.39
Noisy		0.05	0.39
Energetic	0.05		-0.38
Ambitious	0.05		-0.36
Tattle-tale	0.05		-0.35
Stubborn		0.05	0.35
Industrious	0.1		-0.34
Cooperative	0.1		-0.32
Even-tempered	0.1		-0.3
Restless		0.1	0.29

Eigenvalue	%	CHI I II	DF	Prob.	Canon. corr.
1.03	100.0	38.22	18	0.996	0.71
Wilks lambda		F		Prob.	
0.492718		(18, 45)=2.574		0.9948	

Group	Discriminating functions		Estimated pairwise overlap prob.		
	Mean	SD	I	II	
I. Girls	1.673	1.116	1.0	0.1136	4/31
II. Boys	3.671	0.878	0.1816	1.0	5/33

The clustered traits distinguishing the Skolt girls from the boys are only remotely similar to those operating among the Finnish children. The discriminator of the Skolt group is weighted most powerfully by traits measuring attitudes towards school, work habits, and psychic balance, in all of which the Skolt girls are rated more positively. The emphasis within the Finnish group lies on general behaviour traits indicating activity in both a negative and a positive sense. The girls are rated lower.

Thus the basic dynamics and problems which characterize the situation of the whole culture and the male-female roles

TABLE 3
Significance of differences of means on teachers' ratings and discrimination analysis, Northern Finnish girls (I) versus boys (II)

Rating	p on group rated higher		Correlations between discriminating functions and variables
	I	II	
Restless		0.001	-0.6
Short-tempered		0.01	-0.55
Noisy		0.01	-0.54
Boastful		0.01	-0.51
Dissatisfied		0.01	-0.45
Vicious		0.05	-0.44
Pitiless		0.05	-0.44
Quick to take offence		0.05	-0.44
Quarrelsome		0.05	-0.43
Shy, timid	0.05		0.43
Active		0.05	-0.42
Self-assertive		0.05	-0.42
Cautious	0.05		0.4
Is a leader		0.05	0.4
Ready to accuse		0.05	-0.38
Talkative		0.05	-0.35
Likes to go to school	0.1		0.33
Calm	0.1		0.31
Attention-seeking		0.1	-0.3

Eigenvalue	%	CHI I II	DF	Prob.	Canon. corr.
1.086	100.0	37.12	19	0.992	0.7215
Wilks lambda	F			Prob.	
0.479444	(19, 41)=2.343			0.9888	

Group	Discriminating functions		Estimated pairwise overlap prob.		
	Mean	SD	I	II	
1. Girls	0.4392	0.8488	1.0	0.1136	5/30
II. Boys	-1.611	1.127	0.1816	1.0	4/31

distinguish the two sexes within each culture: within the Skolt culture it is adaptation to the new way of life, to school as its transmitter, while within the Finnish group the typical static male-female contrast, dominance-submission or masculinity-femininity, is reflected as a sex-role discriminator among the children.

When compared cross-culturally, avoidance behaviour manifested as fear, ineffectiveness, and dislike of school characterize the Skolt boys, while approach behaviour in the form of activity is typical of the Finnish boys. These

TABLE 4
Significance of differences of means on teachers' ratings and discrimination analysis, Sevettijärvi boys (I) versus Finnish boys (II)

Rating	p on group rated higher		Correlations between discriminating functions and variables
	I	II	
Shy, timid	0.01		-0.61
Energetic		0.01	0.55
Likes to go to school		0.05	0.47
Talkative		0.05	0.43
Flexible		0.05	0.43
Unpersevering	0.05		-0.42
Active		0.05	0.41
Is a leader		0.05	0.4
Short-tempered		0.1	0.38
Dependent	0.1		-0.37
Impolite	0.1		-0.37
Hard-working		0.1	0.34
Retiring	0.1		-0.34
Self-assertive		0.1	0.34
Relaxed		0.1	0.33
Sad, melancholy	0.1		-0.33

Eigenvalue	%	CHI I II	DF	Prob.	Canon. corr.
0.6559	100.0	27.74	16	0.966	0.6294
Wilks lambda	F			Prob.	
0.603884	(16, 47)=1.927			0.9584	

Group	Discriminating functions		Estimated pairwise overlap prob.		
	Mean	SD	I	II	
I. Sevetti boys	-0.1035	0.9687	1.0	0.2052	7/33
II. N. Finland boys	1.492	1.032	0.2199	1.0	4/31

distinguishing traits increase as a function of years at school.

The differences between the girls are relatively small. The Skolt girls experience school as somewhat less pleasant than do the Finnish girls and they are rated somewhat higher in positive social behaviour.

School Achievement (Table 1)

The percentage of Skolt boys who fail to progress from one
grade to the next in classes I-III (follow-up and retro-
spective study of the whole sample) is significantly higher
than that of the Skolt girls and Finnish boys (Skolts: boys
26 per cent, girls 11 per cent; Finns: boys 6 per cent,
girls 3 per cent). Most of the failures occur after the
first year, indicating that readiness for school work among
the Skolt boys is low from the very beginning. The school
grades show the same differences. Within the Finnish group,
the differences in failures and in school grades are in the
same direction as in the Skolt group, but not as marked.
Among the Skolt girls the failures are more frequent, but
the school grades do not differ significantly. The pupils
remaining in the same class for two years are included in
the calculations of the school grades. Thus the longer
school career of the Skolt boys does not serve to raise
their achievements to the same level as those of the other
groups.

DISCUSSION

The results for the most part support our hypotheses, though
the differences in school motivation and achievements between the girls and within the Finnish group were not as
clear as anticipated. The Finnish school system favours
submissive behaviour, and hence the girls are rewarded more
than the boys. This encouragement obviously serves to reduce the differences in question.

Current changes in the role of the Skolt men are fundamental and lead to feelings of insufficiency, with effects
upon the adaptation of the Skolt boys. Poor readiness for
school in the Skolt boys and the inadequacy of a school
system based on the Finnish culture, with instruction in
Finnish, result in low school achievement. This, in turn,
prevents the boys from finding school rewarding, lowers
motivation and self-confidence, and leads to behavioural
disturbances.

The over-all situation of the Lapps is changing, and
the proposed new legislation, once adopted, will allow
better opportunities for development, based on the Lapps'
own culture.

ACKNOWLEDGMENT

The support of the National Board of Education in Finland
is acknowledged with thanks.

SUMMARY

The whole school age group of Skolt children in Sevettijärvi
and a control group of northern Finnish children were studied by means of intelligence tests (WISC), school achievement tests, teachers' and children's ratings (Cattell,
Schaefer). The Skolt boys had more difficulties in adapting
to culture change: intellectual readiness typical of the
school environment, school motivation, and achievement were
poorer than those of the Skolt girls and Finnish boys, and
they showed more behaviour disturbances. Within the Finnish
group the differences were in the opposite direction. The
differences between the girls were small. The results were
interpreted with special reference to differences in role
playing adjustments: the Skolt men are undergoing the most
fundamental changes, with feelings of insufficiency, and
have little chance of influencing the development of the
boys.

REFERENCES

1. Bloom, B.S., Stability and Change in Human Characteristics, Third printing (New York: Wiley, 1966)
2. Dawson, J.L.M., "Theory and research in cross-cultural
   psychology," Bull. Brit. Psychol. Soc., 24: 291-306
   (1971)
3. Forsius, H., "The Finnish Skolt Lapp children. A child
   psychiatric study (academic dissertation)," Acta Paed.
   scand. Suppl., 239 (1973)
4. Hunt, J. McV., Intelligence and Experience (New York:
   Ronald Press, 1961)
5. Mischel, W., Introduction to Personality (New York:
   Holt, Rinehart & Winston, 1971)
6. Seitamo, L., "Das elterliche Verhalten in der Wahrnehmung der Kinder. Abstract in Bericht uber das 4,"
   Internationale Symposium Der Mensch in der Arktis,
   Antrop. Anz. Jg. 33, 2: 114-31 (1971)
7. Seitamo, L., "Intellectual functions in Skolt and
   Northern Finnish children with special reference to
   cultural factors," Inter-Nord., 12: 338-43 (1972)

8. Spindler, L., and Spindler, G., "Male and female adaptations in culture change: Menomini," in Hunt, R. (ed.), Personalities and cultures (New York: Natural History Press, 1967)
9. Wolf, R.M., "The identification and measurement of environmental process variables related to intelligence (academic dissertation)," Microfilmed by Department of Photo-duplication, the University of Chicago Library, 1964

Influence of environment on the physical and psychic development of Skolt Lapp and north Finnish children

HARRIET FORSIUS

The Skolt Lapps living in northeastern Finland form a Lapp minority of about 600 inhabitants. They have left their earlier nomadic style of life and live in small lodgings built by the Finnish state. These buildings have no electric light or other conveniences.

Fishing and reindeer herding remain important, but now income can also be derived from road construction or forestry work. However, the Skolt Lapps live in poorer economic circumstances than northern Finnish families, often having an insufficient food supply, lacking in proteins and vitamins (4).

During the school term, 90 per cent of the schoolchildren live in boarding houses where the food supply and the eating and sleeping habits are regular. However, this way of living differs from their earlier life; Skolt children are used to free outdoor activities not bound by any regular hours, such as fishing and walking in the woods.

All Skolt Lapp children under 15 years of age were investigated in 1967-68, using the methods of child psychiatry (1), and they were compared with a sample of Finnish children living under similar circumstances (Table 1). A follow-up study was made in 1974.

TABLE 1

	Skolt Lapps	Finnish
No. of children 0-14.9 years		
Boys	74	48
Girls	70	62
Total	144	110
Mean age (years)	9.2	8.8
No. of families	37	28

RESULTS

Physical Health

Fifty-one per cent of the Skolt children were considered in poor health. Recurrent infections, especially ear infections, and a poor general condition with low nutritional status were often seen. The corresponding proportion for the Finnish children was 26 per cent ($p < 0.001$).

Psychomotor Development

In infancy and at preschool age, psychomotor development was approximatley the same for both groups. However, the Skolt school boys showed a significantly poorer motor proficiency (Oseretsky's test) than both the Lapp girls and the Finnish boys and girls (Figure 1). Detailed study of the different components of the test (static co-ordination, dynamic co-ordination of the hands, dynamic co-ordination

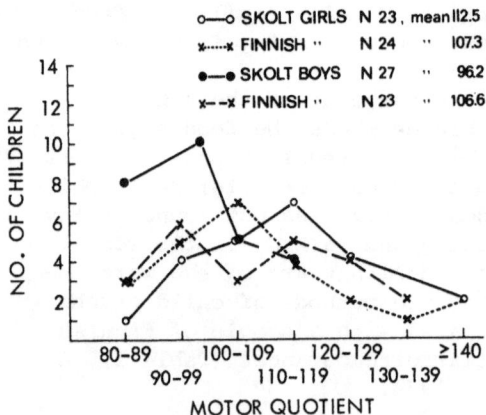

Figure 1   Oseretsky test of motor proficiency, for children aged 7 to 13 years

of the whole body, speed of movements, simultaneous movements, and differentiation of movements) revealed that the
Skolt boys exhibited a poorer performance than the other
groups throughout, apart from static co-ordination (balance)
where they reached the same performance as the Finnish
groups.

This difference is not the result of a lack of physical
training, since the Skolt boys were at least as physically
active as the Finnish boys. One explanation might be that
neurophysiological maturation takes place later in the
Skolt boys than in the Finnish boys. The Skolt boys, admittedly, also showed less co-operation during the test, but a
statistically significant difference of performance persisted even after the cases who would not co-operate were excluded from the calculations.

Follow-up Investigation of Motor Proficiency

A small sample of eight Skolt boys and eight Skolt girls
were retested with the Oseretsky test in the spring of
1974. The performance level in general, and especially
among the girls, had fallen throughout. This is partly due
to the fact that the structure of the test favours younger
age groups, but partly also to the teen-age slackness of
the girls and their lack of interest in physical exercise
(Figure 2). As for the boys, it was found that many showed
a higher degree of maturation in their behaviour.

Physical Growth

A corresponding "maturation" is also observable in the
growth curve of these boys. The longitudinal growth curves
of all boys were below the 50 percentile level of the normal growth curve for Finnish children. Three boys, however,
have changed "channels" in the last two years, moving one
"channel" upwards (Figure 3).

Similarly for the girls, all growth curves are below
the 50 percentile level. Here, however, no growth spurt at
the age of 14 to 15 years is visible in the same way as
for the boys.

According to Lewin the growth-rate of the Skolt children
is less than that of the Finnish children from the first
year of life. Their height at the age of 14 to 15 years is
about 8-9 per cent below that of Finnish children (5).

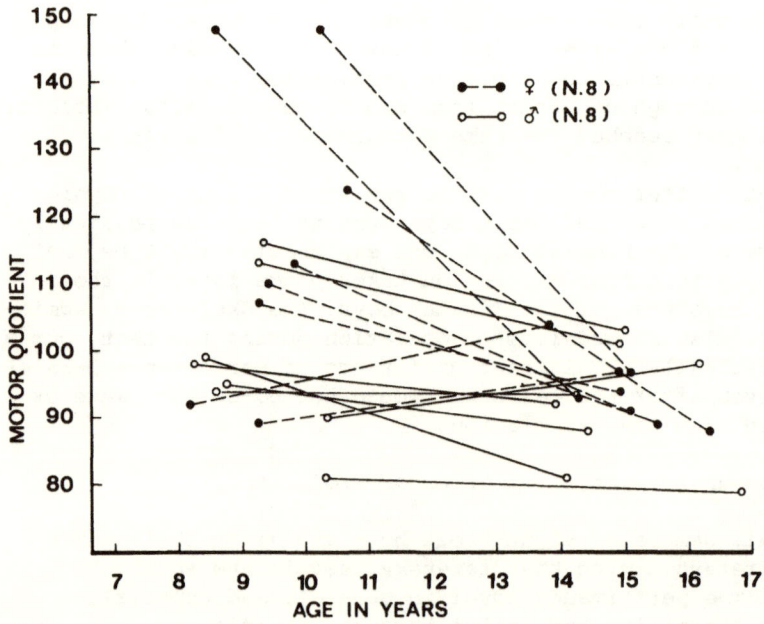

Figure 2   Oseretsky motor tests in the same individuals, 1968 and 1974

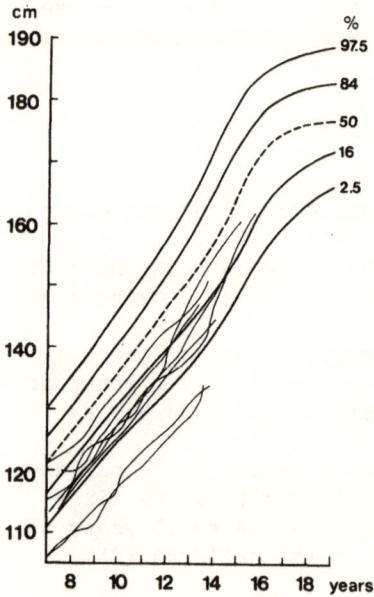

Figure 3   Growth curves for Skolt boys

"Emotional Maturity"

An indication of emotional "immaturity" was that the Skolt
boys showed poorer co-operation than the Finnish boys in the
different test situations. Similarly the attempt to assess
the "psychic disturbances" on the basis of the psychiatric
observation, the number of nervous symptoms, and the appraisal of the parents showed that the highest percentage of
"disturbed" individuals, 37 per cent, was found among the
Skolt boys, whereas the figure for the Finnish boys was 31
per cent. The figures for girls were 16 and 23 per cent, for
Skolt and Finnish girls, respectively.

The fact that there are almost twice as many disturbed
Skolt boys as Skolt girls is apparently due not only to the
greater immaturity of the Skolt boys, but also to the fact
that less is expected from the girls than from the boys.
This again depends on various cultural factors and is reflected in other psychological traits as well (6a, b).

Enuresis Nocturna

Nervous and psychosomatic symptoms, including enuresis nocturna, occurred on average in equal number (2 per child) in
both groups. The frequency of enuresis nocturna was, however, significantly higher among both the Skolt boys, 27.4
per cent against 4.8 per cent among the Finnish boys, and
the girls, 14.9 and 2.1 per cent respectively. This was interpreted as being partly due to a greater neurophysiological immaturity among the Skolt children.

CONCLUSION

It can be said that there are environmental factors apparently influencing the psychic and physical development of
the Skolt Lapp children. The principal negative factors are
the poorer economic circumstances which, in turn, are responsible for the poorer food supply and adverse living conditions. This negative influence is manifested in the higher
frequency of somatic diseases, slower longitudinal growth,
and higher incidence of enuresis nocturna among the Skolt
Lapp children. Furthermore, the Skolt boys showed a weaker
motor proficiency as measured by the Oseretsky test and a
greater emotional immaturity compared with the Skolt girls
and the Finnish children. Low stature was also more noticeable among the Skolt boys than the girls.

These last findings support the theory that boys are more sensitive than girls to negative factors in the environment (2, 3).

Positive factors in the environment of the Skolt Lapp children include the flexible and permissive manner of the Skolt parents in bringing up their children, without which the Skolt children would presumably show many more behavioural disturbances, considering that they are living under continuous pressure from the surrounding Finnish majority.

SUMMARY

All children under 15 years of age belonging to the Skolt Lapp tribe in the northeast of Finland have been investigated using the methods of child psychiatry. Negative environmental factors such as adverse economic circumstances and poor nutrition are considered partly responsible for their poorer physical health, slower physical growth and neurophysiological immaturity, leading in turn to poorer motor proficiency, greater emotional immaturity, and a higher incidence of enuresis nocturna when compared with a control group of Finnish children. Positive factors are the flexible and permissive manner of the Skolt parents in bringing up their children; this supports the Skolt children in their difficulties in adapting to the culture of the surrounding Finnish majority. The Skolt Lapp boys showed more disturbances in behaviour and development than the girls, which supports the theory that boys are more sensitive than girls to negative environmental factors.

REFERENCES

1. Forsius, Harriet, "The Finnish Skolt Lapp children: a child study," Acta Paediat. scand. suppl., 239 (1973)
2. Graffer, M., and Corbier, J., "Contribution à l'étude de l'influence des conditions socio-économiques sur la croissance et le développement de l'enfant," Courrier XVI: 1-25 (1966)
3. Greulich, W.W., "A comparison of the physical growth and development of American born and native Japanese children," Am. J. Phys. Anthropol., 15: 489-515 (1957)
4. Hasunen, Kaija, and Pekkarinen, Maija, "The dietary intake of the Finnish Skolt children," Third International Symposium on Circumpolar Health, Yellowknife, NWT, 8-11 July 1974

5. Lewin, T., Karlberg, J., Skrobak-Kaczidsky, J., Land-
   ström, T., and Nordström, U., "Tillväxtens, den adulta
   ålderns och åldrandets morfometri hos samer." Unpublished
   monograph (1971)
6. (a) Seitamo, Leila, "Das Elterliche Verhalten in der
   Wahrnehmung der Kinder," Abstract in Bericht über das IV
   Internat Symp. Der Mensch in der Arktisch, W. Lehmann,
   (ed.), in Anthropol. Anz., 33: 114 (1971)
   (b) "Psychological adaptation of Skolt Lapp children to
   culture change," Third International Symposium on Circumpolar Health, Yellowknife, NWT, 8-11 July 1974

Mental health in northern Finland

E.J. VÄISÄNEN

A survey of comparative psychiatric epidemiology was carried
out in the region of northern Finland during the period
1970-72. A stratified random sample of 250 men and women
aged 15 to 64 years was selected to include in each group
three representatives from centres of population, and two
representatives from rural areas. The findings were compared with identical data for the southern Finnish town of
Uusikaupunki, and a rural community of Kalanti. The material
for investigation consisted of 16,415 people, of whom 1,000
were selected; data suitable for research were obtained from
991 of the group. The results are based on clinical interviews. To confirm the reliability of the findings, each of
the interviewers drew a random sample of 50 persons from one
area and compared their diagnoses (Table 1). Although the
results for the two observers seemed similar, since one of
the research team worked mainly in the north of Finland and
the other in the south, it was thought desirable that each
interview a fifth of the sample in the other's area. In addition to the clinical interviews, respondents filled out
Cornell Medical Index questionnaires, and they were given
two psychological tests, the projective Zulliger-test and
Wartegg's test "filling in the picture." Respondents were
divided into five diagnostic categories developed by Alanen
and co-workers (1). The prevalence figures are shown in

TABLE 1
The result of a preliminary interview, conducted by the two
observers on subjects from the same area (figures are percentages)

Diagnosis	Observer E.V. (n = 49)	Observer V.L. (n = 50)
Healthy persons	46	44
Milder neurotic disorders	34	34
Neuroses	16	18
Character disorders	2	2
Borderline cases	0	2
Psychoses	2	0
Total	100	100
Female	58	48
Male	42	52
Age-group under 44	52	68
Age-group over 44	48	32

TABLE 2
Psychiatric epidemiology in four areas of Finland (all data expressed
as prevalence per 1,000 inhabitants*)

Disorder	ST	SR	NT	NR	Total
Mild neurotic disorders	385	320	425	368	383
Neuroses	168	195	153	210	182
Character disorders	85	82	43	43	60
Borderline cases	7	5	8	4	6
Psychoses	30	13	8	10	15
Total of clinical disorders	290	295	212	267	263
Mild psychosomatic disorders	435	400	623	605	531
Severe psychosomatic disorders	85	59	54	66	67
Total of psychosomatic disorders	520	459	677	671	598

* ST = Uusikaupunki, N = 300, northern town; SR = Kalanti and
Uusikaupunki mlk, N = 200, northern rural area; NT = Kemijärven kpla,
N = 300, southern town; NR = Kemijärven mlk, N = 200, southern rural
area.

Table 2. There seems no significant difference between findings in northern and southern Finland and the results are
generally consistent with data from other parts of the world
(2,3,4).

The Cornell Medical Index results were generally consistent with those attained by clinical interview (Table 3), although there was misdiagnosis of both sick and healthy (x^2 = 44546, $P < 0.001$).

The best point in time for a field investigation seems June and July, because seasonal factors play an active role at other times. In the north of Finland, people have conspicuous psychosomatic and depressive symptoms in August and September, passing in October. Neurotic disorders seem most frequent among the fourth and third social strata, while the second is the healthiest. More severe disorders (psychoses and borderline cases) occur more frequently then expected among the first and fourth social strata. As to psychosomatic disturbances, the third social stratum seems to fare the worst.

Disturbances occur most often in individuals with frequent unemployment. Psychic disturbances are seem particularly in the poorly educated, and increase with age. Neurotic disorders occur more frequently than expected from the age of 35 onwards, and disturbances more severe than neuroses from the age of 45 onwards. Unmarried people have poor mental health, severe disorders afflicting them more often than expected. On the other hand, disturbances at the neurotic level are more common among married people. Psychic disorders are most common in marriages which are unbalanced and psychosomatic disorders prevail in balanced marriages. If there is a history of psychotic disturbances in close relatives, the respondents tend to develop disturbances more

TABLE 3
Results of the CMI health questionnaire on the 867 individuals interviewed in relation to psychiatric diagnoses. This table has been made by combining psychiatric data into a two-class distribution: A, healthy persons and those with only milder disorders; B, persons with clinical disorder

Psychiatric interview	Cornell Medical Index (%)		
	Healthy persons	Sick persons	Total
A. Healthy persons	74.0	26.0	100 (N = 629)
B. Sick persons	26.9	73.1	100 (N = 238)
Total	61.0	39.0	100 (N = 867)

x^2 = 44.546; DF = 1; p <0.001.

severe than neuroses, but if the psychotic disorders are found only in distant relatives, then respondents seem more liable to show neurotic disturbances. Suicide, misuse of drugs or alcohol, and neurotic disturbance among relatives are other adverse findings. This would seem to imply there is a genetic predisposition to neuroses and more severe disturbances.

The findings of this study are comparable with those of other studies; 28.4 per cent of the Finnish population suffer from some form of psychiatric disorder. According to the Leighton research team, 23.4 per cent of the population of midtown Manhattan, Stirling County, and Yorupa, Nigeria show psychiatric disorders.

ACKNOWLEDGMENT

This study was supported by the Social Insurance Institute of Finland.

SUMMARY

A socio-psychiatric study was carried out in north Finland during 1970-72. A population of 500 was selected at random to include five women and five men from each age group 15 to 64 years old, 500 persons altogether. This population was matched with a comparable population selected from southern Finland. A psychiatric interview, the Cornell Medical Index questionnaire and the psychological tests of Wartegg and Zulliger were used. Prevalence figures per 1,000 of the population were: mild neurotic disorders, 425 from the town and 368 from the rural area (compared with 385 from southern Finland); neurotic disorders, 153 and 210 (168 and 195); character disorders, 43 and 43 (85 and 82); borderline cases, 8 and 4 (7 and 5); psychoses, 8 and 10 (30 and 13); milder psychosomatic disorders, 623 and 605 (435 and 400); and psychosomatic disorders, 54 and 66 (85 and 59).

REFERENCES

1. Alanen, Y.O., Rekola, J.K., Stewen, A., Takala, K., and Tuovinen, M., "The family in the pathogenesis of schizophrenic and neurotic disorders," Acta Psych. scand., V, 42, Suppl. 189 (1966)

2. Leighton, A.H., Lambo, T.A., Huges, C.C., Leighton, D.C., Murphy, J.M., and Macklin, D.B., "Psychiatric Disorders Among the Yoruba," A Report from the Cornell-Aro mental Health Project in the Western Region, Nigeria (New York: Cornell University Press, 1963)
3. Leighton, D.C., Harding, J.S., Macklin, D.B., Macmillan, A.M., and Leighton, A.H., The Character of Danger, Psychiatric Symptoms in Selected Communities. The Stirling County Study of Psychiatric Disorder and Socio-cultural Environment (New York: Basic Books Inc., 1963)
4. Srole, L., Langer, T.S., Michael, S.T., Opler, M.K., Rennie, T.A.C., and Leighton, A.H., Mental Health in the Metropolis, The Midtown Manhattan Study 1 (New York: McGraw-Hill Book Company, 1962)

Psychiatric consultation and social work at a secondary school for Eskimo, Indian, and Aleut students in Alaska

ELINOR B. HARVEY

Although early identifications with parents and others are part of normal development (13), transient identifications at a later stage of development can also become permanent features of the child's personality. A capacity to make temporary identifications remains after childhood, particularly during adolescence (7,8,10). Teachers, dormitory staff in a boarding school, and peers serve as models for these identifications (4, 6).

This epitomizes the basis for the work of the mental health team at Mt Edgecumbe School (5). A Bureau of Indian Affairs secondary boarding school near Sitka, Alaska, its native student population includes Eskimo, Aleut,* Athabascan,* Haida, and Tsimpshian, as well as Tlingit Indians,

* Information about the Athabascan and Aleut students is not within the scope of this paper.

TABLE 1
1972-73 Mount Edgecumbe students, classified by ethnic origin

	Number	Per cent	
Eskimo	259	66	
Aleut	30	9	
Athabascan	40	11	
Tlingit	43	12	Total
Haida	7	2	southeast
Tsimpshian	5	1	Alaskan Indian 15%
Total	384	100	

coming from homes with differing languages,* customs, and
mythology (Table 1).

PSYCHIATRIC-SOCIAL WORK PROGRAM

The psychiatric-social work program at Mt Edgecumbe School
was established to aid the students, aged 13 to 23, with
the impact of vast cultural changes, plus the ordinary and
extraordinary psychological difficulties of adolescents.
Prior to the advent of the mental health team, there were as
many as two suicidal gestures a week among the girls. The
team comprises a part-time psychiatric consultant and two
social workers who are in the dormitories from 1:00 to
10:00 p.m. daily.

Student Problems Engendered by Cultural Change

The majority of the 400-600 students come from 178 isolated
Eskimo villages, some with a population of 150 or less
(Table 2). A second group comes from communities large
enough to support high schools, that is, the larger conglo-
merate† Eskimo or southeast Alaskan Indian villages. Fami-

---

* Among the Eskimo, for example, there are many differences and dialects. People from Barrow speak Inupik, while
people from Bethel speak Yupik; they either cannot understand or have great difficulty in understanding each other.
    † A conglomerate village is a heterogeneous community of
some 2,000 population, mainly migrants from different smaller villages, in contrast to the isolated village with a
long-standing permanent population.

TABLE 2
Mount Edgecumbe student Eskimo population by size
of village of origin

	Number	Per cent
Small village	222	85
Large conglomerate village	37	15
Total	259	100

lies or teachers in these larger villages may consider it
best that a student with personal or social problems receives secondary education away from home; some young people
choose boarding school as an alternative to jail. Also
available and chosen by some students are the boarding home
programs in the larger cities of Alaska, and regional boarding schools closer to home.

Transfer to the boarding school involves an abrupt transition from a close family and village culture to the culture and environment of a school in a larger community (1).
Most come from the treeless arctic tundra, while this school
is set in the mountainous rain forest near Sitka.

Student Problems According to Symptom

Disruptive behaviour while intoxicated.
The largest problem group during the five-year study consisted of students referred for disruptive behaviour while intoxicated. They were primarily southeast Indian students
and Eskimo students from the large conglomerate villages
(Table 3).

It is postulated that southeast Alaskan Indian students
(3,9,16) are more prone to manifest their problems by an
outward show, such as by drinking. Their cultural heritage
is one of relative boldness and competitiveness, in contrast to the repression of negative feelings required by
the harsher life of the Eskimo. The proportion of drinkers
among southeast Indian students was high in comparison to
their numbers in the total student population.

As for the students from the larger conglomerate villages, it is postulated that their acting out behaviour is
based on the following dynamics. Prior to their family
move from a smaller and more intact village, there was already a loosening of ties with the traditional culture,
Eskimo, Aleut, or Athabascan. This allowed new identifications, especially for the children and adolescents, when

TABLE 3
Drinking problem by ethnic origin, based on the 70
students referred for drinking during a representative
school year

	Number	Per cent of the 70 students
Eskimo*	31	44
Southeast Alaskan Indian*	23	33
Athabascan	14	20
Aleut	2	3
Total	70	100

* Although the Eskimo students comprise 66 per cent of
the student population, they represent 44 per cent of
the problem drinkers; the southeast Alaskan Indian
students, although 15 per cent of the student population, represent 33 per cent of the problem drinkers.

TABLE 4
Eskimo drinking problem by size of village of origin,
based on the number referred for drinking during a
representative school year

	Number	Per cent
Eskimo - small village	15	48
Eskimo - large conglomerate village	16	52
Total	31	100

Note: Although 85 per cent of the Eskimo student
population derives from the small villages, only 48
per cent of the Eskimo problem drinkers come from these
villages. Fifteen per cent of the student population
comes from the larger conglomerate villages, and 52 per
cent of the Eskimo problem drinkers come from these
villages.

the family moved to the larger and mixed community where
the existing population looked well established. Since the
"well settled" neighbours were themselves suffering from
difficulty in adapting to cultural changes and privations,
frequently demonstrating their pain in alcoholism and semi-
delinquent behaviour, it is not surprising that the new
arrivals identified with such aggressive qualities, and
that a number of students with this background continue the
aggressive behaviour at boarding school. This is particularly

true when such a student finds himself acting out for his group in the dormitory.

Anxiety and depression. The next largest group referred were students from smaller, more intact and isolated Eskimo villages. They were referred to the mental health team primarily for anxiety and depression, 25 and 20 per cent respectively of the referred group, albeit 13 and 10 per cent of the total student population. Their traditional background has necessitated group and individual co-operation; competitiveness and outward expressions of anger could not be allowed (12, 15). Many of the students seen for anxiety or depression will deny any possibility of anger in a situation where anger would be appropriate (in the interviewer's eyes). If we accept the theory that depression is most often anger turned against oneself, these students are prime candidates for depressive episodes.

Suicidal gestures. A group previously large and worrisome consisted of those making suicidal gestures. All were girls (Table 5). Some 85 per cent were Eskimos, although they comprise only 66 per cent of the school population. In contrast, only 10 per cent were of the southeast Indian group, which accounts for 15 per cent of the school population. The Athabascan Indian students made 5 per cent of the suicidal gestures, although they comprise 11 per cent of the school population.

The female Eskimo students appear to follow the traditional pattern of the older female generation (2), with no "out" for the expression of negative emotions, such as the channelling of aggression into the hunting enjoyed by boys and men. The girls thus become masochistic, with depression and suicidal gestures. In the villages, completed suicides also appear to have become more prevalent among adolescents

TABLE 5
Female suicidal gestures by ethnic origin

	Number	Per cent
Southeast Indian	3	10
Athabascan	1	5
Eskimo	16	85
Total	20*	100

* This number comprises the last 20 that have occurred at the school; all are female.

during the past decade.* The marked reversal of the previously high suicide gesture rate at Mt Edgecumbe School we
attribute to: (1) an intense attempt to improve the identity of staff and students, and (2) the ready availability of
the mental health team to students and staff.

STAFF CONSULTATION

Services offered the dormitory staff by the mental health
team include in-service training, problem-oriented conferences, and courses in adolescent psychology and dormitory
management that can be applied towards college credits.
Case conferences involve teachers, dormitory staff, guidance
counsellors, and school clinic personnel; in addition to
helping staff understand problem students, these regular
meetings promote trust and, consequently, collaborative efforts among staff members (14).

The academic staff is primarily Caucasian, but the dormitory staff is composed almost entirely of local southeast
Alaska Indian people whose education is at the high school
level. They have remained low on the status and pay scale,
even after years of experience (11). Prior to the advent
of the mental health team, resentment smouldered because of
lack of advancement possibilities. These people could not
confront the administration with their needs since confrontation was culturally frowned upon. Only within the past
year have they learned to ask for what they need. The administration has responded by arranging a regular meeting
time to hear complaints, suggestions, and recommendations,
and a career ladder approach has been instituted to allow
advancement to dormitory manager.

In the past, the native dormitory staff projected attitudes of discouragement, frustration, and helplessness.
Their change in attitude, we postulate, has provided the
students with positive models of identification.

ACADEMIC CHANGES

Academic changes instituted by staff and administration include: (1) courses appropriate to the student cultures, such
as native land claims, native arts, crafts, anthropology,

* "Study of suicides in the Alaska native population,"
paper presented by Robert Kraus at the 1972 Alaska Science
Conference in Fairbanks, Alaska.

TABLE 6
Number of expulsions, drop-outs, suicidal gestures,
by year

	Expulsions	Drop-outs	Suicidal Gestures
1968-69	27	52	35
1969-70	15	40	20
1970-71	12	36	8
1971-72	4	12	4
1972-73	12	20	2

archaeology, and history; (2) individualized instruction in
some courses; (3) career-oriented programs for the last two
years of school; (4) special education, with considerable
mobility in or out of the department. College courses, including classes at a local junior college, have always been
available.

Over the past five years, these changes have been associated with sharp decreases in the expulsion rate, drop-out
rate, and suicide gestures (Table 6).

CONCLUSIONS

Educating students to cope with change is a vital part of
the Alaskan secondary school program. The small villages
continue to alter in many ways as the children return from
school and as there is traffic with bigger communities,
loosening identity ties rooted in the culture.

The work of the mental health team is predicated on
strengthening the identity of students and staff, utilizing
the thesis that adolescent students will use staff, especially native staff, as models of identity. Central to the
project has been "teaching" through the experience of preventive and crisis intervention services that there are viable alternatives to outwardly destructive or masochistic
modes of behaviour.

ACKNOWLEDGMENT

My thanks are due to my co-workers at Mt Edgecumbe School -
Louis Gazay and Bennett Samuels.

SUMMARY

The attitudes of staff members, most particularly native

staff (the term native [as used in Alaska] refers to Eskimo, Aleut, and Indian people), form the models of identity for students; when staff attitudes can be modified to feelings of strength and hopefulness, these are likely to become the attitudes of the students. Staff identity can be strengthened through constant in-service training using a variety of methods reflecting staff needs. With such methods, it has been possible to lower markedly the drop-out, expulsion, and suicide-gesture rates at a secondary boarding school over a five-year period.

REFERENCES

1. Bloom, D., "Psychiatric problems and cultural transitions in Alaska," Arctic, 203-15 (Sept. 1972)
2. Brill, A.A., "Piblokto or hysteria among Peary's Eskimos," J. nerv. ment. Dis., 514-20 (1913)
3. Burland, C., North American Indian mythology (England: The Hamlyn Publishing Group, Ltd., 1965)
4. Erikson, Erik H., Childhood and Society (New York: W.W. Norton, 1950)
5. Harvey, Elinor B., and Samuels, Bennett, "The mental health worker as agent of change in an educational setting," Paper presented at the 50th annual meeting of the Am. Orthopsychiatric Assoc., New York, 1973
6. Harvey, Elinor B., Samuels, Bennett, and Gazay, Louis, "Educational models in a secondary boarding school provided via the social work and psychiatric program," Paper presented at the Southwest Regional Meeting of the Am. Orthopsychiatric Assoc., Galveston, 1972
7. Jacobson, Edith, The Self and the Object World (New York: International Universities Press, 1964)
8. Kohut, Heinz, Analysis of the Self (New York: International Universities Press, 1971)
9. Krause, Aurel (translated by Erna Gunter), Tlingit Indians (Seattle, Wash.: University of Washington Press, 1956)
10. Lampl-de-Groot, Jeanne, "Ego ideal and superego," in The Psycho-analytic Study of the Child, Vol. XVII (New York: International Universities Press, 1962)
11. Murphy, J., and Leighton, A., Approaches to Cross Cultural Psychiatry (Ithaca, NY: Cornell University Press, 1965)
12. Oswalt, Wendell H., Alaskan Eskimos (San Francisco, Calif.: Chandler Publishing Co., 1967)

13. Sandler, Joseph, "On the concept of superego," in The Psycho-analytic Study of the Child, Vol. XV (New York: International Universities Press, 1960)
14. Stanton, Alfred H., and Schwartz, M.D., Mental Hospital: A study of institutional participation in psychiatric illness and treatment (New York: Basic Books, 1954)
15. Vanstone, J., Point Hope, an Eskimo Village in Transition (Seattle, Wash.: University of Washington Press, 1962)
16. Willard, Mrs. Eugene S., Kin-da-shon's Wife (New York: Revell, 1892)

"Experience statements" of Alaskan native high school students

J. BLOOM, B. MENDELSOHN, and W. RICHARDS

How does it feel to be a native high school student in Alaska? Traditionally, workers in the helping professions have taken descriptive data from their clients for the purpose of developing general dynamic or socio-cultural theories to explain personal statements. We* have noticed a poignant eloquency in many personal statements, and have thus concentrated on developing techniques to stimulate expression for the purpose of improving therapeutic relationships in a cross-cultural setting.

The purpose of this study is to present the method, giving illustrations of personal statements, and to assess the general usefulness of such an approach.

* Alaska Area Mental Health, USPHS-IHS, has offered a variety of mental health services to schools throughout the state since 1966, depending on requests from local communities. The team includes professionals and native paraprofessionals, and works closely with the Alaska Native Health Board in developing programs and contracting with native groups to run their own programs.

ALASKAN HIGH SCHOOLS

Native students often attend school far away from home, in
boarding or dormitory settings, because of the unavailabil-
ity of local schools. There are currently some 4,800 rural
students (grades 9-12), with a projected increase to 5,700
by 1976. Cultural groups include Eskimos, Aleuts, Athabas-
cans, and Tlingits. Usually, the students go to village
schools through the eighth grade, but get their secondary
school education in a large town or city.

A multiplicity of state and federal agencies, health-
provider groups, and consumer boards attempt to plan and
deliver services to the students, with relatively poor academic and socio-emotional results. Students are usually not
well screened before entering school, leading to inappropriate placement with high drop-out and transfer rates. School
staff may be comparatively untrained in cross-cultural education. Differences of language and culture transience of
non-native staff, and long distances separating key people,
make communication and co-ordination difficult. Many students have partial hearing loss from otitis media - adding
to the problems of communication.

Because of chronic funding problems, there are usually
scant counselling services for students, and there is some
concern that available funds are being mismanaged. Native
leaders are quoted: "Even if we released the (boarding home)
money, we would still be funding programs that are destroy-
ing our children."

School officials are often defensive because of heavy
criticism, and are reluctant to have outside mental health
consultants observing less than ideal school situations. Native students usually resist any attempt by counsellors to
define their difficulties as "mental problems," pointing out
that it is the school system that has the problem. They may
be unco-operative if they sense any attempt by a counsellor
to analyse or study them.

In such a system, it is important to have methods for
gathering information about a student's health needs that
are non-threatening, free of jargon or "analysis," and are
culturally relevant.

EVOLUTION OF AN EXPERIENTIAL APPROACH

We have gradually evolved non-intrusive methods in response
to needs expressed by consumer boards, school staff, and
students. These methods lead to statements in the students'

own words, describing their own experiences from their own
frame of reference.

Forms easily used by para-professionals and largely self-
administered by healthy or disturbed students have been
developed to record this information. Students write down
their experiences, working independently, at their own pace,
without being stigmatized as "mental cases." We use a number
of forms: "story of your life," "draw a dream," "TAT,"
"story knife," "family drawing," "what's happened since last
time," "write a letter," "write about your world."

RESULTS

Sample fragments give some impression of the types of experiential information we obtain.

#1 - Story of Your life
21-year old Tlingit, 12th grade male from S.W. Alaska

Please write down the story of your life, filling up this
page - how you grew up, what your family is like, what
school has been like, any family problems or troubles in
school or any health problems.

"Well to make a long story short I'll start writing how we
live different from different people of Alaska. Our people
put up food for the winter or let me put it this way. They
start in the springtime like we pick seaweed, put them out
in the sun to dry, then put the seaweed in bags or can.
Then the big hunt in the spring is seal. We go hunting for
maybe four-five days and troll same time for King Salmon.
Maybe we would get really lucky for the hunting and trolling. We skin all the seals. Give all the seal meat away to
all the people that live in the village or most of the seal
meat to the old timers that can't go hunting or sick. The
fish that we catch we sell to the Cold Storage.

"Maybe make about couple hundred bucks a trip. The summer
coming up we make fishing in the summer we go scining for
the fishing co. I think we got the bigest fishing fleet in
S.E. Alaska. Hunting trolling all in the fall because everything open then. Winter comes then we eat all the food we
put up. Go hunting for deer until season is close December
31. Do all sorts of things like sports in winter well nothing really talk about our way of living but been prod Indian!"

#2 - Story of Your Life
18-year old Eskimo, 10th grade girl from Central Alaska

"I grew up in a very small town where everybody knows everyone almost by heart. I have eight brothers and sisters back
home now. My family, well, my parents are nice but they
drink a lot which I don't really agree but sometimes I like
it when they drink cause I can do what ever I want to do
like stay out late with friends and just bum around. But I
like my parents anyway.

   "I used to really enjoy school starting from Beginner to
eighth grade. After that I had to go quite a ways to finish
school like coming here. And I don't like it at all cause I
get homesick and the school is too big for me. I don't get
along too well cause there are so many students and yet there
I go to school and be lonely. I hate going to school where
there are too many students and they don't know me and I
don't know them."

#3 - Story of Your Life
13-year old, 7th grade Eskimo girl from N.W. Alaska

"I was born in a town and I was put in a foster home when I
was just a child. I lived with them for about six years and
then Welfare took me away from them and put me in another
foster home. I lived with her in one town for a year and
then we moved to another town and lived with her for another
two years. Then Welfare took me away from her because I was
getting a little too bouncy for her cause she was getting
old. Then when Welfare took me away from her a Welfare officer drove me down to a big city and brought me down to the
children's home and I stayed there until I was ready to go
to another foster home. Then they started to let me visit a
home every week-end and after a while I moved in with them
and I lived with them for one year and three months cause
they got a divorce and I didn't want to live with them. Then
I was put back in the children's home and after a while I
was put in with another couple for about eight or nine
months and didn't like it because I didn't like the way he
handled the family. I can't explain it. I was put back in
the children's home again. Before I moved with that family
I was put in another foster home and I was forced to leave
them because he was a State Trooper and the State said he
was transferred to a village and I couldn't go there cause
there wasn't a Welfare office and if any Welfare officer
wanted to see me, he'd have to drive all the way down to

see me. Then I was put in another foster home. And that's
the story of my life."

DISCUSSION

The four main uses of the experiential information are for
treatment, training, community development, and research.
    1. *Treatment*. The methods used can easily be applied to
groups of students by native para-professionals, making
them appropriate for screening purposes. Surprisingly, students who may be reluctant to talk verbally to school staff
or counsellors are often quite frank in writing down problems. Many students feel "helped" just by the process of ex-
pressing their experiences, and continue to send us letters,
poems, and follow-up stories on a regular basis. The method
allows for a freer flow of pertinent historical data and
emotionally charged material, facilitating the setting-up of
a relevant therapeutic contract.
    2. *Training*. The methods used are easily standardized.
Native para-professionals who would feel uncomfortable with
formal mental status examinations or social histories can
collect much information by these methods. Mental health
concepts can then be discussed, using this information with
a minimum of jargon or abstruse theory, and practical plans
of treatment can be worked out for the para-professionals
to pursue. The mental health professional often learns as
much in this process as the para-professional, as a result
of the cultural knowledge of the para-professionals, and
the discipline required in relating his theoretical knowledge to the concrete experiences at hand.
    3. *Community Development*. The methods described yield
material telling how people see their problems in plain language, and can therefore be used in groups with widely
varying backgrounds. We often organize conferences involving
consumer board members, health providers, and educators, to
discuss the mental health needs of younger people. These
conferences are at various levels, from meetings to plan
treatment for an individual student, to state-wide school
mental health planning sessions. Experiential information
is often productive in mobilizing such groups. Human services provided by community, state, and federal agencies
are most effective when responsive to the totality of an
individual's needs, but each service frequently attends to
only a fragment of the needs. Conference approaches, especially if focused on concrete practical problems and experiences, can help co-ordinate fragmented services and inte-
grate specialist systems.

4. *Research*. Many native people criticize "western research" and "white middle class" concepts of mental health.
"We should study the studiers" is a frequent comment. The
methods we are using seem more acceptable to many native
people, since they stick to the experiences of native people
in their own words. The material we obtain often points to
social and cultural aspects which seem to play major roles
in shaping the individual's experience. We need research
methods, theoretical models, and methods for delivering psychological services, which take full account of these social
and cultural dimensions.

SUMMARY

This paper describes a method for exploring the inner world
of Alaskan native high school students. Most past research
focused on external measurements like academic success or
failure, or on behavioural measurements, rather than directly on the inner feelings of the student. Examples of material obtained through use of the method are presented, and
uses of the material in treatment, para-professional training, community development work, and research are discussed.

Adaptation to an extreme environment

V. STILLNER and MARIANNE STILLNER

Providing mental health services to a rural environment is
a challenging and often neglected endeavour. This is partially due to the urban professional's reluctance to assume
demanding and often alien life-styles. The US Department of
Health, Education, and Welfare is now addressing this deficiency by designating medical shortage areas and offering
incentives for medical personnel to serve in such areas.
Nevertheless, the recruitment of medical manpower for work
in extreme environments will not be resolved readily. The
training of local practitioners could help alleviate the
critical shortage, but in order to provide relevant and
effective training, professionals will need to leave their
urban "educational citadels" and assume exotic life-styles.

The ensuing psychological, physical, and cultural stresses
have implications for the effectiveness and longevity of
the urban-educated professionals. Effective exchanges between rural "trainee" and urban "trainer" is a reciprocal
process of maturation, requiring the "trainers" to make
sound adaptation to their new environment. This paper describes our stresses in adapting to the extreme environment
of one medical shortage area.

We moved to Bethel, Alaska, in July 1973 to work as the
State's first full-time rural psychiatrist and child psychiatric nurse. This placement of a Public Health Commission
psychiatrist was part of the Alaska Native Mental Health
Service decentralization program. The hiring of a child
psychiatric nurse by the local Native Yukon-Kuskokwim Health
Corporation was a first attempt to offer preventive mental
health services to children.

During our first six months in Bethel, we made serial
tape recordings totalling five hours. These described our
subjective and objective observations. One recording was
conducted in a semi-structured manner by a psychiatric consultant. The others were open-ended. We arranged the content
into three categories: personal-family, socio-political,
and professional. In addition, we each scored ourselves on
the Zung Self-Rating Depression Scale (13) twelve weeks before moving and at eight and sixteen weeks after arriving
in Alaska.

PERSONAL-FAMILY

Our departure from the northeastern United States separated
us from our friends, family, mentors, and an enjoyable environment. We felt guilty at leaving aging parents. Our six-
month-old son was deprived of his grandparents. Seeing our
new home left us lonely and stunned by its strangeness.

The closed physical environment increased our feelings of
alienation. We experienced sensory deprivation. The treeless, excoriated tundra around our tract home presented
visual monotony. Ankle-deep mud from summer rains, poor
roads, and the inability to get away made us feel trapped.

Our behaviour during the first six weeks could be termed
hypomanic. We were constantly engaged in domestic chores
and professional preoccupations; yet we had no motivation
to pursue hobbies. We were not elated. These concerns and
obsessions resulted in decreased family communication and
recreation. Much of our behaviour was consistent with symptoms of depression (12). We experienced initial insomnia

and one of us had terminal insomnia. Both of us experienced
decreased libido. We were subjected to 20 hours of daylight
and constant physical fatigue. Occasional nocturnal doses
of Diazepam (5-10 mg) helped us to sleep.

We began to reverse these symptoms during a week-end visit to a coastal village. This excursion enabled us to transcend our daily environmental stresses and professional demands. Returning, we initiated our only mutual recreational
activity: bi-weekly karate classes. Not only was karate an
excellent physical conditioner, but it also provided an out-
let for the anger, frustration, and aggression that were beginning to accumulate. Another positive contribution to our
adaptation was the enjoyment we experienced in rearing our
son. Observing his maturational progress helped give an objectivity to our stresses.

At 12 weeks one of us made the statement: "I feel like
I've made it, but have lived 10 years in 3 months." It took
approximately another eight weeks before both of us were
functioning at our pre-removal levels.

In examining our motivations for moving to an extreme
environment, we recognize in each of us latent desires to become medical missionaries as a fulfilment of our religious
backgrounds. We were, however, confronted with ambivalent
feelings about introducing our particular psychiatric models
into another culture. Unfortunately, the same forces which
generate a desire to "help" others often result in infanti-
lization of the "helpee." We tried to minimize this problem
by understanding our own urges to help. Conquering the challenges that our environment provided became a strong motivational force in itself. Although it was difficult and
frightening, we developed self-confidence. This was accomplished through a strong familial unit and through gradual
entry into the community by way of native colleagues.

SOCIO-POLITICAL

We left friendships in a highly inbred professional environment. In our new home we felt we were a minority, both
professionally and racially. Living away from the "medical
compound" separated us socially from hospital peers. Socia-
lizing with people of varied backgrounds, training, and
ages was a new experience. Moreover, towns-people scruti-
nized us closely and were cautious of our interests in
"activities of the mind." The confidentiality of our work
made us feel isolated.

The closed nature of the community illuminated all social interactions and their underlying policital ramifications. Much of the subgrouping that we encountered resulted
from socio-political inbreeding of agencies. This made it
difficult to socialize in any group without becoming politi-
cally earmarked. The temptation to be seduced into territorial power struggles frustrated us. Power was the important
commodity in daily exchanges. People assumed that because we
dealt with behaviour and the mind, we would naturally agree
with their social hypotheses, be it the firing of a school
teacher or voting the town "wet" or "dry" in the coming el-
ection. We had numerous invitations from groups to align
with their causes. Because of the political cross-fires
generated by these power struggles, we remained socially
isolated.

PROFESSIONAL

We completed our respective educations in Boston, Massachu-
setts, immediately prior to arrival in Bethel. Thus, the
transcultural, rural exposure presented a first in almost
all aspects of our work. Fortunately, two reconnaissance
visits to Alaska in the nine months preceding our move allowed us to anticipate some of the differences between the
two environments.

As we were the first full-time mental health workers to
live in Bethel, community expectations were high and often
unrealistic about what our specialities could provide. Our
knowledge of the previous years' homicide and suicide rates
provoked a statement recorded at five weeks: "I feel I'm a
lifeguard on a sea of psychoses." Our exposure to violent
behaviour, often alcohol related, fostered a fear of verbal
and physical aggression, including homicide. This fear
lessened as we became familiar with the community's cultural patterns of expression.

Interviewing Eskimo adults and children posed problems
because of our inabilities to understand non-verbal and
facial expressions. Lengthy interviewing through third par-
ty translators frustrated client, translator, and interviewer. Interviews sometimes violated social taboos. Certain words were difficult to translate; quantification and
establishment of temporal relationships seemed to be less
relevant, particularly with adults. Communication with children through play and drawings was less complicated.

The lack of understanding of prevalent norms created
nosological problems. For example, apparent affective

disorders did not respond to intervention with "tricyclics."
Therefore, emphasis was placed on symptom alleviation rather than on diagnosis. Long-term treatment, familiar to us
in our training, was often impossible owing to the migratory
nature of the clients. Job opportunities, medical and legal
needs, and schooling precipitated constant travel from village to town to city. Consequently, short-term therapy had
to be effective in one to three sessions or through written
correspondence.

Proper regimens of psychotropic medications were difficult to prescribe through third parties on short-wave radio.
Initial heavy reliance on psychotropic medication decreased
after we became familiar with the behaviour, thoughts, and
feelings of the people. The establishment of effective native mental health workers also reduced reliance on medication. The training and psychological support of bilingual
mental health workers were difficult because of problems in
the selection of relevant educational content and communication difficulties. However, we soon recognized that the
training of local health workers would bring the best long-
term results. The mental health "trainees" screened out our
irrelevant urban values and focus. They bridged many other
transcultural difficulties. Once we were able to allow these
workers maximum professional freedom, the reciprocal learning process progressed.

COMMENT

Our total immersion in an extreme environment was a painful
maturational process. A number of factors stand out as beneficial to adaptation.

The two pre-removal Alaskan visits enabled us to dispel
some of the fantasies we had about living in Alaska. We
were able to prepare ourselves for the environmental changes. During these visits, we encountered colleagues from
whom we received preparatory information on housing, food,
and clothing. The visits also stimulated self-analysis of
our motives for working in an extreme environment. Our hus-
band-wife competitiveness had to be acknowledged before
isolating ourselves in an area where professional activities
assumed so much time and energy. We became aware of potential stresses to our marriage. Also, we developed a new
awareness of rescue fantasies and delusions of professional
grandiosity. By keeping these notions in check during the
year, we prevented two relatively common side-effects of
frontier living: frequent staff turnover and psychological

"burn-out." In becoming aware of our marital and personal
behaviour, we found the Holmes and Rahe Scale of Life Stress
Units (14) and the Zung Self-Rating Depression Scale (13)
beneficial psychological "thermometers."

A leisurely cross-country move enabled us to recuperate
from the stresses of separation before assuming the new
ones of adjustment. Expanding the move into a vacation gave
us an adventurous interlude. The establishment of our first
trip "out" shortly after our arrival became our psychological "emergency exit." The short trip to an urban area was a
pscyhological "tune-up." Subsequent vacationing in a tropical environment satisfied our sensory deprivation. In addition, fishing, hunting, and camping in the Bethel region
were important adaptational milestones.

Tape-recorded sessions describing our thoughts, feelings,
and experiences enabled us to attain an objectivity that
aided adaptation. Psychometric scales, biochemical measures,
and sleep studies could provide additional investigational
tools for such adaptational experiences.

After three months, our adjustment needs became more
specific. We required activities that helped us transcend
the local stresses. Attendance at professional conventions,
study, and hobbies reminded us of the world at large and
gave our immediate problems a smaller dimension. Communication with past friends and mentors helped greatly. In addition, respiratory viral insults, diurnal changes, and psychological stresses became less overwhelming after we developed an activity to keep physically fit. Professionally,
establishing a relationship with knowledgeable, trusted
consultants provided us with valuable periodic input. The
selection of competent indigenous colleagues helped us develop a reciprocal working relationship and broaden our
clinical skills.

We encountered problems unique to the extreme environment and others that are common human experiences but become magnified where there is an environment with few exits.
Proper anticipation of these stresses can facilitate a good
adjustment to the total environment. Before training of rural manpower can be effective, the urban "trainer" has to
make a good adaptation to his extreme environment.

SUMMARY

The challenges of providing mental health services to a
rural extreme environment seldom acknowledge the personal
adaptation required of urban-trained professionals. We have

described our personal, professional, and socio-policital
experiences in the medical-shortage area of southwestern
Alaska. Serial tape recordings of our subjective observations were made over the first six months of residence. Our
total immersion in an extreme environment has been a painful
maturational process, but has enabled us to suggest a number
of factors helping adaptation. The psychological, physical,
and cultural stresses of adaptation and their resolution
have implications for the effectiveness and the longevity of
the urban-education professional in an extreme environment.

REFERENCES

1. Boag, T.J., "The white man in the Arctic: a preliminary
   study of problems of adjustment," Am. J. Psychiat.,
   109: 6 (1952)
2. Briggs, J., Never in Anger - Portrait of an Eskimo Family (Cambridge, Mass.: Harvard University Press, 1971)
3. Chance, N., The Eskimo of North Alaska (New York: Holt,
   Rinehart and Winston, 1966)
4. Gunderson, E.K., "Adaptation to extreme environments,"
   USN Neuropsychiatric Research Unit Report 66-17: 1-41
   (1966)
5. "Handbook of information for physicians (MD & DO), dentists, optometrists, pediatrists, veterinarians and
   pharmacists entering an agreement to practice in a shortage area," US Department of Health, Education and Welfare publication No. (HRS) 74-11 (Washington, DC:
   Government Printing Office, 1973)
6. Holmes, T.H., and Rahe, R.H., "The social readjustment
   scale," J. Psychosom. Res., 11: 213 (1964)
7. Mullin, C.S., "Some psychological aspects of isolated
   antarctic living," Am. J. Psychiat., 117: 323-7 (1960)
8. Nelson, P.D., "Psychological aspects of antarctic living," Milit. Med., 130: 485-9 (1965)
9. Palmai, G., "Psychological observations on an isolated
   group in antarctica," Brit. J. Psychiat., 109: 364-70
   (1963)
10. Popkin, M.K., Stillner, V., Osborn, O.W., Pierce, C.H.,
    and Shurley, J.T., "Novel behaviours in an extreme en-
    vironment," Am. J. Psychiat., 131: 651-4 (1974)
11. Strange, R.E., "Emotional aspects of wintering over,"
    Antarctic of the United States, 16: 255-7 (1971)
12. US Department of Commerce Bureau of the Census and 1970
    census of Population, general social and economic cha-
    racteristics, Alaska PC (1) - C3

13. Willis, J.S., "Mental health in the North," Med. Serv.
    J. (Canada), 16: 689-70 (1960)
14. Zung, W.W.K., The Measurement of Depression. The Self-
    Rating Depression Scale (Milwaukee Wisconsin Lakeside
    Laboratories, Inc.)

A model for psychiatric education in the North

R.F. KRAUS and R. LYONS

The Pacific northwest, which contains 20 per cent of the
land mass in the United States, is considered to be criti-
cally underserved medically and a demonstration area for
the development of innovative programs in medical education.
The widely dispersed rural populations of the area constitute a particular problem. Examination of physician - patient ratios for Alaska for the year 1968 shows that Alaska
has far less than its share of the United States pool of
physicians. A second problem is one of maldistribution. The
more urban southcentral and southeastern areas have ratios
which compare favourably with National averages, while the
rural sections, predominantly populated by indigenous
peoples, are greatly underserved. A similar situation exists
with respect to psychiatric manpower. Of the 28 psychiatrists in active practice in Alaska during the summer of
1974, 21 were in the city of Anchorage.
     The severity of the physician shortage in the Pacific
northwest is due in part to the fact that Alaska, Montana,
and Idaho have no medical schools. This also affects the
problem of maldistribution. Legislative pressures have
forced most state-supported schools to limit drastically the
number of positions available to out-of-state residents;
moreover, there is a tendency for physicians to cluster in
areas where they have been trained. The Washington-Alaska-
Montana-Idaho (WAMI) program of the University of Washington was organized in response to this problem in 1971. It
had the following objectives: (1) to increase medical school
enrolment in the WAMI states; (2) to improve uneven distribution of physicians in the region; (3) to save tax dollars
by using existing facilities; (4) to provide clinical experience in small communities; and (5) to improve patient

care by providing a better flow of information to outlying
physicians. The University Phase of WAMI offers first-year
basic science instruction at various sites within the four-
state region. The Community Clinical Phase provides clinical instruction in various specialty areas for third and
fourth year students at outlying sites.

The Alaskan program in psychiatry is the only psychiatric community clinical unit in the WAMI program and is an
integral part of the Department of Psychiatry and Behavioral Sciences of the University of Washington. Many of the
social, cultural, and administrative features of Alaskan
psychiatry are unique. The State offers an extraordinarily
wide range of clinical experiences and settings. In order
to bring this range of experiences into relationship with a
single program and utilize maximally psychiatric manpower
which was in short supply, the Alaska chapter of the American Psychiatric Association, to which most of the psychiatrists in the state belong, became the sponsoring body for
the Alaska Community Clinical Unit in psychiatry. This is
the first time that an element of the American Psychiatric
Association has organized itself as a medical faculty and
contracted with a university to provide accredited training. Currently, some sixteen Alaskan psychiatrists hold
clinical appointments at the medical school and provide
training for psychiatric residents and medical students in
the state, both in the University Phase and the Community
Clinical Phase.

SUMMARY

Over-all statistics relevant to the medical manpower shortage in the North are presented with particular reference to
psychiatric physicians. The Washington-Alaska-Montana-Idaho
(WAMI) program of the University of Washington is a unique
experiment designed to meet the medical education needs of
the Pacific northwest. The contribution of the Alaskan psychiatric community to the psychiatric education of medical
students and residents within the WAMI model is reviewed in
terms of background and development of the program, curriculum, and planning principles.

Psychiatric consultation to the eastern Canadian arctic communities

J.D. ATCHESON and S.A. MALCOLMSON

At the request of the federal Department of Health and Welfare, we have had the opportunity of consulting to several communities in the eastern Arctic, including Frobisher Bay, Cape Dorset, and Pangnirtung. Frobisher Bay is some 1,500 miles north of Montreal, and has a population of approximately 2,500 people, of whom roughly 1,500 are native Canadian Eskimo people; it has become a major communications, transportation, and administrative base for the eastern Canadian Arctic, experiencing very rapid growth in the last ten years, with associated changes in housing, the delivery of services, and in political organization. The modern 30-bed hospital has been in operation since 1964. The medical services in Frobisher Bay assume responsibility for consulting and providing direct services to all communities in the Baffin zone through visits arranged by their medical staff and consultants and through the transport of particularly difficult cases to this centre for diagnosis and treatment. Cape Dorset is some 350 miles from Frobisher Bay, with a population of 600 to 700 people, approximately 90 per cent of whom are native Canadian Eskimos. This settlement is the centre of native art which has gained international recognition. Trapping and hunting are also a part of the economy. Pangnirtung has a population of 500 to 600 people, 90-95 per cent of whom are Eskimos. It is some 400 miles from Frobisher Bay. The basis of the economy includes native art productions, tourism, hunting, and trapping.

In terms of understanding emotional disorders, psychiatrists face very unique problems. Specific techniques developed in the south are only partially appropriate and valid in arctic communities, and consultation departs from the traditional medical model. The psychiatrist in the North must subject his observations to careful examination, not assuming an arrogant stance of criticism without knowledge of the specific cultural, ethnic, and developmental problems that a given community is facing. As a person concerned with mental illness, a psychiatrist may be seen as threatening, and it may be assumed he is critical when, in fact, he is attempting to be objective. The psychiatrist, more than any other specialist in medicine, must seek new methods of making his skills appropriate and available. He finds himself involved in the process of cultural erosion and the ongoing cultural clash between the traditional problem-solving methods of the Canadian natives and the non-native Canadian administrators, educators, and other members of the health delivery team.

The non-native members of the community are very sensitive to the problems created by attempting to establish a community based on southern political economic and educational systems. They have often been subjected to the advice of experts and one representing a profession concerned with human mental disability tends to be viewed with alarm if not to be seen as a thinly disguised Gestapo, sent to discover and describe their stresses and the inadequacies of the system they are establishing.

Four differing types of responsibilities of the Arctic psychiatric consultant can be identified:

1. The consultant may be utilized as a medical specialist who examines patients, makes a diagnosis, and undertakes direct case management, as in the following example. A 30-year-old Eskimo female had been actively hallucinating for some three months prior to the consultant's arrival. The patient had been a significant concern to her family and to the community. Subtherapeutic doses of major tranquillizers had been ineffective in reducing the hallucinations and controlling her disturbed behaviour. The patient was seen at the request of the public health nurse. Following assessment in the home, it was decided to admit her to hospital. Here, she was treated with high doses of Chlorpromazine, and subsequently discharged with appropriate arrangements for immediate and long-term out-patient management. The case was managed directly by the psychiatrist, who was available to the nursing staff throughout the patient's stay in hospital; this helped alleviate the anxiety felt by the nursing staff in managing a psychiatric problem.

This fact, together with the success of treatment, helped reduce the apprehension felt by some of the medical staff at the admission of a psychiatric patient to a medical and surgical ward. The case brought together the public health nurses, the medical practitioner, and the in-patient nurses in discussions concerning treatment.

As a result of this experience, the nursing staff requested a seminar on the use of phenthiazines and their side-effects and this further facilitated the acceptance of in-patient treatment for acute psychiatric disorders.

Discussions about the case very quickly forced the medical specialist into a close and reliant relationship with the local practitioner, nurses, and social worker, even though he personally undertook the direct treatment. This is, to a degree, a departure from the composition of consultant teams in southern areas, which usually have a social worker, a nurse, or perhaps a psychologist as members.

2. The second type of consultation involves the consultant with local health and social agencies, with utilization of primary community contacts. The fact that consultants visit reinforces their role as back-up and educative resources personnel. In leaving the primary therapist and the case behind, the consultant forces the primary community contact into total involvement with case management, and by case-centred discussion, development of such staff occurs.

3. The third role of the psychiatric consultant is to discuss with local agencies such broad issues as cultural erosion, alcoholism, incorporation of children into the school system, and the creation of political systems. In this area, the psychiatric consultant must approach his task with considerable humility, recognizing that he must learn about local conditions before pontificating and offering arbitrary decisions as to management.

4. The fourth area in which the psychiatrist has an important role to play is in research and evaluation of therapy. There is a need for hard data on socio-medical problems to replace impressionistic findings. A circumscribed case register would seem a useful tool to assess whether a medical service is influencing the decline or containment of an illness. We were aware that the information collected could only be as valuable as the questions asked, and that the register needed the co-operation of those in the community. Where lines of command stretch halfway across the continent, there may be legitimate suspicion about a research tool that could be used to evaluate local personnel. Although concern was expressed over potential abuse of the privacy and human rights of the native people, this was probably partly a screen for concern about invasion of the privacy and rights of local health workers.

The major lesson learned from attempts to establish such a register was that the instrument might jeopardize other aspects of our relationship with the community.

One of our most significant conclusions is the importance of continuity of service. This seems particularly important in psychiatric care. In order to establish such continuity, the federal Department of Health and Welfare,

in contract with the Clarke Institute of Psychiatry of the
University of Toronto, has established programs in which the
same consultants accompanied by senior residents in psychiatry, plus other consultants in specialties such as speech,
learning disability, education, and psychology, visit the
Baffin zone of the Northwest Territories on a quarterly basis, making their headquarters in the Frobisher Bay area.

This program is now entering its second year. Between
consulting visits, it is hoped that public health nurses
trained in psychiatric nursing will be given the task of
following-up patients, serving as a liaison between the community and the consulting team.

SUMMARY

The general and specific problems of providing psychiatric
consultation to an arctic community are identified. Continuity of consultations is important. Resources for treatment
of psychiatric problems in the local community should include the use of public health nurses for follow-up work.
Consultation of social agencies is also most important.
Problems of evaluation, epidemiological studies, and research into mental health disorders in the arctic communities are discussed.

REFERENCES

1. Hellon, C.P., "Mental illness and acculturation in the
   Canadian aborigines," Canad. psychiatr. Arch., 15: 2
   (April 1970)
2. Boag, Thomas, "Mental health of native people in the
   Arctic," Canad. Psychiat. Arch., 15: 2 (April 1970)
3. Vallee, F.G., "Stress of change in mental health among
   the Canadian Eskimos," Arch. env. Health, 17: 5 (1965)
4. Sampath, H.M., "The characteristics of hospitalized Eskimo patients from the eastern Arctic," Proceedings of
   Killam Workshop on Research Problems in Social Psychiatry of the Eastern Arctic, Memorial University, Newfoundland

Alcohol problems in western Greenland

INGE LYNGE

The delimiting of alcoholism and other alcohol problems is difficult. The "Criteria for the diagnosis of alcoholism" (1) illustrate the complexity of the problem. We are in need of simple operational definitions, particularly when comparing different countries and cultures.

As is usual in psychiatric practice, the present study has assessed the person's total situation, his physical and psychological health and the part that alcohol plays in any disorders that are found. When there have been definite signs of damage by alcohol (such as alcoholic dementia, other alcohol psychoses, alcoholic neuropathy, and cirrhosis) and/or a habitually large consumption has had crucial influence on the individual's life, he has been recorded as suffering from alcoholism.

When episode drinking bouts have resulted in violence, working stress, a change of employment, or mental problems, but there have been no signs of alcohol damage between bouts, such patients have been noted as suspected cases. Persons with a heavy but steady consumption of alcohol that has influenced their living to some extent, and may later cause definite damage, have also been recorded as suspected cases.

The investigation has covered three areas of West Greenland with about 4,000 inhabitants, half of whom were over 15 years of age. Data were gathered in the autumn of 1970. Key personnel from the Health Services with thorough knowledge of the community identified persons with suspected mental disorder or alcoholism. In all three areas, the author made the final evaluation after clinical examination and a study of available medical records. Mental disorders were classified according to WHO's manual and alcoholism or suspected alcoholism was determined as mentioned above.

The figures include only persons born in Greenland who have lived in the area of study for more than six months. The Health Service had less concern with the alcohol problems of Danish-born individuals, and the technique used was not suitable for an examination of alcohol problems among the Danes. However, Danish alcohol consumption while in Greenland is on average 50 per cent higher than that of the Greenlandic people and that of Danes in Denmark (2). The

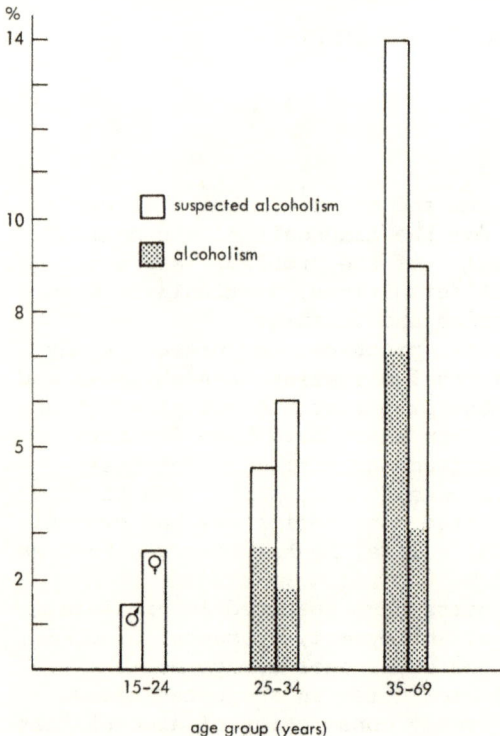

Figure 1 Alcoholism and suspected alcoholism in a Greenlandic population of 1,965 persons 15 years of age or over:
prevalence classified by age and sex as a percentage of the
total population

Danes in Greenland are for the most part socially protected, and their drinking is less likely to cause overt problems than to produce pathological manifestations later in
life - perhaps after they have left Greenland.

Diagnoses by the predominantly Danish Health Service
usually follow Danish middle-class standards; Greenlandic
drinking patterns are instinctively considered more pathological and thus attention is more easily drawn to alcohol
as an essential factor in social and medical problems.

RESULTS

Among 1,965 Greenlandic persons over 15 years of age, there
were 50 cases of alcoholism and a further 75 suspected cases, giving a 6 per cent total prevalence of alcohol

problems. Of the 125 individuals concerned, 64 were men and
61 women. Compared with other (Nordic) countries, the even
sex ratio is remarkable. In the lower age groups, there is
a slight preponderance of women, whereas over the age of
35 years the males predominate (Figure 1). The prevalence
of mental disorders other than alcoholism is shown in Table
1. The persons concerned were not necessarily in a mental
hospital or under out-patient care. Nevertheless, they exhibited symptoms such that they would be considered at least
periodically disabled by mental illness or by alcoholism.
Among the 116 persons with mental disorders other than alcoholism, nearly half (52) had alcohol problems secondary
to the psychiatric disease. Two-thirds of them showed personality disorders, ranging from impulsive actions to in-
troversion, hyper-sensitivity and suspicion. Self-assertive-
ness was often a reason for conflict.

Seventy-three of the 125 persons with alcohol problems
had no conclusive signs of psychiatric abnormalities prior
to the consequences of alcohol use. The 767 households studied were classified according to alcohol consumption and
alcoholism (including suspected alcoholism) by members of
the household (Figure 2). A total of 480 households had
neither large consumption of alcohol nor recorded alcohol
problems. Two hundred and seven households had at least one
member who consumed a large amount of alcohol but no recorded alcoholism. Eighty households had at least one member

TABLE 1
Psychiatric morbidity among 1,965 persons over
the age of 15 years born in Greenland and living
in West Greenland, 1970

Psychosis		26
Organic	7	
Schizophrenic	7	
Manic-depressive	9	
Uncertain diagnosis	3	
Neurosis		30
Personality disorder		39
Non-psychotic symptoms due to organic		
conditions (epilepsy, etc.)		11
Mental subnormality		10
Alcoholism and suspected alcoholism		
without other psych. diagnosis		73
Alcoholism and suspected alcoholism		
as second diagnosis	52	
Total		189

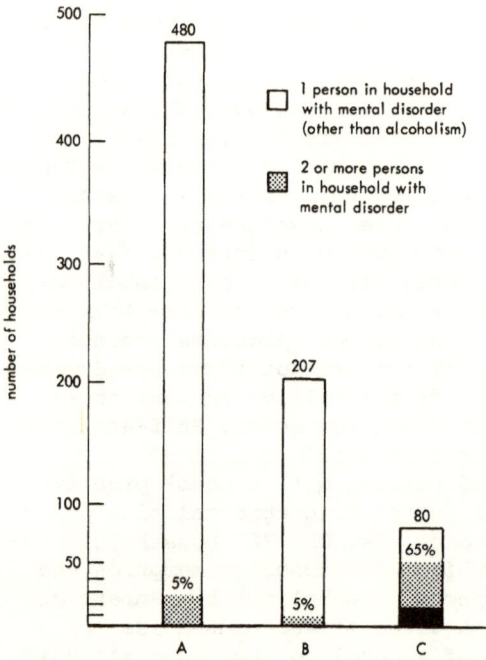

Figure 2 The 767 households studied are here classified
according to consumption of alcohol or alcoholism (including suspected cases) by any member of the household (A,
without great consumption or alcoholism; B, with great consumption but without alcoholism; C, with alcoholism)

with alcoholism (or suspected alcoholism). The hatched
areas at the bottom of the columns show households with at
least one person with a mental disorder besides alcoholism.
The black sections are households with two or more persons
with mental disorder.

In households with alcoholism, there is also a greatly
increased prevalence of mental disorder. It is only in such
households that one finds more than one person with mental
disorder. However, households with a known large alcohol
consumption, but no alcoholism, have no more mental disorder
than households without heavy consumption. One could invert
the problem by saying that it looks as if households with
special psychological problems are the households whose
drinking leads to alcoholism or who classify their members
as alcoholics.

According to Leif Sølling (2), these households had most of the signs of social stress, whereas in households with a high consumption but without alcoholism there was only slightly greater social stress than in households without a large consumption of alcohol.

What use can be made of these results? The Greenlandic Temperance Commission has used them to emphasize that alcohol problems are not isolated phenomena and that they should not be treated in isolation from other social and medical problems (3). Proposals to establish special treatment-institutions for alcoholics were rejected in favour of better utilization of resources within existing social- and health-services as well as other institutions, co-operating in the treatment of multiproblem families and alcoholism.

SUMMARY

A medical survey of alcohol problems has covered some 2,000 persons 15 years of age or more living in West Greenland. Using traditional psychiatric techniques, a prevalence of 6 per cent alcoholism or suspected alcoholism was shown, with little difference between the sexes. There was a slight preponderance of females below 35 years of age, but a large increase among males in the older age groups. The most severe cases were found among males. Of the 767 households studied, about 10 per cent (in all, 80 households) included all cases of alcoholism and most cases of mental disorder. These households also showed most of the signs of social stress, whereas the households with a known large consumption of alcohol but without alcoholism had the same frequencies of mental disorders, and only slightly more signs of social stress than households without a large consumption of alcohol.

REFERENCES

1. National Council on Alcoholism, "Criteria for the diagnosis of alcoholism," Am. J. Psychiat., 129: 127-35 (1972)
2. Sølling, Leif, "Undersøgelse af sammenhaengen mellem alkoholforbrug og social belastning" (Investigation of connection between alcohol use and social stress), Appendix to the final report of the Greenlandic Temperance Commission, The National Council of Greenland, 1971
3. Sølling, Leif, Alkoholforbruget i Grønland (Alcohol use in Greenland) (Copenhagen: Danish National Institute for Social Research, 1974)

Criminal homicide in Greenland

J.P. HART HANSEN

Since World War II, Greenland has experienced explosive
development, with dissolution of the many small hunting
communities and establishment of industrialized settlements.
Once a closed country, communication with other parts of
the world is increasing, and there has been an impressive
influx of Danish workers and administrators. Because of rapid change in the national, racial, social, and economic
character of the small Greenlandic community, there is social and some political unrest with instability. Are these
developments reflected in the pattern of criminal homicide?

In the first half of this century, homicide was excep-
tional in Greenland (1). Earlier, in the pagan days, killings were more frequent (for example, blood-feuds and the
killing of witches). Because of restricted food resources,
other types of intentional killing were also common, as in
other primitive communities. Old and disabled persons were
abondoned to die, and often they asked for this themselves
to avoid burdening their family. Such killings were regarded as acts of compassion, just as were killings of the
mentally ill and children without parents or family.

A forensic enquiry into homicide in Denmark during the
25-year period 1946-70 has allowed comparisons with homicidal criminality in related environments of the North Atlantic area: Greenland, Iceland, and the Faroe Islands.
The investigation covers homicide, violence resulting in
death, abandonment, culpable behaviour during childbirth,
leaving in a helpless situation, and failure to aid those
in distress, provided that death was the consequence of the
act or omission. Cases of unintentional manslaughter and
criminal abortion are not included.

Registration and investigation of such crimes has been
excellent in the countries mentioned with the exception of
Greenland (2, 3, personal data), where a vast territory,
isolated and sparsely inhabited settlements, difficulties
of travelling, and the lack of police and medical officers
have caused many to be closed by the authorities without
proper investigation. However, reporting has improved considerably during the last 15 years.

The total number of cases is limited (Table 1). There
were 45 cases in Greenland from 1946 to 1970, 0.45 per cent

TABLE 1
Victims of criminal homicide and manslaughter in
Greenland, Denmark, Iceland, and the Faroe Is-
lands, 1946-70

	No. of victims	Per cent of all deaths
Greenland	45	0.45
Denmark	892	0.08
Iceland	21	0.07
Faroe Islands	3	0.05

TABLE 2
Area and populations of Greenland, Denmark, Iceland, and
the Faroe Islands

	Area (km^2)	Population in 1970	Increase of population since 1945 (%)
Greenland	2,175,600	46,400	117
Denmark	43,000	4,906,900	22
Iceland	103,000	205,000	42
Faroe Islands	1,400	38,700	22

of all deaths over the same period. Of these cases, three
were non-Greenlanders. Criminal homicide was more than five
times as frequent in Greenland as in Denmark and Iceland
and nine times as frequent as on the Faroe Islands.

The countries mentioned are very different in area,
population, and culture (Table 2). Greenland has the largest area, covering more than 2 million km^2, of which only
about 15 per cent is free of the icecap. Iceland is an island of 103,000 km^2, while the Faroes are 18 small islands
covering 1,400 km^2.

Greenland has been administrated as an integral part of
Denmark since 1953; until then, it had been a colony for
nearly 250 years. Iceland is a republic, and the Faroes are
a self-governing part of Denmark. Greenland is inhabited by
Eskimos, mainly hybridized with Europeans over the centuries. Iceland and the Faroes have very strong ties to the
other Scandinavian countries. Populations are small: in
Iceland little more than 200,000 persons, on the Faroe Islands nearly 40,000. The increase of population since World
War II has amounted to about 22 per cent in Denmark and the
Faroes and 42 per cent in Iceland. Development has been
much faster in Greenland, with an increase from 21,400

inhabitants in 1946 to more than 47,000 in 1970. The culture
of Greenland differs greatly from that of the other countries. Ancestry and present living conditions differ, and
social and economic inequalities are numerous.

The frequency of homicide has increased in Greenland
from 1946 to 1970 (Table 3). This increase is in excess of
the population growth, even taking into account the age
groups most often involved in such cases. However, the rate
of homicide has been relatively constant in Denmark and
Iceland.

In Greenland, 43 per cent of the victims were female,
while in Denmark and Iceland 51 and 53 per cent were female.
Slightly more females are victims of homicide in western
countries, and the opposite is usually the case in less developed countries. In Greenland and Denmark, 67 and 69 per
cent of the culprits were men, while in Iceland not one woman committed homicide, not even so-called "extended suicide" with killing of herself and her children.

The age distribution corresponds with other similar material (4). In Greenland, the youngest perpetrator was a
boy of 12 who killed a little girl after having raped her.

The most frequent motives (Table 4) were revenge, sudden
exasperation over minor disagreements and abondonment (including maltreatment) of children. Only two cases of sexual
killing are recorded in Greenland, and no cases of murder
with intent to rob, though minor thefts have been committed
in connection with some killings. In Iceland, there has
been only one possible sexual murder, incidentally the only
unsolved homicide in Iceland. There are no unsolved homicides in Greenland or the Faroe Islands over the period in
question. It is very difficult to commit homicide in a

TABLE 3
Yearly distribution of criminal homicide (as a percentage)
in Greenland, Denmark, Iceland, and the Faroe Islands,
1946-70

	Greenland	Denmark	Iceland	Faroe Islands
1946-50	4	24	5	0
1951-55	9	23	38	0
1956-60	16	18	19	0
1961-65	38	17	19	0
1966-70	33	18	19	100
Totals	100	100	100	100

TABLE 4
Motives of criminal homicides (as a percentage) in
Greenland, Denmark, and Iceland, 1946-70

	Greenland	Denmark	Iceland
Altercation due to minor disagreements	36	22	24
Abandonment, self-defence	27	6	5
Infanticide	15	4	0
Jealousy	9	12	24
Sexual killing	4	5	5
Family drama	2	34	24
Robbery	0	6	5
Other or unknown	7	11	13
Totals	100	100	100

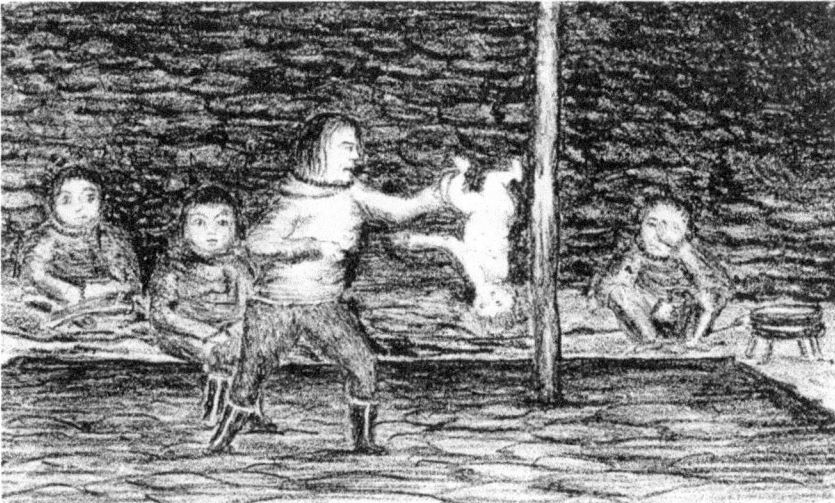

Figure 1 Infanticide in Greenland. Lithograph from the
legend about the Cousins, after a drawing by ARON about
1860, from the archives of the Arctic Institute, Copenhagen

small secluded community without being discovered. Characteristically, the parties involved are related to or know
one another, a situation determined by the limited size and
special structure of the communities.

Infanticide has been rather frequent in Greenland compared with other countries (Figure 1). Since World War II,
no such case is on record in Iceland and the Faroes and it
is impossible to find reports even of newborn babies found
dead in Iceland since the 'twenties. This is remarkable,
as such cases are well known in other countries. Presumably,
in small communities pregnancy is not easily overlooked or
forgotten. The moral attitude to birth out of wedlock might
also be important.

So-called family dramas or extended suicides, when a
parent, most often the mother, kills herself and her children are frequent in Denmark and Iceland. In Greenland, only one such case is on record. This case involved a Danish
woman who was depressed over living in a remote place; she
killed her three-year-old son and tried to commit suicide
(Table 5). In Denmark and Iceland, family dramas are most
often committed by poisoning; in Denmark, carbon monoxide
from kitchen gas has been preferred. Parents want to apply
as little violence as possible. No murder by poison has
been recorded in Greenland.

A rather unique method of committing homicide has been
used in Greenland, where sledge dogs have been involved in
two cases. In one example, a woman was hit on the head by a
stone during an argument with her husband. She was unconscious, and suddenly the husband had the idea that this was
an opportunity to get rid of his wife. He made some skin ab-
rasions so that blood was flowing, and then called some
sledge dogs into the vicinity. In a few minutes, the dogs
killed the woman and ate most of the corpse.

In many countries, it is not unusual that the murderer
commits suicide. Nearly a third (30%) of homicidal killers

TABLE 5
Methods of killing in criminal homicides (as a percentage)
in Greenland, Denmark, and Iceland, 1946-70

	Greenland	Denmark	Iceland
Beating	24	20	33
Stabbing	7	9	14
Shooting	18	14	24
Asphyxia	24	27	5
Poison	0	23	24
Abandonment	18	1	0
Other or unknown	9	6	0
Totals	100	100	100

in Denmark did so. Most were so-called family dramas. Suicide subsequent to homicide was very infrequent (2 per
cent) in Greenland (as were family dramas), though suicide
in itself was at least as frequent as in Denmark. In Iceland, 16 per cent of the perpetrators committed suicide.

Alcohol is a very important factor, being involved in 71
per cent of homicidal cases in Greenland, and 77 per cent
in Iceland. The increasing abuse of alcohol is a great problem in Greenland today, and it goes hand in hand with an increasing frequency of all kinds of criminality, including
homicide. In 1967, 62 per cent of all recorded crimes were
committed under the influence of alcohol (5). In Denmark,
alcohol was involved in 34 per cent of homicides.

DISCUSSION

One very important factor for criminality is the social stability of a community (6). Where the social order is stable,
criminality is low. Iceland and the Faroes have limited
communities, race and culture are uniform, and there is no
significant differentiation into classes and social groupings. Behaviour is uniform and there is a rather high degree of group-control over the individual members of the
community. The social and technological development of Denmark, Iceland, and the Faroes has progressed at a moderate
rate, in contrast with Greenland, where a too rapidly changing society has suffered from social unrest and instability.

SUMMARY

Since World War II, there has been an increased frequency
of criminal homicide in Greenland relative to other North
Atlantic countries. This phenomenon is closely related to
an explosive social development with resettlement, profound
changes in living conditions, social instability, and increasing abuse of alcohol.

REFERENCES

1. Hart Hansen, J.P., "Drab i Grønland 1946-1970,"
   Tidsskr. Grønland, 20: 214-23 (1972)
2. Hart Hansen, J.P., and Bjarnason, O., "Homicide in Iceland 1946-1970," Forensic Sci. (in press)

3. Debes Joensen, H., and Hart Hansen, J.P., "Dráp og
   frásagnir um dráp i Føroyúm," Ann. societ. scient. Faero-
   ensis, 21: 72-85 (1973)
4. Wolfgang, M.E., Patterns in Criminal Homicide (Philadelphia: University of Pennsylvania, 1958)
5. Betaenkning om det kriminalrettige system m.v. i Grønland Copenhagen & Godthåb, 1968
6. Reckless, W.C., cited in S. Hurwitz and Christiansen,
   K.O., Kriminologi II (Copenhagen, 1971), p. 311 ff.

Commentaries

"Childhood, family, and social change in the Canadian eastern arctic," by Hugh Brody (Scot Polar Research Institute,
University of Cambridge, England). Eskimo family life today presents a number of continuities and discontinuities
with the recent past. The administrative phase of southern
intervention has generated important changes: inter-genera-
tional tension, intra-family violence, and altered relations
between husbands and wives. The data on which this paper is
based were accumulated during two years of field work in
the eastern arctic, while living and working with Eskimo
families. The results of the study are tentative: domestic
life in today's Eskimo communities is informed if not largely determined by retreatism and confusion. These two circumstances are surprisingly pervasive, and seem to have
arisen in only very recent years. They are, moreover, both
political and economic in origin. A central, if general,
conclusion is that any account of social change in the region must proceed by considering the degree in which economic and ideological domination have driven people deeply
into the nuclear family. The reconstituted family relationships are explicable by reference to specifiable features
of the larger society.

"Challenges experienced as a bilingual Eskimo in areas of
social services and mental health," by B.G. Beans (Yukon-
Kuskokwim Health Corporation, Bethel, Alaska, USA). I come
from a small village of a population of 350. I graduated
from high school in 1967, went to college and graduated in
1970. There has been an average of 15 graduates from St
Marys per year since 1957. In 1970, I was the third student
to graduate from a four year college. From January 1971 to
May 1972, I worked as a social service aid in the Bureau of
Indian Affairs in Bethel, Alaska. From August 1972 to the
present date I have been working with Yukon-Kuskokwim
Health Corporation, a local non-profit organization delivering health services to Bethel and 57 outlying villages in
the area. I have been working in the Mental Health Department of the Corporation. During the first year we dealt with
community organization and the second year with direct
services, since July 1973. One of the first changes we made
in the department was to change the name to "Ikayuristet
Umyuanek," a term meaning "Helpers of the Mind." The term
"mental health" was not too well received in the community
and people generally shied away. Each counsellor is known
as a singular "Ikayurista."

  Challenges encountered: (a) Making a sociological psychological adjustment: I had difficulty making an adjustment
to working in a large bureaucracy while working with the
bureau. I found it difficult to work with people from villages because I found such impersonality between the Bureau
and those they work for. My work and what I know and learned
as a village person were opposites. (b) Psychological
stress: I underwent psychological stresses generated from
both employer and my own people because of high expectations
due to a degree received. There was a lack of day-to-day
supervision in certain matters that I felt were important.
(c) Ambivalence and frustration on my part resulting from
living and knowing both cultures. Some of my behaviour resulted in reprimand from one and sanction from another.

"Mental illness and behaviour problems in native and immigrant northern Canadians," by A.P. Abbott (Northern Region
Headquarters, Department of National Health and Welfare,
Canada). The picture of mental illness and behaviour problems in the Yukon Territory and Northwest Territories of
Canada is changing. Current problems include: (1) incidence
of major psychoses; (2) aggressive and suicidal behaviour -

particularly in association with alcohol consumption; (3)
changing structure of native communities and family and the
destructive results of such changes; (4) specific problems
of the immigrant northern Canadian, particularly "cabin fever."

"Influence of cultural change on Alaskan health," by F.A.
Milan (University of Alaska, Fairbanks). Culture is an abstract summation of the mode of life of a people and represents the results of a long-time experiment in social living, ecological adjustment, and psychological orientation.
When people of two autonomous cultural systems meet, as
occurred in Alaska 200 years ago, an acculturative situation arises. This includes the entire set of social processes involved in acceptance, rejection, and reorganization
of cultural elements, and affected Europeans minimally and
native Alaskans to a greater extent as they became a poli-
tically, numerically, and technologically subject people.
Barriers to learning existed; the acceptance of an idealized
moral order was required, but political and economic power
was withheld. Traumatic psychological primary drives appeared since the socialization process prepared individuals
for a specific and different behavioural world. Despite the
passing of 200 years, true assimilation - where peoples of
diverse racial origins and cultural heritages occupying a
common territory achieve a cultural solidarity - has not
occurred.

"Suicide in Alaskan natives: a preliminary report," by R.
Kraus and P. Buffler (Department of Psychiatry and Behavioral Sciences, University of Washington, and the Washington-
Alaska-Montana-Idaho (WAMI) Experiment, University of Alaska; Health Sciences Center, Alaska Methodist University).
Suicidal behaviour in American natives is a matter of continuing public health concern. Alaska native is a collec-
tive term. In fact, Alaskan Eskimos, Aleuts, Tlingit, Indians, and Athabascan Indians are historically, culturally,
and linguistically quite distinct. Examination of the suicide incidence, mean age, and population of Alaskan natives
by year in 1950-72 reveals a sharp increase in incidence in
1965-66 which has continued up until the most recent period.
The increase in suicide is characterized by a decreasing
mean age. The suicide rate for Alaskan natives in 1972 was
40.4 per 100,000 per year, with a mean age of 23.7 years.

This rate is in excess of the rates for Alaskan whites,
United States natives, and all races in the United States.
Examination of suicide incidence in Alaskan natives by year
and age group in 1950-72 further clarifies the emergent
pattern of suicide among late adolescents and young adults.
Further analysis of suicide incidence by year and sex and
year and mode shows an over-all male - female ratio of approximately 3:1 and suggests an increased incidence of suicide among young women. Although gunshot continues to be
the most common cause of death, in recent years drug overdose has occurred with increasing frequency. Examination of
the mean age and sex of suicide deaths among Alaskan natives by ethnic groups for intervals between 1950 and 1972
suggests that the pattern is not a uniform one. Significant
intercultural differences in patterning seem to exist.
(Supported in part by National Institute of Mental Health
Grant MH 18749 and MH 23233.)

"Alcohol and the subjective experience of power," by L.
Soelling (National Council of Greenland, Danish National
Institute for Social Research, Denmark). An alternative to
the existing cross-cultural theories of the functions of
alcohol is based on the conception of anxiety. Existing
theories are criticized from an existential perspective in
the tradition of the Danish philosopher S. Kierkegaard and
of modern existential psychology. It is argued that the
conception of anxiety (properly understood) is a key conception for the understanding of any human behaviour, but
not necessarily the most important conception for the
understanding of the drinking of alcohol as behaviour different from other forms of behaviour. It is argued that
the subjective experience of power and the legitimization
of a certain sacred/profane reality through drunken behaviour is central for the understanding of the social functions of alcohol. The discussion is carried through with
special reference to the cultural conflict in Greenland.

"Alcohol abuse and its criminogenic role in Frobisher Bay,
NWT," by H.W. Finkler (International Centre for Comparative
Criminology, University of Montreal, Quebec, Canada). The
destructive nature of alcohol abuse and the Inuit's vul-
nerability to its excessive and hazardous use appear to be
further indications of the strains of adaptation to interaction between Inuit and Euro-Canadian cultures. The

material for the paper was gleaned through observations in
Frobisher Bay in the summer of 1972 during a 12-week period.
An evaluation of cases coming to the attention of socio-
legal control agencies shows a significant correlation of
excessive and hazardous patterns of drinking as a precondition to the initiation of and/or participation in deviant behaviour. Observations have revealed the rising incidence of assaultive behaviour within the family, provoked
or aggravated by alcohol abuse. Similarly, male - female
relationships and traditional concepts of marriage, already undermined by white sexual exploitation of Inuit females, have further deteriorated through a prolonged use
of alcohol. The impact in terms of labelling by the community of those engaged in deviant behaviour aggravated by
the excessive use of alcohol is negligible, except on the
part of some individuals who are usually associated professionally with the agencies of socio-legal or medical control. However, the latter agencies seem to lack over-all
coordination and the mobilization of adequate means to com-
bat the serious ramifications of alcohol abuse. Evaluation
of the existing alcohol education program poses grave
doubts as to its effectiveness.

HEALTH CARE DELIVERY

Evaluation of Alaskan Native Health Service: alternative approaches to meeting basic health needs

S.S.R. HARALDSON

It has been estimated by the World Health Organization that about eighty per cent of the world's total population do not have reasonable access to health services of acceptable standards. In spite of great national and international efforts to solve the problem, the world map of health services still has many blank spots, empty of health services and not yet included in any five-year plan. Thus, something has to be changed, if we are to fulfil even a minimum of what is claimed by the United Nations Declaration of Human Rights (1948).

Reasons for lack of success in reaching unserved populations include geographical inaccessibility and the practice of a nomadic livelihood. Areas may also be treated unfairly because of strained racial, cultural, or political relations. A common denominator of most unserved groups is an extreme limitation of resources - financial, manpower, and physical. Another common factor is a low population density. Many of the groups concerned live in developing countries, which cannot afford to provide services to areas where the accessibility is so poor that utilization and profitability rates are unacceptable (11, 13).

Maldistribution of health services is almost universal, especially in underdeveloped countries. Sparsely populated areas must be included in programs of health planning and assistance, and also in the design of realistic service systems. However, full equalization of medical care is a Utopia that will hardly be achieved in any country, although often promised by political leaders.

The author is consultant to the WHO program "Alternative approaches to meeting basic health needs of populations in developing countries." Concerns of the program include: reasons why certain areas are unfairly treated;

specific problems of geographically less accessible groups
and the nomads of the world; review of non-traditional approaches to health care such as the barefoot doctor scheme
in China.

The author has studied nomadic populations and sparsely
populated areas in some 10 to 15 developing countries in
Africa and southwest Asia. The observations were discussed
by representatives of Arabic countries at a WHO seminar in
Iran in 1973 and recommendations were made regarding health
services for nomadic populations (10). An evaluation of the
Alaska Native Health Service was carried out in 1971 and
1973 (9); parallel studies are planned for Canadian Eskimos
during summer 1974, and for Greenland in 1975, with the objective of comparing services to the three related population groups and exploring the effectiveness of different designs of health service.

Eskimos are found in Greenland (40,000), Canada (15,000),
and Alaska (25,000). Studies of the Eskimo will contribute
to the discussion of alternative approaches to health care.
Techniques that have been instrumental in the success of
Alaskan health services include:

1. Each Eskimo settlement chooses a woman who will serve
as a village health aide. Her initial training of 6 months
to 1 year's duration takes place at a district hospital.
She then starts a clinic in her own village, equipped with
a well-designed drug kit and an appropriate health care
manual.

2. A radio-telephone is used for daily consultation with
physicians at the district hospital.

3. "Bush-pilots" transport emergency cases to the hospital with minimal delay.

Evaluation of the Alaskan Eskimo health service indicated that it fulfilled many of the demands for health services in a sparsely populated area.

EFFECTIVENESS

Launched in 1953 as a tuberculosis control program (1,4,5,
9,12), the Alaska Native Health Service has developed into
a comprehensive system of health services available to all
natives, on the premise that every Alaskan is entitled to
the same assurance of life and health as citizens of more
populous states (12). When the scheme was initiated, education, health, and economics were considered the poorest in
the US. Poverty, cultural clashes with the modern world,
geographic isolation and the adverse physical environment

combined to develop in many Alaskan Natives feelings of
frustration, alienation, and hopelessness.

The coverage provided by today's services is almost total. The utilization rate is high and has become almost independent of distance, since aircraft can reach any settlement.

Diseases such as tuberculosis and anterior poliomyelitis
have been virtually eradicated, but the most dramatic
achievement is the decrease of infant mortality; twenty
years ago, this was about 100 per thousand newborn, but it
has dropped to around 20, the same figure as for the USA as
a whole. This is a remarkable achievement for a sparsely
populated region, and it has few parallels elsewhere in the
world.

EFFICIENCY

The reductions in morbidity and mortality have been attained
at a high price. The average health expenditure per Eskimo
has mounted to around US $700, much of this being attribu-
table to air transportation of personnel and patients.
Specialists regularly visiting the districts from the Anchorage Native Medical Center and public health teams screening
village populations are both expensive but nevertheless important activities. Services to date have focused chiefly on
physical problems, where the results may well justify the
high costs involved. However, it is generally accepted that
substandard housing contributes to a high incidence of en-
vironmentally related problems, such as respiratory diseases,
otitis media, rheumatic diseases, skin diseases, accidents,
and even mental disorders.

As in other arctic countries, otitis media is still a
serious scourge, the control of which is given a high priority. Urbanization is creating a new flora of socio-medical
problems, including alcoholism, suicide, and other mental
disorders, family break-up, and venereal diseases. Methods
for the control of these problems are underdeveloped and
current dollar investment is insufficient for their solution. However, the new socio-medical challenges have provoked two projects, each assisting Eskimo districts: the
Yukon-Kuskokwim Health Corporation and the Norton Sound
Health Corporation. Both are tackling health problems
through non-traditional methods, based on an extended participation of local villagers.

LESSONS FROM ALASKA

"Latitude-thinking" may hamper a sound exchange of experience between tropical and arctic populations. Human health problems are surprisingly similar in disparate regions and are only influenced to a minor extent by the climate, even if an extreme climate, hot or cold, has necessitated the development of a specialized human culture.

Compromises have to be accepted when designing and providing health service under extreme conditions. Full geographical equality will continue to be an Utopian ideal. However, it is important to set a lower limit to planned services.

Low population density reduces the accessibility and utilization of health care services and thus gives a poor cost/benefit ratio. Service to a scattered population is inevitably costly.

Some features of the Alaskan Native Health Service could, beneficially, be copied in other places, However, lesser national resources may make expensive air evacuation of emergencies wishful thinking. Some details of the Alaskan scheme are efficient without being costly:

1. The infrastructure of health services in sparsely populated areas should be based on a village health service in which the local people co-operate.

2. The training of village health aides should not reach a level where "brain drain" will be a risk. The village health aide has a double loyalty, to her own people who have chosen her, and to the health authorities and supervisors who have given her training. Her special training and her family situation encourage her to remain at her post.

3. The manpower problems of developing countries and of sparsely populated areas include a shortage of trained personnel, disproportion between different categories of personnel, geographic maldistribution favouring urban areas, and a heavy turnover of personnel. It is impossible to solve these problems by applying traditional service models with university trained staff; such an approach is prohibitively expensive and leads to a brain drain, with a high staff turnover in remote areas. Auxiliaries are the realistic alternative, including the whole range from the medical assistant (East Africa) and dental therapist (Canada), to the village health aide, all with less than full professional qualifications.

The barefoot doctor of the Peoples Republic of China is initially chosen by the villagers for training; he lives

in his village and is linked by telephone to an area medical
care team (14). This approach has some similarities to the
Alaskan village health aide system and the Papua/New Guinea
system with "aid posts orderly."

4. Regular supervision including use of a radio-telephone
is an inexpensive and efficient means of raising both the
quality of health services, and the morale of personnel workers in remote areas.

5. Technical developments can bring physical problems
rapidly under control, but urbanization creates new and
less readily solvable socio-medical problems such as suicides, alcoholism, and venereal diseases.

Rapid technical development brings with it the risk of
"overprotection," and calls for more cautious advancement,
a "hurry slowly" attitude, while watching for emerging
socio-medical disorders.

SUMMARY

Health services of sparsely populated areas are often insufficient, owing to shortage of manpower and funds, maldistribution of services, and disproportion between different
categories of personnel. Specific accessibility-utilization
rates have to be considered in planning services for scattered populations. Shortsighted cost-benefit considerations
should not be overemphasized. Alaskan Eskimos have adequate
services at a high cost; these include a village health
aide with drug-kit and "fool-proof" instructions, daily consultation with hospital physicians by radio-telephone, air
evacuation of emergencies by "bush-pilots," and regular
supervision by the district nurse and DMO. The Alaskan experience is recommended as a model for other sparsely populated areas.

REFERENCES

1. Alaska Area Native Health Service: Alaska Area program
   plan, FY 1973-FY 1977
2. Elliott, K., "Meeting world health needs - the doctor
   and the medical auxiliary," World Hospitals, 9: 3 (1973)
3. Fendall, N.R.E., Auxiliaries in health care (Baltimore:
   Johns Hopkins Press, 1972)
4. Fleshman, J.K., "Disease prevalence in the Alaskan Arctic and Subarctic," Alaska Medicine (June 1971)
5. Fortuine, R., "The development of modern medicine in
   SW Alaska," Alaska Medicine (April 1971)

6. Haraldson, S.R.S., "Socio-medical conditions among the Lapps in northernmost Sweden," Svenska Läk.tidn., 59: 2829 (1962)
7. Haraldson, S.R.S., "Appraisal of health problems and definition of priorities in health planning," Ethiop. Med. J., 8: 37 (1970)
8. Haraldson, S.R.S., "Aspects on development of health services in pastoral areas in Ethiopia," Ethiop. Med. Assoc. (1970), Duplicated report
9. Haraldson, S.R.S., "Evaluation of Alaska Native Health service. Report on a study trip 1972/73," Alaska Medicine, 16: No. 3 (1974)
10. Haraldson, S.R.S., "Report on WHO Seminar in Shiraz, Iran: Health problems of nomads," WHO project EMRO 4004 (1973), Duplicated report
11. Haraldson, S.R.S., "Health planning in sparsely populated areas," Dissertation, Gothenburg, Sweden (1973)
12. Parran, Th. et al., "Alaska's health - a survey report to the US Dept. of Int. by the Alaska Health Survey Team (Pittsburgh: Graduate School of Public Health, 1954)
13. Second International Symposium on Circumpolar Health, Oulu, Finland (1971)
14. Sidel, V.W., "The barefoot doctors of the People's Republic of China," New Engl. J. Med. (June 1972)

Comparison of health care in Alaska and Scandinavia

BETTY PRICE

Despite similarities in geography, Scandinavia and Alaska differ climatically; this affects transportation, communications, sanitation, and the frequency of communicable diseases.

The Scandinavians have a more unified approach to health care delivery, with a blend of local direction and national financing and standard setting. This contrasts with the pluralism of the Alaskan providers of health services.

Both regions, responding to rising costs, seek to emphasize ambulatory care. Alaska shows greater interest in

exploring the role of para-professionals. There is a fundamental difference in the currently acceptable level of
health-care taxation in the two regions.

This report compares some aspects of health care in the
Scandinavian countries and in Alaska. Background factors
will be considered first, followed by a look at some facets
of current health care delivery. Finally, convergent and
divergent trends in these two northern regions will be discussed.

Geographically, the two locales are similar in latitude,
in their extensive coastline, in their rugged terrain, and
in having limited land fit for cultivation. However, significant climatic differences affect transportation, communication, and the character of medical problems. Alaska con-
tends with widespread permafrost, while in Scandinavia the
moderating effect of the Gulf Stream permits farming far
north of the Polar Circle. The contrast in transportation
is highlighted by comparing the daily ships between Bergen
and Kirkenes in Norway and the single annual visit of the
supply ship to Barrow in northern Alaska. Similarly, northern Scandinavian communities are linked by a network of
roads - a resource as yet lacking in Alaska. The Alaskan
permafrost causes difficult engineering problems in the
provision of safe drinking water and satisfactory waste
disposal. Hepatitis, shigellosis, and other contagious illnesses indicate that these difficulties have not yet been
resolved. Communication difficulties in northern Alaska
have led to exploration of the potential benefits of satellite telecommunications.

Demographically, the older populations of Scandinavia
contrast with the youthful Alaskan populace, with its mean
age of 23 years. Both areas have important ethnic minorities: the Lapps in Scandinavia, and the Eskimos, Indians,
and Aleuts in Alaska. Both regions have previously suffered
severely from tuberculosis and still contend with a heavy
toll from accidents. Infectious diseases continue to cause
severe medical problems in Alaska while the Scandinavians
are concerned mostly with degenerative conditions.

Socio-economically, the low rate of unemployment in
Scandinavia (e.g., 0.6 per cent in Norway) is vastly different from that of Alaska, where a nominal 10 per cent
average rate of unemployment masks a much greater prevalence in some communities and at some times of the year.
The Scandinavian nations have a far more homogeneous population since World War II than that of Alaska.

In health matters, there is a fundamental philosophical difference. Scandinavians agree that people's health is a social responsibility, and accept that all should have similar access to care; Alaskan health care systems are pluralistic and are not predicated upon a comparable acknowledgment of public responsibility.

Scandinavians seek to blend local responsibility with national financing and standards. This approach is reinforced by the national health insurance program, which finances most medical care. Health care in Alaska is provided by multiple sources: the private sector, State public health nurses and sanitarians, and federal government personnel, functioning primarily through the Indian Health Service, and military agencies. Both areas utilize public resources in the North, since a viable economic base is lacking for privately employed physicians.

Scandinavia follows the European tradition of separate medical staffs for hospitals and ambulatory care, whereas the Alaskan physician usually treats his patient both inside and outside the hospital.

Health planners in northern Europe benefit from a tradition of well-kept records and statistics, which are much less readily available in Alaska.

A comparison of health care delivery in the two regions shows some important trends. In both regions, the inflationary rise in medical costs has led to measures to deemphasize the hospital and foster ambulatory care. Scandinavians have proceeded further in differentiating patients with medical and domiciliary needs. Another trend, common to both localities, is the coming together of medical and social service personnel in health centres.

There remain important areas where Alaska and the Scandinavian nations have chosen different routes of health care. Thus, Sweden has nationalized its pharmacies and has placed all physicians on salary, with equal pay for equal training and experience. Swedish doctors now have a work week much shorter than before initiation of the salaried medical service. There is no sign of this kind of development in Alaska. The Scandinavian countries have invested heavily in preventive dentistry, with free dental care for children, a concept which has not yet been accepted in Alaska. The higher level of industrialization in Scandinavia is expressed also in greater sophistication in occupational health.

In Alaska, there has been keen interest in the role of the para-professional, who may relieve the physician of part

of his duties. Scandinavians do not seem to share this
point of view, preferring to create more physicians if
necessary. These may suffer, at times, from lack of support
personnel. Lastly, there seems a basic difference in the
level of taxation which the public is willing to accept to
to pay for health protection. Scandinavians have proven
willing to accept extremely heavy taxation to ensure security against illness. Alaskans do not seem ready to allow
such a level of taxation for health care.

In conclusion, each region has developed innovative approaches to its challenges in health-care delivery. International comparisons can provide the stimulus for further
improvements in health care, providing that useful techniques seen elsewhere are suitably adapted to local circumstances.

ACKNOWLEDGMENT

This study was undertaken with the support of a WHO travel
fellowship.

Alaska native regional corporations and community mental health

J.D. BLOOM and W.W. RICHARDS

The Alaska Native Land Claims Settlement Act of 1971 (1)
set in motion vast changes in the lives of Alaska's Indians,
Eskimos, and Aleuts. Twelve regional corporations were established to receive and administer the benefits of the
settlement (Figure 1). The business corporation receives
the great amounts of money and land which are part of the
settlement. Operating as a holding and investment company,
it attempts to conserve and enlarge the worth of the corporation and, consequently, the value of the stock owned by
individual native persons in their region. The non-profit
branch of the corporation has entirely different goals,
being concerned with such issues as health, education, and
welfare. Their aim is to work with existing government

Regional corporation

Business corporation — Non-profit corporation

Investment   Land management   Exploration   Health   Education   Social service

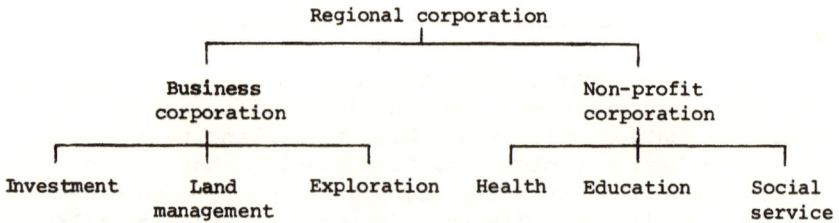

Figure 1   Post-Land Claims Settlement Act: simplified diagram of regional corporation structure in Alaska

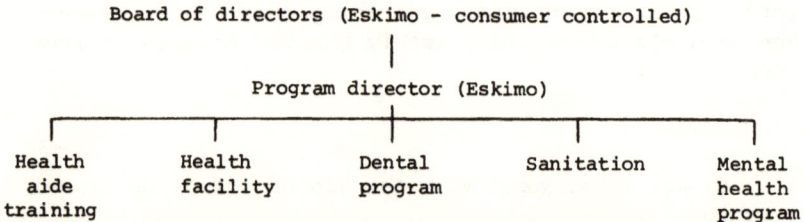

Board of directors (Eskimo - consumer controlled)

Program director (Eskimo)

Health aide training   Health facility   Dental program   Sanitation   Mental health program

Figure 2   Health corporation structure (Model - Yukon-Kuskokwim Health Corporation, Bethel, Alaska)

agencies whether federal, state, or local to improve the delivery of service to people in the regions. This is no small task, given the multiplicity of poorly co-ordinated agencies from every level of government which have some responsibility for the lives of Alaska natives.

Figure 2 provides a closer look at the structure of the health corporation: the model for these health corporations was two OEO funded corporations begun in the late 1960s. Both the Yukon-Kuskokwim Health Corporation in Bethel and the Norton Sound Health Corporation at Nome were originally funded to speed up the training of village health aides. They have subsequently developed programs in many areas of need and have taken on advisory, management, and regulatory powers in their regions. As fully funded native consumer-controlled boards they were tailor-made to fit into the structures of the developing regional corporations.

Mental health programs have been one need the health corporations have had to face. The mental health service in rural towns and villages historically has been very meagre. At the time of statehood in 1959 it was generally "assumed" that the State of Alaska would be responsible for the mental health of all Alaskans, while the Indian Health Service of the United States Public Health Service would be responsible for the physical health of Alaskan Indians, Eskimos, and Aleuts. In 1966, the Indian Health Service funded a small mental health project to "supplement" the efforts of the state government. At the present time, the Indian Health Service program has a budget of about $300,000.00, with its major focus on mental health para-professional training and decentralization of service components of field stations. Both of these goals fit closely with the wishes of developing health corporations. To date, state programs have been located centrally, with small clinics in the larger cities of Anchorage, Fairbanks, and Juneau. Most of the state's efforts have been directed to the maintenance of two hospitals, one for the mentally ill in Anchorage and another for the mentally retarded in the town of Valdez.

It can be seen that the health corporation provides the most plausible vehicle for the development of local mental health service by region. The health corporation has ready-made consumer boards, native staff leadership, and is part of an organization in which the vast majority of people in the region are actual stock holders. It represents a true experiment in community control and community mental health.

The structure is thus one of native-controlled regional health corporations, which in the mental health fields can receive monies from various governmental or private sources in order to develop meaningful programs for their region. As mentioned above, several of the health corporations have been in existence since 1968, but others have not been organized for more than six months to a year. Several of the health corporations have a great deal of money, but some are as yet totally without funds. Even in "older" programs, the mental health component has a history of no more than two years. Structures are therefore tentative and unstable, but nonetheless the potential for development is there. The ultimate success of the corporations will depend on two major factors: the ability of staff to work in very complicated and often ambiguous areas, and the quality of outside advice sought by the corporations.

One could make a long list of potential pitfalls for the developing structures, but we will focus rather on positive developments that have already taken place. Both the Yukon-Kuskokwim and the Norton Sound Health Corporations have had mental health programs for two years. Their thrust has been aimed at on-the-job training of Eskimo mental health workers. Combined funding from several federal agencies has allowed an Indian Health Service psychiatrist to be assigned as team leader to a group of people working in the town of

Bethel. Bethel is a transitional town of 3,000 people, and many of the population are suffering very serious social and emotional problems (2,3,4). The Bethel team works intensively with the Indian Health Service Hospital and in the Bethel grade school, Eskimo mental health workers serving along with outside professional workers.

In contrast with Bethel, the Nome project is village based. The Nome corporation decided to start its mental health programming by hiring three Eskimo mental health workers to work with the village people, an approach not previously explored. While something is known about the mental health of city and town people, virtually nothing has been discovered about traditional native society and the problems common in villages. The question has practical importance, for in many of these villages the traditional elements of Eskimo society are still viable. We may expect different corporations to develop differing styles of program, but certain consistent needs will persist across corporation lines, particularly in the areas of training, grantsmanship, and the need for on-the-spot professional team members to work with the local people.

It was assumed until very recently that the indigenous healer or shaman had been virtually abolished earlier in the century by organized religion and medicine. However, a renaissance of native cultural traditions has accompanied the political organization necessary to achieve the Land Claims settlement. This has given people confidence to talk about the "old" ways and healing practices as they exist in some areas today. People have begun to come forward and speak of themselves as Eskimo doctors, describing folk theories and cures. If the present direction continues we will soon learn a great deal more about healing practices as they currently exist in the villages.

There remain great gaps between plan and programs, between what is good sense and what really happens. Nevertheless, this short paper is written with tempered optimism. For the first time in our experience, Alaska has theoretically sound structures to tackle the problem, to get a grip on government, and bring about a totally new mental health program. Replacing the "migrant" worker with a local person, replacing English-speaking therapists with bilingual staff, moving the seat of power closer to the people, and developing true consumer boards are all big steps in the right direction. The next five years will tell us if the promise will come to fruition.

SUMMARY

The development of mental health services to Alaskan natives is reviewed. Particular attention is paid to the impact of the Alaska Native Land Claims Settlement Act. This
has led to the development of native corporations, which
are planning and carrying out innovative regional mental
health programs.

REFERENCES

1. Alaska Native Claims Settlement Act: US House of Representatives Report No. 92-746, December 1971
2. Ervin, A.M., "Conflicting style of life in a northern
   Canadian town," Arctic, 22: 90-105 (1969)
3. Hippler, A., Barrow and Kotzebue: An exploratory comparison of acculturation & education in two large Northwestern Alaska villages (Minneapolis: University of
   Minnesota Press, 1969)
4. Lubart, J.M., "Psychodynamic problems of adaptation -
   MacKenzie Delta Eskimos," Ottawa: MacKenzie Delta Research Project, Dept. of Indian Affairs and Northern Development, 1970

Inception of a "grass roots" mental health delivery system

R.A. FEIGIN

Norton Sound Health Corporation (NSHC) is a non-profit, Es-
kimo-controlled and consumer-oriented organization whose
goal is to meet the emerging health care needs of some 5,000
Eskimos in Western Alaska. The 5,000 people represent different levels of acculturation, and owing to isolation, they
have several dialects. Nome, the largest community, has
some 2,000 Eskimos, and the surrounding villages range in
size from 80 to 500 people. Acculturation has been rapid
and basic patterns such as family size (increased with improved health care) and economic needs have changed. The
majority of families depend on subsistence food gathering.
Children are generally educated in their villages until the

eighth grade and then transferred to boarding schools. This
has resulted in an alarming proportion of mental disturbances, including an "epidemic" of suicide during the period January to November 1973. There were 41 attempts and 10
successful suicides among the 10 to 30 age group. The current tendency for suicide in the younger age groups has also been noted by Kraus (personal communications); it is a
dramatic and shocking change from the traditional pattern
of Eskimo suicide, where older people helped death along
when they became a burden on their families. Alcohol, drugs,
and related problems are also very prevalent, especially in
Nome itself.

Traditionally, people with severe emotional illness were
tolerated unless they caused much interference with the necessary pattern of life. Then, they might have been killed
or ostracized. Presently, Western civilization has provided
a means of dealing with the severely disturbed community member through psychiatric clinics and hospitals. However, the
person who has problems in adjusting to day-to-day living
falls outside the domain of usual medical practice, and unfortunately is not always adequately dealt with by the Eskimo culture, especially during the present period of transition.

Within this framework, Norton Sound has developed what
appears an excellent and progressive health care system
that has recently turned its attention to the area of mental health. The reasons for delaying work in this area are
complex. The topic - even the words "mental health" - denotes a subject not usually dealt with by Eskimos. Private
feelings, emotions, and conflicts have not been subjects for
discussion. But, paraphrasing a quotation from a board
meeting: "Since Eskimos have decided to kill themselves,
maybe we had better find out what is happening."

A directive to explore the areas of mental health and
illness was given with the mandate that indigenous people
be utilized in the delivery of services and an attempt be
made to use traditional methods. Prospective workers were
interviewed by the village councils, emphasizing the need
to have somebody acceptable to the people among whom they
would be working. Three workers were eventually picked.

The author was in Alaska for a transcultural elective
during his second year of psychiatric residency, and was
asked to help the NHSC develop its mental health delivery
system. It was decided that the most impact would be accomplished if available time was applied to the training of
workers. The task was difficult: how does one determine

what is mental health and who needs help, and who should do
the determining, the treating, and the training?

TRAINING: PERSONNEL AND CONTENT

The most appropriate course seemed to listen to trainees
talking about their problems and to elicit if and how they
had attempted to deal with them. A common theme among the
trainees was their strong concern to help and a sensitivity
to the needs of their people. Some basic characteristics
were shared - among them, the ability to listen attentively
and non-judgmentally, give concerned advice, share personal
experiences, and maintain confidences. We came prepared to
teach the trainees these concepts, but the first days'
planned sessions were abandoned as unnecessary. The term
mental health was discussed, and a consensus emerged that
"mental health" had to do with "crazy" and people who
"wouldn't take it right." The trainees preferred to be
called Family Service Workers - shying away from references
with a "mental" label.

The bulk of the three weeks was spent discussing trouble-
some problems in which the trainees had been involved. We
encouraged sharing of different orientations towards helping. As common problem areas were identified, they were discussed through a role playing approach which at times produced a great deal of frustration, as the workers realized
we didn't possess needed solutions. Problem areas identified
included: marriage and family communication, child abuse
and children in general, jealousy towards successful people,
feelings of rejection and lack of self-confidence, as well
as depression, violence, and the relations of all the above
to alcohol and suicide.

None of the trainees had specific knowledge of how people
with problems were dealt with traditionally, but we heard
many stories passed on from old to young that served as a
guide in dealing with life situations. There were also some
discussions of the grieving process and how a change in the
traditional patterns of dying at home sometimes prolonged
depression. The three workers felt that many of the problems
that develop related to a tendency among Eskimos to keep
feelings and problems to themselves; their approach should
thus be to encourage talking out of problems before they
built up.

It became evident that much anxiety existed related to
meeting expectations of themselves and other villagers. If
this anxiety were allowed to continue unchecked we could
ultimately lose the workers' services. Because of this, we

became most directive and supportive, suggesting certain
limitations of role which they could alter as their clinical
knowledge improved and they became more comfortable in the
exercise of their responsibilities.

As we became better acquainted with the trainees, and
their knowledge of problems and culturally acceptable methods of helping, we were able to adjust our goals as
"training people." We were also able to learn, because we
recognized the need to listen and not rush in with suggestions pertinent to western mental health which had little
bearing at Norton Sound. But for all our listening and patience, we still talked too much and asked too many questions
for our trainees' tastes.

At the end of the three week session, a conference involving state and local level consultants was held to explain where we were with the program and to obtain advice.
Exposure to the very verbal western proceedings was intended also to provide necessary insights for the Family Service Workers when dealing with other western conferences.

FUTURE DEVELOPMENT

Future training will help the trainees provide a full range
of social services by developing natural skills and becoming better acquainted with many public agencies. It will be
necessary to pay particular attention to appropriate utilization of consultants - keeping the delicate balance necessary to encourage independent decision-making. Various
consultants will be available on a monthly basis, providing
training through discussion of cases, and the workers will
be able to communicate with Nome or each other using tapes,
letters, or telephone. Ultimately, it is hoped that trainees will be able to obtain college credits for their work,
enabling upward mobility if desired.

Much work remains in Nome itself, particularly in organizing the existing system of helping programs. Little co-
operation exists among the many local social agencies, and
patient-clients can misuse them, so that they sometimes un-
wittingly foster dependence rather than independence. Once
a director for the mental health program is picked, it will
be his or her task to organize the various services with
the goal of developing a more comprehensive approach to
people with problems. This should serve a dual purpose:
(1) providing better over-all care, and (2) serving as a
training ground by exposing mental health workers to a multiplicity of disciplines. This will in turn provide further

opportunity to educate the non-native professional as he or she gathers impressions and culturally relevant information from the native health workers.

CONCLUSION

A planned mental health system must make involvement of the community serve a primary goal and an important part of the health corporations' total philosophy. In keeping with this aim, mechanisms must be included to allow community feedback in the planning of new programs, to facilitate on-going operations, and ultimately to educate villagers to make use of the various services provided. A culturally relevant understanding of mental health may be one way of facilitating the development of village and Eskimo pride and in turn dealing successfully with the changing cultural values of a changing world.

Within the above framework we can see some answers to important questions asked earlier. It will ultimately be the people themselves who determine the problem areas. Problems will be treated by peers with training that will enable them to utilize both Eskimo and Western therapeutic modalities and personnel. Administered with care, such a program has the potential to draw from two cultures rather than imposing the values of one on another.

ACKNOWLEDGMENT

I would like to acknowledge the help and friendship of Caleb Pungowyi, Tommy Ongtooguk, James Hahn, Carol Perron, Allen Soosuk, Marilyn Dexter, and Rosena Lockwood, the rest of the NHSC staff, and many others.

Consultant–general practitioner interaction in a northern university clinic*

M.M. MORISON and D.G. FISH

Universal medical care insurance has been in effect in Canada for a number of years. The removal of the economic barrier, however, does not guarantee equal availability of medical services to all Canadians. There is an increasing tendency for physicians to locate in larger, urban areas, and in order to ensure the provision of care to residents of "remote" areas, governments are exploring alternatives to the traditional "free enterprise" system of medical practice. Recognizing that individual physicians attracted to remote areas are likely to be transient, new arrangements tend to be institutionally based, with an emphasis on continuity of service rather than on continuity of personnel.

The practice of medicine continues to be organized in a way that reinforces the independence and decision-making power of the individual practitioner. In providing continuous care to remote areas, however, the planning, organization, recruitment, and administration of facilities and personnel becomes the responsibility, not of the individual practitioner, but rather of an institution. As a result, the traditional role of the primary physician is fundamentally altered. The University of Manitoba's Northern Medical Unit exemplifies the conflicts that arise when traditional physician practice is brought into a complex institutional setting.

The Northern Medical Unit, based in Churchill, began operation in July 1970 under the auspices of the Faculty of Medicine, University of Manitoba. The Unit is staffed by four salaried general practitioners, a social worker, a dentist, and other support personnel. In addition, there is a scheduled rotation of visits by a full spectrum of specialists drawn from the teaching faculty of the University of Manitoba. The 40-bed Fort Churchill General Hospital functions as the base hospital for the Unit. Patients needing treatment not available in Churchill are evacuated to the teaching hospitals in Winnipeg. Medical services are provided for both the Churchill area (population approximately 3,000) and the Keewatin District of the Northwest Territories (population 3,500). The area is characterized by

* Research supported by National Health Grant 606-7-228.

a harsh climate and flat treeless landscape; its population includes "whites," Métis, Chipewayan, Cree, and Eskimo.

The university's interests in undertaking this responsibility were, first, to provide continuous medical care to a previously underserviced area; second, to provide on-going education to resident practitioners; third, to increase awareness among the visiting specialists of medical problems in the North; and, finally, to provide a remote health care facility for medical training and research.

The original intention of the authors was to evaluate the effect of the university on the socio-economic development of the area and the local population's attitudes towards health services. During the course of the research, it became apparent that of equal interest to the sociologist and the planner of remote care facilities were difficulties arising from the organization of medical personnel to meet the objectives of continuing care, education, and research. The emphasis in this paper is thus on the interaction between the resident general practitioners and the visiting consultant-specialists.

The information presented is based on: (1) structured interviews with twenty-eight consultants (representing twelve specialty areas) who had been to Churchill at least twice; (2) structured and unstructured interviews with the general practitioners; and (3) participant observation. All data were collected between July 1970 and June 1973. The results will be used first to describe the characteristics of the consultants and general practitioners, and second to contrast the situation of the Northern Medical Unit with conventional practice in the three areas of education, policy-making, and referral.

CHARACTERISTICS

Northern Medical Unit consultants who had been north at least twice represent the specialty areas of obstetrics and gynaecology, psychiatry, paediatrics, ENT, respirology, surgery, orthopaedics, radiology, cardiology, anaesthesiology, ophthalmology, and clinical psychology. Most of these consultants have a long-term commitment to the Unit and to the area it serves. At the outset, many were personally asked by the Director to help develop the Unit and they feel a responsibility to remain involved. Many have had previous experience with medical care in remote areas and consider that its importance has been overlooked until now by both university and government. Most of the

consultants define their prime responsibility as the delivery of a high quality medical service.

Since July 1970 sixteen general practitioners have
stayed in Churchill for an average of about one year. Most
are recent medical school graduates. They are attracted to
Churchill by the opportunity to practice in a remote area
with the reassurance of supporting services from a tertiary
centre and concomitant expectations that the consultants
will provide opportunity for on-going education. The relative transience and inexperience of the general practitioners compared to the consultants accentuate the divergent expectations of the two groups with respect to education,
policy-making, and referral.

EDUCATION

While it is traditional for consultants to perform a teaching role in university settings, both the general practitioners and the consultants feel this function has been
overlooked in the Northern Medical Unit. The reasons the
consultants suggest for paucity of on-site education include "tourist and noblesse oblige" attitudes of some consultants, a strong service orientation, lack of time, and
a high turnover of general practitioners. The general practitioners attribute the problem to a lack of interest of
the consultants in teaching, and see university standards
being used to delimit their areas of competence.

POLICY-MAKING

In conventional practice, decisions with respect to patient
care, staffing, and organization are made by the practitioners involved in primary care. Policy for the Northern Medical Unit, however, is formulated largely in Winnipeg by the
Director and consultants. Thus, the consultants are more
than specialists to whom the general practitioners can refer; they also influence policies related to patient care
and operation of the Unit. For example, the limitations on
elective surgery were determined by the Director and his
consultants. Also, the Director and his consultants participated in the initial architectural planning for the Community Health Centre. However, the general practitioners were
not involved in either of these policy-related activities.

REFERRALS

In the private sector, the relationship between general
practitioners and specialists is fairly well defined. General practitioners are free to refer to the specialist of
their choice; they accept or reject the advice of the specialist, and expect to be closely informed about their patient's progress. The institutionalized structure of the
Northern Medical Unit places restraints on these traditional arrangements: (1) the general practitioners in Churchill
do not have a free choice of specialists to whom they may
refer or from whom they may seek consultation; (2) patients
needing specialist attention are often evacuated to Winnipeg and remain out of contact with their general practitioner who may receive only scanty progress reports; (3)
conflicts over evacuation decisions may be referred to the
Director for resolution; (4) consultants touring the Keewatin may usurp the primary care role, referring patients
to general practitioners in Churchill; (5) the extended
contact of the specialists with the Keewatin and their continuing interest in patients they have seen results in a
situation where consultants may be perceived as being better known to the population than are the general practitioners.

CONCLUSIONS

Our research indicates that a hierarchically arranged medical care system administered from the outside and under the
auspices of a university carries with it some latent dysfunctions. These arise from specific aspects of the organization: (1) there is a conflict between the physician's
self-definition as an independent practitioner and the hierarchical structure within which he is expected to work;
(2) there is a lack of clear authority relations; and (3)
there is a lack of a mutually agreed definition of the role
of the consultants.

The handling of this confusion over roles has changed as
the Unit has developed. As recruitment from the University
of Manitoba teaching hospitals has increased, the time required for consultants and general practitioners to know
and trust one another has declined. Initially, the general
practitioners tended either to adapt individually or to
complain. More recently, they have become a cohesive group
and, as such, are in a position to negotiate changes.

The Northern Medical Unit has achieved its primary objective of providing continuous medical care to a previously underserviced area. The institutional conflicts outlined are not meant as criticism, but rather reflect the lack of clear definition of authority relations and a subsequent confusion over roles. There is an inherent conflict between the traditional independence of the practice of medicine and the hierarchical arrangements necessary to ensure continuity of care in remote areas without continuity of personnel. Thus, it is perhaps optimistic to expect immediate change in physician practice patterns even within a university setting.

SUMMARY

The University of Manitoba, Northern Medical Unit in Churchill, Manitoba, was established in 1970 to provide continuous general practitioner coverage and scheduled visits by university affiliated consultants to residents of Churchill and the Keewatin District of the NWT. Interviews and participant observation over a three-year period show that although the Northern Medical Unit model succeeds in providing general practitioner and consultant services to the North, there are problems inherent in its implementation. The general practitioners and consultants hold divergent expectations with respect to the teaching and service roles of the consultants, authority relationships, and the responsibility for policy development. These differences are aggravated by the stability and experience of the consultants compared with the relative transience and inexperience of the general practitioners. The nature, then, of the consultant-general practitioner interactions indicates the potential instability of an institutionalized model of delivery.

The impact of two-way audiovideo satellite communication and a computerized health records system on the management of a rural arctic health program

J.M. ARMBRUST

On 30 May 1974 the United States National Aeronautics and Space Administration (NASA) launched the sixth in a series of experimental communications satellites. The placement in space of this satellite enables it to "view" a portion of Alaska. NASA thus invited the Indian Health Service of the US Department of Health, Education and Welfare to submit a proposal for utilizing audio and video communication in the delivery of health care. Until April 1973 pre-launch planning indicated that the communication beam would cover southeastern and southcentral Alaska. However, NASA then determined that the shadow of the satellite's beam would focus on more of central and southeastern Alaska. At the same time, IHS was requested to design an experiment utilizing this new technology. Over the last few years, the US government has involved the beneficiaries of its Alaska health program very actively in the design and control of that program, However, in the present instance, this was not so, owing partially to late notice of the satellite's "shadow change" and partially to the late notice IHS received from its parent agency to proceed in project design. In consequence, it was necessary to convince the people who were to benefit from this newest technology of the benefits of participation after the crucial decision had been made.

The purpose of the experiment was to evaluate the capability and usefulness of two-way audiovideo, satellite-enabled communications to support the provision of high quality comprehensive health care to a rural Alaskan population. The experiment is unique because it utilizes a satellite as the communications medium, it focuses on a rural delivery system, and a computerized problem-oriented health record system has been instituted in the same IHS service area.

The Tanana Service Unit of the IHS covers approximately 388,000 square kilometres of interior Alaska populated by some 10,000 Athabascan Indians. The health care focal point

is a 26-bed acute care hospital at Tanana, an earlier transportation centre and village approximately 220 kilometres
west of the city of Fairbanks.

Three health centres make up the next level of care. They
are located in Galena, a village 250 kilometres west of
Tanana, Ft Yukon 390 kilometres to the northeast of Tanana,
and Fairbanks.

Ft Yukon is staffed by a registered nurse who functions
as a nurse-practitioner. Galena is staffed by three types
of health professionals: a public health nurse, a physician's assistant, and a community health aide. Fairbanks,
because of its size and the shift in population to the urban centre, is staffed by two physicians.

Each of the other 24 communities in the area has one or
more community health aides who usually are the first to
see the patient as he starts through the health care system
of rural Alaska.

At the other extreme is the IHS Medical Centre in Anchorage, 500 kilometres to the south of Tanana. It is staffed
by specialist physicians whose prime responsibility is to
provide medical centre care on a referral basis.

The community health aide makes daily contact with the
doctors at Tanana. Action may be recommended at the village
level or arrangements may be made for the referral of the
patient, either to the health centres at Galena or Ft Yukon,
or if dictated by the patient's condition or availability
of transportation, to Tanana or Fairbanks for evaluation by
a physician. Once in Fairbanks or Tanana, the patient may
be further referred to the medical centre in Anchorage.

The new experiment provides two-way audiovisual communication between Galena, Ft Yukon, Fairbanks, and Tanana. The
Anchorage Medical Centre has two-way audio communication
with the other sites but is only able to receive video. At
Galena, a health aide conducts telemedicine consultations
with the doctor in Tanana. At Ft Yukon, the consultation is
between a clinical nurse and the doctor. Thus, the applicability of television communication is being assessed for
two types of non-physician health care providers.

The physician at Tanana can also control the camera at
other health centre sites. This enables full screen eye
examinations and wide angle observation of the whole examining room. Heart, lung, and abdominal sounds can be transmitted via an electronic stethoscope. X-rays can also be
transmitted by focusing on the actual film. The physician
can direct and then observe the results of palpation and
percussion. Meanwhile, the appropriate consultant in Ancho-

rage can also observe transmissions and offer consultation
as necessary.

The computerized health record system is an Alaskan adaptation of a system in existence elsewhere in the IHS.
Each person in the Tanana area who has been a patient of
the Alaska IHS system has a computer record which is available on demand in each of the facilities noted. The data
include basic demographic information, a list of active
health problems, an immunization record, a list of active
prescriptions, and all past encounters both in-patient and
out-patient. State public health nurses and some non-IHS
physicians are participating in this part of the experiment.
The computer record is normally transmitted via the ATS-1
satellite, but can also be passed over long-distance telephone lines which are available in all participating communities.

Reliable two-way audio communications are still a key
issue in rural Alaska. This is especially true of the Tanana area, where atmospheric and geographic characteristics
combine to make single side band radios worthless. Tele-
phones are found in the experiment villages only. Thus, before the ATS-1 satellite came into use, the vast majority
of area villages felt they had no communication with a doctor. Satellite communication has now become a way of life.

Future investigation will look at such things as referral patterns, frequency of transportation, and utilization of various facilities both with and without the video
satellite; eight specific clinical criteria have also been
selected and modified to see if care can be improved through
use of video-satellite technology. Several constraints have
limited current utilization of the video satellite. By previous international agreement, the satellite will be moved
to India after nine months. Thus, little long-term impact on
clinical care is expected. The satellite is available only
three hours per week, and for this reason its main application is in specialty care, usually post-operation or post-
hospitalization.

These are just some of the impacts of a new technology
upon the health care delivery system. A more detailed analysis will be possible after the experiment's conclusion.

SUMMARY

The purpose of an audiovideo satellite experiment is described, together with features of the Tanana area health
care system. Adaptation of a new method of health care

evaluation is reported, together with features of a computerized health record. Practical constraints on the project
are discussed.

Involvement of natives in health care

E.M. BOESEN

EARLY HISTORY

The development of the health service and the involvement
of natives in health care are closely knit with the history of Greenland over the past 250 years. From the time
when the first medically trained person entered the country until 1953 (when a referendum changed the status of
the land from a colony to a country) Greenlanders have experienced health care as a miracle - if something went
wrong, you expected nothing - but sometimes fate was changed
either by the Angakok or the doctor.

The first doctor came to Greenland in 1726. He and his
followers created in the local population some knowledge of
possibilities for help if health failed. As it had been an
honour to assist the Angakok, so now assisting doctors gave
the individual status. The register of the medical administration in Godthaab has certain cards on natives employed
by the health service, with their professional status
classed as "Clean female." There are none functioning in
this capacity today, but some still live at the outposts of
Eastern Greenland where they served in their working years.

The name "clean female" indicates very simply the prime
quality a doctor sought in native women who assisted in
health care delivery.

THE MIDWIFE

In the middle of the last century the professional title
began to change, and in 1856 we have records of the first
"midwife-aids" (Fødselshjaelpere). There were no midwives,
but the meagre training these dedicated women received on
the job made them capable of doing better than the ordinary

woman when delivering babies. In spite of all hardships,
the population of Greenland grew, and more skilled people -
doctors and other Danes - settled in the country. Greenlanders also felt an increasing urge to travel overseas; among
those who ventured into the unknown around 1900 was a woman
who returned to her home settlement of Holsteinsborg four
years later as a fully trained nurse and midwife. In 1910,
she was joined by the first Danish nurse to be employed in
Greenland.

Around the middle of this century, the school of midwifery (Jordemoderskolen) at the university hospital in
Copenhagen accepted 30 entrants per year; it became the rule
that one of these students could be from the Faroe Islands
and one from Greenland, if recommended by the local health
authorities. Most of the Greenlanders thus trained returned
to Greenland to practice, so that by 1965 there was a fully
trained midwife at all the 17 district hospitals. At present, the school in Copenhagen has 300 applicants for every
30 places, and the Greenlander faces a tougher game generally, as her co-students often have a general education to
the 13th grade, while hers is somewhere between the 7th and
10th grades.

The birth rate of Greenland plateaued in 1967 and the
number of deliveries has now stabilized. Deliveries take
place in the district hospitals, and thus a total of 17 to
20 midwives seems adequate. We have debated how we may fare
if the Danish training of midwives is exchanged for the
Anglo-Saxon way (where a fully trained nurse specializes as
a midwife); so far, we have not reached any useful conclusions, because fully trained nurses of Greenlandic origin
are few and needed in many other fields. More skilful midwives would be an asset. Many of the reasons for high infant mortality have been corrected, but the rate per thousand, 80 in 1967, is still around 45 today as compared with
17 in Denmark.

Until recently, prevention has not been emphasized sufficiently at the school for midwives. Public health nurses
seldom saw the mother until she returned from hospital with
the baby. The prenatal period and the postpartum time in
hospital are thus two areas on which we must now focus. Recently, the interaction between midwife, public health
nurse, maternity ward personnel, doctors, and the mother-
to-be has been stepped up in Godthaab. However, the cobweb
which should secure the rearing of "wished-for" babies is
still very fragile, as replacements of personnel are frequent, and the needed interaction is endangered.

THE NURSE

Greenlanders at the moment fill between 15 and 20 of about
150 nursing positions in Greenland. Some 20 work in Denmark
- primarily because they have married and settled there.
There are posts for 17 public health nurses - one in each
municipality and two in Godthaab - but unfortunately not
all are filled, since public health nurses are scarce in
Denmark, too. At the moment, one public health nurse is a
Greenlander, another graduates in 1974 and a third is expected to graduate in 1975.

LOCAL TRAINING PROGRAMS

The backbone of the health service was and still remains
the group of 185 midwife-aides or (as they have been called
since 1966, when their program was changed) community
health aides (Sundhedsmedhjaelpere). Early in this century,
the district doctor and his head-nurse took in suitable
girls for a three year training program; this was mainly
practical, and theory came as a final touch - if at all!
Most hospitals developed a manual and over the years instruction was formalized to the point that a girl trained
in one hospital could function satisfactorily in another
hospital along the coast if she moved (a rare thing for a
long time).
    In 1958, a new 90-bed district hospital was opened in
Egedesminde. The well-qualified head-nurse (who speaks
Greenlandic) started an intensive training program. This
was at once recognized by both the authorities and the
Greenlanders. Girls with more than seven years of general
schooling were admitted; if more mathematics or Danish was
required, this was arranged, but it was not considered all
important, if in other respects they proved hard working
and interested. Within the first year, the students were
evaluated and also evaluated themselves on their suitability
for this type of work. Those who could cope with their studies and wanted to proceed were eligible for a grant from
the ministry for Greenland, enabling them to go to Denmark
for advanced training in one of several fields: nursing,
midwifery, administration of linen etc. at hospitals, or
general administration of hospitals. They could also train
in office work at various levels. The sound idea behind
this was that during their year in Egedesminde the girls
had seen these various possibilities, had tried them out,
and to a certain extent had made up their own minds on a

career. If they finished their training in Denmark, there were jobs waiting for them back home, but they could also work in Denmark, since their training was recognized there. Between 1958 and 1968, seventy girls went to Denmark; by 1968, 30 had graduated, 20 were still studying, and 20 had quit because of academic difficulties or marriage. Those ineligible to go to Denmark remained in Egedesminde. Here, they received - like girls at other hospitals along the coast - a training which made them capable of functioning very well in their chosen field, in some cases better than those who went to Denmark. It was not necessarily the most clever who went overseas, but rather the most courageous, or perhaps even the thickest-skinned!

As general schooling in Greenland improved, those with adequate general education became eligible for immediate acceptance at schools in Denmark and the evaluation in Egedesminde came to an end.

A remodelled program started in 1966. It is still a three-year program, but offers extended theory. A total of 1,350 lessons is given over the three years, about a half being devoted to Danish, mathematics, physics, and chemistry.

By 1970, a new school-building was opened in Godthaab which has a 200-bed but not too modern hospital. The students "live in" during the first two years. In Egedesminde there were rooms for 12 new students a year; these facilities are now used for third-year students from Godthaab and elsewhere. The school in Godthaab has beds for 46 - 13 double rooms for first-year students and 20 single rooms for second-year students. Around 20 students have been admitted every year, with a drop-out rate of 30 to 35 per cent. This is unfortunate, especially for the girls themselves.

Although the students are taught medication and midwifery, their qualifications are not recognized in Denmark. If the girls want to work in Denmark, they are classified as nurses' aides, whereas in Greenland they are recognized as nurse-assistants. To protect them, Danish-trained nurses' aides cannot work in Greenland.

Whenever possible, a student who has completed her training and is interested in public health work is posted to work with a public health nurse. In the outposts, the Sundhedsmedhjaelper (community health aide) is on her own, directed by the local district doctor either by phone or regular monthly visits. Home nursing was taken up in Godthaab just last year, and luckily enough a Greenlander was interested. We hope that in the future the community health aide will be recognized for work in this field.

What are the prospects? Many Greenlanders want home-rule. This is likely to come within the next five years. Greenlandic society will most likely have neither money nor desire to pay people from outside unless absolutely necessary. Doctors will be in short supply for many years, but Greenland is likely to be able to produce other personnel - maybe not to a so-called Danish standard - but certainly to a happy Greenlandic one.

SUMMARY

Non-native doctors have been present in Greenland since 1726 and any community of more than 70 people was required to have a person trained by a physician in delivery and other procedures. From 1900, the most suitable were sent to Denmark to train as midwives and/or nurses; the first nurse in Greenland was thus a Greenlander who graduated in 1904. Since 1950, there has been a population explosion and a vast escalation of health personnel and budgets. By 1970, both tuberculosis and the birthrate were brought under control, and facilities were developed for training health personnel in a western frame. The first Greenlandic doctor returned to practice in 1974, and it is now suggested that responsibility for the health service should be assumed by the provincial authorities in the 1980s.

Native community health auxiliaries: developments in northern Canada, 1973–4

HOPE SPENCER

The "Report of the Task Force on Community Health Auxiliaries" offered a challenge to Northern Region, Medical Services, to train indigenous people to work at the grass roots level, in the homes and the communities of which they are a part. Accordingly, it was decided to initiate an educational approach geared to the unique needs of the north and its people, emphasizing public health and problems of a changing life-style.

Joint meetings were held at all staff levels including Community Health Auxiliary Workers. The agreed long-term goals were (1) increased consumer consultation on health needs and increased community involvement in health programs; (2) increased emphasis on public health; and (3) acceptance of the Community Health Auxiliary Worker as an equal and vital member of the health team.

Because of the vastness of the area served by the northern region of Canadian Medical Services and differences between the ethnic groups above and below the tree line, two courses were held, at Fort Simpson, near Yellowknife, NWT, and at Pangnirtung on Baffin Island. The latter course was conducted largely in the Eskimo language.

Indian communities sent seventeen participants (as they were called, rather than students) to the course in Fort Simpson; the Northwest Territories Department of Education also sent three Home Management trainees, to increase their knowledge of preventive health. Inuit communities sent nine participants and an interpreter to the course in Pangnirtung. These participants came from as far afield as Burwash Landing and Grise Fiord, representatives of a land stretching from Alaska to Greenland. For five weeks, the participants worked together in "learn-by-doing" situations in order to prepare themselves as members of a community health team. All twenty-nine successfully completed their course.

The courses are part of a one-year apprenticeship. They are the beginning of a long-range program in which Community Health Representatives will become as essential a part of the local health team as the nursing staff.

The involvement of native leaders was very important in carrying out this program. In the Pangnirtung course, we were fortunate to include a representative of the Inuit Association who, among her contributions, worked with the participants in listing Eskimo beliefs on ways of treating illness. This information is now available to nurses new to the North.

The participants learned by doing. They learned about "germs" by using a microscope, about garbage problems by visiting the dump, about first aid by practice sessions, about nutrition by preparing foods such as seal liver for babies. They taught each other to run movie projectors and video receivers. They made stencils and posters for mass media campaigns. They learned to take pictures which could be used in teaching slide sets within their home communities. The participants themselves taught many of the lessons, having previously worked through the factual information

with the consultants. It is planned that some of these
Community Health representatives will return to help teach
the next class.

The Hamlet Council of Pangnirtung and their Health Committee took a keen interest in the participants and their
progress, joining the course from time to time, welcoming
them to their meetings, and inviting them into their homes
and to social events. This helped to make the course a
happy one. As one participant wrote to a friend, "Everyone
is happy and is having lots of fun in every course. Everything is to help people."

At these courses proud, and capable native people grew
in stature, giving evidence of real leadership potential.
There is hope that this is the beginning of a long-term program bringing Community Health representatives into the
"Northern Health Team" to the benefit and well-being of
their people.

SUMMARY

Two experimental courses for Community Health representatives permitted an increasingly dynamic teaching/learning
process to evolve. The representatives were viewed as essential members of the health team, and their training
placed increased emphasis on public health and community involvement. Twenty-nine participants were sent to two courses, both held north of the 60th parallel. The process used
was "learning by doing." In addition, the participants were
encouraged to share in the teaching, to prepare themselves
for their subsequent role in the community.

Indian and Eskimo health auxiliaries

ALICE K. SMITH

A program for the preparation of Indian and Eskimo Health
Auxiliaries began in 1961. Short-term goals were: (a) to
encourage the participation of local people in health activities of their communities by involving them in initiating, planning, and carrying out programs; (b) to give professional health workers an opportunity to become more effective by providing a link with the local community; and
(c) to increase the number of active health workers in the
field. The long-term goal was to assist the Indian and Eskimo people in Canada to reach and maintain standards of
health and living conditions comparable to those enjoyed by
the remainder of the Canadian population.

HISTORY OF PROGRAM 1961-72

The first Community Health Auxiliary course was held at
Norway House, Manitoba, under the joint sponsorship of the
Department of Indian Affairs and the Medical Services
Branch of the Department of Health and Welfare Canada.
"Months before the commencement of the course a Regional
Planning Committee designated the areas where candidates
were to be selected, provided the facilities for training
and looked after administrative details. The program was
explained to Medical Services and Indian Affairs Branch
staff and Band meetings were called to explain the program
to the communities. All interested persons were invited to
submit applications. The Chiefs and Councillors (local government) were asked to recommend four applicants from
those who applied. The final selection of candidates was
made by the Regional Planning Committee ... there were eleven students in the first course - four women and seven
men." (1)
    The course had three parts. Firstly, there was a two-
month orientation period which candidates spent in their
respective communities under the guidance and supervision
of field nurses.
    "The formal training period that followed initial orien-
tation concentrated on teaching techniques, the use of
teaching aids, and basic health knowledge, including germ
theory, nutrition, and first aid. Field trips were taken

in order to observe conditions in native communities and to
gain experience in holding public meetings. After six weeks
of general health education, the candidates were divided into groups, the women attending discussions on public health
nursing subjects under the direction of a public health
nurse, the men receiving two weeks in practical sanitation
training from the Regional Sanitarian." (2)

LAY DISPENSERS

Persons known as Lay Dispensers were employed by the Department for many years. Some were Indian and Eskimo people
but many were non-native missionaries, teachers, traders,
or RCMP personnel. All lived in small outlying communities.
They were people who could be depended upon, with a minimum
of instruction, to dispense certain drugs safely. They were
geared to the environment and facilities available, and
learned to use wise judgment in communicating information
on health and sickness problems to nurses and doctors at
the nearest nursing station or hospital.
    Training programs for Lay Dispensers were undertaken in
1969 and the name of the graduates was changed from Lay
Dispenser to Community Aide. As many Indian and Eskimo
people as possible were recruited. They were employed as
part-time workers on call at any hour of the day or night,
often working many more hours than the time for which they
were paid. At times, they found their training was inadequate for the tasks with which they were faced.
    By 1971, a marked increase in the number of Community
Health Worker trainees coming from widely differing geographic, economic, and social conditions made training more
difficult and in some instances the quality suffered. It
also became difficult to provide sufficient encouragement
and support for the large number of new graduates. Other
problems included a high turnover of nursing staff in some
outlying areas, and an awakening interest in self-determi-
nation among many Indian bands. Despite progress in many
respects, the role of the Community Health Worker became
confused and frustrating, particularly in the case of more
recent graduates.

COMMUNITY HEALTH AUXILIARY TASK FORCE STUDY, 1972

A task force to study the Community Health Auxiliary situation was established in 1972 to recommend policy for the
direction, training, and employment of Community Health

Auxiliaries and to outline medium and long-range implementation plans.

The task force of four members - a sociologist (Chairman), a health educator, a nurse, and a physician - visited all Medical Services Branch Regions in Canada. A total of 174 Medical Services' personnel were interviewed, including Community Aides and Community Health Workers, as well as the nurses with whom they work.

Discussions were also held with ten Provincial and Territorial Indian Associations, and other community leaders, the Department of Indian Affairs and Northern Development, Provincial, Territorial, and local government officials, Manpower and Immigration officials, universities, Community Colleges, and other educational bodies. Finally, the task force visited the United States Indian Health Service, Washington, DC, where they spoke with fourteen senior staff members, a number of whom were Indian people.

The Task Force Report (2) contains 83 recommendations, a number of which support fully the original objectives laid down in 1961. Personnel policies including socio-economic factors are pursued in some detail. The major focus is on the course itself, the functions of its graduates, organizational factors, and methods of continuing education. Pertinent recommendations include:

1. In the conduct of community health activities, the Indian and Northern Health Services should orient health professionals and allied workers to the local culture and to Community Health Auxiliary Programs. In particular, nurses who are to be field guides and supervisors of auxiliary personnel should be well prepared for this specific task.

2. Two Community Health Auxiliary roles should be established: (a) a Community Health Representative (CHR) whose main orientation is toward the community; and (b) a Family Health Aide (FHA) whose main orientation is toward the individual and the home.

3. The principle of career development be recognized in Community Health Auxiliary employment and that four levels of employee be established: (a) the probationary CHR and the probationary FHA; (b) the fully qualified CHR and the fully qualified FHA; (c) the Community Health Auxiliary Co-ordinator who would operate at a district or zone level; and (d) the Community Health Auxiliary Adviser who would operate at a regional level. Formerly, first level auxiliary health personnel positions had always been dead-end positions.

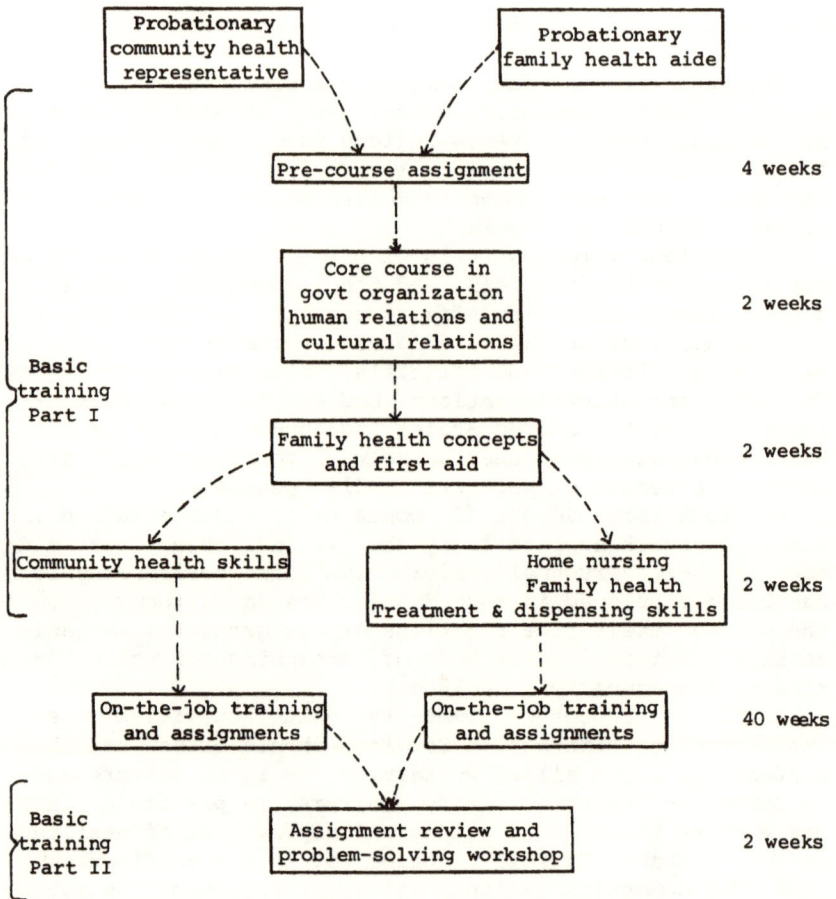

Figure 1   Flow chart for probationary year training

4. There should be a basic training year for probationary Community Health Auxiliaries (see Figure 1), consisting
of: (a) a four-week pre-course assignment in the trainee's
home community under the supervision of the Community
(Public) Health Nurse or Nurse-In-Charge; in areas where
there is no resident nurse, a portion of the time should be
spent in a community with a nurse; (b) six-weeks of Part I
basic training comprising (i) a two-week core course common to CHRs and FHAs and offered also to community leaders,
other community workers, Health Liaison Officers and Indian
and Northern Health Services' personnel; (ii) a two-week
health concept and first aid course; common to CHRs and
FHAs and offered to Health Liaison Officers; (iii) a two-

week community health skills course for CHRs; and a two-week home nursing, family health treatment and dispensing course for FHAs; (c) forty-weeks of on-the-job training; (d) two-weeks of Part II basic training, including on-the-job assignment review, workshops in community health, problem-solving, and reinforcement of Part I basic training.

5. Advanced training should be offered in one or two-week units designed to provide CHRs and FHAs with the skills and knowledge to conduct a broad range of more specialized tasks in response to community needs, and to equip auxiliaries to deal with a variety of health and social problems. Completion of two one-week units or one two-week unit of advanced training once every second year should be a condition of continued employment.

6. The Senior Consultant, Health Education, in consultation with Regions, should pursue the feasibility of educational institutions offering advanced training units for Community Health Auxiliaries, with students receiving credits towards established course requirements in the health professions.

SUMMARY

The history of Indian and Eskimo health auxiliaries is outlined, and pertinent recommendations from the 1972 Community Health Auxiliary task force study are summarized. Appropriate career structures and training program are indicated for both community health representatives and family health aides.

REFERENCES

1. Martens, Ethel G., Public Health Auxiliary Workers in Community Development (Medical Services Branch, Health and Welfare Canada, 1964)
2. Task Force Report on Community Health Auxiliaries, Medical Services Branch, Health and Welfare Canada, 1972

Experience in the clinical training of nurses for isolated northern regions

SUE M. MILLER

In 1972, the Canadian federal government sponsored six pilot projects in the nurse practitioner field. The object was to offer additional university training appropriate to situations faced by nurses in isolated northern regions. Five of these programs are still operational and are collaborating to complete a core curriculum.

The University of Alberta, Edmonton, as one of the participants, holds two four-month courses per year and is now completing its fifth program. As of February 1974, 33 students had graduated. The average age of the students was 31 years, with a range from 23 to 49 years. The group included 11 midwives, one public health nurse, and four students with a B.Sc.N. degree. Three students had no previous experience of the North, but the average experience was 24 months (range 4 months to 10 years).

The course included initial tests, a lecture period, a period of clinical experience, further tests, and a final group of seminars. The lectures and initial testing covered 7 weeks, and the rotating clinical experience, a total of 12 weeks (Figure 1). The students in the first course were not pre-tested so our analysis of data is restricted to the three subsequent courses. Variables examined were: (a) knowledge of surgical techniques, (b) adult physical examination, (c) adult and paediatric simulated patient, (d) written examinations (Paediatrics, Obstetrics, General Medicine, and Surgical topics)

Using dogs, students were trained to suture various types of lacerations, to perform an intravenous cutdown and a thoracentesis. A surgeon was present to relate this experience to the clinical setting. Further practical experience in suturing was gained in the emergency rotation and some students had opportunities to help with cutdown procedures on patients.

The general adult physical examination was marked adhering to a strict key to minimize variation in evaluation (Table 1). Two sets of marks were given - one for perform-

	MON	TUES	WED	THURS	FRI
2 1/2 WKS	LECTURE			PRE TEST	
3 WKS	CLINICAL				
1 WK					
1 WK					
3 WKS					
1 WK					
3 WKS					
3 WKS					
1 1/2 WKS					

LECTURE - 7 WKS (PLUS TEST)   CLINICAL - 12 WKS

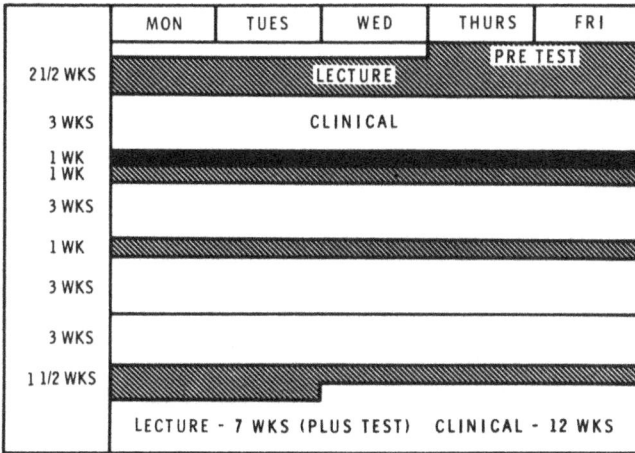

Figure 1   Illustrating the format of the course

ing a procedure, the other for doing it adequately. No partial marks were given.

Simulated patient situations where the person playing the role of the patient (adult) or parent (paediatrics) follows a detailed key regarding history were used (Table 2). The physical findings and laboratory data were available on specific questioning (paediatrics) or given to the student (adult) who was then required to reach a differential diagnosis and suggest appropriate management.

Pre- and post-test scores were based on identical material, although post-testing was more extensive. The results (Table 3) are shown as class averages for courses II, III, and IV; however, these parallel individual results fairly closely. The analysis was useful in finding both areas where the students were initially weak and areas where teaching was ineffective. The pre-testing also helped the students to see their learning needs. Prior knowledge of clinical topics was relatively consistent from one course to another. The average improvement also was gratifying and showed a consistency in teaching from course to course.

The necessity of delineating the core material so that evaluation could be more reliable led to a series of workshops among the five courses. Conclusions will be detailed in the form of behavioural objectives, as illustrated by

TABLE 1
Objective marking scheme for examination of ears, adult physical key

Procedure	Performance of procedure		Technique of examination	
	Possible marks	Marks awarded	Possible marks	Marks awarded
External ear and auditory canal	1		1	
Drum	2		2	
Hearing	2		2	
Total	5		5	

TABLE 2
Example of marking scheme for simulated patient

I.	Identification	
	13-month-old male child	2
II.	Chief complaint	
	diarrhea and vomiting	2
	for 3 days	2
III.	History of present illness	
	Well until 6 months of age	2
	Formula - had been Similac	2
	Solids (cereal, meat, veg., fruit) at 6 weeks	2
	Since 6 months, BMS* vary from 2 to 5 mushy BMS/day	4
	Never tarry, no blood or mucus	4
	Appetite very good - can't fill him up	4

* BMS = blood and mucus containing stools

TABLE 3
Scores of three classes for initial and final tests, with improvement in marks over the course (class average, in per cent)

	Pre-test	Post-test	Improvement
II	40.83	74.00	33.17
III	39.71	74.30	34.30
IV	34.70	65.70	31.00

two examples: to know that the peak incidence of bronchiolitis is found in chidren less than 2 years of age; to recognize increased respiratory rate, indrawing without stri-
dor, inspiratory rales, and expiratory wheeze as signs and
symptoms of bronchiolitis.

The lecture blocks (1 week each) were interspersed with
clinical rotation where possible. The necessary backgound
material was covered near the beginning of the course and
lecturers were chosen not only for specialist knowledge,
but also for their experience of the work. Further seminars
were included during clinical rotation. One week consisted
of a live-in seminar on alcoholism and psychiatric problems, held at an alcoholism treatment centre.

The clinical periods, each three weeks in duration, ran
concurrently and the students rotated through them in pairs.
The medical rotation was at the Charles Camsell Hospital,
which has a high proportion of Indian and Eskimo patients.
It focused mainly on adult history taking and physical examination. Evaluation and management of common medical
problems were also taught. Although some of the students
had much field experience, they initially found difficulty
in completing an adequate physical examination and describing their findings. Thus, this was seen as a vital part of
the course.

The paediatric rotation again focused initially on history taking and physical examination. Common paediatric
problems were covered in seminars. Experience in starting
intravenous medication and doing lumbar punctures was emphasized.

The rotation through the emergency room gave students
opportunity to assess patients, suture lacerations, and
read common X-rays.

In Obstetrics and Gynaecology, ante-natal care assessment of risks and monitoring of labour was stressed. Since
northern policy is to evacuate all primiparous and other
high risk pregnancy patients to hospital, no attempt was
made to develop proficiency in the delivery of such patients.

Teaching in laboratory procedures, practical and preventive dentistry, and surgical techniques was interspersed
with the Emergency and Medical rotations.

At the present time, a proposal for objective evaluation
of the nurses who have returned to the field is being prepared, based on the behavioural objectives of the core curriculum. Our subjective impression is that the course has
improved both the nurses' handling of situations and their
confidence and so has prolonged their average stay in the

North. However, we hope to confirm this when the objective
evaluation becomes available.

SUMMARY

In 1972, the Canadian government sponsored pilot projects
at six universities aimed at providing further clinical
training for nurses in isolated northern regions. Five of
the projects are still operational and are collaborating to
produce a core curriculum. The courses are of four months'
duration and at the University of Alberta are divided into:
(1) pretest, (2) lecture block, (3) clinical rotation, (4)
post-test periods, and (5) a week of seminars on alcoholism
and psychiatric problems in the North. Particular emphasis
is placed on history taking and physical examination. Common
problems are discussed with a view to helping the nurses
decide between the urgent case requiring evacuation and
those less urgent. The nurses are also given guidelines for
better handling of cases in the nursing station. Clinical
rotations are three weeks each (Obstetrics and Gynaecology,
Medicine and Out-patient, Emergency, and Paediatrics).
Technical skills (suturing, intubation, beginning IV's and
LP's) are also taught. There are eight students per course;
four courses have been completed. Extensive pre- and post-
testing has shown significant results. Field evaluation is
presently being anticipated jointly for all five programs.

The outpost nurse: role and activities in northern Canada

HARRIET E. FERRARI

Outpost nurses in northern Canada are the prototype of the
nurse in an expanded role. They are primary care workers in
the broadest and best sense, combining treatment with a
public health approach and incorporating health promotion
into their daily routine. They function as agents of change
by being aware of community needs and resources and working
with community leaders to meet community, family, and individual needs. This paper will discuss the area served, special problems the nurses face, and the actual work they do.

AREA SERVED

Outpost nurses serve that region of Canada north of the 60° parallel, including the islands of the Arctic Archipelago. There are rugged mountains on the west, a harsh and craggy coast on the east, and the "barrens" in between, a treeless expanse of rock, tundra, muskeg, and water. About 56,000 people including Indians, Eskimos, Métis, and Caucasians of many ethnic origins are grouped in settlements of 50 to 10,000 people. The diversity of language, life-style, and culture adds complexity to the role of the outpost nurse as she seeks to influence health behaviour. Having to work through interpreters requires considerable patience and a system of checks to ensure that the intended message is getting across. Building rapport and trust also takes time and a true interest in the people as individuals and families with acceptance and understanding of cultural and conceptual differences.

Out of the geography and climate of the North, two major problems arise - transportation and communication. All transport, whether by air, water, or land, is beset by the uncertainties and vagaries of weather and rugged terrain. Often, the evacuation of patients is delayed because of transportation difficulties. Communication by radio, radiotelephone, and telephone is subject to interference from atmospheric conditions, mineralization, intervening land masses, and technical breakdowns. Consultation with a physician in times of acute illness or injury is vital, but on occasion the nurse must still rely on her own experiences and judgment owing to problems of communication.

ORGANIZATION

The Medical Services Branch of the Department of National Health and Welfare, Canada, in conjunction with the Yukon and Northwest territorial governments, is responsible for the delivery of health care to the North. In addition, there are some private physicians and dentists and a few municipal and mission hospitals.

Medical Services Branch has its head office in Ottawa, with a Regional office for the Northwest Territories region in Edmonton, Alberta, and a newly formed Yukon regional headquarters in Whitehorse. Further decentralization divides the Northwest Territories region into four zones. Each zone is supervised by a physician or Zone Director who reports to the Regional Director in Edmonton, who, in turn,

reports to Head Office in Ottawa. Each zone also has one
or two nursing officers who are responsible to the Zone Director for the nursing activities within the zone.

FACILITIES

Hospitals

Hospitals are situated in the major population centres such
as Whitehorse, Frobisher Bay, and Inuvik. They vary in size,
but are relatively fully equipped and are staffed by teams
of doctors, one of whom is a surgeon. The catchment area is
large, and the doctors travel great distances to visit outlying nursing stations.

Nursing Stations

Nursing Stations are located in settlements with populations
of from 150 to approximately 1,000 people. There are currently about forty of these facilities, each staffed with
1 to 4 nurses. A typical station consists of out-patient
facilities, in-patient beds, and living quarters for the
nursing staff. The nurse is responsible for the total functioning of the station - the janitor, housemaid, clerk, and
interpreter all work under her supervision. When there are
problems with the sewer, the water supply, or the electrical power, the nurse must assume responsibility for correcting these problems.

Health Centres

In settlements where there are facilities for care of the
sick, health centre nurses provide a generalized public
health nursing program with the emphasis on preventive
medicine, health promotion, and rehabilitation.

Health Stations

Health stations are basic facilities provided in small
communities, under the supervision of a local resident who
has had some training and operates with the help of a
treatment manual and radio-telephone contact with a nurse
or doctor. A nurse from the nearest nursing station or
health centre visits these satellite communities once or
twice a month.

REFERRALS AND MEDICAL SPECIALIST VISITS

Patients who require treatment beyond the scope of the
health services in the North are referred to major hospitals in southern Canada. One of these is the Charles Camsell Hospital in Edmonton, the chief referral centre for
the Western Arctic.

In recent years, several university teaching hospitals
have become involved in the provision of health services to
the North. Many patients are referred to these hospitals.
Also, regular visits are made by medical specialists to
provide consultation services and teaching for the medical
and nursing staff. Referrals, including preparation of case
histories and transportation arrangements, are handled by
the nurse and she also assumes responsibility for follow-up
treatment and surveillance.

COMMUNITY HEALTH REPRESENTATIVES

About twenty-five native residents have received basic
training in health subjects and health promotion techniques.
They work in their home communities, under the supervision
of the nurse, as full members of the health team, providing
a vital liaison between the native community and the health
services. Nurses participate in the training program and
during the orientation period and the CHRs educational
year (page 596) the supervising nurse provides additional training, encouragement, and guidance, including the
CHR in the in-service programs, staff discussions on program planning and implementation.

FUNCTIONS OF THE OUTPOST NURSE

The outpost nurse functions as a general practitioner, diagnosing, treating, giving emergency care, and supervising
chronic care and rehabilitation. She practises independently and interdependently with the physician and other health
team members who may be hundreds of miles away. She often
performs procedures commonly held to be the prerogative of
physicians, such as suturing, IVs, cutdowns, delivery of
babies, prescribing of medications, and pulling teeth in an
emergency. The Medical Services now has a special training
program for nurses where advanced clinical skills can be
acquired (page 596).

As well as the daily treatment clinic, the outpost nurse
conducts the public health nursing program consisting of

maternal and child care, school health (including surveillance of the school environment - lighting, heating, hygiene, and safety), communicable disease control, mental
health, chronic disease care, accident prevention, and nutrition counselling, while always integrating health teaching and promotion. Environmental aspects of community health
also come under the surveillance of the nurse. She works
with the local health committees, the CHR, the visiting
EHO, health educator, and zone director, to work out practical improvements that will make the community a healthier
place in which to live.

Several special clinics are held on a regular basis, such
as prenatal, postnatal, well-baby and immunization, chronic
disease, and follow-up. The emphasis is on preventive medicine and health counselling. Home visiting is an important
function, as such contacts make possible the integration of
individual care with a family perspective and allow health
teaching more relevant to home conditions.

The outpost nurse's other skills must include taking X-
rays and gleaning some information from them, physical and
psychosocial data collection and assessment, growth and
developmental assessment, interviewing and observation, and
treatment and management of common physical and psychosocial
deviations from health. She performs these functions on a
one-to-one basis, but always with a family-community viewpoint. On the community level, the nurse functions as a resource person, working with health committees on alternative solutions to health problems and helping people plan
and implement the approach they choose.

CONCLUSION

The challenge for the outpost nurse is to render a high
standard of health care despite the difficulties of distance, communication, transportation, inclement weather,
and the psychological effects of isolation. While practising
in many ways as a general medical practitioner, she remains
primarily a nurse, combining the "curing" function of the
physician with the "caring" role of the nurse.

The quality of the care currently provided is shown by
the improvements in mortality and morbidity statistics for
the North. To quote but two examples: the infant mortality
rate has been gradually but steadily improved from 60.9
per 1,000 live births in 1968 to 27.8 in 1973. The incidence of tuberculosis, also, has declined from 194 in 1969
to 53 in 1973. Much remains to be done, but improvements in

the health status of Canada's Northerners have been made -
by such fruits may outpost nurses be known.

SUMMARY

Outpost nurses in northern Canada provide treatment and
public health services, with a heavy emphasis on independent judgment. The outpost nurse must function as a general
practitioner, diagnosing, treating, giving emergency care,
supervising chronic care and rehabilitation. She often performs procedures commonly held to be the prerogative of the
physician such as physical assessments, suturing, IVs, cutdowns, delivery of babies, and prescription of medications.
A population of 56,000 people (including Indians, Eskimos,
Métis, and Caucasians) is scattered throughout 1.3 million
square miles north of the 60° parallel. Facilities include
hospitals, nursing stations, health centres, and health
stations. The challenge for the outpost nurse is to render
a high standard of health care despite the difficulties of
distance, communication, transportation, inclement weather,
and the psychological effects of isolation.

Physicians' assistants in Alaska

D.K. FREEDMAN

Physician's assistants (PA) are a recent addition to the
long list of health workers who give technical support to
the physician. Historically, nurses and school teachers
pioneered the way in native villages of Alaska where physicians were rarely seen. Gradually, public health nurses
and volunteer native health aides became the main providers of health care in Alaskan villages. The PA has emerged
over the past decade in the US and over the last four years
in Alaska. The original intent was to increase physician
productivity.

In Alaska, the public health nurse (PHN) has provided
medical care, preventive health services, social services,
and counselling, in addition to utilizing medical standing
orders. Consequently, the respective roles of PHN and PA

have become somewhat blurred.

TITLE, DUTIES AND EMPLOYERS

The term physician's assistant is synonymous with "physician extender, physician's associate, and medex." Special types of physician's assistants are developing in Alaska; for example, those who assist orthopaedic surgeons and paediatricians. For several years, training programs in other parts of the United States have been producing such categories of trained personnel as the assistant to the primary care physician, orthopaedic physician's assistant, and urologic physician's assistant. Similarly, the nurse practitioner, the nurse midwife, and the paediatric nurse practitioner function with, but not necessarily under, the supervision of a physician. Some PAs work for private physicians. Others are in public medical clinics, public health programs, or in private practice themselves. In Alaska, a paediatric nurse practitioner has opened an office for the practice of paediatric nursing. However, complex diagnostic and curative problems are referred to the paediatrician, with whom she shares office space.

The duties of the above-named include medical history taking, diagnostic services, on-going care for chronic disease and pregnancy patients, care of acute diseases and injuries, rehabilitation services, health maintenance, and health services to the community at large.

To delineate further the tasks performed by a primary care physician's assistant, I would point to his use of technical skills. The execution of medical standing orders provides another range of proficiency involving every system in the body. Numerous routine patient-care tasks are performed, such as dressings and suture removal. Diagnostic and therapeutic procedures are also undertaken, although physicians determine the degree of proficiency of the PA prior to assigning responsibility for specific procedures such as the diagnosis of otitis media, hypertension, muscle strain, and the need for suturing. Finally, complete records of all patient encounters are maintained by the PA.

Physicians in private practice are the most common employers of PAs, especially those in general or family practice and specialists such as paediatricians, oto-laryngologists, orthopaedic surgeons, and general surgeons. Several federal agencies such as the Indian Health Service and the National Health Service Corps also utilize PAs.

LEGALIZATION

Two years ago the Alaska Statutes were amended to permit
PAs to perform functions previously limited to physicians.
The legal conditions were simple. The physician had to be
fully responsible for the acts of the PA whom he employed
and had to report his name to the State, with the date of
hiring and release.

In several instances, the PA has been stationed in a remote community visited by the physician every week or two.
However, telephone or radio contact is maintained as needed,
24 hours a day. The legislature avoided defining what constitutes a PA. Wisdom dictated that some experience should
be gained prior to providing rigid regulations concerning
training requirements, or detailed medical procedures which
would be permitted or prohibited.

Earlier this year, after only two years' experience, the
law establishing PAs was repealed, and replaced with a requirement that the State Medical Board establish regulations
spelling out the conditions under which PAs could be utilized and the type of training and experience required.

GEOGRAPHICAL DISTRIBUTION

The State of Alaska has an area of 600,000 square miles.
Travel time and costs of travel for health care are thus
major considerations, and the optimal use and location of
clinics, physicians, public health nurse practitioners,
community health aides, physician's assistants, and others
is a concern and responsibility not only of the health professions, but also of official agencies.

Unfortunately, the appearance of PAs in remote areas is
slow. We know of two each in Kenai and Bethel; and one in
each of the smaller communities of Palmer, Sitka, Nome,
Haines, Unalaska, Yakutat, and Galena. Some 90 per cent
work in the two largest cities, Anchorage and Fairbanks.
The total number of PAs in Alaska is currently 45. Half of
these are associated with private medical clinics, or with
medical institutions, and the remaining half are affiliated
with individual practicing physicians in different parts of
the State.

Other examples are to be found in a remote mining camp
accessible only by air, and a small community reached by
ferry or air. With the onset of construction of the oil
pipeline in Alaska and with the establishment of some 30
construction camps along the route, PAs are being placed in

these remote areas, between Valdez and Prudhoe Bay. As many
as 40 PAs are scheduled for the next few years.

SIGNIFICANCE FOR THE FUTURE

Council on Medical Education of the American Medical Association has developed a Joint Review Commission on Education
Programs for PAs. National guidelines for certification of
the various categories of PAs have been established, and
since May 1972 over 50 educational programs have been accredited by the Commission.

The cost of health care is enormous and is rising rapidly. Increasing use of non-medical health workers is thus
inevitable. By 1985, it is estimated that 100 to 150 PAs
will be functioning in Alaska. They will work primarily in
public clinics, with private physicians, and in remote
permanent stations along the pipeline. In addition, many
specialists will utilize specially trained assistants, such
as the orthopaedic PA. In the villages, native Alaskans
will be serving in the role of primary health care provider,
as the major part of a health team. Their training will be
more broadly based than that of the PA. It will also be in
tune with native needs, customs, conditions, and desires.

Carlson and Athelson, writing on this matter in the
Journal of the American Medical Association, 7 December
1970, observed: "Perhaps it would be well ... to recognize
the entry of Physician's Assistants in this initial phase
as a frankly expedient, even a stopgap measure, calculated
to meet immediate needs while the basic reorganization and
'rationalization' of the health system proceeds toward more
long-range solutions. The physician's assistant can be expected to adapt and adjust to coming changes as they take
place, just as the physician presumably will. Thus, the
physician's assistant category should be regarded as part
of a dynamic, continuously evolving health system, and not
as a rigidly codified formulation of tasks conforming to
established modes of practice ..."

One may question the development of supports and crut-
ches for a system of health care which appears to be obso-
lescent. However, in the old system, the MD, the nurse, and
the assistant knew their respective roles. Now, the US is
in a transitional stage when national health insurance is
being readied, and many of these titles and categories are
less distinct. We are, we hope, moving towards a more ra-
tional system, in which roles, titles, and relationships,
including that of the consumer, will be classified. Never-

theless, with 150 PAs, 200 community health aides, mental
health workers, dental health aides, ophthalmology aides,
and alcoholism counsellors, one must anticipate a certain
amount of "doctor shock," superimposed upon cultural shock!

SUMMARY

The nomenclative duties and employers of the physicians'
aides are discussed. After a two-year period of legaliza-
tion by the State of Alaska, it is now the responsibility
of the State Medical Board to specify conditions under
which a PA may operate. Unfortunately, the appearance of
PAs in rural Alaska is slow, and currently 90 per cent are
concentrated in Anchorage and Fairbanks. In the next decade, the oil pipeline, rising health costs, and a possible
national health insurance scheme will lead to further changes in the PA with clarification of his role and an increase
in numbers.

The WAMI program: a three-year progress report on

regionalized medical education in the north

W.W. MYERS, REBECCA A. SILLIMAN, R. B. LYONS,
and M.R. SCHWARZ

The education and training of physicians in the United
States has become, to a large extent, the responsibility of
individual states. Within this context, the problems of
health manpower shortages and the maldistribution thereof
have important implications for states without medical
schools. The prohibitive cost of building new medical
schools plus lack of a sufficient population base to justify such facilities ha~ led the states of Alaska, Montana,
and Idaho to join wit.. Washington in an experiment in medical education (WAMI, an acronym for the four states involved).

Since its establishment in the autumn of 1971, WAMI has
focused its attention on two phases: university and clinical. In Alaska, approximately ten students in each of the

last three years have obtained their first semester of medical school training at the University of Alaska (Fairbanks).
The university faculty, staff of the Arctic Health Research
Center, the Fairbanks medical community, and visiting resource persons from throughout the state and the University
of Washington have provided the students with essentially
the same curriculum as their fellow students in Seattle.
After one or two semesters, they have joined their class-
mates in Seattle for the remainder of their basic science
training.

During the clinical phase, third and fourth year students and residents receive training in Family Medicine and
Psychiatry in Kodiak and Anchorage, respectively. Other Community Clinical Units (CCU) are being considered for Alaska
and eleven other CCUs are found in the other WAMI states.

The Commonwealth Fund of New York provided an initial
grant and, after the first year of operation, the Bureau of
Health Resources Development of the United States Department of Health, Education, and Welfare provided additional
support. In 1974, the legislatures of each of the four
states appropriated funds for the project. It is anticipated that by 1975 the states, including Alaska, will assume
full financial responsibility for the WAMI program. This
will make it economically more feasible for the University
of Washington to admit to its School of Medicine a greater
number of students from Alaska, Montana, and Idaho, thus
directly addressing the medical manpower problem in those
states.

The complementary problem of physician maldistribution
has been approached on the hypothesis that students trained
in rural areas are more likely to practise in such settings
than those trained in urban areas. Three different mechanisms are being employed to increase rural experience. The
first is in the university phase. WAMI students at the
University of Alaska elect to work with local Fairbanks
physicians at least one morning each week; they observe the
operation of a private practice, experience on-call duty
at the local hospital, and attend local medical society and
scientific meetings. Most participate in a week-long field
experience designed to allow them to observe rural Alaska
health care in action. In addition, a course in Rural
Health has been added to the curriculum; general problems
of rural health are discussed with emphasis on Alaska. The
course explores the providers of health services, consumer
influences, and factors that influence the impact of those
services. Situations and programs relatively unique to

Alaska are emphasized; for example, the Native Land Claims Settlement Act, the Trans-Alaska Pipeline, the Public Health Service Community Health Aide Program, the Native Health Corporations, and the State Department of Health and Social Services.

As a second mechanism, community clinical units offer clinical exposure to rural practice. Here, the students treat patients, see special problems, and observe professionals working in non-urban environments.

Finally, summer work-study opportunities are provided under such agencies as the Public Health Service. Ten of thirty students who have participated in the university phase at the University of Alaska have worked throughout the state in hospitals, clinics, and villages.

One might legitimately ask at this point whether the WAMI program is achieving its goals. It is much too early to document its impact in providing manpower for rural practice. The first students will graduate in 1975. To evaluate the basic science training, the scores from the National Boards Part I and a system of testing common to all sites and the University of Washington have been employed. Scores from such examinations reveal no significant difference in performance between WAMI and Seattle students.

The WAMI educational activities provide certain "spin-off" advantages to the local communities. In Fairbanks, the WAMI faculty has organized and helped to teach accredited continuing education courses for nurses in coronary care, paediatric nursing, and pathophysiology. Several physician assistants have also taken these courses, receiving academic credit from the Alaska Methodist University School of Nursing in Anchorage. Thus, an additional function of WAMI has been to provide an academic home for accreditation purposes.

WAMI has also been involved with the Tanana Health Authority (see page 581) in providing additional training for Community Health Aides. During the summer of 1974, three students visited several villages in the interior of Alaska, endeavouring to broaden the Health Aides' knowledge of common respiratory diseases and to increase their expertise in obtaining diagnostic information. The students developed a better understanding of the people, the environment, and the culture in these villages.

The medical community of Fairbanks is enthusiastic about the presence of the medical students. Several of the physicians present clinical sessions. Others teach portions of the basic science courses, and the students receive membership in the Fairbanks and Alaska State Medical Associations.

The academic year 1974-75 marks the beginning of a full year Alaska WAMI program. With this development come new challenges, new complexities, and new ideas. The launching of the ATS-6 satellite in May 1974 provided a new experimental arena. Throughout 1974-75, the two-way audiovisual capabilities of the satellite will permit both the Seattle and Fairbanks faculties to present lectures live with immediate feedback from students over 1,000 miles away. As an extension of this philosophy of innovation, negotiations with the University of Washington School of Dentistry and the Washington State University School of Veterinary Medicine have begun, with the ultimate goal of involving them in WAMI.

One of the most important factors allowing WAMI to develop so successfully in such a short period of time has been the support given by both students and faculty. The students value close professorial and peer associations, the opportunity to "get their feet wet" in clinical medicine, and the chance to be a part of "Bush" life for a few days. Because the class is small, students are encouraged to undertake special projects as well as to seek assistance with individual academic questions. The faculty also benefits from the close association with students occasioned by the small classes, and the added curricular offerings help expand the academic program at the University of Alaska.

SUMMARY

Faced with the increasing cost of medical education, physician shortages, and the maldistribution thereof, the states of Washington, Alaska, Montana, and Idaho joined in a cooperative regional medical education experiment (WAMI, an acronym for the four states involved). Based at the University of Washington School of Medicine in Seattle, the program provides medical students with both basic science and clinical training in rural settings. The program began in 1971, and objective evaluation of student progress over the subsequent three years indicates that it has been a success. Problems of accreditation and funding have not been solved completely, but the enthusiasm of the staff, students, and medical community, plus the quality of the education received, point to an optimistic future for WAMI.

Commentaries

"The changing health picture in Canada's north," by H.B.
Brett (Medical Services, Northern Region, Edmonton, Canada). Cultural, ethnic, and language differences affect the
state of health of the northern people not only in terms
of physical status but in terms of mental well-being and
"quality" of life. Diseases such as tuberculosis, and venereal disease, infant morbidity and mortality, and some
categories of mental illness have multifactorial causes.
Innovative approaches to the present health care system include the training of native para-medical personnel in
various areas of endeavour in the health field.

"The economics of health care delivery in south-central
Alaska," by R. Fortuine (USPHS, Alaska Native Medical Center, Anchorage, Alaska, USA). The Alaskan Native Medical
Center is the unit of the US Indian Health Service with the
direct responsibility for health care of the Alaskan natives of south-central Alaska. The area served includes not
only the Greater Anchorage area, but a number of smaller
towns and some 35 remote native villages. Besides offering
full hospital and ambulatory services at Anchorage, the
Medical Center sends its physicians on approximately semi-
annual field trips to the villages. It also contracts with
numerous private physicians and small hospitals in outlying
areas for care of the natives. There is no direct cost to
the patient for these services.

"The use of a travelling ophthalmic technologist in the
provision of ophthalmological care in a remote, sparsely
populated region," by T.W.D. Grant and H.A. Rose (Department of National Health and Welfare, Northern Region, Mackenzie Zone, Yellowknife, NWT). An attempt has been made
to meet the ophthalmological needs of the population of
the Mackenzie Zone of the Canadian Northwest Territories by
the use of a well-trained ophthalmic technologist who tra-
vels to each of the small, widely separated communities. He
carries out the necessary refraction tests and screens patients selected by the local nurses for ocular disease and
/or motility problems. Patients requiring treatment or further investigation are referred to the supervising

ophthalmologist, who provides instructions by phone or radio, sees them on a subsequent visit, or, if indicated, has
them evacuated to the well-equipped treatment centre in
Yellowknife. Some of the advantages of this program are:
(1) Communities are visited on a regular schedule with
reasonable frequency by the same personnel. This provides
a continuity of service by the same persons who come to
know the patients and their problems well. (2) The skills
and training of the ophthalmologist are more effectively
used by enabling him to spend most of his time at the
treatment centre where adequate medical and surgical facilities are available. (3) Standardized, centralized records
are kept which are identical with those in the patient's
home community. This results in quick and easy availability
of information when required. It is suggested that the use
of well-trained paramedical personnel may be of significant
value in the provision of adequate medical care to widely
dispersed population groups in the far north.

"Supervision at a Distance: ophthalmic paramedicals in remote areas," by H.T. Wyatt, H. Rose, and D. Grant (University of Alberta and Department of National Health and Welfare, Northern Region). Ophthalmic paramedicals provide a
service system for widely scattered population groups in
the Northwest Territories. However, supervision at a distance presents difficulties because the number of people
screened for eye disease as falsely positive and falsely
negative has not been measured. This problem has been investigated at one settlement by having all patients presenting for eye examinations seen first by the ophthalmologist.
Comparison of results allowed the merits of the paramedical
to be measured in terms of sensitivity (under-referral) and
specificity (over-referral). It was concluded that acceptable standards of performance can be defined in these
terms. Failure to achieve standards of sensitivity will result in the neglect of patients needing treatment. Failure
to achieve standards of specificity will unnecessarily increase the work load of visiting ophthalmologists. By systematic sampling of performance in this way a means of controlling paramedical working standards and of providing a
continuing paramedical education should be obtained.

"Alaskan native health in the space age," by L. McGarvey
and M. Richardson Wilson. Paper not submitted.

"Organizational peculiarities of medical insurance of the Soviet Antarctic Expedition," by A.L. Matusov (Department of Polar Medical Researches AARI, Leningrad, USSR). The peculiarities of polar expeditions demanded special requirements of the state of health of the participants in the SAE. Therefore, a new list of medical contraindications for selecting the participants was worked out in 1973. When selecting the SAE participants their specialty and type of activity as well as participation in various polar expeditions were taken into account. Medical examination determines the suitability for participation and provides an opportunity to investigate the state of health to discover the initial forms of disease and to determine treatment. All the polarmen undergo systematic dispensary control together with necessary clinical and laboratory investigations. Information obtained about wintered-over polarmen is registered on a "Medical Polarman Card." The dispensary method of medical-prophylaxis during the winter and a sanitary-hygienic program (prevention of sunshine deficiency, vitamin and metabolic regulation, pharmacological prophylaxis, etc.) provide for prevention of factors promoting the occurrence of dynamic diseases, lowering morbidity, and improving work capacity. The analyses carried out during SAE's and drifting "North Pole" expeditions (1965-72) have made it possible to determine the distribution and frequency of diseases as well as their character.

"Native consumer participation in federal health services in Alaska," by J.F. Lee and R. Singyke (Alaska Area Native Health Service, US Public Health Service, USA). Traditionally the role of government has been to decide on, plan, and carry out services for those it has legislatively been directed to serve. Six years ago the Alaska Native Health Service began to develop a milieu to make possible the meaningful involvement of Alaskan natives in policy determinations which affected their health program. Gradually a strong Native Health Board formed and acquired a considerable body of knowledge on health matters and expertise in dealing with health problems. The Alaska Native Health Board is the official statewide health arm of the 12 native regional corporations, established as a result of the Native Land Claims Settlement Act of 1971. Each region, in turn, has its own regional health board, composed of a cross-sectional membership representing the communities of the region. These health boards relate to the service units of

the Alaskan Native Health Service in their particular region as participants in planning, policy-making, and the
evaluation process. The evolution of native consumer involvement has progressed steadily, but not without uncertainty and difficulty at times. The experience has been a
new one for both sides, with new ground constantly being
broken. Our future roles and changes in the health care
system are being worked out step by step, influenced by external factors such as economic, social, and technical development, governmental policy, and the land claims settlement, exerting various effects. There is no doubt that the
native health consumer is now contributing to shape the future of things in the health services arena in Alaska.

"Use of physician assistants in rural Alaska," by T.S.
Nighswander (National Health Service Corps, Anchorage, Alaska, USA). To improve the quality of health care in rural
Alaska, the National Health Service Corps has placed three
physician assistants as primary health care providers in
isolated areas of the state. The back-up physician and medical facility are 200 to 800 miles distant. The assistants
are operating remote out-patient medicine departments and
they have available routine laboratory and x-ray facilities.

"Role and function of itinerant public health nurses in rural Alaska," by A.C. Bruce and M.E. Crawford (Division of
Public Health, Department of Health and Social Services,
Juneau, Alaska). The primary health care team consisting of
itinerant nurses, doctors, and resident community health
aids is a strategy used in the delivery of health services
to the more remote areas of Alaska. The itinerant public
health nurse has a unique role as a member of this team.
One of the last of the generalists in this era of speciali-
zation, the itinerant public health nurse combines some of
the basic skills of the paediatric and medical nurse practitioner with a public health approach toward health maintenance and health promotion. A recent survey of the functions and training needs of the itinerant nurses reveals
their role is influenced by many factors including health
needs and resources, local attitudes and expectations, federal and state legislations, environmental determinants,
and agency objectives. Itinerant public health nurses, historically, are among the forerunners of the nurse practitioners in the USA, and their role could become a model in
providing health care services to widely scattered, sparse
populations in other states and countries.

PUBLIC HEALTH AND ARCTIC ECOLOGY

Resource exploitation and the health of western arctic man*

K.R. REINHARD

I first ventured into the Arctic about 22 years ago, to study the natural history of infectious diseases. At the outset, I held the common belief that the native people of the Arctic, in their prehistoric state, had no serious health problems and that major disease problems were primarily the result of contamination caused by Euro-American adventurers and immigrants. The target was completely susceptible, and the imported microorganisms were irresistible.

Before long this stereotype faded. We found very little clinical poliomyelitis in the native Alaskan population at a time when it was epidemic among urban non-natives. Serological studies revealed the common pre-existence of naturally acquired immunity in the native people of western central and northern Alaska. Entero-viruses were recovered repeatedly from native populations with no clinical evidence of infection. Acute otitis media could be aborted and recurrent or chronic otitis prevented if prompt medical treatment was provided. Measles no longer occurred in total-community epidemic form, but were maintained endemically. The epidemiology of tuberculosis suggested not population hypersusceptibility, but rather inadequate health services with widespread undetected and untreated "open" cases. This was confirmed when a few years of intensive casefinding, hospitalization, and ambulatory chemotherapy and chemoprophylaxis drastically reduced the prevalence of this disease. The spectrum of diseases experienced by arctic populations is generally no different from that of temperate zone populations. Why, then, has so much disease been present for so many years? And how had the great problems been generated? This is not merely a "Host vs Parasite" issue; other environmental factors have been at work.

* A more extensive narrative with a full bibliography can be obtained on request to the author.

The aboriginal people of the Arctic were originally highly adapted groups, making the most of an area of relatively
low biological productivity. Populations were, of necessity,
small and diffuse, limited by the ecology. The large and
concentrated populations existing in the Arctic today sub-
sist on the resources of more southerly areas. In the aboriginal state, famine was an ever-present threat, precipitated by unusual weather or changes in animal migration. If
resources were overutilized, renewal was slow. As a consequence, a nomadic or semi-nomadic mode of existence was developed.

Early explorers describe nosebleeds, "scrofulous" skin
diseases and boils, dysentery, neurological disorders, a
high infant mortality, snowblindness and other ophthalmias,
pulmonary diseases, lousiness, and injuries among arctic
natives. Several accounts describe pulmonary disorders that
could have been tuberculosis; for example, Zagoskin men-
tions "consumption" among Kuskokwim people who had had
little contact with the outside world. Most observers agreed
that the arctic people were relatively healthy in their aboriginal state, although subject to early senility. The
greatest dangers to individual and public welfare were un-
toward natural events, and if there were great epidemics
before the advent of the Euro-American, we have no record of
them.

In the past 20 years, ecological and sociological concepts have infiltrated epidemiology, and it has become clear
that social and economic deprivation and depressed or poor
health are directly related. How do such concepts relate to
the health status of native Alaskans? How can social and
economic deprivation become established among a hunting and
gathering society? The answer is simple: if natural resources are depleted, and are not replaced by adequate alternative resources, then the people are deprived of subsistence just like a person without cash or credit in an industrialized society. When Euro-American commerce and industry extended to Alaska, to appropriate renewable and non-
renewable resources, it entered into direct competition with
the native people.

THE FUR TRADE

While native commerce had been based on local exchange,
Euro-American activities involved exploitation and removal
of resources for the benefit of distant shareholders and
consumers. Unregulated exploitation of the Aleutian Islands

by Russian adventurers brought not only despoilment of resources, but also the massacre of native people who resisted the adventurers. Under the Russian-American Company,
homicidal activities were reduced, but the land from the Yukon to the southeast archipelago was denuded of its rich
fur resources. Often, the native people participated, either
by impressment or out of desire for trade items.

The US-sanctioned monopoly which succeeded the Russian-
American Company appeared no better in its treatment of indigenous people. Skins were bought with script, which could
be spent only at the company store, at its prices, and
early treatment of the fur seal resources was an ecological
disaster. It is a miracle that the fur-seal rookeries were
able to become re-established and that the sea otter did
not become extinct.

As a result of exploitative commerce, the arctic Americans were deprived of primary sources of the traditional
clothing needed for protection against their rigorous environment. The excessive kill also depleted food sources
and the native people began to substitute commercial articles such as textiles, guns, steel knives, axes, and metal
cookware for home-made clothing, utensils, tools, and wea-
pons. Skills needed to make the traditional items faded and
the people became dependent upon commerce for the necessi-
ties of life. However, there is no evidence that the depletion of fur resources, per se, caused increased death and
disability among the Alaskan population.

WHALE, WALRUS, AND SEAL

The major portion of the aboriginal population lived in the
maritime regions. In western and southern Alaska, fish and
marine mammals were important to the support of human life.
North of Norton Sound, marine mammals were more important
than fish, while in the Bering Sea Islands and along the
Arctic coast, whales, walruses, and seals provided most of
the subsistence. Land mammals were also available, but were
utilized much less along the coast than in the interior.

In the first part of the nineteenth century, the whaling
industry reached the North Pacific. Whalers derived from
the large San Francisco fleet moved into the Bering Sea
and Arctic Ocean, taking large harvests until the last two
decades. Then, low catches, decreasing demand, and multiple
shipwrecks caused a rapid decline of the industry. The last
commercial whaling effort in the American Arctic took place
about 50 years ago.

TABLE 1
Whale and walrus products, 1874-91 (from report of Govt.
of Alaska 1892)

Year	Oil (bbl)*	Bone (lb)	Ivory (lb)**
1874	10,000	86,000	7,000
1875	16,300	157,800	2,540
1876	2,800	8,800	7,000
1877	13,900	139,600	74,000
1878	9,000	73,300	30,000
1879	17,400	127,000	32,900
1880	23,200	339,000	15,300
1881	21,800	354,500	15,400
1882	21,100	316,600	17,800
1883	12,300	160,200	23,100
1884	20,373	295,700	5,421
1885	24,884	451,038	6,564
1886	37,200	304,500	2,850
1887	31,714	564,802	875
1888	15,774	303,587	1,550
1889	12,834	231,981	1,506
1890	14,890	231,232	4,150
1891	12,228	186,250	1,000

* Petrof estimates that the average yield of oil per
  whale was 40 bbl.
** Petrof estimates that the average yield of ivory per
  walrus was 5 lb. He estimated further that 7 out of
  10 walruses hunted in the open sea were lost after
  being shot.

Catches in the nineteenth century greatly exceeded the
levels of sustained yield. In addition to whales, many
thousands of walrus were taken for ivory and oil. Depletion
was so drastic that nearly 100 years after the peak activity of the whaling industry, none of the affected animal
populations has fully recovered. As with the fur trade, native people were motivated to hunt beyond their subsistence
needs, obtaining baleen and ivory to trade against store
items that had become part of their life-style. The advent
of the repeating rifle and bomb lance further aggravated
the wastefulness of hunting. Table 1 indicates the rise and
eventual fall of the whale-walrus harvest.

Within a couple of decades of the advent of intense commercial whale and walrus hunting in the Bering Sea, Chukchi
Sea, and Arctic Ocean, the maritime native population of
those areas declined substantially, stimulating concerned
comment from members of Arctic expeditions. A massive famine killed at least half the people of St Lawrence Island
and depopulated three of four communities in 1879-80.

TABLE 2
Salmon pack, 1883-1908

Year	Canned (cases)*	Salted (bbl)
1883	36,000	
1884	45,000	
1885	75,000	
1886	120,700	
1887	190,200	
1888	439,273	
1889	703,963	
1890	671,000	6,390
1891	688,332	7,300
1892	789,294	9,000
1893		
1894	646,345	21,000
1895	675,041	32,011
1896	619,379	5,502
1897	949,645	10,000
1898	909,538	17,388
1899	1,000,000	15,000
1900	1,098,000	24,922
1901	1,529,569	30,000
1902	2,690,000	
1903	2,400,000	
1904	1,910,000	
1905	1,131,312	
1906	1,500,000	
1907	2,146,000	
1908	2,000,000	

* A case consisted of 48 one-pound cans.
  Excerpted from Reports of the Governor
  of Alaska.

In recent years there has been a resurgence of walrus
populations and some recovery of the whale population, but
the future size and use of these resources remain to be
seen. Meanwhile, welfare programs have helped the people
eat, albeit a "flour and sugar" diet of limited nutritive
value.

SALMON

The salmon fisheries of northwestern United States and
western Canada were sufficient to supply world demand in
the mid-1800s. However, when those fisheries were depleted,
the industry moved north into Alaska (Table 2). Some rivers were completely depleted of salmon by dams or cross-
nets. Fish-traps decimated runs of salmon headed into rivers

for spawning. Canneries competed for control of the catch
and often bought more than could be canned or salted.

Until the establishment of salmon canneries, the maritime natives had taken the brunt of resource deprivation,
but with the rise of commercial salmon fishing, the river
peoples also suffered a severe setback. Their subsistence
had never been as secure as that of the coastal people, for
they had to depend upon seasonal runs of fish and relatively inefficient (but conservatory) means of catching them.
Large land mammals were an unreliable additional resource,
since their migration routes shifted from one year to another. Each family had to catch, dry, and cache a number of
tons of fish during the runs.

IMMIGRATION

At the end of the nineteenth century, the Gold Rush brought
a flood of Europeans, Euro-Americans, and Orientals, seeking
a quick fortune in the great river valleys and some coastal
areas. Immigration doubled or tripled the population com-
peting for natural resources, and caused severe inflation.
The native people had little buying power to compete for
commercial items they had come to depend upon; Indian communities which had experienced fishing failures could not
afford flour, sugar, blankets, or ammunition at the inflated prices. The traditional resources of the native people
remain greatly depleted, with no hope for early renewal,
and they have not been made partners in the new economy to
the extent that they can be self-supporting; in recent
years only welfare programs have enabled most of the rural
native people to survive.

CHANGES IN WAYS OF LIVING

While their environment was suffering drastic change caused
by exploitation, the way of living was also changed in a
more subtle fashion by the pressures of the dominant Euro-
American "culture." The drift towards commercial procure-
ment of food, hunting equipment, and household articles was
discussed above. Many of the items available from the trading post were labour-saving, but not all were well adapted
to arctic life. Foods were high in calories but low in essential proteins, vitamins, and other essential nutrients,
and high in price. Repeating arms ammunition increased the
monetary cost of food gathering and caused decimation of
animal populations. Alcoholic liquors blighted the lives of

a substantial portion of the native population, both physically and psychologically.

The establishment of fixed trading posts, church missions,
post offices, and schools gradually brought an end to the
semi-nomadic life. The copying of housing from the dominant
culture slowly terminated the use of housing made from local materials. Poverty then determined that families would
live most of the year in crowded, poorly ventilated, one-
room cabins or shacks, which were hard to keep in repair.
The low-grade, permanent housing was inferior, sanitation-
ally, to that of the semi-nomadic life, for temporary shelters were open to the cleansing effects of the natural elements between times of use. Native Alaskan communities became rural slums, with ill-nourished people living in crowded quarters, without adequate sanitation or protection
from accumulating pollution and rigorous elements. Concentration of the population greatly aggravated the problems
of hunting and gathering and fostered high rates of communicable diseases such as tuberculosis.

Many people of Euro-American extraction respected and
loved the Alaskan native people and worked towards their
betterment - admittedly, not always with the right methods,
but certainly with the right motivation. But over-all, the
intruding society was incredibly arrogant and intolerant
of the "ways of the savages." The government took a custo-
dial stand. Euro-American society disparaged the native
life-style and held up the "way we do it in the States."
Some early military ventures were for tactical reconnoi-
tering - to gauge the potential resistance of the native
houses to small arms or cannon fire. Among the missionaries, too many purveyed damnation, Euro-American mores, and
a pietistic philosophy rather than the Gospel of Grace.
Traders robbed, cheated, and intimidated the natives. Such
treatment by a dominant culture inevitably degrades the
self-image of an overwhelmed people. Is there any wonder
that mental health problems are serious among Alaskan natives, and that the current, tardy release of the native
people from intellectual and cultural tyranny brings with
it overreaction and militancy?

HEALTH AFTER EURO-AMERICAN CONTACT

Devastating epidemics were introduced by seafarers and immigrants, including outbreaks of smallpox, measles, dysen-
try, influenza and other respiratory diseases, gonorrhoea,
and syphilis. As the population gained experience of these

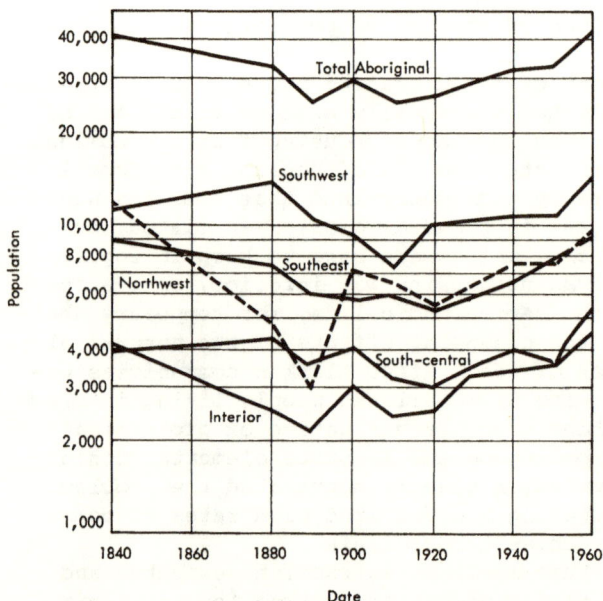

Figure 1   Regional growth of aboriginal populations of Alaska, 1840-1960 (from *Alaska's Population and Economy*, by George W. Rogers and Richard A. Cooley (University of Alaska, Economic Series, Publication No. 1, Volume 1, 1963))

diseases, and vaccination was introduced, mortality decreased. But lethal epidemics contributed strongly to the decline of the native population in the western American Arctic during the nineteenth century. Figure 1 shows the fluctuations caused by these factors and those cited earlier.

By the latter half of the nineteenth century, tuberculosis had become hyperendemic - or perhaps epidemic - among the native population. The disease did not sweep the country dramatically, like smallpox or influenza, nor did it decimate villages in weeks like measles. But by the late 1800s, it existed throughout the territory and took a constant, heavy toll of life. As recently as 1960 one could see many households that comprised re-knitted fragments of families broken up by deaths from tuberculosis. The entrenchment and emergence of tuberculosis as the principal infectious cause of mortality correlates well in time with the increasing disjointment of the native economy and way of life.

"LEVELS OF DISADVANTAGEMENT" CAUSED BY DISRUPTIVE FACTORS (ESTIMATED)

severe

AGGREGATE CHANGE IN LIFE STYLE

moderate

FUR EXPLOITATION

WHALE & WALRUS EXPLOITATION

slight

SALMON EXPLOITATION

IMMIGRATION & INFLATION

| JURIS-DICTION | PRIVATE RUSSIAN ENTERPRISE | RUSSIAN-AMERICAN COMPANY | U.S. MILITARY | DISTRICT DEPT. of INTR. | TERRITORY |

YEAR 1750   1800   1850   1900

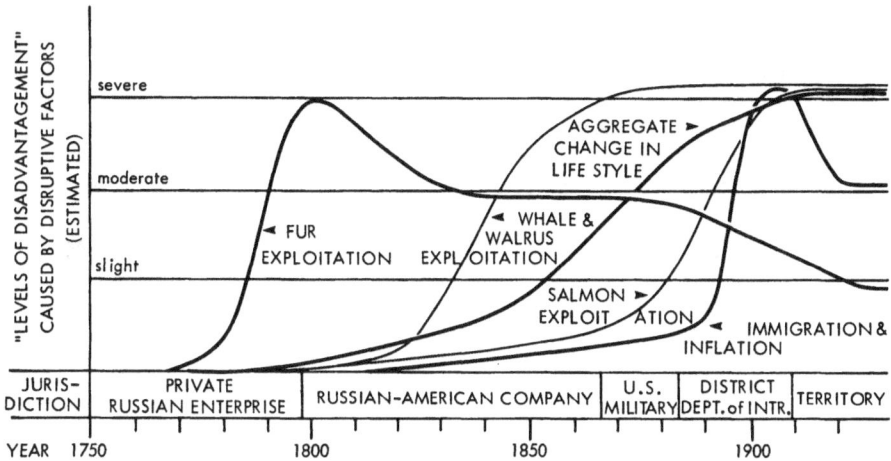

Figure 2   Estimate of effects of disruptive ecologic events
on the health and security of Alaskan natives (the curve
for immigration and inflation increases again greatly in
1940-45 and after 1950)

THE CURRENT SITUATION

The current patho-ecological status of the Alaskan native
people is little different from that of disadvantaged people
in more southerly climes. Communities have first decreased
in number and then grown in size. The initiation of midwifery and immunization programs some 30 years ago greatly
reduced foetal wastage and infant and childhood mortality.
For many years, the native population has been increasing
at a rate about four times the US national average (Figure
2). An aggressive control program has greatly reduced the
morbidity and mortality rate from tuberculosis. Current
health problems include iron deficiency anaemia, diarrhoeal
disease, otitis media, "common colds," enterovirus infections, bronchitis and pneumonia, and, above all, psychosocial problems and accidents. To these we should add an in-
definable amount of malnutrition. A bourgeoning population
is beset with health issues that cause disability rather
than death. The disabling diseases aggravate social and
economic problems, while needs continue to out-distance
efforts to provide services.

THE ROAD TO IMPROVEMENT

Efforts to improve the health of the native people started
after the close of World War II. Medical services were expanded greatly, both for hospitalization and ambulatory
care. Recently, regional health corporations (page 615)
have given the native people themselves a voice in health
policy.

Notwithstanding these desirable efforts, it is unlikely
that Alaskan native people will enjoy a health status
equivalent to that of the general population until economic
and social disadvantages are corrected.

EPILOGUE

At this period in history, knowing the ecological and sociological aftermath of unbridled commercial and industrial
exploitation, we are not entitled to point an accusing fin-
ger at the exploiters of centuries past who thought they
were dipping into inexhaustible resources. Today a multitude
of people foresee, at least partly, the ecological results
of commercial and industrial exploitation, yet the latter
continues with ever greater avariciousness. Even now a new
commercial exploitation of a non-renewable resource is
underway in Alaska, and it is difficult to predict what this
will mean eventually to the Arctic environment and the
health of its population. The settlement of the Alaskan native claims brings with it more imponderables. Can the new
land holdings become bases for the development of local industrial economies capable of ending deprivation among Alaskan native people, or are they merely the beginning of another kind of disadvantaged living "out on the reservation"?

SUMMARY

The high prevalence of disease among residents of the western Arctic, starting in the first half of the nineteenth
century and extending through the first half of the twentieth century, appears to have been caused primarily by external, commercial exploitation of the resources necessary
for subsistence of the indigenous people. This has been
complicated by incomplete industrialization of the native
economy, increasing urbanization, great surges of immigration, and economic inflation. The net results have been a
defacto pauperization of most of the indigenous population
and degradation of their life-style, producing greatly

increased morbidity and mortality with social depression.
Current health problems among the indigenous racial stocks
of Alaska are now similar to those prevalent among the disadvantaged people of more densely populated temperate zones.
Increased medical service activity has substantially reduced morbidity and mortality, but health problems remain
more severe among Alaskan natives than among the non-native
population. Socio-economic disadvantagement seems a prime
cause of the continuing problems; therefore, the attainment
of good general health depends on the establishment of social parity and a sound economic base of support.

Housing and sickness in South Greenland:
a sociomedical investigation

O. BERG and J. ADLER-NISSEN

The housing situation in Greenland has been much improved
during recent years by intensive house building - especially
in the towns. Yet many households still live in houses of a
size, quality, and furnishing far beneath the required quality of a population, which for long periods of the year
needs not only a climatic shelter but also a natural frame
for all indoor activities.

   We shall present here an analysis of data collected by
interviews and observations of families in South Greenland,
examining the relation between the housing situation and
the incidence of illness. Our hypothesis is that the incidence of certain diseases, such as the common cold, gastroenteritis, tonsillitis, and otitis, is influenced by the
housing situation, partly along physical lines and partly
because of crowding. According to our hypothesis, badly
equipped or overloaded houses will show a higher incidence
of illness than houses physically well equipped and uncrowded.

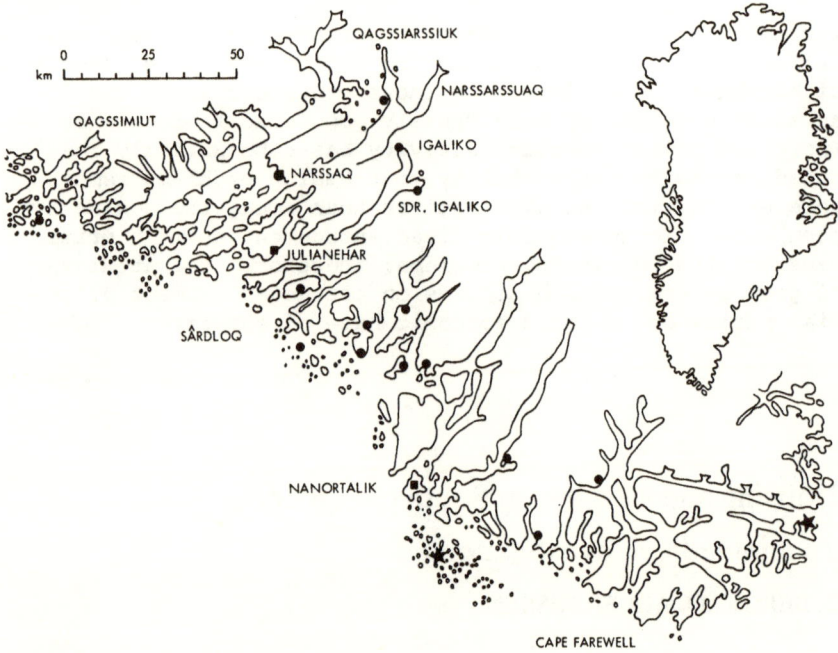

Figure 1 Map of South Greenland

POPULATION - DESCRIPTION AND DATA COLLECTION

The population includes 286 Greenland households with children under 16 years living at home. Two hundred and thirty-
eight households of 1268 persons were interviewed, all
living in Narssaq and Julianehab municipalities: 151 households with 779 persons in the town of Narssaq; 39 households
with 216 persons in two inshore-fishery trading stations at
the Davis Strait; 32 households with 181 persons on three
sheep-farming trading stations in-fiord; and 16 households
with 92 persons in 15 sheep-farming settlements along the
same deep fiords (see Figure 1).

Seven of 9 households not interviewed in the rural district were away from home (at summer-fishing grounds and the
like) whereas two could not be reached because of bad
weather. In the town of Narssaq, 39 households were not
interviewed: 13 because of departure, 19 because of refusal,
and 7 because of shortness of time. Narssaq town was surveyed in the summer of 1969 and the rural district in the
summer of 1970. Data include four main facts: the physical
structure of the house; the incidence of illness in the

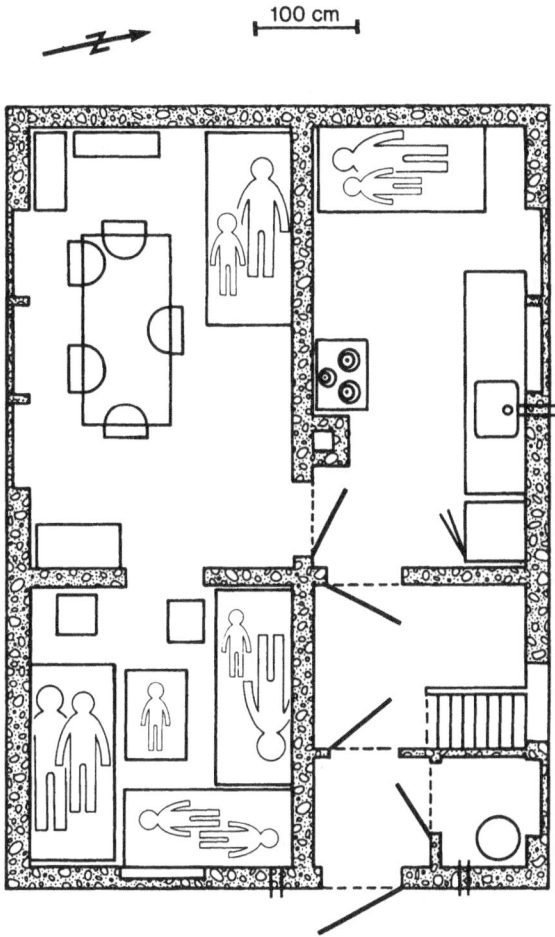

Figure 2   Household of four adults and seven children in an old-style house in an inshore fishery trading station (net area 26 m^2, kitchen included)

household; the family structure, occupation, and income; and the contents of the house (1, 2).

Data include the complete measurements of the house, from the plan of the rooms even to the size and placing of the furniture; likewise the arrangement of the kitchen, the larder, tools, fuel, clothes, and linen were noted, together with use of the house, including who is sleeping where and with whom.

Among the 151 households in Narssaq town there were 44
with 1 bed, 13 with 2, and 2 households with 3 beds in
which 2 or more children were sleeping - corresponding with
at least 152 children. At the same time there were 19 households with 1, and 3 with 2 beds, in which at least one
grown-up and at least one child were sleeping. Only about
half of the 433 children from the town material were sleeping in their own beds. About half of the 151 households had
at least one bedroom with 4 or more occupants, a little
more than a fourth had one bedroom with 5 or more, and hardly a tenth had a bedroom with 6 or more occupants (Figure
2).

Each person was characterized as to age, sex, education,
occupation, income, and incidence of illness during the past
12 months. The registration of diseases is based partly
upon the district medical officer's notes, and partly upon
the memory of the person interviewed (usually the housewife).
Interviews were conducted by one of the authors (Berg), who
speaks Greenlandic so that an interpreter was not needed.

HOUSING INDICES

A housing quality index has been developed to measure qualities of the house. Crowding has also been calculated as a
"day burden index," and a "night burden index."

SELECTION OF DISEASES

Attention has been focused on frequently occurring diseases
likely to be affected by housing - the common cold, gastroenteritis, tonsillitis, and otitis media. We have information on the number of cases, and the number of persons affected over the past 12 months.

HOUSING QUALITY INDEX

The following elements are included: the kind of dwelling
(one-family house, flat, two-, or four-family house), the
water supply (water installed or carried), the distribution
of water indoors (water pipe - none), personal hygiene facilities (in private - not), toilet conditions (water closet or earth closet - none), kitchen conditions (dining-
kitchen - ordinary kitchen), heating of the house (conveni-
ence in operation), heating of the house (distribution in
the rooms), porch area ($m^2 \geq$ or < number of rooms + 1).

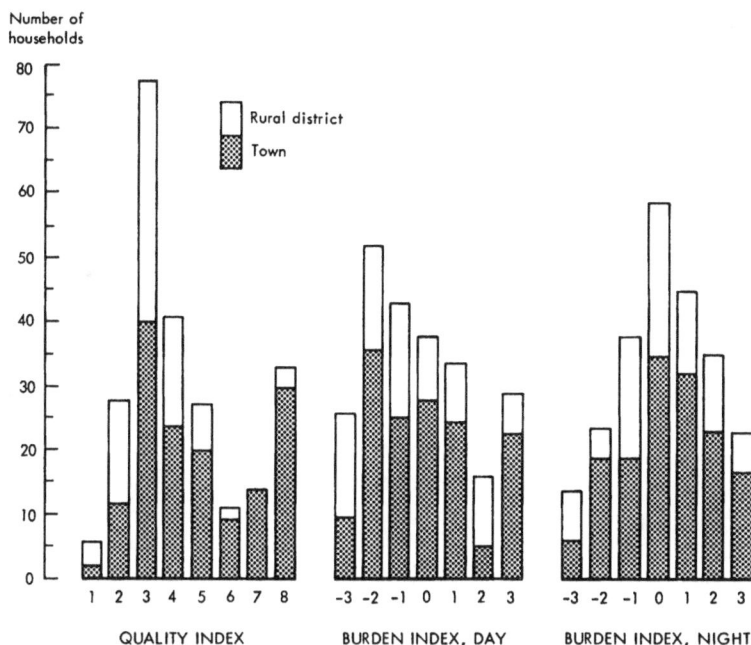

Figure 3   238 households related to three different house indices

The potential score is from 0 to 9, and the actual range from 1-8 (Figure 3).

With regard to the common cold, there are no significant deviations from the zero-hypothesis (assuming no connection), when speaking of numbers of persons affected. The number of cases, however, shows a clear decrease with increase of the housing quality index. This relation is evident for individual age groups too, especially for children (0-6 years and 7-15 years). Product/moment correlation coefficients (4), however, are not exceptionally high. The relation between index and number of cases with colds per occupant of the household is -0.17, and for number of persons affected per occupant, it is -0.12.

For gastroenteritis, there is no relationship between the index and the number of cases or the number of persons affected.

For tonsillitis, there is a significant ($P < 0.05$) relationship with numbers of cases, but a non-significant relationship for persons affected.

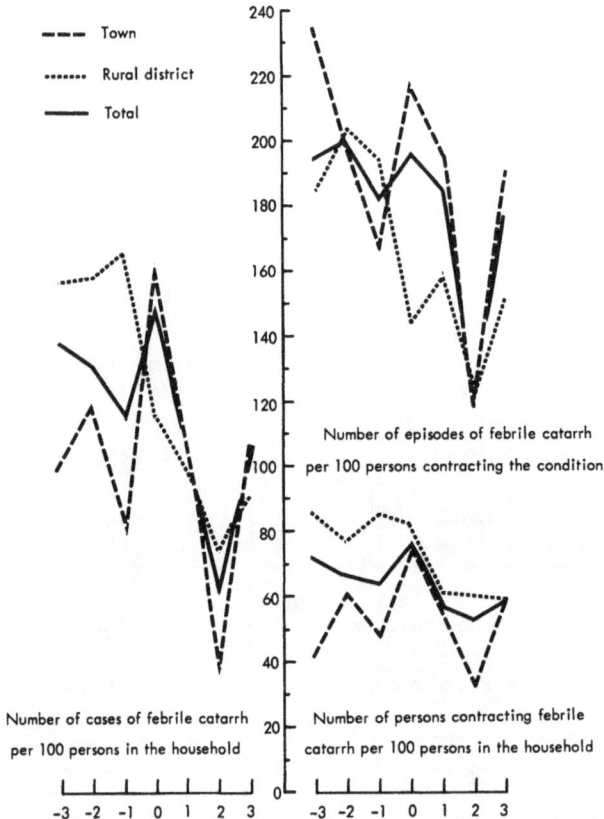

Figure 4   Relation between incidence of febrile catarrh and
"day burden index" (number of people living in house during
day)

For otitis media, there is a marked decrease in the number of cases with increase of the housing index; the relation is significant, and the correlation coefficient -0.14.
For the number of persons affected, the trend is less evident, the relation being insignificant, and the correlation
coefficient only -0.09.

DAY BURDEN INDEX

This index includes the following factors: persons per
living room (sleeping room and kitchen dining room included), square metre living room per person, and square metre
porch per person. Each part of the index is rated -1, 0 or
+1, giving an over-all score ranging from -3 to +3.

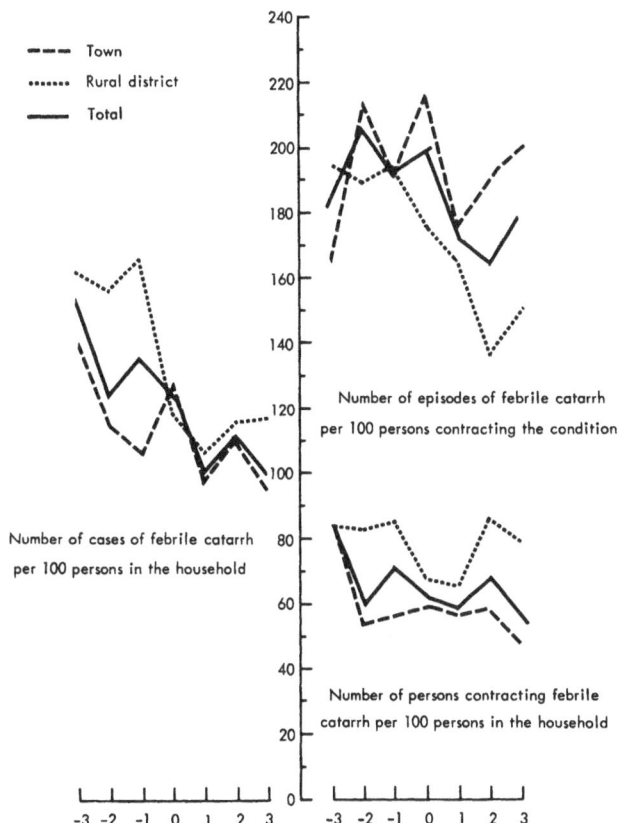

Figure 5   Relation between incidence of febrile catarrh and "night burden index" (number of people sleeping in house during night)

The distribution of cold frequencies in towns, rural districts, and the total is seen in Figure 4. The number of cases decreases as the index rises, both for the rural district and the total, while in the town there is an increase around an index value of 0. A corresponding trend is seen for the number of persons affected. Correlations are, respectively, -0.14 and -0.07, significant for the number of cases.

Other diseases show some correspondence with altered index values. Gastroenteritis shows a U-shaped relationship, with high frequencies around index values of -3 and +3 (19.9 respectively 20.6), and a low frequency when the index is zero (4.2). This is also true in the town, both for numbers of cases and persons affected - all three values

being significant. Tonsillitis shows a decrease as the index increases but an index value of +3 seems an exception
to this rule with a very high frequency of infection (25.3).

Otitis media is less common as the index increases, the
relationships for the number of cases both in town and in
total being significant. The number of persons affected decreases too, but insignificantly.

NIGHT BURDEN INDEX

This index shows how the house is used by night. It takes
account of the following factors: number of persons sleeping per room, number of persons per blanket on the floor,
and cubic metres of air per person in the bedroom with the
largest number of occupants. Each component of the index is
allocated points from -1 to +1, giving a possible score
from -3 to +3 (Figure 3).

The frequency of colds (Figure 5) shows a tendency to decrease as the index increases, both in town and in the rural district, though most evident in the latter. All three
categories are significant. The correlation coefficient for
the number of cases in all 238 households is -0.12. No
trend is evident for the number of persons affected or for
the number of cases per 100 persons affected.

Gastroenteritis, tonsillitis, and otitis media show no
trends with respect to this index.

SUMMARY

The incidence of disease has been mapped for 1268 persons
in 238 Greenlandic households over a 12 month period. Indices of housing quality and crowding by day and by night
have also been developed, and correlations explored between
certain infectious diseases and housing conditions. All
three indices are related to the occurrence and persistence
of the common cold, although correlation coefficients are
rather low. Otitis media is affected by housing quality and
by day- but not night-time crowding. Gastroenteritis and
tonsillitis are less obviously affected by housing.

REFERENCES

1. Berg, O., Tidsskrift. "Grønland," 2: 11-16 (1973)
2. Berg, O., and Adler-Nissen, J., Tidsskrift. "Grønland,"
   3: 102-11 (1973)

3. Christensen, V., Boligforhold og børnesygelighed (Copenhagen: Munksgaard, 1956)
4. Hellevik, O., Forskningsmetode i sosiologi og statsviten-
   skap (Oslo: Universitetsforlaget, 1971)

Community attitudes and perception of waste management problems at Resolute, Northwest Territories

F.J. TESTER

Well-organized health care delivery systems, advanced technology, and thoughtful planning of northern communities
will not in themselves solve the waste management and public health problems of isolated settlements in the Canadian
Arctic. Well-designed systems only function effectively
when they are understood by, and receive enthusiastic support from their users. Willingness of the individual to
solve a particular problem depends upon his understanding
of the problem. There is a relationship between the intensity of attitudes towards an environmental problem and
willingness to act (1). A more complete understanding of
the attitudes and perception that northern people have of
waste management problems is thus essential. The research
reported here examines the attitudes of a random sample of
18 Inuit residents of Resolute, NWT.

THE COMMUNITY

Resolute village has a population of about 220. South camp,
approximately one mile away, contains facilities used by
the Ministry of National Defence and the Department of the
Environment. The airstrip, a motel, and facilities for
various oil and exploration companies are located several
miles to the north. The island is extremely barren and
covered with limestone and sandstone gravels. A new townsite, integrating the Inuit village with "North and South"
camps, is presently being constructed (2).
    The Inuit village is located on an open beach and is ex-
posed to north-westerly winds. Temperatures range from an
average low of -29°F in February to an average high of

40°F in July. At present, water for the community is
trucked from Char Lake. Moretta Lake and Resolute Lake are
nearer, but receive sewage effluent from "North" camp.
Sewage pollution in Moretta Lake appears to have increased
greatly (3).

The beach ridges at Resolute contribute significantly to
waste management problems. During the summer months, water
collects in pools along the ridges and these in turn fill
with tin cans, paper, barrels, and raw sewage from improper-
ly handled disposal bags. There are no running water or sewage systems in Resolute. A community dump is located one
quarter of a mile to the west of the village. During the
summer of 1973, the dump stretched 300 yards along the
beach and varied in width from 15 to 40 yards. It had not
been covered for over a year and only portions had been
burned. North-westerly winds carry odours and loose papers
from the dump to the village.

All homes in the village are of plywood-frame construction, and ventilated by holes four inches in diameter that
penetrate the exterior walls. A dusty gravel road runs
through the centre of the community, carrying considerable
vehicular traffic to the nursing station.

PROCEDURE

An "instrument package" was designed to reveal attitudes
towards waste management, public health knowledge, problems
of waste management, and ideas about waste management. Cultural problems of the undertaking were recognized to be much
as in cross-cultural studies of mental health and anthropology (4). The instrument package was translated into sylla-
bics, field tested, and modified as necessary.

A random sample of 18 residents were interviewed in
their homes. The age range was from 15 to 57 years, with a
mean of 31.5 years; eleven females and seven males were
seen. Interviewing was usually done in the dialect of the
villagers by Miss Lilly Kyak, a resident of Pond Inlet,
Baffin Island, but in some cases where the respondent was
known to me and had a command of English, I was responsible.
Interviews were casual and lasted from one to two hours. In
the case of some older residents, questionnaires were left
with respondents who could later reply verbally or in
written form.

RESULTS

Where applicable, responses are reported as a percentage of
those answering a particular question. Unfortunately, not
all respondents answered all questions. A high percentage
(46 per cent) of subjects had received no formal education.
A considerable proportion (36 per cent) stated that they
planned to leave Resolute; however, a similar proportion
(36 per cent) had not visited other communities since taking
up residency in Resolute.

Attitudes to Community and Domestic Cleanliness

Respondents were asked to comment on the cleanliness of
their community and homes (Tables 1 and 2), its importance,
the magnitude of difficulties encountered, and whether or
not they thought more effort could be made to keep the community clean. While 36 per cent of respondents had not visited other communities, only 11 per cent indicated they had
no basis for comparing community cleanliness (Table 2).
Other respondents indicated that while they thought Resolute
was cleaner, they did not really know what problems were
being experienced by other communities. The majority of
respondents indicated that personal and community cleanliness were important (Tables 3 and 5). However, while the

TABLE 1
Perceived cleanliness of Resolute

Very clean	10%
Fairly clean	0
Clean	20
Fairly dirty	40
Very dirty	30

TABLE 2
Perceived cleanliness of Resolute
in comparison with other communities

A lot cleaner	22%
A little cleaner	11
About the same	33
A little dirtier	22
A lot dirtier	0
Don't know	11

TABLE 3
Perceived importance of community cleanliness

Definitely important	56%
Important	33
Neither important nor unimportant	11
Not important	0

TABLE 4
Perceived magnitude of the problem
of keeping the community clean

A big problem	40%
A small problem	10
Not a problem	50

TABLE 5
Perceived importance of personal facilities
that are easy to keep clean

Definitely important	78%
Important	11
Neither important nor unimportant	0
Unimportant	0
Definitely not important	11

TABLE 6
Perceived magnitude of the problem
of keeping individual homes clean

A big problem	40%
A small problem	20
Not a problem	40

majority of respondents (70 per cent) indicated that Resolute was a dirty community (Table 1), about half of the
respondents did not feel that keeping the community and
homes clean constituted much of a problem (Tables 4 and 6).
A majority of respondents (67 per cent) felt that more
could be done to keep the community clean.

Public Health Knowledge

A high percentage of respondents indicated that a clean
community (78 per cent) and a clean home (88 per cent) were
important to personal health. However, there was considerable

confusion as to why a clean community and home were important. Some said a clean home and community were comfortable
to live in. Others replied that the health nurse had told
them cleanliness was important, but that they didn't understand why. Typical responses were: "We heard from nurses
that clean is important to health. An Eskimo never used to
get sick twenty or thirty years ago, even when they used to
be dirty. I don't know why." "In the house we eat and we
always live here and sleep here. It is good for health. In
old days we didn't really know about it and we never used
to have something to clean up house and we never used to
know that we have to keep it clean because of sickness until
white man told us that unclean is unhealthy. That time in
old days we never used to clean up anything and we never used
to get sick and we used to be strong, even old people. But
now we are easy to get sick now, even when we are clean like
I was told. I try it. It doesn't work out."

Thirty-three per cent of respondents indicated they had
never received any instruction in public health or personal
hygiene. The majority of these were males.

Problems of Waste Management

Respondents indicated that the two greatest problems in
keeping the community clean were the use of uncovered waste
barrels outside the houses and the accumulation of seal carcasses on the beach. Other difficulties included the dusty
road which bisects the community, garbage which blows into
the village from the dump, and the burying of sewage bags
and garbage in the snow during the winter.

Domestic problems included a lack of running water and
the fact that most homes were too small relative to family
size. Respondents also mentioned the lack of bath tubs or
showers, the use of paints and finishes which are difficult
to keep clean, the presence of poorly designed porches
which let in dust and snow, and the lack of storage space.

Ideas about Waste Management

Respondents indicated that unpleasant and annoying odours
originated from garbage cans and from carcasses left on the
beach. Personal property was hard to look after, owing to
a lack of proper storage and work facilities, and this contributed to waste management problems. The majority anticipated improved waste management and public health conditions once the new townsite was completed, but 30 per cent

of respondents were not optimistic that the situation would improve.

Recommendations to improve community and household clean-liness included the provision of running water and larger homes with more storage space, the use of paints and materi-als that were easier to clean, and the collection of gar-bage directly from receptacles built into community dwell-lings. It was also suggested that public health education relevant to waste management be directed towards the men of the community as well as the women.

DISCUSSION

Many residents of Resolute do not travel to other communi-ties and a high proportion have little or no formal educa-tion. Instruction in the basic prinicples of public health and waste management seems critical to the health and wel-fare of such native northern Canadian populations. An ex-change of ideas relevant to waste management, public health, community planning, and housing design would do much to im-prove community spirit and pride. Such an approach should relate to northern people in a personal way, and be under-stood by all - regardless of educational background. Re-search has demonstrated the visual memory of native nor-thern people (5, 6). Video-tape replay units could thus play a valuable role in the public health education of nor-thern people.

Respondents were often confused as to the underlying reasons for cleanliness. Thus, they indicated that keeping their homes and the community clean was not a problem. How-ever, elaborations on this response indicated a problem of attitudes: "It is no problem ... people just don't care to do anything about it." Positive attitudes cannot develop in an atmosphere of misunderstanding.

Many of the problems discussed relate to the provision of adequate housing and community planning. It is therefore essential, if "defeatist" attitudes towards public health problems are to be avoided, that native northern people be involved maximally in both community development and the development of public health education programs.

It is also important that male residents of isolated settlements receive public health education. The men were responsible for the carcasses on the beach and for irregu-larities in the collection and disposal of the community's sewage and garbage.

CONCLUSIONS

Waste management and public health problems in the north
are compounded by confusion about the relevance of these
problems. The use of video tape and the involvement of native northerners in educational programs is recommended,
with particular attention to education of the male residents
of arctic communities. Existing designs of housing and community planning practices contribute significantly to waste
management problems in the Canadian North. Native northerners and public health officials should play a more important role in housing design and northern community planning.

ACKNOWLEDGMENT

The invaluable assistance of Miss Lilly Kyak in both field
work and the translation of information is gratefully acknowledged.

SUMMARY

Attitudes towards waste management and public health problems have been examined in a random sample of 18 Inuit residents of Resolute, NWT. Seventy per cent of respondents
indicated that Resolute was not a clean community, although
only 23 per cent thought it dirtier than other settlements
with which they were familiar. Twenty-two per cent thought
that community cleanliness and proper waste management were
not important to their health or well being.
  Respondents over 30 years of age showed some confusion
about the relationship between community cleanliness and
public health. The majority of respondents who indicated
they had never received any public health education were
males. Carcasses left on the beach by (male) community
hunters were thought a prime cause of bad odours and represented a significant health problem. It was suggested
that public health education be directed towards the hunters and trappers of the community. Community nurses can
more readily direct information towards females, and to
this point the health education of the male population has
been neglected. Respondents suggested that elimination of
open garbage cans, the use of shiny washable paint in homes,
and installation of running water and sewers would do much
to promote community cleanliness.

REFERENCES

1. Boldt, E.D., Frideres, J.S., and Stephens, J.J., "Perception of pollution and willingness to act," Alternatives, 2: 31-6 (1973)
2. Bissett, D., Resolute, and area economic survey, Department of Indian Affairs and Northern Development, 11 (1967)
3. Eedy, W., "Human impact on the Canadian Arctic: A literature review." First Preliminary Version of a Report to the Water Subcommittee of the National Research Council (Canada). Associate Committee on Scientific Criteria for Environmental Quality
4. Murphy, J.H., and Leighton, A.H., Approaches to Cross-Cultural Psychiatry (New York: Cornell University Press, 1965)
5. Kleinfeld, Judith,"Visual memory in village Eskimo and urban Caucasian children," Arctic, 24: 132-8 (1971)
6. Bland, L., Perception and Visual Memory of School-age Eskimos and Athabascan Indians in Alaskan Villages (Anchorage, Alaska: Human Environmental Resource Systems Monographs, 1, 1970)

Preventive measures against venereal diseases

G.Å. OLSEN

Few infectious diseases are cured so easily and efficiently as the venereal diseases (VD). The paradox of VD is that, nevertheless, the problem is out of control today. This applies especially to the developing areas; the arctic regions of Greenland, Canada, and Alaska unfortunately confirm this beyond dispute.

Depending on our background, we can all mention a number of environmental factors which dispose to the present VD situation in the Arctic. But it is not only a question of behaviour and environment. We must ask whether Public Health measures have been sufficiently modified to deal with the present epidemiological situation.

Asymptomatic but highly infectious venereal diseases have been the subject of considerable concern (2, 9), especially

because of urbanization and population mobility which create
an increasing pool of unrecognized asymptomatic infections.
This results in additional diagnosis, treatment, reporting,
and time consuming contact-tracing. The efficiency of the
latter is well known to persons dealing with VD. The growing
pool of unrecognized infection is probably the crucial epidemiological reason for unsuccessful efforts to control
sexually transmitted diseases. What possibilities do we have
to bring the invisible part of the iceberg to light? The answer seems a more extensive use of preventive measures - individual prevention and community-motivated screenings of
groups at special risk. We cannot wait for a possible vac-
cine to be developed.

Individual voluntary prevention could include both the
use of condoms and control examination for asymptomatic infection. The first possibility - the condom - is traditionally included in every Health Education program. This is
done in a world that uses highly efficient anticonceptional
products - hardly the best basis for a public relations
operation aimed at motivating additional use of a product
considered unacceptable by many consumers. Other possibilities for individual prevention include vaginal preparations
with antibacterial activity (3) and the intra-uterine device which liberates copper ions, but the value of these
is not yet known. One final type of individual prevention
is the voluntary check-up for asymptomatic venereal disease.
This, however, implies a high level of health information.
Appropriate motivational programs are currently in operation in Denmark and will be initiated in Greenland in the
autumn. We hope this motivation will reach the target
group, but for the moment this is only a hope. So let us
therefore turn to the last sheet anchor - community-motivated screening procedures.

Recent research in the United States (1) indicates that
screening for venereal diseases in gynaecological wards,
family planning clinics, and the like is less expensive per
case diagnosed than traditional examination, contact-
tracing, and so forth. Cost/effectiveness naturally varies
according to the prevalence of VD. Nevertheless, the en-
couraging results to date strongly suggest a pilot investigation, particularly as the cases diagnosed by such screenings are almost all of the asymptomatic type, and thus lead
to a reduction of the pool of infection.

Meanwhile, in areas with particularly high rates of sy-
phylis and gonorrhoea, such procedures will be insufficient
to produce major improvements. In such areas, we must take

further advantage of the epidemiological features of these
diseases. Experience from Greenland (8) has shown that a
small minority accounts for the majority of gonorrheal infections. The prevalence of undetected disease is extremely
high in this group. Control examinations a few months after
treatment have shown that 20 to 35 per cent were reinfected
(7). This is indeed a high risk group. Preventive re-exami-
nations have thus been utilized in the southern part of
Greenland for the last 3½ years (7). In spite of imported
reinfections from neighbouring areas without preventive campaigns, we have succeeded in reducing the incidence by one-
third, and the prevalence by 50 to 80 per cent. Re-examina-
tions were performed by a special team. Unfortunately, manpower and economics make it impossible to re-establish such
teams today.

Meanwhile, it should be possible to obtain equal prevention through a rationalization of control measures. Let us
consider to what extent traditional medical practice is relevant to the problem. After treatment of a patient with
syphilis, we prescribe a number of serological control examinations varying according to the stage in which the disease is diagnosed. We know that a patient recently infected with syphilis has an increased risk of being infected
with gonorrhoea because syphilis is cured if the recommended
doses of penicillin have been used. In the case of gonorrhoea, we recommend a treatment that cures around 95 per
cent of uncomplicated infections, and re-examine the patient two or three times to determine whether he is cured
or not.

To my mind, this is an irrational approach. Why not design a treatment appropriate to the sensivity pattern of
the gonococcal strains in the area, in order to ensure that
all uncomplicated infections are cured. By doing so, the
reason for control examinations will be switched to a test
for re-infection - a preventive test. Dependent on the legal provisions in a given area, we are then able to consider the time when it would be relevant to test for re-infection. A proposal for preventive measures against VD in
Greenland is currently under consideration. This proposal
is based upon the experience of preventive clinics in Greenland, together with sexological interview-studies among the
youth of Greenland (8). The principles are as follows:
1. A gonorrhoea treatment with a failure rate below 1 per
cent has been designed. The recommended therapy is either
parenteral benzyl-penicillin-natrium (5 mill. units) or
pivampicillin (2.1 g orally) combined with probenecid (1 g).

2. Regional gonococcus laboratories will be created with a capacity to serve neighbouring districts. This phase is currently in operation in Greenland.

3. A person treated for gonorrhoea will abstain from immediate control examinations or will be content with one. However, he will return for preventive examinations for gonorrhoea and syphilis 4 or 8 months later.

4. Gonococcal culture examinations will be carried out along with serological tests for cure after treatment for syphilis.

Benefits of the proposed program should include: (1) earlier diagnosis of VD from the pool of asymptomatic infections, thus limiting the dissemination of infection within a community; (2) limitation of complications and late manifestations of VD; (3) increased likelihood of revealing partially cured syphilitic infections caused by gonorrhoea treatment (4); (4) limitation in the breeding of less sensitive gonococcal strains (5, 6); (5) reduction in the prevalence and incidence of VD, perhaps by 50 per cent or more, without an increase in the load on manpower and budgets.

The proposal has two major psychological benefits. First, examinations can be performed by the local primary health workers. Secondly, the target groups, through their co-operation in the project, will be the ones who improve control and reduce the risk of infection for other youngsters.

Although designed for Greenland, these ideas may have relevance to VD control in other areas suffering from the impact of extreme development.

SUMMARY

Public Health measures against gonorrhoea and syphilis should take into account that lack of symptoms are an outstanding feature of both diseases. For this reason, preventive screehing procedures should be extended. A preventive scheme currently proposed for Greenland (7) may have practical application in other areas. The following advantages of the proposal may be listed:

1. Earlier diagnosis of VD from the pool of asymptomatic infections, thus limiting the extent of complicated or late manifestations.

2. Increased likelihood of detecting partially cured syphilitic infections caused by gonorrhoea treatment.

3. Limited breeding of less sensitive gonococcal strains.

4. Reductions in the prevalence and incidence of VD without increasing the load on manpower and budgets.

On the basis of previous experience, a 50 per cent reduction in the incidence of VD in Greenland may be anticipated when the proposal has been implemented for two years.

REFERENCES

1. Blount, B.A., "A new approach for gonorrhoea epidemiology," Am. J. Publ. Health, 62: 710-12 (1972)
2. Handsfield, H.H., Lipman, T.O., Harnisch, J.P., Tronca, E.T., and Holmes, K.K., "Asymptomatic gonorrhoea in men," New Engl. J. Med., 290: 117-23 (1974)
3. Lee, T.Y., Utidjian, H.M.D., Singh, B., and Cutler, J.C., "Potential impact of chemical prophylaxis on the incidence of gonorrhoea," Brit. J. vener. Dis., 48: 376-80 (1972)
4. Olsen, G., "Consumption of antibiotics in Greenland, 1964-1970, II.   Effect of coincidental administration of antibiotics on early syphilitic infections," Brit. J. vener. Dis., 49: 27-9 (1973)
5. Olsen, G.A., "III. Effect of coincidental administration of antibiotics on gonorrhoeal infections," Brit J. vener. Dis., 49: 30-2 (1973)
6. Olsen, G.A., "IV. Changes in the sensitivity of N. Gonorrhoeae to antibiotics," Brit. J. vener. Dis., 49: 33-41 (1973)
7. Olsen, G.A., "Epidemiological measures against gonorrhoea. Experience in Greenland," Brit. J. vener. Dis., 49: 130-4 (1973)
8. Olsen, G.A., "Sexual behaviour among the youth of Greenland, sociomedical aspects" (English summary) (Copenhagen, Denmark: Institute of social medicine, publ. 4, 1974)
9. Pariser, H., and Marino, A.F., "Gonorrhoea - frequently unrecognized reservoir," Southern Med. J., 63: 198-201 (1970)

Cannikin nuclear explosion: human surveillance

CAROLYN V. BROWN

In November 1971 the Atomic Energy Commission (AEC) carried
out a five-megaton underground nuclear explosion at Amchitka Island (Figure 1). Two previous explosions took place on
Amchitka, (equivalent to 80,000 tons of TNT) in 1965 and
1969 (one megaton).

It was thus decided to assess the radioactive burden of
Cesium-137, Strontium-90, Tritium, and Iron-55 among the
native people of Atka, a small island about 200 miles from
Amchitka. About 85 Alaskan native people of Aleut heritage
live in Atka. Their ages range from infancy to over 75
years. The main livelihood is from fishing, and over 75 per
cent of their food comes "from the land." The only non-Aleut
people are school teachers, whose term of duty varies from
one to two years. The island is visited monthly by a US
Navy tug carrying mail, supplies, and passengers. Medical
care is provided by a Community Health Aide trained by the
Alaska Area Native Health Service Community Health Aide Program. Itinerant visits are made by the Alaska Department of
Health and Social Services Public Health Nurse and by the
US Public Health Service physician. Emergency and evacuation
care is provided by the US Navy, based at the nearby island
of Adak. Measurements of radionuclides were made prior to
the Cannikin explosion in September 1971, and again about
one year after the explosion, in order to determine if the
people nearest Amchitka carried a radioactive burden different from other groups located elsewhere in the United
States.

METHODOLOGY

Urine and blood samples were collected from 53 people currently on Atka in September 1971. The urine samples were
tested for Cesium-137 and Tritium. Blood samples were tested for Iron-55, and all teeth extracted by the itinerant
US Public Health Service dentist were submitted for assay of
Strontium-90. Patients were questioned whether they wore a
watch with an illuminated dial to obviate false recordings
in Tritium levels. Blood samples were centrifuged and serum
taken from the clot. All samples were then mailed air express to an analytical laboratory in Las Vegas. Immediately

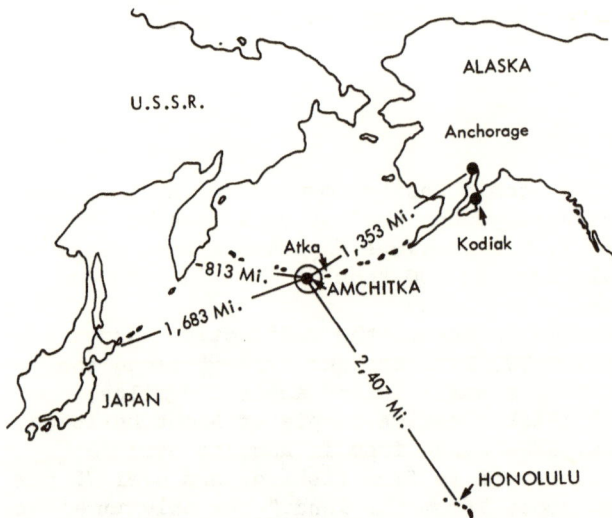

Figure 1   Site of Cannikin explosion, Amchitka, Alaska

prior to the Cannikin explosion, the people at Atka also
participated in whole body counting for radioactivity (1).
One year after the explosion, a repeat assessment was made
of blood and urine from 37 of the Atka people previously
tested. At this time a determination was made of the relative amounts of food obtained "from the land" and from the
local store. The indigenous foods eaten were reindeer, seal,
crabs, clams, halibut, salmon, trout, bass, Japanese perch,
ptarmigan, duck, goose, eider duck eggs, petruska and moss-
berries. At this point, 36 people from Akhiok, a village
some distance between Anchorage and Atka, were invited to
participate in the testing for radionuclides. Akhiok is on
the southern point of Kodiak Island, and has a population
of about 130 Aleuts. The people have a fishing economy and
obtain some of their food "from the land." This village was
chosen to determine whether relative distances from Amchitka altered the radioactive burden.

   Lastly, 33 persons who visited a hospital out-patient
department in Anchorage were invited to participate in the
testing. Anchorage is a cosmopolitan city of 160,000 people,
with commodities available to other American cities of
similar size. There is minimal opportunity to gather food
"from the land." We selected every tenth person who came to
the out-patient desk (a) who was of at least one-quarter
native heritage, (b) who did not have an acute illness,

(c) who had lived in Anchorage at least one year, and (d) who agreed to participate in the testing. Reports of the findings to date have been given to the village council and people of Atka and Akhiok.

RESULTS

Results of urine analyses for Cesium-137 and Tritium in September 1971 and October 1972 indicate radioactive burdens similar to those of persons from near the Western Environmental Research Laboratory testing area in Nevada, with no significant elevations of either Cesium-137 or Tritium. The Strontium-90 analysis of teeth has yet to be completed.

In 1971, the people of Atka had slightly elevated Iron-55 levels compared to known norms. However, the deviations were extremely small relative to the maximum allowable concentration as presently understood. There was no significant difference in the Iron-55 levels of Atka people between 1971 and 1972. Lower levels of Iron-55 were found in Akhiok and even lower levels in Anchorage. We think this may be due to diet. The people at Atka ate more than 75 per cent of their food "from the land." At Akhiok, the proportion was approximately one-half, and in Anchorage about 25 per cent.

DISCUSSION

There is no evidence to date that the people of Atka, Akhiok, or Anchorage have a dangerously increased radioactive loading of their bodies. This is consistent with AEC reports that the Cannikin vault has been contained with no leakage of radioactivity.

The small increase in Iron-55 among the people tested may imply that food eaten "from the land" has had more exposure to atmospheric "fallout" from previous tests. The high levels of Iron-55 among salmon in the Pacific Northwest ocean has not yet been clarified (2). Nevertheless, the consumption of fish at Atka and Akhiok (and less in Anchorage) may account for the small but significant elevation of Iron-55 levels among those persons tested.

Further investigation of the elevated Iron-55 in fish would seem appropriate. As atmospheric detonations decrease in frequency, it will also be of value to follow the high levels of these radionuclides among the people of Alaska.

SUMMARY

The Cannikin nuclear explosion was a five-megaton underground explosion conducted by the US Atomic Energy Commission
(AEC) on Amchitka Island on 6 November 1971. This report
concerns blood and urine surveillance of people at Atka, the
closest native village to Amchitka (200 miles). Three weeks
before the explosion, blood and urine samples from 53 of 85
natives were analysed for Cesium-137, Fe-55, and Tritium. An
estimate was also made of the amount of indigenous foods
used by the people. One year later, tests were repeated on
35 of the initially sampled population of Atka, and 35 people
on Kodiak Island were similarly tested. As controls, 35 native out-patients without acute disease were tested at an Anchorage hospital. Levels of the radionuclides tested did not
approach dangerous levels as presently understood. The relationship between radionuclide levels and consumption of indigenous foods requires further study.

REFERENCES

1. Fort, C.W., and Wruble, D.T., Off-site radiological safety
   for the Cannikin event November 6, 1971. US Atomic Energy
   Commission. US Environmental Protection Agency (Las Vegas,
   Nevada, September 1972), pp. 1-25
2. Jenkins, C.E., "Radionuclide distribution in Pacific salmon," Health Physics, 17: 507-12 (1969)

The significance of reports of mercury in
various body tissues

A.D. BERNSTEIN

When I first became involved in the mercury situation we
were confronted by headlines such as "MERCURY POISONS FOUR
CREE INDIANS. Four Cree Indians from a northern Quebec reserve recently spent one week in Montreal's Queen Mary
Veterans' hospital where they were treated for mercury
poisoning." This, of course, was not the case. The four

Indians concerned were investigated for possible mercury
poisoning. Blood mercury levels were "elevated," but no clinical signs were found. As a matter of fact, Canada has no
proven case of organic mercury poisoning from eating fish.

Population investigations have now been carried out in
three areas of Canada to evaluate the effects of environmental organic mercury, in northwest Quebec (1), in northwest
Ontario (4), and in northwest Canada (2).

Our investigation in northwest Quebec was initiated in
1971 as the result of an ecological study carried out by
some university students. In studying the effluents from a
pulp and paper plant on the Bell-Nottaway river system, the
students noted fish mercury levels ranging to three parts
per million (ppm). They then tested the blood of 29 Waswani-
pi Indians from the communities of Matagami and Miquelon,
downstream on this river system, and noted whole blood mercury levels ranging to 135 parts per billion (ppb), with an
average level of 55 ppb.

It was thus felt necessary to carry out more extensive
testing in the area. It had been reported that the mercury
content of fish in Mistassini Lake, northeast of the Was-
wanipi area, was also quite high, so that some testing was
also carried out among the Mistassini band of Indians.
Field test results were summarized in Table 1. Altogether,
over 300 persons of all ages had blood samples drawn for

TABLE 1
Results of field tests in northwestern Quebec

	Matagami, Waswanipi Band	Miquelon, Waswanipi Band	Mistassini, Mistassini Band
Blood mercury			
No. of persons tested	79	141	181
No. with >100 ppb	10	3	9
Highest value recorded	306 ppb	148 ppb	155 ppb
Mean	41.0 ppb	21.6 ppb	36.8 ppb
Hair mercury			
No. of persons treated	11*	56*	
Highest value recorded	44.9 ppm		
No. of physical examinations	49 full**	69 screening 29 full*	None
No. of electromyograms and maze performance tests	11**	56**	None
No. of visual field examinations	8**	None	19*

* r = 0.82 with blood values.
** No significant findings.

mercury determinations by atomic absorption. Twenty-two had
whole blood mercury levels greater than 100 ppb, and the
highest reading was 306 ppb. Many of these individuals also
had hair specimens collected for mercury determination by
an atomic absorption method. There was a good correlation
(0.82) between hair and whole blood mercury levels.

Approximately half these people had clinical testing
done, 78 undergoing complete history and physical examinations, and 69 undergoing a screening battery of simple tests
for neurological dysfunction. Sixty-seven persons also underwent electromyography and maze performance testing. There
were no clinical findings suggestive of organic mercury excess.

There was some relationship between an individual's stated fish consumption and his blood mercury level. Individuals with blood levels over 100 ppb admitted to fish consumption more than once per week, whereas the majority of
individuals stated that their fish consumption was once per
week or less. However, the value of such statements was reduced, since the group had previously been warned to reduce
their fish consumption. More significantly, children who had
attended schools in towns away from home for the previous
two years or more had whole blood mercury levels of 0, with
one exception who had a whole blood mercury level of 21 ppb.

In the second phase of this investigation, five individuals from Matagami, four of whom had previously demonstrated blood mercury levels of greater than 100 ppb, underwent
extensive evaluation at the Montreal Neurological Hospital
(Table 2). In addition to routine hospital tests, detailed
neurological examinations, electromyograms, nerve conduction
studies, electroencephalograms, audiograms, visual field

TABLE 2
Mercury levels of five Indians from Matagami, P.Q., admitted to
Montreal Neurological Hospital between 8 and 11 February 1972

Subject No.	Birth date	Blood mercury level (ppb)			Hair mercury level (ppm)
		June 1971	Aug. 1971	Feb. 1972	Feb. 1972
1	1914	227 rbc 17 plasma	187	43	29.2
2	1921	-	306	105	58.7
3	1909	73	127	23	20.8
4	1933	-	172	111	49.6
5	1895	-	-	11	16.8

determinations, blood cytogenetic studies, and blood and
hair mercury level determinations were carried out. Again,
there were no clinical findings suggestive of organic mercury excess.

More detailed studies of fish subsequently revealed mercury levels ranging to a maximum of 4.44 ppm in the Waswani-
pi area and to 0.84 ppm in the Mistassini area (unpublished
data, Environment Canada).

In northwest Ontario, attention was focused on the Ojib-
way Indian communities of Grassy Narrows and White Dog, located downstream of a pulp and paper complex and a chlor-
alkali plant on the Wabigoon-English River system. In these
waterways, fish mercury levels of 27 ppm have been reported
(3). In one lake, the average mercury levels of burbot were
reported as more than 12 ppm (unpublished data, Ontario
Ministry of Natural Resources). These levels are considerably higher than those found in most other waterways serving traditional native communities in Canada.

Blood mercury levels in these communities for the years
1970 and 1972-73 were higher than in those of northwest
Quebec (Table 3).

In the spring of 1973, six individuals with blood mercury levels greater than 100 ppb (Table 4) underwent evaluation at the Health Sciences Centre in Winnipeg. The evaluation was similar to that carried out at the Montreal Neurological Hospital, except that it included more extensive
biochemical testing, and electronystagmographic studies.
Again, no evidence of mercury intoxication was found.

The Ontario Ministry of Health recommended that fish
from the Wabigoon-English River system not be eaten. Despite this, fish still are consumed regularly by many in
these communities, according to information volunteered by
residents. A federal task force (4) felt that the most
serious consequences of the mercury situation lay in the
economic, social, and cultural fields, and they recommended
that a program of socio-economic development for the two
communities be instituted as a matter of priority.

A third study in northwest Canada determined whole blood
mercury levels in small samples of persons living in selected communities of British Columbia, Alberta, the Yukon,
and the western part of the Northwest Territories between
August 1972 and March 1973 (Table 5). Levels tended to be
low in British Columbia, Alberta, and the Yukon; in the
western part of the Northwest Territories they were somewhat higher, but still essentially within acceptable limits.

TABLE 3
Comparison of blood mercury levels for northwestern Ontario and north-western Quebec

Community	No. of persons tested	No. > 100 ppb	Highest value recorded (ppb)	Mean (ppb)
White Dog, Ont.				
1970	35	3	159	46.4
1972-73	70	7	289	52.0
Grassy Narrows, Ont.				
1970	61	17	385	77.4
1972-73	49	12	222	62.5
Matagami, P.Q.				
1971	76	8	306	44
Miquelon, P.Q.				
1971	146	3	148	21.5
Mistassini, P.Q.				
1971	198	9	155	36.7

TABLE 4
Mercury levels in six Indians investigated in Winnipeg
(clinical examination in spring of 1973)

	January 1973 ppb Hg(total), blood	Spring 1973* ppb Hg (total), blood	ppm Hg, hair
Case 1	107	78	45
Case 2	126	55	22
Case 3	172	82	24
Case 4	125	46	20
Case 5	289	91	43
Case 6	126	162	24

* May or June.

Data soon to be reported on levels in Saskatchewan are consistent with figures for British Columbia and Alberta (C.A.R. Dennis, personal communication). The reasons for the higher levels in the Northwest Territories are not readily apparent, but are being looked into by Environment Canada. It is known, however, that in the Northwest Territories special efforts were made to test individuals who spent much time outside of their settlement, fishing, hunting, and trapping. However, in Fort Liard those who spent much time away from their settlement were "out in the bush" when testing was carried out. Thus the individuals tested there were "urbanized" and probably relied mainly on

TABLE 5
Average levels of mercury (ppb) in each community
(T, target; C, control)

Community	Mercury average	No. of blood samples	
Alberta			
Ft. McKay	7.64	20	T
Janvier	14.22	20	T
Conklin	9.00	20	T
Beaver Lake	7.97	20	T
Saddle and Frog	9.59	24	T
Gift Lake (Whitefish)	5.98	20	C
McLeod River	5.30	20	T
British Columbia			
Squamish	5.45	20	T
N. Vancouver	5.02	20	C
Pemberton	6.15	21	C
Masset	7.27	20	T
Metlakatla	8.75	14	T
Kitselas	5.75	6	C
Kitsumkalem	6.56	13	C
Kitimat	8.23	16	T
Hazleton	5.91	22	T
Tachie	10.89	22	T
Takla	10.42	20	T
Necoslie	11.47	20	T
Lilloett	6.57	22	T
Lower Nicola	6.20	20	T
St. Mary's	5.03	21	T
Trail	5.98	20	C
Aquatsino	6.14	19	T
Ucluelet	7.43	20	T
Ladysmith	9.54	14	T
The Yukon			
Dawson	5.24	22	T
Old Crow	5.61	22	T
Whitehorse	9.37	20	C
Carcross	7.57	10	T
Burwash	11.57	10	T
Carmacks	9.34	20	T
The Northwest Territories			
Aklavik	16.37	20	T
Tuktoyaktuk	37.76	20	T
Holman	34.01	23	T
Coppermine	19.39	20	T
Yellowknife	14.80	21	C
Detah	20.76	3	T
Ft. Rae	15.00	19	T
Snowdrift	20.79	23	T
Fort Franklin	34.79	12	T
Fort Liard	6.86	15	T

store-bought foods. Fort Liard had the lowest average mercury level of any Northwest Territory community. The Yukon
communities were tested before those of the Northwest Territories, and there is some uncertainty as to the type of individual generally sampled in these communities.

All of the above investigations are generally consistent
with testing carried out in other countries (5, 6). We may
thus conclude that: (1) in northern Canada, some moderately
elevated blood mercury levels have been found; (2) there is
a relationship between fish consumption and mercury levels;
(3) no clinical findings suggestive of organic mercury excess have been detected; (4) Grassy Narrows and White Dog,
Ontario, deserve special attention and are, in fact, at the
centre of clinical surveillance measures for mercury in
Canada.

DISCUSSION

Could it be that by eating sufficient fish or other "native
foods," one may sustain somewhat elevated tissue mercury
levels? Can it also be that such levels are tolerated through
adaptation or interaction? An example of the latter phenomenon would involve selenium, which is found in significant
amounts in certain species of fish such as tuna; ingestion
of selenium can modify the toxic effects of mercury.

Several years ago, "high" levels of mercury were found in
the livers of seals caught near Rankin Inlet, NWT. Eskimos
in that area, who apparently considered raw seal liver a
delicacy, were advised not to eat the liver. Now, however,
it is known that the greater part of mercury in liver is inorganic, which is significantly less toxic than the methylmercury found in fish. It appears that the seal has an enzyme system that degrades methylmercury to inorganic mercury.

In the future, great caution must be exercised in making
pronouncements on practical matters such as fish consumption on the basis of laboratory findings alone. Fish is an
extremely important source of protein for many native Canadians and fishing is a significant component of their traditional way of life. More attention must be paid to the individual than to his laboratory results.

ACKNOWLEDGMENTS

Blood analyses were performed by the Federal Fisheries and
Forestry Department, Montreal, and hair analyses, electromyography, and maze testing by the University of Michigan.

SUMMARY

In northwestern Quebec, over 300 Indians from Matagami,
Miquelon, and Mistassini had blood mercury determinations
carried out. Field clinical testing was completed on approximately half this number. Twenty-two individuals had blood
mercury levels greater than 100 ppb, the highest being 306
ppb. There were no clinical findings suggestive of organic
mercury excess; however, there appeared to be a relationship between fish consumption and blood mercury levels. Five
residents of Matagami, four of whom had previously shown
blood mercury levels greater than 100 ppb, subsequently
underwent extensive hospital evaluation. No significant
clinical findings were detected. In addition, six Indians
from Grassy Narrows and White Dog, Ontario, all with blood
mercury levels greater than 100 ppb, underwent similar extensive hospital evaluation. Again, there was no evidence of
organic mercury intoxication. Blood levels of mercury were
determined in small samples of persons living in various
communities of northwest Canada. Levels were low in British
Columbia, Alberta, and the Yukon; although somewhat higher
in the Northwest Territories, they remained essentially
within acceptable limits.

REFERENCES

1. Bernstein, A.D., "Clinical investigation in Northwest
   Quebec, Canada, of environmental organic mercury effects,"
   Presented at International Symposium: Recent Advances in
   the Assessment of the Health Effects of Environmental
   Pollution, Paris, 24-28 June 1974 (proceedings to be
   published)
2. Environment Research Consultants Ltd., Level of Mercury
   in the Blood of Persons Living in Selected Communities
   in Alberta, British Columbia, the Yukon and Northwest
   Territories (North Vancouver, British Columbia, 1973)
3. Fimreite, N., and Reynolds, L.M., "Mercury contamination
   of fish in Northwest Ontario," J. Wildlife Management,
   37: 62-8 (1973)

4. Final Report, Task Force on Organic Mercury in the Environment: Grassy Narrows and White Dog, Ontario (Ottawa:
Health and Welfare Canada, 1973)
5. Skerfving, S., "Methylmercury exposure, mercury levels in
blood and hair, and health status in Swedes consuming contaminated fish," Toxicology, 2: 3-23 (1974)
6. den Tonkelaar, E.M., Van Esch, G.T., Hofman, B.,
Schuller, P.L., and Zwiers, T.H.L., "Mercury and other
elements in blood of the Dutch population," Presented at
International Symposium: Recent Advances in the Assessment of the Health Effects of Environmental Pollution,
Paris, 24-28 June 1974 (proceedings to be published)

Mercury content of Iglooligmiut hair

M. HENDZEL, JUDITH E. SAYED, O. SCHAEFER, and J.A. HILDES

Because there is little information on mercury residues in
hair, particularly in northern populations, it was decided
to analyse samples from an Eskimo population located at
Igloolik, NWT (69° 10' N latitude, 83° 59' W longitude).
An initial 28 samples were analysed for total mercury and,
in addition, for selenium, because of the relationship between these two elements (1). The Freshwater Institute
regularly analyses fish products for both selenium and mercury, but the methods used were thought suitable for hair.
It was thus agreed to test the reliability of the mercury
method by collaborating with another laboratory able to
perform neutron activation analysis. Mercury data obtained
on the first 28 samples proved interesting and an additional
104 samples were analysed. Selenium data, however, could not
be correlated with corresponding mercury levels and selenium analyses were thus terminated after completion of the 28
samples.

METHOD

The method of mercury analyses used was "cold vapour"
flameless atomic absorption. A 80 to 120 mg sample of hair
was weighed into a graduated digestion tube and a mixture

of 1 ml concentrated nitric, 4 ml concentrated sulphuric, and 0.5 ml of fuming nitric acid was added. Standards (100, 200, 300, 400 ng of Hg as $HgCl_2$) and two reagent blanks were prepared at this time and taken through the entire procedure with the samples. The tubes containing samples, standards, and blanks were placed in an aluminum block which was heated to 170° C and maintained at this temperature overnight to effect digestion. When digestion was complete, that is the samples were clear and colourless, they were removed from the block, cooled, and brought to a constant volume (25 ml) with distilled water.

The analysis from this point on was essentially that of Armstrong and Uthe (2). The instrument used was a Perkin Elmer 403 Atomic Absorption Spectrophotometer fitted with a mercury lamp and flowthrough cell. An aliquot of the sample was mixed with reductant solution, ionic mercury being reduced to the atomic state with stannous sulphate and partitioned into the gaseous phase. This phase passed into the flowthrough cell and absorbed an amount of light from the mercury lamp proportional to the amount of mercury in the sample. Necessary dilutions used a 4:1 mixture of water and acid to ensure that the matrix of the samples closely approximated that of the standards.

Selenium was determined by fluorometry, using the method of Hoffman, Westerby, and Hideroglou (3). Sample weights of 60 to 400 mg were used.

The majority of samples used in this study were washed, using a non-ionic detergent, air-dried, and desiccated prior to analysis. Sample size allowed 23 samples to be re-analysed for mercury on an "as received" basis. The mean mercury content of washed samples was approximately 8 per cent higher than that of unwashed samples, a finding similar to that of a previous study (4). Although the difference between washed and unwashed samples was statistically significant, it was not considered biologically significant. Accordingly, data obtained on the "as received" samples has not been adjusted to compensate for this difference.

Twenty-two samples were analysed for mercury by neutron activation analysis. There was good agreement with atomic absorption results, although figures obtained by neutron activation were generally higher. This is quite often the tendency with neutron activation as compared with other methods (L.H. Hecker, personal communication to authors).

TABLE 1
Mercury levels in hair of male population, Igloolik, NWT

Age group (years)	Number of samples	Mean of group (ppm)	Maximum of group (ppm)	Minimum of group (ppm)
0.5-10.5	4	5.62	9.55	2.28
10.5-20.5	5	36.4	94.7	2.70
20.5-30.5	15	15.0	38.7	3.99
30.5-40.5	11	12.3	30.9	4.37
40.5-50.5	5	8.93	13.0	5.80
50.5-60.5	8	9.16	18.3	4.98
60.5-70.5	3	7.43	8.64	6.05
70.5-80.5	1	12.0		

TABLE 2
Mercury levels in hair of female population, Igloolik, NWT

Age group (years)	Number of samples	Mean of group (ppm)	Maximum of group (ppm)	Minimum of group (ppm)
0.5-10.5	5	9.18	17.5	1.94
10.5-20.5	10	27.9	109	2.36
20.5-30.5	29	15.5	93.7	3.77
30.5-40.5	17	15.7	42.5	4.61
40.5-50.5	7	14.4	42.7	5.90
50.5-60.5	10	20.7	97.3	5.47
60.5-70.5	4	9.94	10.5	9.30

RESULTS AND DISCUSSION

Mercury was found in all 134 samples, ranging from a low of 1.94 to a high of 109 ppm. Table 1 shows data for the male population. The number of males sampled was 52, with an overall mean of 13.8 ppm. Table 2 shows data for the female population. The number of females sampled was 82, with an overall mean of 16.9 ppm. The means of both groups are higher than the US norm of 1 to 3 ppm (Hecker, personal communication) and higher than the safety limit of 6 ppm reported in a Finnish Study (5).

Figure 1 shows the distribution of the male and female populations between four arbitrary concentration groupings. Approximately 4 per cent of the Eskimos had levels greater than 60 ppm. This is considered the level at which toxic symptoms may appear (5). Maxima occurred in the 10-20 age group for males and in the 10-30 and 50-60 age groups for females.

MALE VERSUS FEMALE POPULATION

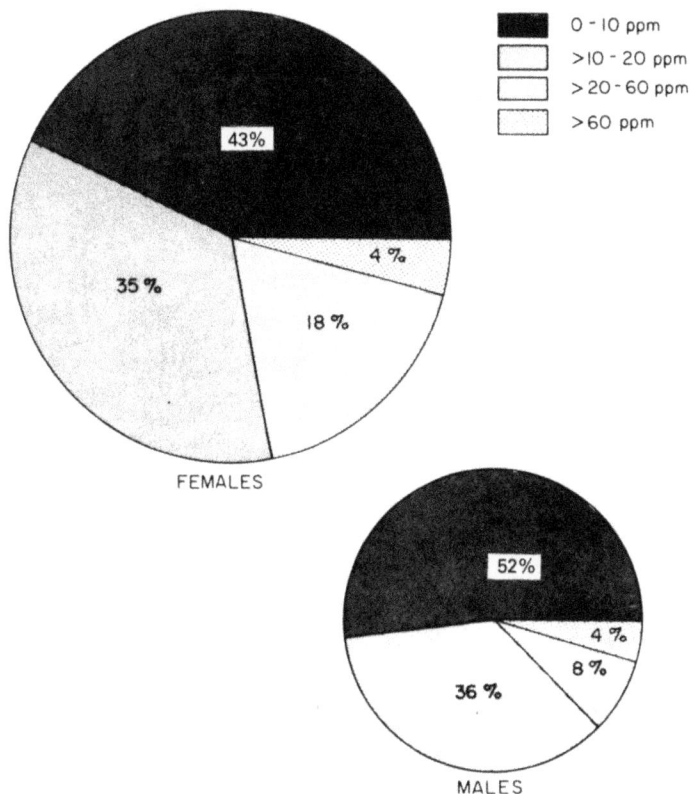

Figure 1   Distribution of male and female population according to mercury levels found in hair samples

Table 3 compares selenium and mercury data on 28 samples.
The mean selenium concentration was 2.53 ppm, with individual means of 1.15 ppm for males and 3.95 ppm for females.
Levels ranged from 0.69 to 18.5 ppm. No published data could
be found on selenium levels in human hair. Five control samples were thus analysed (4 males, 1 female); the mean was
0.90 ppm for the males (range from 0.75 to 1.11 ppm), with
a result of 0.77 ppm for the female. There was no apparent
relationship between mercury and selenium levels and selenium analyses were thus terminated.

It is difficult to explain the high mercury levels found
in this study. Information is not available as to the mercury content of the foods consumed by Iglooligmiuts.

TABLE 3
Mercury and selenium content of hair,
Igloolik, NWT

Age (years) and sex	Hg level (ppm)	Se level (ppm)
66 M	7.59	1.46
63 M	8.64	1.66
58 M	4.98	0.74
55 M	7.41	0.84
48 M	13.0	0.90
42 M	8.39	1.93
37 M	30.9	0.90
31 M	9.84	0.91
27 M	10.8	1.26
21 M	38.7	0.88
19 M	64.7	1.41
14 M	10.5	1.26
10 M	7.89	1.01
5 M	2.75	0.96
65 F	10.5	18.5
65 F	9.54	1.19
55 F	5.85	3.28
55 F	11.9	0.76
42 F	9.02	0.69
41 F	10.9	0.99
36 F	24.3	1.72
33 F	19.2	1.04
29 F	9.38	0.91
22 F	3.45	0.83
13 F	15.1	1.18
13 F	58.9	5.27
9 F	15.5	1.37
5 F	6.81	17.5

There is a possibility of external contamination from various hair preparations, but again there is no information to substantiate this. Nor is there any known industrial mercury contamination in that region. Therefore, it may be stated that the hair of Igloolik Eskimos generally has higher levels of mercury than that of Americans but the reason for this remains unknown. Clinical data do not indicate symptoms related to mercury poisoning.

ACKNOWLEDGMENTS

Neutron activation analyses were carried out by Dr Lawrence Hecker of the University of Michigan. The authors also wish to acknowledge the assistance of A. Beal, J. Harding, and

A. Rieger with the laboratory analysis.

SUMMARY

Frontal hair from unselected male and female subjects aged
1 to 71 years was analysed for total mercury, using flameless atomic absorption, and for selenium by fluorometry. The
mean mercury concentration in 134 samples was 15.7 ppm (13.8
ppm for males, 16.9 ppm for females, with a range from 1.9
to 109 ppm). The mean selenium concentration of 28 samples
was 2.53 ppm (1.15 ppm for males, 3.95 ppm for females, with
a range from 0.69 to 18.5 ppm). Mercury levels were higher
than expected, and five subjects had readings > 60 ppm,
which is considered the level at which toxic symptoms may
appear; nevertheless, a full medical history and examination
showed no indication of mercury toxicity in any of the subjects.

REFERENCES

1. Ganther, H.E., Goudie, C., Sunde, M.L., Lopecky, M.J.,
   Wagner, P., Sang-Hwan, Oh, and Hoekstra, W.G., "Selenium:
   relation to decreased toxicity of methyl mercury added
   to diets containing tuna," Sci., 175: 1122-4 (1972)
2. Armstrong, F.A.J., and Uthe, J.F., "Semi-automated determination of mercury in animal tissue," A.A. Newsletter,
   10: 101-3 (1971)
3. Hoffman, I., Westerby, R.J., and Hideroglou, M., "Precise
   fluorometric microdetermination of selenium in agricul-
   tural materials," J.A.O.A.C., 51: 1039-42 (1968)
4. Benson, W.W., and Gabica, J., "Total mercury in hair
   from 1000 Idaho Residents - 1971," Pestic. Monit. J.,
   6 (2): 80-3 (1972)
5. Sumari, P., Partanen, T., Hietala, S., and Heinonen,
   O.P., "Blood and hair mercury content in fish consumers.
   A preliminary report," Work-environm.-hlth, 9: 61-5
   (1972)

Commentaries

"Public health engineering research in northern Canada," by Jack W. Grainge (Department of Environment, Edmonton, Canada). Distinct differences are required in public health engineering in the north, which result from a variety of factors, including the long cold winters, frost heaving soils, permafrost, and poor community planning. Design engineers who do not fully understand these complex problems usually resort to conservative engineering, which may not produce the most useful systems. Sometimes pipelines are laid above ground unnecessarily. In this position, they occupy valuable space, restrict the routing of roads and other land development, and sometimes fail to serve near-by residences with a gravity sewer. One study of particular interest concerns the excellent treatment provided to sewage effluent that is discharged to swampland. One of the most significant advances in northern public health engineering can be made in the construction of water mains and sewers.

"Sewage collection in northern Alaska," by D.R. Rogness and W.L. Ryan (Indian Health Service, Anchorage, Alaska). The Indian Health Service is a unit within the United States Public Health Service and is responsible for improving the health of all Indians and Alaskan natives in the United States. As part of this program, the Sanitation Facilities Construction Branch of the Indian Health Service's Office of Environmental Health plans, designs, and constructs water, sewer, and refuse facilities in Indian communities and Alaskan native villages. Since the beginning of the construction program in 1959, community sewer systems have been constructed in over 40 native villages throughout Alaska. In constructing these systems, particularly in arctic areas, many unique problems are encountered. Four completely different types of sewer systems have been used by the Indian Health Service in Alaskan native villages: conventional gravity systems, pressurized systems, vacuum systems, and haul systems. The conventional gravity system has been modified by using insulated pipes and manholes and providing automatic flushing devices at deadends or other sections with low flow where freezing might occur. The pressure sewage collection system lends itself well to frost-susceptible areas where shifting of pipes might cause reverse grades in

a conventional system. The vacuum sewage collection system
has the attractive characteristics of the pressure system
and the additional advantages of very low water use and
lower operating costs. Haul systems are used mainly in areas
where economic conditions prevent the construction of any
type of piped system. An evaluation to determine which type
of system to use in a particular situation must include detailed assessment of the physical and economic conditions
under which the system will operate.

"Hygienic evaluation of climatic conditions in Far Northern
settlements and problems of urban planning," by A.P.
Shitskova and L.F. Tulyakova (Moscow Erisman Institute of
USSR). In developing scientific foundations for the optimi-
zation of living conditions of the Far Northern population
a significant place is taken by hygienic criteria of urban
planning. Studies have primarily been carried out in Norilsk.
Techniques of physiological-hygienic investigation have made
it possible to evaluate climatic conditions by changes of
human physiological functions, in particular thermoregula-
tion. Comparison of meteorological and physiological data
shows that strong winds account for most significant discomfort. The investigation has established easily tolerable
conditions and uncomfortable conditions for different coefficients of anti-wind protection. Comparison of the above
findings with actual speeds of winds has helped in choosing
the most effective types of building in terms of wind protection: small settlements where houses are erected closely
along the perimeter without gaps between them, or blocks of
dwelling houses overlapping each other producing an obstacle
for winds. In the above types of settlements there are 67%
of easily tolerable combinations of air temperature and wind
speed, which gives six months of easily tolerable weather
conditions out of nine months of cold.

"Persistence of human faecal-borne bacteria on the tundra,"
by L.A. White and M.R. Spence (Defence Research Establishment Suffield, Ralston, Alberta, Canada). The staging and
bivouac areas employed by Canadian Forces Exercise New
Viking at Ft. Churchill, Manitoba, were examined for evidence of fouling of ground by human excrement and bacteria
normally present in the excrement. One major bivouac area,
near Stygge Lake, was studied in detail. Examination of
latrine sites, both on and beneath the surface, indicated

that weathering, at least over the subarctic summer and a
portion of the winter, does not result in complete elimination of the groups of microbes employed as indicators of
human faecal pollution (total and faecal coliforms and
faecal streptococci). Runoff from latrine sites apparently
does not cause additional fouling of ground.

"Assessment of the potential health hazard in accumulations
of mercury in Alaskan marine mammals," by William A. Galster
(Institute of Arctic Biology, University of Alaska, Fairbanks). Accumulations of mercury frequently exceed safety
standards by as much as a hundredfold in the tissues of the
fur seal, harbour seal, and polar bear and less frequently
in the sea lion, ringed seal, walrus, and bearded seal in
seas near Alaska. The potential health problems are assessed
through observation of absorption, transport, accumulation,
and excretion in mink. Differences in tissue concentrations
in populations of marine mammals in waters near northern
and southern Alaska and Siberia are used to implicate areas
of apparently high geological input of mercury.

LIST OF CONTRIBUTORS

Adler-Nissen, J.: Institute of Hygiene, University of Copenhagen, Copenhagen, Denmark

Allen, C.: Defence and Civil Institute of Environmental Medicine, P.O. Box 2000, Downsview, Ont., Canada

Andersen, K.L.: International Biological Program, Human Adaptability Project, Scandinavian Section, Oslo, Norway

Andersson, R.: Department of Medicine, Örnsköldsviks Hospital, Örnsköldsvik, Sweden

Armbrust, J.M.: U.S. Public Health Service, Alaska Area Native Health, Tanana Service Unit, Fairbanks, Alaska, USA

Atcheson, J.D.: Clarke Institute of Psychiatry, Toronto, Canada

Bang, H.O.: Clinical Chemical Department, Aalborg Hospital North, Aalborg, Denmark

Baxter, J.D.: Department of Otolaryngology, McGill University, Montreal, Canada

Berg, Lisbet: School Medical Service, County of Copenhagen, Denmark

Berg, O.: Institute of Hygiene, University of Copenhagen, Copenhagen, Denmark

Bernstein, A.D.: Health and Welfare Canada, Medical Services, Ottawa, Canada

Berry, J.W.: Department of Psychology, Queen's University, Kingston, Canada

Bloom, J.D.: Langdon Psychiatric Clinic, Anchorage, Alaska, USA

Boesen, E.M.: Sundhedsmedhjaelperskolen, boks 601, Godthåb, Greenland

Brett, B.: Northern Medical Services, Health and Welfare Canada, Edmonton, Canada

Brodovsky, D.: Northern Medical Unit, University of Manitoba, Winnipeg, Canada

Brown, Carolyn V.: Alaska Area Native Health Service, Box 7-741, Anchorage, Alaska, USA

Brown, G.W.: 3140 Wesleyan Drive, Anchorage, Alaska, USA

Bryngelsson, C.: Department of Radiology, University of Helsinki, Finland

Cameron, D.G.: Montreal General Hospital, Montreal, Canada
Cass, E. Elizabeth: Box 688, Fort Smith, NWT, Canada
Charlton, K.M.: Animal Pathology Division, Agriculture
   Canada, Animal Diseases Research Institute, Ottawa,
   Canada
Cooper, K.E.: Division of Medical Physiology, University of
   Alberta, Calgary, Canada

Draper, H.H.: Department of Food Science, University of
   Illinois at Urbana-Champaign, Urbana, Ill., USA
Duchek, M.: Department of Urology, University of Umeå, Umeå,
   Sweden (Present address: Department of Urology,
   Karolinska Sjukhuset, Stockholm, Sweden)
Dyerberg, J.: Clinical Chemical Department, Aalborg Hospital
   North, Aalborg, Denmark

Edgren, J.: Department of Radiology, IVth Department of
   Medicine, Helsinki University Central Hospital, Helsinki,
   Finland
Eidus, L.: Bureau of Bacteriological Diseases, Laboratory
   Centre for Disease Control, Health and Welfare Canada,
   Ottawa, Canada
Eriksson, A.W.: Institute of Human Genetics, Free University
   of Amsterdam, Amsterdam, The Netherlands
Eskola, M.-R.: Folkhälsan Institute of Genetics, Population
   Genetics Unit, Helsinki, Finland

Falkmer, S.: Department of Pathology, University of Umeå,
   Umeå, Sweden
Feigin, R.A.: Department of Mental Health Sciences,
   Hahnemann Medical College, Philadelphia, Pa., USA
Fellman, J.: Folkhälsan Institute of Genetics, Population
   Genetics Unit, Helsinki, Finland
Ferrari, Harriet E.: Regional Nursing Officer, NWT Region
   Medical Services, Health and Welfare Canada, Edmonton,
   Canada
Finell, B.: Nordic Council for Arctic Medical Research,
   Oulu, Finland (Present address: Muurola Hospital, Toton-
   vaara, Finland)
Fish, D.G.: Department of Social and Preventive Medicine,
   University of Manitoba, Winnipeg, Canada
Fitzgerald, E.J.: Department of Radiology, Charles Camsell
   Hospital, Edmonton, Canada
Forsius, H.: Department of Ophthalmology, University of
   Oulu, Oulu, Finland
Forsius, Harriet: Department of Paediatrics, University of
   Oulu, Oulu, Finland

Freedman, D.K.: Division of Public Health, Department of
Health and Social Services, Pouch H06, Juneau, Alaska,
USA
Freeman, R.S.: Department of Parasitology, School of Hy-
giene, University of Toronto, Toronto, Canada
Fugelli, P.: Institute of Work Physiology, Oslo, Norway

Godin, G.: Department of Environmental Health, School of Hy-
giene, University of Toronto, Toronto, Canada
Granberg, P.O.: Urological Research Laboratory, Karolinska
Sjukhuset, Stockholm, Sweden
Greidanus, P.: Northern Medical Research Unit, Medical Ser-
vices, Health and Welfare Canada, Edmonton, Canada
Grzybowski, S.: Department of Medicine, University of
British Columbia, Vancouver, Canada

Hansen, J.P. Hart: University Institute of Pathological Ana-
tomy, Copenhagen, Denmark
Hansson, Hasse: Department of Prosthetic Dentistry, Faculty
of Odontology, University of Göteborg, Göteborg, Sweden
Haraldson, S.S.R.: Department of Education and Training,
Scandinavian School of Public Health, Göteborg, Sweden
Harvald, B.J.: Medical Department B, Odense University Hos-
pital, Odense, Denmark
Harvey, Elinor B.: P.O. Box 1427, Juneau, Alaska, USA
Hasunen, K.: Department of Nutrition, University of Helsin-
ki, Helsinki, Finland
Hendzel, M.: Freshwater Institute, 501 University Crescent,
Winnipeg, Canada
Hildes, J.A.: Northern Medical Unit, University of Manitoba,
Winnipeg, Canada
Hjørne, N.: Clinical Chemical Department, Aalborg Hospital
North, Aalborg, Denmark
Hobart, C.W.: Department of Sociology, University of Alberta,
Edmonton, Canada
Hodgkin, M.M.: Bureau of Bacteriological Diseases, Labora-
tory Centre for Disease Control, Health and Welfare
Canada, Ottawa, Canada
Hofer, P.-Å.: Department of Pathology, University of Umeå,
Umeå, Sweden
Holubowsky, M.: NWT Region, Medical Services, Health and
Welfare Canada, Edmonton, Canada

Isokoski, M.: Department of Public Health Sciences, University of Tampere, Tampere, Finland

Itoh, S.: Shionogi Research Institute, Fukushima-ku, Osaka, Japan

Jamieson, J.: Department of Parasitology, School of Hygiene, University of Toronto, Toronto, Canada
Jamison, P.L.: Department of Anthropology, Indiana University, Bloomington, Ind., and US/IBP Human Adaptability Coordinating Office, The Pennsylvania State University, University Park, Pa., USA

Katz, S.H.: Departments of Orthodontics and Anthropology, University of Pennsylvania; W.M. Krogman Center for Research in Child Growth and Development; and Eastern Pennsylvania Psychiatric Institute
Kaznacheyev, V.P.: Siberian Branch of the Academy of Medical Science, Novosibirsk, USSR
Kirjarinta, M.: Folkhälsan Institute of Genetics, Population Genetics Unit, Helsinki, Finland
Koch, E.A.: Department of Radiology, Charles Camsell Hospital, Edmonton, Canada
Kraus, R.F.: Department of Psychiatry and Behavioral Sciences, School of Medicine, University of Washington, Seattle, Wash., USA

Lehmann, W.: Institute of Human Genetics, University of Kiel, Kiel, W. Germany
Leung, D.: Northern Medical Research Unit, Medical Services, Health and Welfare Canada, Edmonton, Canada
Lewin, T.: Institute of Human Anatomy, University of Göteborg, Göteborg, Sweden
Linderholm, H.: Department of Clinical Physiology, University of Umeå, Umeå, Sweden
Ling, D.: School of Human Communication Disorders, McGill University, Montreal, Canada
Lobban, Mary C.: University Medical Clinic, Montreal General Hospital, Montreal, Canada (Present address: Clinical Research Centre, Harrow, Middlesex, England)
Lozovoy, V.P.: Siberian Branch of the Academy of Medical Sciences, Institute for Clinical and Experimental Medicine, Novosibirsk, USSR
Lupin, A.J.: Division of Otolaryngology and Head and Neck Surgery, Charles Camsell Hospital, Edmonton, Canada
Luukka, P.: Folkhälsan Institute of Genetics, Population Genetics Unit, Helsinki, Finland
Lynge, Inge: Greenland Health Service, Psychiatric Department, Queen Ingrid's Hospital, Godthåb, Greenland

Lyons, R.B.: The WAMI Experiment, University of Alaska,
   College, Alaska, USA

Malcolmson, S.A.: Clarke Institute of Psychiatry, Toronto,
   Canada
Martin, J.D.: 406 Lambert St., Whitehorse, NWT, Canada
Masnick, G.S.: Department of Population Sciences, Harvard
   University, Cambridge, Mass., USA
Mattsson, B.: Department of Psychiatry, University of Umeå,
   Umeå, Sweden
Mayhall, J.T.: Faculty of Dentistry and Department of Anthro-
   pology, University of Toronto, Toronto, Canada
McLean, D.M.: Division of Medical Microbiology, University
   of British Columbia, Vancouver, Canada
Medd, L.M.: Northern Medical Unit, University of Manitoba,
   Winnipeg, Canada
Mendelsohn, B.: Langdon Psychiatric Clinic, Anchorage,
   Alaska, USA
Metayer, M.: Cambridge Bay, NWT, Canada
Miller, Sue M.: Department of Paediatrics, University of Al-
   berta, Edmonton, Canada
Morison, M.M.: Department of Social and Preventive Medicine,
   University of Manitoba, Winnipeg, Canada (Present address:
   Department of Clinical Epidemiology and Biostatistics,
   McMaster University Medical Centre, Hamilton, Canada)
Mussell, W.J.: P.O. Box 90, Chilliwack, B.C., Canada
Myers, W.W.: WAMI Medical Education Program, University of
   Alaska, Box 95753, Fairbanks, Alaska, USA

Nijenhuis, L.E.: Central Laboratory of the Netherlands Red
   Cross Blood Transfusion Service, P.O. Box 9190, Amsterdam
   W, The Netherlands

O'Hara, W.: Defence and Civil Institute of Environmental
   Medicine, P.O. Box 2000, Downsview, Ont., Canada
Olsen, G.Å.: Rudolph Berghs Hospital and Institute of Social
   Medicine, University of Copenhagen, Copenhagen N, Denmark

Palva, A.: Department of Otolaryngology, University of Oulu,
   Oulu, Finland
Palva, H.L.A.: Department of Medicine, University of Oulu,
   Oulu, Finland
Palva, I.P.: Department of Medicine, University of Oulu,
   Oulu, Finland (Present address: Department of Medicine,
   University of Kuopio, Kuopio, Finland)

Patton, J.F.: U.S. Army Research Institute of Environmental
   Medicine, Natick, Mass., USA
Pekkarinen, M.: Department of Nutrition, University of Hel-
   sinki, Helsinki, Finland
Pollak, B.: Montreal Chest Hospital Centre, Montreal, Canada
Porsild, R.: 406 Lambert St., Whitehorse, NWT, Canada
Price, Betty: Alaskan Department of Health and Social Servi-
   ces, Section of Community Health, Pouch HO6C, Juneau,
   Alaska, USA

Rantakallio, P.: Department of Public Health, University of
   Oulu, Oulu, Finland
Reinhard, K.R.: Office of Research and Development, Indian
   Health Service, Tucson, Ariz., USA
Richards, W.W.: Alaska Area Native Health Service, Box 7-741,
   Anchorage, Alaska, USA
Rode, A.: Department of Environmental Health, School of Hy-
   giene, University of Toronto, Toronto, Canada (Present
   address: DNIA Laboratory, Igloolik, NWT, Canada)

Sahi, T.: Department of Public Health Science, University of
   Helsinki, Helsinki, Finland
Salokannel, S.J.: Department of Medicine, University of Oulu,
   Oulu, Finland
Sampath, H.M.: Memorial University, St John's, Nfld., Canada
Sayed, Judith E.: Department of Paediatrics, University of
   Manitoba, Winnipeg, Canada
Schaefer, O.: Northern Medical Research Unit, Medical Servi-
   ces, Health and Welfare Canada, Edmonton, Canada
Schwarz, M.R.: School of Medicine, University of Washington,
   Seattle, Wash., USA
Sedov, K.R.: Irkutsk State Medical Institute, Irkutsk, USSR
Seitamo, L.: Department of Paediatrics, University of Oulu,
   Oulu, Finland, and Department of Psychology, University
   of Jyväskylä, Jyväskylä, Finland
Shephard, R.J.: Department of Environmental Health, School
   of Hygiene, University of Toronto, Toronto, Canada
Silliman, Rebecca A.: School of Medicine, University of Wash-
   ington, Seattle, Wash., USA
Skrobak-Kaczynski, J.: Laboratory of Environmental Physio-
   logy, Oslo, Norway
Smith, Alice K.: Nursing Services, Medical Services Branch,
   Health and Welfare Canada, Ottawa, Canada
Smith, Marcia C.: Maternal and Child Health, Medical Servi-
   ces, Health and Welfare Canada, Ottawa, Canada

Spady, D.W.: Department of Paediatrics, University of Alberta, Edmonton, Alta., Canada

Spencer, Hope: Regional Health Educator, NWT Region Medical Services, Health and Welfare Canada, Edmonton, Canada

Stillner, Marianne: Yukon-Kuskokwim Health Corporation, Alaska Native Hospital, Bethel, Alaska, USA

Stillner, V.: Yukon-Kuskokwim Health Corporation, Alaska Native Hospital, Bethel, Alaska, USA

Styblo, K.: Department of Medicine, University of British Columbia, Vancouver, Canada

Sundberg, S.: Folkhälsan Institute of Genetics, Population Genetics Unit, Helsinki, Finland

Tabel, H.: Animal Pathology Division, Agriculture Canada, Animal Diseases Research Institute, Ottawa, Canada

Taylor, W.C.: Department of Paediatrics, University of Alberta, Edmonton, Canada

Tester, F.J.: Environmental Sciences Centre, University of Calgary, Calgary, Canada

Thomas, G.W.: International Grenfell Association, St Anthony, Nfld., and Department of Surgery, Memorial University, St John's, Nfld., Canada

Titley, K.C.: Department of Paedodontics, Faculty of Dentistry, University of Toronto, Toronto, Canada

Väänänen, M.: Department of Public Health, University of Oulu, Oulu, Finland

Väisänen, E.J.: Clinic of Psychiatry, University of Oulu, Oulu, Finland

van den Berg-Loonen, E.: Central Laboratory of the Netherlands Red Cross Blood Transfusion Service, P.O. Box 9190, Amsterdam W, The Netherlands

van Loghem, E.: Central Laboratory of the Netherlands Red Cross Blood Transfusion Service, P.O. Box 9190, Amsterdam W, The Netherlands

Virtaranta, K.: Folkhälsan Institute of Genetics, Population Genetics Unit, Helsinki, Finland

von Bonsdorff, C.: Folkhälsan Institute of Genetics, Population Genetics Unit, Helsinki, Finland

Wallenberg, L.R.: Urological Research Laboratory, Karolinska Sjukhuset, Stockholm, Sweden

Wedin, B.: National Defence Research Institute, Sundbyberg, Sweden

Williams, J.H.: International Grenfell Association, St Anthony, Nfld., and Department of Pathology, Memorial University, St John's, Nfld., Canada

Winblad, B.: Department of Pathology, University of Umeå,
    Umeå, Sweden
Woolf, C.: Northern Medical Unit, University of Manitoba,
    Winnipeg, Canada

INDEX OF AUTHORS

www.ingramcontent.com/pod-product-compliance
Lightning Source LLC
Chambersburg PA
CBHW030448210326
41597CB00013B/589